Smart Nanomaterials Technology

Series Editors

Azamal Husen, Wolaita Sodo University, Wolaita, Ethiopia

Mohammad Jawaid, Laboratory of Biocomposite Technology, Universiti Putra Malaysia, INTROP, Serdang, Selangor, Malaysia

Nanotechnology is a rapidly growing scientific field and has attracted a great interest over the last few years because of its abundant applications in different fields like biology, physics and chemistry. This science deals with the production of minute particles called nanomaterials having dimensions between 1 and 100 nm which may serve as building blocks for various physical and biological systems. On the other hand, there is the class of smart materials where the material that can stimuli by external factors and results a new kind of functional properties. The combination of these two classes forms a new class of smart nanomaterials, which produces unique functional material properties and a great opportunity to larger span of application. Smart nanomaterials have been employed by researchers to use it effectively in agricultural production, soil improvement, disease management, energy and environment, medical science, pharmaceuticals, engineering, food, animal husbandry and forestry sectors.

This book series in Smart Nanomaterials Technology aims to comprehensively cover topics in the fabrication, synthesis and application of these materials for applications in the following fields:

- Energy Systems—Renewable energy, energy storage (supercapacitors and electrochemical cells), hydrogen storage, photocatalytic water splitting for hydrogen production
- Biomedical—controlled release of drugs, treatment of various diseases, biosensors,
- Agricultural—agricultural production, soil improvement, disease management, animal feed, egg, milk and meat production/processing,
- Forestry—wood preservation, protection, disease management
- Environment—wastewater treatment, separation of hazardous contaminants from wastewater, indoor air filters.

Santosh Kumar Rath · Vagish Dwibedi ·
Azamal Husen · Nadeem Akhtar
Editors

Nanomaterials for Drug Delivery and Neurological Diseases Management

Springer

Editors
Santosh Kumar Rath
School of Pharmaceuticals and Population Health Informatics
Faculty of Pharmacy, DIT University
Dehradun, India

Azamal Husen
Wolaita Sodo University
Wolaita, Ethiopia

Vagish Dwibedi
University Institute of Biotechnology
Chandigarh University
Punjab, India

Nadeem Akhtar
CBS Bio Platforms Inc.
Calgary, AB, Canada

ISSN 3004-8273 ISSN 3004-8281 (electronic)
Smart Nanomaterials Technology
ISBN 978-981-97-0310-4 ISBN 978-981-97-0308-1 (eBook)
https://doi.org/10.1007/978-981-97-0308-1

This Springer imprint is published by the registered company Springer Nature Singapore Pte Ltd.
The registered company address is: 152 Beach Road, #21-01/04 Gateway East, Singapore 189721, Singapore

Paper in this product is recyclable.

Preface

World Federation of Neurology (WFN) has shown keen interest in the environment and its relation to neurological diseases. In 2018, WFN promoted the awareness of environmental challenges with the slogan 'Clean Air for Brain Health' on World Brain Day. A survey made by the collaboration of WHO and WFN noticed that neurological disorder in the world is a global burden of disease and environmental pollution is a major threat in increasing neurological diseases burden in the world. Several drugs as used in Oncology, Neurology and Psychiatry in recent times but none of them can promise the complete curing of Epileptic, Alzheimer or Parkinson's diseases. However, the side effects seem to be more day by day. Epilepsy and seizure disease is the most common serious chronic neurologic disease, affecting more than 50 million people of all ages, genders, ethnic backgrounds, and geographic locations worldwide. Hence to improve therapeutic effects and reduce their side effect active drug molecules accumulate in the disease site for a prolonged period with high controllability. Drug delivery approaches and nanoformulation technologies are much more acceptable for transporting therapeutics in the body safely and can achieve the desired therapeutic effect. At present, the nanomaterial-based drug delivery vehicles are really helpful in finding new routes of administration by diverse nano-based formulation techniques as targeted therapy for the treatment and management of neurological disorders.

This book aims to provide necessary information on the current scenario of different neurological diseases and is also well focussed to depict how the present nano-drug delivery approach is the best alternative solution of treatment to specific neuro or brain diseases. This book also intends to motivate researchers and the general public to align themselves towards sustainable growth through modern delivery techniques.

This collective work is distinct because of our focus on diverse nano-based drug delivery technologies which are high-throughput, reliable, pioneering, and applicable to researchers of different countries despite their socio-economic conditions. Our book will enliven the up-to-date technologies and ideas, and should invoke researchers and innovators to take ahead the current inter-disciplinary knowledge for more advancement and effective management of various neurological problems which is a serious global issue. This Book will improve the current state of knowledge and should invoke researchers and innovators to take ahead the current inter-disciplinary knowledge into technologies that are readily available and effectively minimize hazards associated with neurological disorders. Chapters have been divided into three main sub-sections.

(A) A fundamental study on nanomaterial-, nanocarrier- and nanoformulation-based drug delivery in neurological diseases management.
(B) Nano-drug delivery therapy—a novel approach towards common neurological disorders.
(C) Novel nano-delivery strategies in targeted neurological diseases management.

Dehradun, India — Santosh Kumar Rath
Punjab, India — Vagish Dwibedi
Wolaita, Ethiopia — Azamal Husen
Calgary, Canada — Nadeem Akhtar

Contents

Editors and Contributors

About the Editors

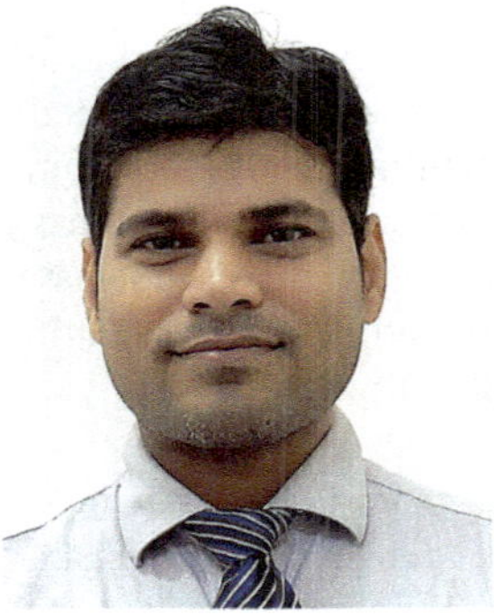

Santosh Kumar Rath is a medicinal and natural product chemist with more than 10 years of experience in research, academia, and industry. Rath received his doctorate from AcSIR at CSIR-Institute of Minerals and Materials Technology (CSIR-IMMT), Bhubaneswar, India. Presently he is working as Assistant Professor in Pharmaceutical Chemistry at the Department of SoPPHI, Faculty of Pharmacy, DIT University, Dehradun, Uttarakhand, India. Formerly, he worked as an Associate Professor and Research Head at the Department of Pharmaceutical Chemistry, Danteshwari College of Pharmacy, Jagdalpur, Chhattisgarh, India (2020–2022). He also worked as Research Associate (CSIR-RA) in the School of Chemistry & Biochemistry at Thapar Institute of Engineering & Technology, Patiala, India (2018–2020). He received Research Associateship from CSIR in 2018 and Senior Research Fellowship (ICMR-SRF) from ICMR, New Delhi, India in 2013. He did research at the CSIR-Indian Institute of Integrative Medicine (CSIR-IIIM), Jammu, India. He has many publications to his credit, published more than 32 research papers in highly reputed international journals, as well as 10 book chapters three edited books, and 2 Indian patent. His area of research is Natural Product Chemistry and Organic Synthesis, in which he is expertise in the isolation, identification, and characterization of bioactive secondary metabolites, and structural modification of major chemical constituents from plants as well as fungal sources. He is acquainted with various chromatographic techniques such as column, Preparative TLC, and HPLC for separating and purifying compounds. He is well aware of the interpretation of spectroscopic data, viz., 1D and 2DNMR, MASS, IR, etc. His research involves multistep synthesis of biologically active synthetic and/or natural product-based hybrid scaffolds for lead identification in special targets for neurological disease, cancer, HIV, Covid-19, and infectious diseases. His research mainly focuses on synthesizing novel P-gp and bacterial efflux pump inhibitors, besides synthetic modifications of the bioactive natural products for better activity/minimize toxicity profiles. Currently, he is developing new synthetic methodologies for the C-H functionalization of heterocycles and other medicinally relevant molecules. He contributed substantially to many research projects and is also having collaborative research work with many other research groups. The contributions, dedication, and brilliance of Dr. Rath in the area of natural product drug discovery and organic synthesis are truly commendable. His contributions aim to serve as an inspiration to all scientific fraternity and inculcate scientific temperament to others to think innovatively.

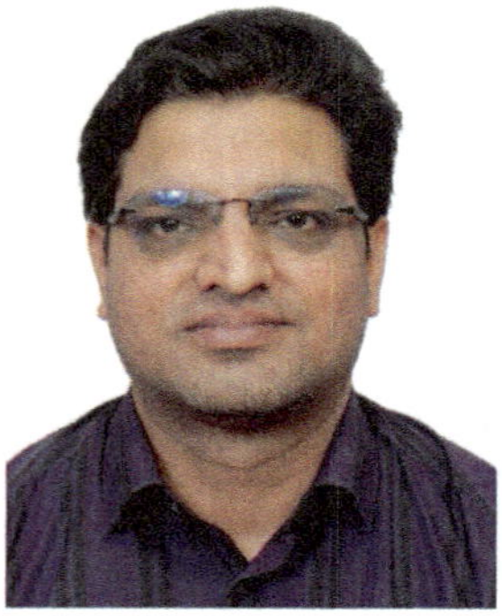

Vagish Dwibedi did his B.Sc. from Lucknow University, Lucknow, Uttar Pradesh, and Ph.D. from Thapar Institute of Engineering and Technology, Patiala, India. Dwibedi is an academician and researcher with more than 8 years of experience in biotech research and development. He has carried out research projects and consultancy work in the areas of plant-microbe interaction/bioassay-guided drug-discovery and development, food security/sustainable agriculture and waste water treatment. Presently he is working as Assistant Professor at University Institute of Biotechnology, Chandigarh University, Gharuan Mohali, Punjab. Formerly, he was worked as Research Scientist at Agpharm Bioinnovations LLP incubated at Thapar Institute of Engineering & Technology, Patiala, India. He was also Winner in Down select competition-DST-Lockheed Martin-Tata Trust_IIGP 2.0 (2k18) (India Innovation Growth Programme 2.0) Innovation ID: IIGPUIBSUNB (The award carries financial support up to 25 Lac INR.). His work is directed towards the development of screening platforms for different biological activities such as anti-microbial, anti-oxidant, anti-cancer, or finding novel molecules that interfere in the mechanism of development of diseases such as Alzheimer Dementia (AD), Parkinson disease (PD), Obesity, Anti-gout (arthritis) and type 2 diabetes. He is also interested in food security, which predominantly involves the exploitation of plant-microbe interaction to combat abiotic stress and post-harvest preservation to enhance the shelf life of fresh crop/horticulture produces. He has published more than 25 research papers in various national and international journals and published 2 Indian patent.

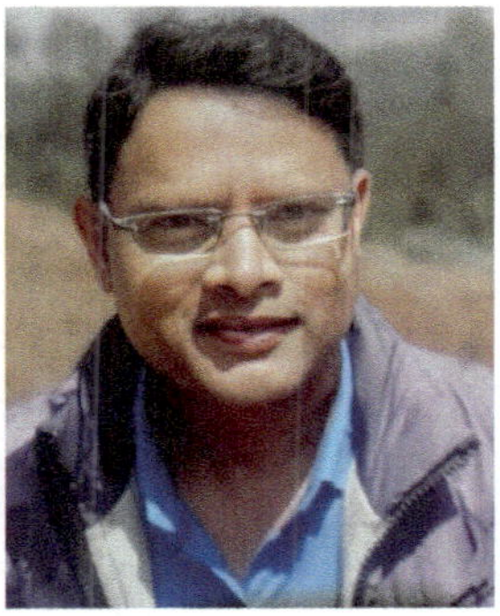

Azamal Husen is presently working as a Professor at Sankalchand Patel University, Visnagar, India; and Adjunct Professor at Graphic Era (Deemed to be University), Dehradun, Uttarakhand, India. He is also working as an Invited Professor at University Putra Malaysia, Selangor, Malaysia. Previously, he served as Professor and Head of the Department of Biology, University of Gondar, Ethiopia; and worked as a Foreign Delegate at Wolaita Sodo University, Wolaita, Ethiopia. He also worked as a Visiting Faculty of the Forest Research Institute and the Doon College of Agriculture and Forest at Dehradun, India. His research and teaching experience of 25 years encompasses biogenic nanomaterial fabrication and application; plant responses to nanomaterials; plant adaptation to harsh environments at the physiological, biochemical, and molecular levels; herbal medicine; and clonal propagation for improvement of tree species. He has conducted research sponsored by the World Bank, the National Agricultural Technology Project, the Indian Council of Agriculture Research, the Indian Council of Forest Research Education, and the Japan Bank for International Cooperation. Husen has published extensively (over 250) and served on the Editorial Board and as reviewer of reputed journals published by Elsevier, Frontiers Media, Taylor & Francis, Springer Nature, RSC, Oxford University Press, Sciendo, the Royal Society, CSIRO, PLOS, MDPI, John Wiley & Sons, and UPM Journals. He is on the advisory board of Cambridge Scholars Publishing, UK. He is a fellow of the Plantae group of the American Society of Plant Biologists, and a member of the International Society of Root Research, Asian Council of Science Editors, and International Natural Product Sciences. He is Editor-in-Chief of the *American Journal of Plant Physiology*, and a Series Editor of *Exploring Medicinal Plants* (Taylor & Francis Group, USA); *Plant Biology, Sustainability, and Climate Change* (Elsevier, USA); and *Smart Nanomaterials Technology* (Springer Nature, Singapore). He has been achieved the distinguished honour of being recognized as one of the "World's Top 2% Scientists" for the year 2022, and again for the 2023 by Stanford University, USA. This recognition has also been prominently featured in the Elsevier Data Repository.

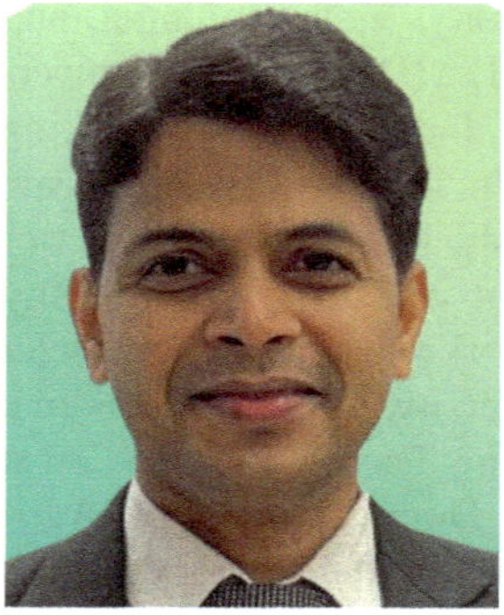

Nadeem Akhtar a scientist, is currently making significant strides in the animal health and longevity sector for a leading Canadian company, CBS Bio Platforms Inc. His impressive background demonstrates that he has held a variety of important positions in academia and research throughout his career. Akhtar was a Research Associate at the University of Guelph, Canada, where the objective of his work was to improve companion animal's health in order to promote a superior and more health-conscious lifestyle. Prior to assuming this position, he excelled as a postdoctoral researcher at the Department of Chemical Engineering, University of Waterloo, Canada (2019–2021) and the Department of Animal Biosciences, University of Guelph, Canada (2015–2019). His accomplishments in the National Eligibility Test (NET-2010) and Graduate Aptitude Test (GATE) in Life Sciences (2010) and Biotechnology (2011) further emphasize his academic excellence. He earned his Ph.D. from the esteemed Department of Biotechnology at the Thapar Institute of Engineering and Technology in India. His scientific contributions are nothing short of remarkable, with over 27 articles published in peer-reviewed international journals as well as 12 book chapters and two edited books. His abilities extend to patent accomplishments, as he has one granted patent to his name. In addition to his research, he has shown his dedication to knowledge advancement by serving as a reviewer for prestigious journals such as RSC Advances, the Journal of Applied Microbiology, Scientific Reports, and Poultry Science. His career exemplifies dedication and excellence, demonstrating his invaluable contributions to the fields of animal science and biotechnology. His journey continues to motivate and shape the global scientific landscape.

Contributors

Shekhar Agnihotri Department of Agriculture and Environmental Sciences, National Institute of Food Technology Entrepreneurship and Management, Kundli, Sonepat, Haryana, India

Manzar Alam Centre for Interdisciplinary Research in Basic Sciences, Jamia Millia Islamia, New Delhi, India

Nemat Ali Department of Pharmacology and Toxicology, College of Pharmacy, King Saud University, Riyadh, Saudi Arabia

Faiyaz Ahmad Ansari Department of Medicine, Government Medical College and Hospital, Purnea, Bihar, India

Md. Meraj Ansari Centre for Pharmaceutical Nanotechnology, Department of Pharmaceutics, National Institute of Pharmaceutical Education and Research, Mohali, Punjab, India

Namita Badoniya Department of Pharmacy, Banasthali, Rajasthan, India

Aman Bhushan University Institute of Engineering and Technology (UIET), Panjab University, Chandigarh, India

Jagadeesh Chandra Bose University Institute of Biotechnology, Chandigarh University, Mohali, India

Aleena James Chirayimmel University Institute of Biotechnology, Chandigarh University, Mohali, India;
School of Biosciences and Technology, Vellore Institute of Technology, Vellore, India

Cleona Elizabeth Mary DCruz Department of Pharmaceutics, Goa College of Pharmacy, Panaji-Goa, India

Amit Kumar Dubey Parasite Immunology Lab, Division of Microbiology, Indian Council of Medical Research (ICMR)-Rajendra Memorial Research Institute of Medical Sciences (RMRIMS), Bihar, India;
Department of Pharmaceutics, School of Pharmaceutical and Population Health Informatics (SoPPHI), DIT University, Dehradun, India

Vagish Dwibedi University Institute of Biotechnology, Chandigarh University, Mohali, Punjab, India;

Institute of Soil, Water and Environmental Sciences, Volcani Research Center, Agricultural Research Organization, Rishon Lezion, Israel;
Dr. B. C. Roy College of Pharmacy and AHS, Durgapur, West Bengal, India

Debasis Gantayat School of Pharmaceuticals and Population Health Informatics, Faculty of Pharmacy, DIT University, Dehradun, Uttarakhand, India

Namita Gupta Department of Pharmacy, Banasthali, Rajasthan, India

Tapasvi Gupta Department of Pharmacy, Banasthali, Rajasthan, India

Tripti Halder School of Pharmaceuticals and Population Health Informatics, Faculty of Pharmacy, DIT University, Dehradun, Uttarakhand, India

Narayan Hemnani University Institute of Pharmacy, Faculty of Technology, Pt. Ravishankar Shukla University, Raipur, Chhattisgarh, India

Nazrul Islam Department of Chemistry, Jawahar Lal Nehru College, Chakradharpur, West Singhbhum, Jharkhand, India

Rudhvi Jain Department of Biotechnology, Thapar Institute of Engineering and Technology, Patiala, Punjab, India;
Department of Biochemistry and Molecular Biology, Faculty of Life Sciences, Tel-Aviv University, Tel-Aviv, Israel

Sahil Jain Department of Biochemistry and Molecular Biology, Faculty of Life Sciences, Tel-Aviv University, Tel-Aviv, Israel

Gursharan Kaur University Institute of Biotechnology, Chandigarh University, Mohali, India

Rehan Khan Department of Nano-Therapeutics, Institute of Nano Science and Technology, Mohali, Punjab, India

Lalit Kumar Department of Pharmaceutics, National Institute of Pharmaceutical Education and Research, Hajipur, Bihar, Vaishali, India

Priyanshu Kumar School of Pharmaceutical & Population Health Informatics, Faculty of Pharmacy, DIT University, Dehradun, Uttarakhand, India

Shubham Kumar University Institute of Biotechnology, Chandigarh University, Mohali, Punjab, India

Jyoti Kumari Parasite Immunology Lab, Division of Microbiology, Indian Council of Medical Research (ICMR)-Rajendra Memorial Research Institute of Medical Sciences (RMRIMS), Bihar, India

Shweta Kumari University Institute of Biotechnology (UIBT), Chandigarh University, Mohali, Punjab, India

Sudip Kumar Mandal Dr. B. C. Roy College of Pharmacy and AHS, Durgapur, West Bengal, India

Samta Manori Advanced Functional Smart Materials Laboratory, School of Physical Sciences, Department of Physics, DIT University, Dehradun, UK, India

Shashank Shekher Mishra School of Pharmaceutical & Population Health Informatics, Faculty of Pharmacy, DIT University, Dehradun, Uttarakhand, India

Zamurrad Nayab Department of Biotechnology, Science College Patna, Patna University, Patna, Bihar, India

Nidhi University Institute of Biotechnology, Chandigarh University, Mohali, Punjab, India

Easha Pandey Department of Pharmacy, Banasthali, Rajasthan, India

Ravi Parashar University Institute of Pharmacy, Faculty of Technology, Pt. Ravishankar Shukla University, Raipur, Chhattisgarh, India

Neha Pathak Department of Pharmacy, School of Medical Allied Sciences, GD Goenka University, Sohna, Gurugram, India

Yashwant Pathak USF Health Taneja College of Pharmacy, University of South Florida, Tampa, FL, USA;
Faculty of Pharmacy (Adjunct Professor), Airlangga University, Surabaya, Indonesia

Payel Mal School of Pharmaceuticals and Population Health Informatics, Faculty of Pharmacy, DIT University, Dehradun, Uttarakhand, India

Shilpi Prasad Siddhi Vinayaka Institute of Technology and Sciences, Bilaspur, Chhattisgarh, India

Shraddha Singh Raghav School of Pharmaceutical and Population Health Informatics (SoPPHI), DIT University, Makkawala, Dehradun, Uttarakhand, India

Kuldeep Kumar Raina M.S. Ramaiah University of Applied Sciences, Bangalore, India

Anupama Rajput University Institute of Biotechnology, Chandigarh University, Mohali, India

Palak Rana University Institute of Biotechnology, Chandigarh University, Mohali, India

Saumya Rastogi School of Pharmaceutical & Population Health Informatics, Faculty of Pharmacy, DIT University, Dehradun, Uttarakhand, India

Santosh Kumar Rath School of Pharmaceuticals and Population Health Informatics, Faculty of Pharmacy, DIT University, Dehradun, Uttarakhand, India

Abhishek Rawat School of Pharmaceutical & Population Health Informatics, Faculty of Pharmacy, DIT University, Dehradun, Uttarakhand, India

Reetika Rawat Department of Pharmacy, Banasthali, Rajasthan, India

Syed Shadab Raza Laboratory for Stem Cell and Restorative Neurology, Department of Biotechnology, Era's Lucknow Medical College and Hospital, Sarfarazganj, Lucknow, Uttar Pradesh, India

Sibasankar Sahu School of Pharmaceuticals and Population Health Informatics, Faculty of Pharmacy, DIT University, Dehradun, Uttarakhand, India

Sipu Kumar Sahu School of Pharmaceuticals and Population Health Informatics, Faculty of Pharmacy, DIT University, Dehradun, Uttarakhand, India

Kangkan Sarma School of Pharmaceutical and Population Health Informatics (SoPPHI), DIT University, Makkawala, Dehradun, Uttarakhand, India

Manu Sharma Department of Pharmacy, Banasthali, Rajasthan, India

Sheelu Sharma PDUNIPPD, Delhi University, New Delhi, India

Sonia Sharma University Institute of Biotechnology, Chandigarh University, Mohali, India

Rupesh Kalidas Shirodkar Department of Pharmaceutics, Goa College of Pharmacy, Panaji-Goa, India

Prashant Shukla Department of Pharmacy, UPES School of Health Sciences and Technology, University of Petroleum & Energy Studies, Dehradun, Uttarakhand, India

Ravi K. Shukla Advanced Functional Smart Materials Laboratory, School of Physical Sciences, Department of Physics, DIT University, Dehradun, UK, India

Devendra Sillu Department of Biotechnology, Thapar Institute of Engineering & Technology, Patiala, Punjab, India;
Environmental Science and Engineering, Guangdong Technion – Israel Institute of Technology (GTIIT), Shantou, China

Jasdeep Singh University Institute of Biotechnology, Chandigarh University, Mohali, Punjab, India

Lakhveer Singh School of Pharmaceutical & Population Health Informatics, Faculty of Pharmacy, DIT University, Dehradun, Uttarakhand, India

Niva Singh Parasite Immunology Lab, Division of Microbiology, Indian Council of Medical Research (ICMR)-Rajendra Memorial Research Institute of Medical Sciences (RMRIMS), Bihar, India

Prayas Singh Advanced Functional Smart Materials Laboratory, School of Physical Sciences, Department of Physics, DIT University, Dehradun, UK, India

Shubhankar Kumar Singh Parasite Immunology Lab, Division of Microbiology, Indian Council of Medical Research (ICMR)-Rajendra Memorial Research Institute of Medical Sciences (RMRIMS), Bihar, India

Palak Singhal Department of Human Genetics, Inselspital, Bern University Hospital, University of Bern, Bern, Switzerland;
Department of Biomedical Research, University of Bern, Bern, Switzerland

Sneha Rani Parasite Immunology Lab, Division of Microbiology, Indian Council of Medical Research (ICMR)-Rajendra Memorial Research Institute of Medical Sciences (RMRIMS), Bihar, India

M. Sudhakara Reddy Department of Biotechnology, Thapar Institute of Engineering & Technology, Patiala, Punjab, India

Preeti K. Suresh University Institute of Pharmacy, Faculty of Technology, Pt. Ravishankar Shukla University, Raipur, Chhattisgarh, India

Arya Swati SGT College of Pharmacy, SGT University, Gurugram, Haryana, India

Babita Thakur University Institute of Biotechnology, Chandigarh University, Mohali, Punjab, India

Mohammad Waseem Department of Pharmaceutical Sciences, University of Maryland Eastern Shore School of Pharmacy, Princess Anne, MD, USA

Abbreviations

AChE	Acetylcholinesterase
ALS	Amyotrophic Lateral Sclerosis
APIs	Active Pharmaceutical Ingredients
APP	Amyloid Precursor Protein
ASOs	Antisense Oligonucleotides
AuNPs	Gold Nanoparticles
BBB	Blood-Brain Barrier
BCSFB	Blood-Cerebrospinal Fluid Barrier
BM NPs	Biogenic Magnetic Nanoparticles
BMP	Bone Morphogenetic Protein
CAA	Cerebral Amyloid Angiopathy
CDR	Controlled Drug Release
ChAT	Choline Acetyltransferase
CNS	Central Nervous System
CPP	Cell-Penetrating Peptide
DDS	Drug Delivery Systems
DMTs	Disease-Modifying Treatments
DWCNTs	Double-Walled Carbon Nanotubes
ECM	Extracellular Matrix
EGCG	Epigallocatechin-3-Gallate
EGFR	Epidermal Growth Factor Receptor
EOF	Ease of Functionalization
GABA	Gamma-Aminobutyric Acid
GSS	Gerstmann-Straussler-Scheinker Syndrome
IONP	Iron Oxide Nanoparticle
LCST	Lower Critical Solution Temperature
LFS	Large and Functional Surfaces
MAPT	Microtubule-Associated Protein Tau
MBP	Myelin Basic Protein
MPS	Mononuclear Phagocytic System
MSNs	Mesoporous Silica Nanoparticles

MWCNTs	Multi-Walled Carbon Nanotubes
NFAT	Nuclear Factor of Activated T Cells
NFTs	Neurofibrillary Tangles
NMDAR	N-Methyl-D-Aspartate Receptor
NMR	Nuclear Magnetic Resonance
NTB	Nose-to-Brain
PEG	Polyethylene Glycol
PICALM	Phosphatidylinositol-Binding Clathrin Assembly Protein
PNIPAM	Poly(N-isopropylacrylamide)
PPMS	Primary Progressive Multiple Sclerosis
PTDs	Protein Transduction Domains
RMT	Receptor-Mediated Transcytosis
SAVR	Surface Area-to-Volume Ratio
SLNs	Solid Lipid Nanoparticles
SORL1	Sortilin-Related Receptor 1
SPIONs	Superparamagnetic Iron Oxide Nanoparticles
SPMS	Secondary Progressive Multiple Sclerosis
TDD	Transdermal Drug Delivery
TfR	Transferrin Receptor
TLE	Temporal Lobe Epilepsy
TLR9	Toll-Like Receptor-9
TREM	Triggering Receptor Expressed on Myeloid Cells
TRH	Thyrotropin-Releasing Hormone
VEGF	Vascular Endothelial Growth Factor
αSN	α-Synuclein
β-CD	β-Cyclodextrin

A Fundamental Study on Nanomaterials, Nanocarriers and Nanoformulation-Based Drug Delivery in Neurological Diseases Management

Nanocarriers for Drug Delivery: General Characteristics

Devendra Sillu, M. Sudhakara Reddy, and Shekhar Agnihotri

Abstract The escalating pace of disease transmission has prompted scientists to embark on innovative approaches to enhance the therapeutic efficacy of modern drugs. Several barriers present in the human body limit the overall efficiency of directly administrated therapeutics. The heterogeneous nature of these barriers across patient populations presents another crucial obstacle to designing a universal solution. The concept of precision therapeutics, which involves tailoring interventions based on the individual patient's pathology, has gained considerable attention but lacks practical affordability on a global scale. Nanomaterials have gained significant attention as potential drug delivery systems owing to their exceptional properties, including high drug loading capacity and ease of administration. However, the administration of any foreign materials, including nanomaterials, may activate the inherent immune response to clear out them. To bypass the defence system and deliver drug molecules at specific target sites, nanomaterials with specific physicochemical properties have been utilised. An in-depth understanding of physicochemical characteristics of nanomaterials is imperative for developing effective nanocarriers capable of surmounting both physical and biological hurdles, ultimately leading to enhanced therapeutic outcomes. The present chapter provides a comprehensive overview of the most frequently encountered barriers in utilizing nanomaterials as drug carriers, ranging from physical to biological hindrances. The chapter elucidates how manipulating the physicochemical attributes of nanocarriers can serve as a powerful tool to circumvent these barriers, leading to improved drug delivery efficacy. Finally,

D. Sillu · M. Sudhakara Reddy
Department of Biotechnology, Thapar Institute of Engineering & Technology, Bhadson Road, Patiala, Punjab 147004, India

D. Sillu
Environmental Science and Engineering, Guangdong Technion – Israel Institute of Technology (GTIIT), Shantou, China

S. Agnihotri (✉)
Department of Agriculture and Environmental Sciences, National Institute of Food Technology Entrepreneurship and Management, Kundli, Sonepat, Haryana 131028, India
e-mail: agnish@niftem.ac.in

S. K. Rath et al. (eds.), *Nanomaterials for Drug Delivery and Neurological Diseases Management*, Smart Nanomaterials Technology,
https://doi.org/10.1007/978-981-97-0308-1_1

the future prospects of employing nanocarriers in drug delivery applications are discussed.

Keywords Nanocarriers · Drug delivery · Barriers · Physicochemical properties · Modifications

1 Introduction

Multiple factors such as lifestyle changes, environmental degradation, aging population, and genetic predisposition have contributed to an unprecedented surge in life-threatening diseases. This has concomitantly increased the demand for active pharmaceutical ingredients (APIs), leading to a significant rise in the production of drugs [1]. Drugs are employed for diagnosis, prevention, cure, or mitigation of harmful diseases to restrict the causalities incurred. Drugs can be designed to affect the structure or functions of the body part affected by these diseases in a target specific manner. The direct administration of drugs however pose many challenges e.g. limited solubility, uncontrolled release rate, lower viability, and low tissue/cell specific actions [2]. Advanced therapeutics based on peptides, proteins, oligonucleotides, and DNA constitute an important class of APIs to treat life-threatening diseases due to their ability to target specific cellular pathways, exhibit high potency, and low toxicity. These APIs too exhibit low bioavailability and are prone to degrade in biological fluids [3]. Conventional drugs used widely for oral or injectable administration have a critical drawback in terms of optimal formulation [3]. The general approach to improve their bioavailability is through increasing the surface area per particle. The size reduction process, however reduces the API's performance especially in case of biomolecules. In addition, smaller drug particles are extremely difficult to stabilize and isolate. Moreover, this strategy does not prevent biomolecules from enzymatic and acid-catalyzed degradation.

The use of non-therapeutic structures as delivery vehicles for drugs is a viable strategy to improve their bioavailability and shielding from body fluids-led degradation [4, 5]. These carriers are biocompatible tools assisting the transport of molecules for pharmaceutical, cosmetic, and nutraceutical applications to specific targeted sites [6]. These carriers provide controlled drug release, enabling the dose precision as per the respective medical need. Specific drug delivery systems are designed which are capable of targeted and regulated release of drugs, hence improving the overall effectiveness of the drug for intended tissues/cells [6]. The delivery of specific therapeutic concentration of drug to the disease causing cells while preserving its biological viability is of utmost importance when selecting any drug carrier. Commonly investigated drug carriers include liposomes, niosomes, polymeric micelles and microparticulates [7, 4].

Drug delivery systems are generally classified based on the interaction between drug and carrier or their release style. For instance, in the matrix drug delivery system, the drug is released through pores of matrix [8]. The semipermeable membrane acts as key controller in case of reservoir systems [9], while degradation of the material is the major drug releasing mechanism in degradable drug delivery systems [10]. The release of drug under the influence of osmotic pressure change instigates the unloading of the concerned drug in osmotic pump systems [11]. The type of drug delivery system is dictated via the choice of material used for design of drug delivery system. The selection of an appropriate material with unique physicochemical properties presenting it as a biocompatible and efficient carrier for drugs is the most crucial step for the system to move on to the implementation techniques and clinical trials steps.

The conventionally used drug carriers often have associated implications such as limited biodistribution, and intracellular trafficking issues [12]. Nanotechnology could help overcome the limitations of conventional drug delivery systems in a systematic manner [13, 12]. Engineered nanomaterials have demonstrated noteworthy potency to improve disease diagnosis and treatment specificity [14]. A wide range of nanomaterials (Inorganic, Organic and Polymer-based) have been investigated for designing of drug delivery systems [12]. This chapter focuses on the key aspects associated with nanomaterials that help them to overcome different physical and biological barriers, presenting them as a viable option instead of conventional drug delivery systems.

2 Nanomaterial as Drug Carriers

Efficacy of drugs delivery systems is directly correlated with the particle size; therefore nanomaterial carriers with appropriate size can easily enhance their effectiveness. Nanomaterials owing to their unique intrinsic properties such as high surface to mass ratio, high loading capacity, and quantum properties have been employed for designing of drug delivery systems [15]. The primary goal for using nanocarrier systems is to attain the following goals in drug delivery:

- Faster delivery of drug
- High specificity for disease causing cells/tissues
- Reduced toxicity
- Superior biocompatibility and viability.

Owing to their small size and large surface area, nanocarriers demonstrate increased solubility resulting in enhanced bioavailability. The small size of nanocarriers facilitates the transportation of these carriers through various barriers [16].

Taking into consideration that nanomaterials, be it synthetic or natural, are considered as foreign particles by the human body, hence understanding how the body reacts when nanoparticles comes in contact with the cells/tissues is most important [17, 15]. Effective biodistribution and targeted delivery is a difficult task as drug carriers have to clear both physical and biological barriers which include shear forces, protein adsorption and clearance by the immune system [18]. These barriers restrict the efficacy of the carriers to reach the targeted therapeutic site and release of drug. The state of these barriers is often different in healthy and ill individuals as well as for different individuals, further making it difficult to generalize the carrier.

2.1 *Barriers in the Way*

The barriers faced by nanocarriers depend on various factors such as the route of administration, physicochemical properties of nanocarriers, disease type, and disease stage [19]. The administration route of nanocarriers is a major factor that can influence the biodistribution. This may also amend the final fate and efficacy of nanocarriers. Numerous studies in the recent past have explored the role of administering means on the overall impact of nanocarriers. Local delivery method though can overcome some of the key barriers; however, their on ground execution is limited due to the involvement of invasive procedures and complex techniques. Moreover, local delivery methods are generally preferred in diseases where the exact target sites are known such as solid cancers or traumatic injuries. Systematic administration on the other hand is a preferred approach where pathology is unable to detect the exact target site [20].

The nanocarriers can be introduced in the human body via direct injection, inhalation or oral intake. Oral delivery methods are widely used for drug administration, however, in case of nanocarrier based targeted delivery the gastrointestinal tract acts as a barrier limiting their efficiency [21]. In case of oral administration, nanocarriers generally rely on endocytosis and subsequent exocytosis to cross the gastrointestinal tract. Nanocarriers with passive diffusion act as a major releasing mechanism, and the passage through the endothelium is limited by concentration gradients and P-glycoproteins.

Inhalation has also been reported to improve delivery of nanocarriers. Different types of pulmonary administration such as intratracheal instillation, intratracheal spraying and intranasal instillation, result in different rates of nanocarrier accumulation and heterogenous distributions [22]. These administration methods avoid exposure to systematic circulation, thus bypassing hepatic first-pass metabolism and accumulating effectively in lung and lymph node as compared to intravenous delivery [23]. Despite their advantages, inhalation of nanocarriers is not considered as a full proof administration method as it is affected by the physical barriers such as mucus and pulmonary surfactants. The unpredictable levels of these physical barriers across patients depending upon the concerned disease also restrict the application of this approach [24, 25]. Intranasal administration has been explored for nanocarriers loaded drug delivery to the brain, as it bypasses the blood–brain barrier (BBB) and limitation associated with systematic administration [26]. Factors including dose volume, patient condition, and mucus are some of the key obstacles to the intranasal route [27, 28]. There is a dire need to further optimise these methods to formulate proper administration route with consistency and accuracy.

Most of the clinically approved nanocarriers are either intratumourally or intravenously administered, however alternative routes must be explored to deliver better efficacy [29, 17]. In a nutshell, knit picking an optimal administration route might result in more desirable distribution which would definitely improve the targeting ability and specificity of nanocarriers.

After entering the systemic circulation, nanomaterial-protein interaction is the forefront line of defence system before movement to different body parts [30]. Clearance of nanocarriers from blood circulation happens by interaction with the mononuclear phagocytic system (MPS) or reticuloendothelial system [19, 31]. The phagocytic cells i.e., macrophages take up nanocarriers and accumulate them in the spleen and liver [32, 18]. Interaction with MPS, apart from resulting in clearance of nanocarriers can also cause toxicity as these cells trigger immune response resulting in inflammation or tissue damage [33, 34]. During circulation mechanistic parts such as excretion, blood flow, and coronas also have significant impact on the overall efficacy of the nanocarrier [14]. The impact majorly depends on the physiochemical properties of the nanocarrier used.

Once in circulation, extravasation is the first step for a nanocarrier to reach the intended target site [35]. Extravasation can be altered by changing the physicochemical properties of the nanocarriers. Adsorption via blood capillaries facilitates the distribution of nanocarriers in the lymphatic system. The key functions of this process include fluid recovery which involves filtration of fluids from blood capillaries. Another function is to impart immunity via eliminating dangerous entities. While recovering the excess fluid, the system also picks up foreign objects (cells, chemicals, drugs etc.), and when these fluids are introduced into the blood stream, the lymph nodes detect foreign objects, and macrophages will engulf and clear it from the body. This function tends to be a critical issue while administrating drug via nanocarriers.

The haemodynamics experienced by nanocarriers also significantly influence the distribution and drug delivery. After entering the human body, nanocarriers experience fluctuating flow rates of bloodstream which might induce shear stress [36, 37]. This could result in damaging the carrier structure and releasing drug abruptly before reaching the target site. These strong forces can also strip the surface coatings/functionalities and prevent nanocarriers from interaction with vessel walls, thus eliminating the chance to reach the target site [19, 35].

Local distribution of nanocarriers is gravely affected by the additional barriers such as biofilms and mucus [21, 38]. Mucus is basically a polymeric slimy substance, where the distances between the neighbouring polymer links control the mesh pore size. The mesh size can vary from 10 to 1000 nm, hence size selection of nanocarriers becomes a key aspect while intending for specific applications [38]. The characteristic features such as composition, mesh size, hydration thickness of the mucus barrier and viscoelasticity fluctuate throughout body depending on its physiological location making it a complex environment for nanocarrier delivery. In addition to filtration based on size, mucus can also trap nanocarriers via non- specific interactions, resulting in rapid clearance from epithelial surfaces [21].

Physical barriers which limit the efficiency of nanocarriers for drug delivery include tight junctions among the endothelial and epithelial cells of the BBB (in intravenous delivery) and the gastrointestinal tract (in oral delivery) [39]. To influence central nervous system (CNS), nanocarriers need to use receptor-mediated endocytosis by endothelial cells of the BBB [40, 31, 34]. However, heterogeneity of plasma membrane transporters on endothelial cells, present a hurdle for nanocarriers to cross BBB [41]. Some of the highly expressed transporters such as glucose transporters help nanocarriers transport to attain some common target sites [42]. However their efficiency to deliver appropriate dose of drug loaded varies. Overall, the BBB is seen as a great obstacle for systemically administered nanocarriers to reach targeted cells of CNS [43].

Even after reaching the target site, nanocarriers have to face the local microenvironment, where change in chemical conditions or formation of physical barriers could influence their physical properties and the drug release profile. For example, the gastrointestinal tract has areas of extreme pH and presence of specific enzymes that might induce the degradation of nanocarriers [21]. The gastrointestinal microenvironment depends on the diet, disease states, and patient pathologies, resulting in unpredicted reaction with the nanocarriers in different individuals [44]. Variation of pH in case of tumours also hinders the general formulation of universal nanocarriers [45]. Specific nanocarriers have been developed in recent times that are environment responsive [39, 46]; such nanocarriers can be used after earlier contemplation of the local microenvironment.

Apart from the general barriers, cellular heterogeneity also has impact on the overall efficacy of the nanocarrier [47]. The cellular variations within different organs/target sites and among patients depend on the characteristics of an individual. Younger cells are capable of anchoring high concentration of nanocarriers as compared to older cells. Furthermore, drug-resistant cells add on to the cellular heterogeneity that makes nanocarrier delivery even complex. Both cell type and phenotypes results in cellular heterogeneity creating diverse barriers for nanocarriers. The innovative nanocarriers design approaches can assist in surpassing these unavoidable barriers.

In case of solid tumours, the vasculature, interstitial fluid pressure and extracellular matrix (ECM) density may act as barriers limiting the permeation and penetration of nanocarriers [19, 48, 49]. The microenvironment of the tumour dictates the final fate of nanocarriers, such as heterogeneous vasculature which might facilitate nanocarrier accumulation via the leaky vessels a phenomenon often referred to as the enhanced permeation and retention (EPR) effect [50]. The heterogeneity of vasculature depends on the individual patients' factors such as age, genetics, lifestyle and even previous antitumour treatments [50, 51, 34]. Hence to select an appropriate nanocarrier for the tumour, individual patient must be assessed for determining the potential of EPR effect. Reports have suggested that mechanisms such as immune cell interactions, protein coronas and molecular mechanisms also play important roles for nanocarrier accumulation in tumour [52]. Furthermore, tumour microenvironments might instigate cells' overproduction or generation of altered ECM components that result in a dense ECM which physically hinders nanocarrier delivery [49]. Specifically tagged nanocarriers can be used to assess the level of the EPR effect at the tumour site.

Additionally, decreased interstitial fluid drainage in tumour vasculature prevents nanocarrier perfusion. The increased intertumoural interstitial pressure in such cases averts most tumour cells from interacting with nanocarriers [48, 33]. Limited perfusion is also an obstacle for nanocarriers used for delivery in brain, as even after crossing the BBB nanocarriers often fail to permeate the tissue because of the limited extracellular space and non-specific adherence to the ECM [53, 54].

Over the time, various modifications in the characteristic features of carrier nanomaterials have been investigated to improve the efficacy of nanomaterial based drug delivery [19]. The key characteristics having the most significant impact on the fabrication of efficient nanocarrier systems are discussed below.

2.2 *Impact of Shape and Size*

The morphological attributes i.e., size and shapes are the key parameters which influence the perspective of the defence system towards the nanocarrier used. The overall loading and release profile of drugs are directly influenced by the by the size; as particles' size get smaller, their surface area to volume ratio gets larger resulting in higher loading of drug. Moreover, in case of smaller particles the drug molecules would be closer to the surface of the particles that would lead to faster drug release [55]. Hence, utilizing nanoparticles with higher surface area to volume ratio are preferred as drug carriers; however, toxicological aspect of these carriers must be monitored. As discussed previously, the size of the nanomaterials dictates their biological fate, as the immune system (vascular and lymph systems) filters out the foreign particulates. Particles with size >200 nm activate the lymphatic system and are removed from circulation quicker [56]. Whereas, nanocarriers with overall size less than 10 nm are eliminated by the kidneys [57]. Hence, considering the reported literature nanomaterials of size around 100 nm are optimum carriers for high drug loading, passing the BBB and deliver sufficient amount of drug.

Previous studies have demonstrated that particles of 100 nm size have 2.5 fold higher uptake by the cell system as compared to particles with 1 μm diameter. The uptake gets even shortened with increase in particle size as a particle of 10 μm exhibits 6 times lesser uptake by the cells [58]. These parameters also affect the distribution, toxicity and targeting ability of the nanocarrier system inside the human body. For instance, it's because of their ultra-small size that they are capable to pass through the blood brain barrier (BBB), and deliver medication for diseases that were previously difficult to treat [43, 26]. These parameters can be easily moulded in case of nanomaterials providing an edge over other delivery methods. This also provides opportunity to realize new targets and more control over drug distribution.

Distribution of nanocarriers in organs is a size-dependent phenomenon, as small nanocarriers can easily cross capillary walls, contrary to large size nanocarriers [34, 18]. Highest accumulation of nanocarriers is often found in the liver and spleen [19, 57]. In some cases, size-dependent distribution of nanocarriers is also affected by the pathological environments. One such case is the presence of larger intracellular gaps in tumour vasculature, where even large nanocarriers can easily transport through the gap [18]. Overall, extravasation results in a non-specific distribution of nanocarriers, and this presents a translational challenge for applications that require specific localization of nanocarriers.

With respect to the haemodynamics factor, large size particles (microscale) have rather high probability of localizing to the vessel walls, and non-spherical particles demonstrated greater margination with the adhesion of white blood cells to the walls of damaged blood vessels [35]. Shapes such as ellipsoids, discoid shapes and nanorods with higher aspect ratios have demonstrated superior localization to blood vessels than spherical shapes [35, 42, 59]. The key reason behind this phenomenon is flow-induced rolling of different shapes, which is equally affected by the aspect ratio of the particle [19]. This might seem as the appropriate choice at this point that non-spherical particles with high ratio can resolve all the issues; however architecture dependent drag forces can still rip nanocarriers from the cell membranes if they lack binding affinity [60].

Nanocarrier curvature and aspect ratio are also important features for selection of appropriate nanocarrier. Shape variation can be a viable approach for avoiding uptake by phagocytic cells as triangular and rod-shaped nanocarriers are frequently captured by phagocytic cells as compared to star shaped or spherical nanocarriers [61, 62]. On the other hand, rod shaped nanocarriers are reported to cause more inflammation in macrophages [63].

In case of oral administration, smaller nanoparticles might avoid transport across the epithelial barrier and perform intestinal permeation through tight junctions [64]. Nanocarriers with large surface area are considered for oral route as there are increased numbers of interactions with the gastrointestinal tract, which would facilitate the efficient delivery of the drug [65]. The nanocarriers with size around 100 nm are reported to be optimal for gastrointestinal applications as compared to lower or higher size [65, 66–69]. Rod shaped nanocarriers generally perform better than spherical shaped nanocarriers, credited to the fact that rods internalize into epithelial cells efficiently as compared to spheres [70, 71]. However, only this aspect does not ascertain effective delivery as only a small portion of these nanocarriers undergo exocytosis [72].

2.3 Impact of Surface Properties

Surface characteristics of the carrier can also influence the performance of nanomaterial-based drug carriers [73]. The interaction of drug molecules with the nanomaterial surface can be easily controlled by surface functionalization of nanomaterials, such as introduction of specific groups or targeting ligands. These functionalities prevent aggregation, improve biodistribution, increase stability, and instil efficient receptor binding, thus improving the overall pharmacological effects of the drug [74, 75]. Incorporation of reactive sites is another class of modifications that can improve the overall efficiency of the nanocarrier.

While selecting the surface properties, the first and foremost important aspect to consider is the safe entrance of the nanocarrier into the human body. Since, nanomaterials can be easily recognised by the defence system as a foreign entity, they will be flushed out as the body's natural immune response. Hydrophobic particles have high affinity towards blood components and are thus easily cleared out by the lymphatic system [76]. Considering this simple point, using hydrophilic particles for drug delivery is considered as a viable option, as they will remain in the human system for a longer period of time, thus increasing their chances to attain the set goals. Coating the nanomaterials with polymers or surfactants has been widely used technique to modulate the hydrophilic nature of the nanocarriers. Various polymers such as polyethylene glycol (PEG), polyethylene oxide, polyoxamer, poloxamine, and polysorbate 80 have been used for such applications [77, 78].

PEG is a relatively inert hydrophilic polymer which inhibits the binding of plasma proteins that may induce degradation, secretion and clearance. Furthermore, PEGylation prevents the drug leaching from the nanocarrier and improve circulation time by altering the solubility. This feature presents the PEGylated nanomaterials as relatively stealth, however this does not completely prevent recognition by macrophages or other cells of the immune system [79, 80, 14]. Prior PEG exposure can prompt the production of anti-PEG antibodies that can induce rapid flushing out of PEGylated nanomaterials [81, 82]. This means even the first dose of PEGylated nanocarriers might not be able to circulate for a long period [83, 84]. They are also reported to contribute to uncommon but severe allergic reactions [85, 86].

Although the safe entry of drug nanocarrier can be envisaged by practise of various approaches, however the aggregation of these nanocarriers inside the human body is yet another critical issue that requires undivided attention. Owing to their large surface area, nanomaterials tend to agglomerate under physiological conditions. As discussed before, the administration route of nanocarriers directly influences their final fate, for example polymeric nanocarriers injected intravenously accumulate primarily in the liver and spleen, whereas if subcutaneously or intranodally injected, they are more likely to accumulate in local lymph nodes [87]. These approaches can be used in several immunotherapeutic applications where there is an immediate need to deliver drug to the lymphatic system thus avoiding the systemic circulation [88]. Nanomaterials such as dendrimers, quantum dots, and micelles form agglomerates easily as compared to others. Scientists have developed strategies to restrict aggregation, such as coatings with capping agents, and alteration of zeta potential [51].

The overall charges on the nanocarriers also affect the clearance from blood circulation. The immune system tends to rapidly clear out cationic nanocarriers as compared to anionic or neutral nanocarriers [19, 41]. The cationic nanocarrier may anchor to the negatively charged tumour ECM, reducing the permeation of nanocarriers [89, 18]. Stiffer nanomaterials are highly prone towards the clearance mechanism associated with the mononuclear phagocytic system (MPS) or reticuloendothelial systems [90, 91].

While circulating in the blood stream the interaction between the nanocarriers and biomolecules present in the blood is inevitable. The interaction with these biomolecules specifically proteins and lipids results in the formation of a corona on the surface of nanocarriers [92, 50, 93]. The physicochemical characteristics of the nanocarrier and the type of biomolecule both affect the composition of the corona. Furthermore, the modified surface properties may encourage corona formation via charge specific interactions [31]. The formed corona then will dictate the distribution and stability of the nanocarriers [92, 34]. For instance, if the corona contains ligands for pattern recognition receptors the nanocarrier can be flushed out by the innate immune system [34]. Scientists have been exploring the area of how the specific corona biomolecules alter nanocarriers' distribution and tissue- specific targeting. Various surface functionalization and cloaking approaches have been explored till date to improve the specificity and offer protection from the immune system.

Non-specific distribution of nanocarriers can be side-lined by attaching targeting moieties on their surface. These moieties could be antibodies, transferrin, folate, transporters and specific ligands [94–96]. These moieties anchor with molecules on the target cell's surface, via ligand–receptor, enzyme–substrate or antibody–antigen—mediated interactions [47]. Density of targeting moieties, ratio of receptors to ligands, and the number of interactions needed to overcome the initial energy barrier for nanocarrier uptake are some of the involved parameters that must be considered thoroughly [41]. Active targeting resulting from these target moieties may also improve the nanocarrier distribution in the human body part affected by disease [74]. Despite all the advantage, the critical shortcoming of the active targeting method is fluctuation of targeting moieties (disease markers) which vary among diseased cells within a patient as well as among patients [57, 47]. Scientists have been scrutinizing engineered antibodies as target moieties; however their combination with nanocarriers often results in increased interaction with MPS, thus rapidly clearing the nanocarriers from the system [57].

Less specific targets such as broadly expressed transporters have been explored as replacement of antibodies, which may reduce the overall immunogenicity [41]. However they might result in off-target delivery, which occurs if target properties are expressed by both diseased and healthy cells. The wide distribution of diseased cells throughout normal cells would further complicate the situation and might even result in allergic reactions [97, 47, 50, 31]. Current clinical studies have demonstrated that approximately 5% of systemically administered nanocarrier dose reached CNS, which reduced to a lower portion on the targeted cells [40, 31]. Hence, target moiety selection is a personalized process which requires time before execution of the actual process, and is not widely used as the ideal solution currently.

In case of gastrointestinal applications, size and shape have rather limited impact on improving the overall efficacy; hence active targeting methods have also been explored to attain passive diffusion across the gastrointestinal tract. Charge on nanocarrier surface can influence the efficacy of nanocarrier, for instance negatively charged nanocarriers demonstrate enhanced intestinal permeation as compared to positively charged nanocarriers. Negatively charged nanocarriers are transported via opening of tight junctions, instead of transport across the epithelial barrier via cellular uptake. Transferrin coated nanocarriers have been used for transepithelial movement in the intestine. This strategy can be used for disease causing overexpression of the transferrin receptor in the intestine such as the colon cancer and irritable bowel disease [68]. However formation of corona in gastrointestinal fluids results in formation of mucus that coats the endothelial surface, thus restricting the interactions between nanocarriers and the intestinal walls [98, 21]. These barriers depend on the patient diet and pathologies making it even hard for generalizing the possible solutions for achieving therapeutically desired biodistribution by oral delivery [99, 14].

Another commonly employed strategy to generate stealth nanocarriers is through platelet membrane cloaking, which reduces cell uptake and avoids the activation of the macrophage- based immune system [100]. However, nanocarriers may still be recognised by other defence system components [101]. Platelet membrane cloaked nanocarriers features the ligands present on native platelet, hence can mediate the adhesion with collagen resulting in affinity towards the targeted injury site and accumulation near stimulated platelets [102].

Summarizing the properties, the size of the nanomaterials should be in the range where it is large enough to avoid leakage into blood capillaries, and small enough to have a high surface area for high drug loading and release. Appropriate modification must be considered to improve the safe entry and avoiding aggregation. Overall the discussed approaches can be implemented for formulation of an appropriate nanocarrier for efficient drug delivery.

2.4 Additional Aspects

Nanomaterial design strategies are another aspect which has been investigated for improving the overall stability of the drug loaded nanocarrier [19]. The interaction between the compositional material and environment dictates the stability as well as performance of the nanocarrier. Lipid and polymer based nanomaterials often suffer from instability and aggregation both in circulation and in storage. The robustness can be instilled by introducing various lipids and cholesterol functionalities on lipid based nanomaterials [103, 104]. Cross-linking techniques are employed to increase the stability of polymer nanomaterials [105, 106]. For improving storage and transport stability lyophilisation is used [103].

Apart from morphological characteristics of carrier (size/shape and surface properties), efficient drug loading/release profile are also an important aspect of the nanocarrier. As through modulating morphological feature one can assure the safe entrance of drug to tissues in the body and increased the stability of the intended drug, however if the drug amount released in the system is not apt the whole process becomes insignificant. The release of drug from the nanocarrier is a complex phenomenon that relies on various parameters such as pH, temperature, drug solubility, desorption of the surface-bound or adsorbed drug, drug diffusion through the nanomaterial matrix, and the combination of erosion and diffusion processes [107, 108].

The release profile primarily depends on the nature/type of nanomaterial used as drug carrier. Commonly used nanostructures are nanocapsules or nanospheres.

Nanocapsules are homogeneous systems, where the drug is encapsulated in a polymer reservoir. Diffusion through the polymer layer is the key mechanism for drug release; thus drug diffusibility through the polymer matrix is the determining factor. Interaction between drug molecules and polymer component can alter the diffusibility of the drug; the issue can be resolved by using auxiliary agents along with the polymer component. The auxiliary agents form a barrier which restricts the direct interactions between drug molecules and polymer facilitating greater release of the drug at targeted sites [109]. In contrary, nanospheres are homogenous systems where drug and polymers are present in a micelle formation [110]. Drug molecules are uniformly distributed through the matrix system, and erosion of the matrix is the key mechanism behind the release of drug molecules. The weekly attached drug molecules on the nanocarriers are released rapidly in the starting, followed by a sustained release of strongly anchored drug molecules [111].

3 Conclusion

Nanotechnology as a multidisciplinary science has facilitated the development of novel treatment and diagnosing modalities. Employment of nanocarriers for safe and targeted drug delivery has emerged as a consistently growing research field. The vast array of nanomaterials synthesised in recent times has provided scientists with viable alternatives to the conventionally used drug carriers. The unique physicochemical properties of nanomaterials facilitate their effective use for targeted delivery of active pharmaceutical ingredients. Nanomaterials, considering their easily modifiable features have opened up new doors for providing customizable and safer treatment option. The treatment of neurological diseases is a critical area that requires immediate scientific attention. Recent advancements into synthesis and functionalization of nanomaterials could possibly lead us to generate efficient drug carriers for this purpose. The chapter provides insights into physicochemical properties of nanomaterials that must be taken into consideration before utilising them for drug delivery specifically in case of neurological diseases. Ultimately, through the manipulation of size and surface properties, it may be possible to deliver drugs for a longer period of time with sustained release, and greater precision in difficult to access tissues.

References

1. Sheingold BH, Hahn JA (2014) The history of healthcare quality: the first 100 years 1860–1960. Int J Africa Nurs Sci 1:18–22
2. Onoue S, Yamada S, Chan H-K (2014) Nanodrugs: pharmacokinetics and safety. Int J Nanomed 9:1025
3. Rostami-Hodjegan A, Tucker GT (2007) Simulation and prediction of in vivo drug metabolism in human populations from in vitro data. Nat Rev Drug Discov 6(2):140–148

4. Trucillo P (2021) Drug carriers: classification, administration, release profiles, and industrial approach. Processes 9(3):470
5. Zhang J, Saltzman M (2013) Engineering biodegradable nanoparticles for drug and gene delivery. Chem Eng Prog 109(3):25
6. Such GK, Yan Y, Johnston APR, Gunawan ST, Caruso F (2015) Interfacing materials science and biology for drug carrier design. Adv Mater 27(14):2278–2297
7. Sercombe L, Veerati T, Moheimani F, Wu SY, Sood AK, Hua S (2015) Advances and challenges of liposome assisted drug delivery. Front Pharmacol 6:286
8. Patel H, Panchal DR, Patel U, Brahmbhatt T, Suthar M (2011) Matrix type drug delivery system: a review. J Pharm Sci Biosci Res 1(3):143–151
9. Yang W-W, Pierstorff E (2012) Reservoir-based polymer drug delivery systems. J Lab Autom 17(1):50–58
10. Fu Y, Kao WJ (2010) Drug release kinetics and transport mechanisms of non-degradable and degradable polymeric delivery systems. Expert Opin Drug Deliv 7(4):429–444
11. Singh K, Walia MK, Agarwal G, Harikumar SL (2013) Osmotic pump drug delivery system: a noval approach. J Drug Deliv Ther 3(5):156–162
12. Sultana A, Zare M, Thomas V, Kumar TSS, Ramakrishna S (2022) Nano-based drug delivery systems: Conventional drug delivery routes, recent developments and future prospects. Med Drug Discov 100134
13. Mitragotri S, Lammers T, Bae YH, Schwendeman S, De Smedt SC, Leroux JC, Peer D, Kwon IC, Harashima H, Kikuchi A (2017) Drug delivery research for the future: expanding the nano horizons and beyond, vol 246. Elsevier, pp 183–184
14. Mitchell MJ, Billingsley MM, Haley RM, Wechsler ME, Peppas NA, Langer R (2021) Engineering precision nanoparticles for drug delivery. Nat Rev Drug Discov 20(2):101–124
15. Rizvi SAA, Saleh AM (2018) Applications of nanoparticle systems in drug delivery technology. Saudi Pharm J 26(1):64–70
16. Kohane DS (2007) Microparticles and nanoparticles for drug delivery. Biotechnol Bioeng 96(2):203–209
17. Hua S, De Matos, Maria BC, Metselaar JM, Storm G (2018) Current trends and challenges in the clinical translation of nanoparticulate nanomedicines: pathways for translational development and commercialization. Front Pharmacol 9:790
18. Wilhelm S, Tavares AJ, Dai Q, Ohta S, Audet J, Dvorak HF, Chan WCW (2016) Analysis of nanoparticle delivery to tumours. Nat Rev Mater 1(5):1–12
19. Blanco E, Shen H, Ferrari M (2015) Principles of nanoparticle design for overcoming biological barriers to drug delivery. Nat Biotechnol 33(9):941–951
20. Gehr P, Zellner R (2019) Biological responses to nanoscale particles. Springer
21. Ensign LM, Cone R, Hanes J (2012) Oral drug delivery with polymeric nanoparticles: the gastrointestinal mucus barriers. Adv Drug Deliv Rev 64(6):557–570
22. Wu L, Rodríguez-Rodríguez C, Cun D, Yang M, Saatchi K, Häfeli UO (2020) Quantitative comparison of three widely-used pulmonary administration methods in vivo with radiolabeled inhalable nanoparticles. Eur J Pharm Biopharm 152:108–115
23. Zhong Q, Merkel OM, Reineke JJ, da Rocha SRP (2016) Effect of the route of administration and PEGylation of poly (amidoamine) dendrimers on their systemic and lung cellular biodistribution. Mol Pharm 13(6):1866–1878
24. Cone RA (2009) Barrier properties of mucus. Adv Drug Deliv Rev 61(2):75–85
25. Dong W, Ye J, Zhou J, Wang W, Wang H, Zheng X, Yang Y, Xia X, Liu Y (2020) Comparative study of mucoadhesive and mucus-penetrative nanoparticles based on phospholipid complex to overcome the mucus barrier for inhaled delivery of baicalein. Acta Pharm Sin B 10(8):1576–1585
26. Wechsler ME, Ramirez V, Julia E, Peppas NA (2019) 110th anniversary: nanoparticle mediated drug delivery for the treatment of Alzheimer's disease: crossing the blood–brain barrier. Ind Eng Chem Res 58(33):15079–15087
27. Bruinsmann FA, Richter Vaz G, de Cristo Soares Alves A, Aguirre T, Raffin Pohlmann A, Stanisçuaski Guterres S, Sonvico F (2019) Nasal drug delivery of anticancer drugs for the treatment of glioblastoma: preclinical and clinical trials. Molecules 24(23):4312

28. Musumeci T, Bonaccorso A, Puglisi G (2019) Epilepsy disease and nose-to-brain delivery of polymeric nanoparticles: an overview. Pharmaceutics 11(3):118
29. Anselmo AC, Mitragotri S (2019) Nanoparticles in the clinic: an update. Bioeng Transl Med 4:e10143
30. Mu Q, Jiang G, Chen L, Zhou H, Fourches D, Tropsha A, Yan B (2014) Chemical basis of interactions between engineered nanoparticles and biological systems. Chem Rev 114(15):7740–7781
31. Schwartz Jr S (2017) Unmet needs in developing nanoparticles for precision medicine. Future Med 12:271–274
32. Park HS, Nam SH, Kim J, Shin HS, Suh YD, Hong KS (2016) Clear-cut observation of clearance of sustainable upconverting nanoparticles from lymphatic system of small living mice. Sci Rep 6(1):27407
33. Nizzero S, Ziemys A, Ferrari M (2018) Transport barriers and oncophysics in cancer treatment. Trends Cancer 4(4):277–280
34. von Roemeling C, Jiang W, Chan CK, Weissman IL, Kim BYS (2017) Breaking down the barriers to precision cancer nanomedicine. Trends Biotechnol 35(2):159–171
35. Cooley M, Sarode A, Hoore M, Fedosov DA, Mitragotri S, Gupta AS (2018) Influence of particle size and shape on their margination and wall-adhesion: implications in drug delivery vehicle design across nano-to-micro scale. Nanoscale 10(32):15350–15364
36. Hosta-Rigau L, Städler B (2013) Shear stress and its effect on the interaction of myoblast cells with nanosized drug delivery vehicles. Mol Pharm 10(7):2707–2712
37. Jarvis M, Arnold M, Ott J, Krishnan V, Pant K, Prabhakarpandian B, Mitragotri S (2018) Detachment of ligands from nanoparticle surface under flow and endothelial cell contact: assessment using microfluidic devices. Bioeng Transl Med 3(2):148–155
38. Witten J, Ribbeck K (2017) The particle in the spider's web: transport through biological hydrogels. Nanoscale 9(24):8080–8095
39. Caldorera-Moore M, Ramirez V, Julia E, Peppas NA (2019) Transport and delivery of interferon-α through epithelial tight junctions via pH-responsive poly (methacrylic acid-grafted-ethylene glycol) nanoparticles. J Drug Target 27(5–6):582–589
40. Saraiva C, Praça C, Ferreira R, Santos T, Ferreira L, Bernardino L (2016) Nanoparticle-mediated brain drug delivery: overcoming blood–brain barrier to treat neurodegenerative diseases. J Control Release 235:34–47
41. Kou L, Bhutia YD, Yao Q, He Z, Sun J, Ganapathy V (2018) Transporter-guided delivery of nanoparticles to improve drug permeation across cellular barriers and drug exposure to selective cell types. Front Pharmacol 9:27
42. Da Silva-Candal A, Brown T, Krishnan V, Lopez-Loureiro I, Ávila-Gómez P, Pusuluri A, Pérez-Díaz A, Correa-Paz C, Hervella P, Castillo J (2019) Shape effect in active targeting of nanoparticles to inflamed cerebral endothelium under static and flow conditions. J Control Release 309:94–105
43. Alyautdin R, Khalin I, Nafeeza MI, Haron MH, Kuznetsov D (2014) Nanoscale drug delivery systems and the blood–brain barrier. Int J Nanomed 9:795
44. Oliva N, Carcole M, Beckerman M, Seliktar S, Hayward A, Stanley J, Parry NMA, Edelman ER, Artzi N (2015) Regulation of dendrimer/dextran material performance by altered tissue microenvironment in inflammation and neoplasia. Sci Transl Med 7(272):272ra211–272ra211
45. Kruse CR, Singh M, Targosinski S, Sinha I, Sørensen JA, Eriksson E, Nuutila K (2017) The effect of pH on cell viability, cell migration, cell proliferation, wound closure, and wound reepithelialization: in vitro and in vivo study. Wound Repair Regener 25(2):260–269
46. Ruan S, Cao X, Cun X, Hu G, Yi, Zhou, Zhang Y, Lu L, He Q, Gao H (2015) Matrix metalloproteinase-sensitive size-shrinkable nanoparticles for deep tumor penetration and pH triggered doxorubicin release. Biomaterials 60:100–110
47. Nag OK, Delehanty JB (2019) Active cellular and subcellular targeting of nanoparticles for drug delivery. Pharmaceutics 11(10):543
48. Dai Q, Wilhelm S, Ding D, Syed AM, Sindhwani S, Zhang Y, Chen YY, MacMillan P, Chan WCW (2018) Quantifying the ligand-coated nanoparticle delivery to cancer cells in solid tumors. ACS Nano 12(8):8423–8435

49. Zan Y, Dai Z, Liang L, Deng Y, Dong L (2019) Co-delivery of plantamajoside and sorafenib by a multi-functional nanoparticle to combat the drug resistance of hepatocellular carcinoma through reprograming the tumor hypoxic microenvironment. Drug Delivery 26(1):1080–1091
50. Scheetz L, Park KS, Li Q, Lowenstein PR, Castro MG, Schwendeman A, Moon JJ (2019) Engineering patient-specific cancer immunotherapies. Nat Biomed Eng 3(10):768–782
51. Sykes EA, Dai Q, Sarsons CD, Chen J, Rocheleau JV, Hwang DM, Zheng G, Cramb DT, Rinker KD, Chan WCW (2016) Tailoring nanoparticle designs to target cancer based on tumor pathophysiology. Proc Natl Acad Sci 113(9):E1142–E1151
52. Sindhwani S, Syed AM, Ngai J, Kingston BR, Maiorino L, Rothschild J, MacMillan P, Zhang Y, Rajesh NU, Hoang T (2020) The entry of nanoparticles into solid tumours. Nat Mater 19(5):566–575
53. Nance EA, Woodworth GF, Sailor KA, Shih T-Y, Xu Q, Swaminathan G, Xiang D, Eberhart C, Hanes J (2012) A dense poly (ethylene glycol) coating improves penetration of large polymeric nanoparticles within brain tissue. Sci Transl Med 4(149):149ra119–149ra119
54. Wadajkar AS, Dancy JG, Roberts NB, Connolly NP, Strickland DK, Winkles JA, Woodworth GF, Kim AJ (2017) Decreased non-specific adhesivity, receptor targeted (DART) nanoparticles exhibit improved dispersion, cellular uptake, and tumor retention in invasive gliomas. J Control Release 267:144–153
55. Buzea C, Pacheco II, Robbie K (2007) Nanomaterials and nanoparticles: sources and toxicity. Biointerphases 2(4):MR17–MR71
56. Prokop A, Davidson JM (2008) Nanovehicular intracellular delivery systems. J Pharm Sci 97(9):3518–3590
57. Hoshyar N, Gray S, Han H, Bao G (2016) The effect of nanoparticle size on in vivo pharmacokinetics and cellular interaction. Nanomedicine 11(6):673–692
58. Desai MP, Labhasetwar V, Walter E, Levy RJ, Amidon GL (1997) The mechanism of uptake of biodegradable microparticles in Caco-2 cells is size dependent. Pharm Res 14:1568–1573
59. Uhl CG, Gao Y, Zhou S, Liu Y (2018) The shape effect on polymer nanoparticle transport in a blood vessel. RSC Adv 8(15):8089–8100
60. Khor SY, Vu MN, Pilkington EH, Johnston APR, Whittaker MR, Quinn JF, Truong NP, Davis TP (2018) Elucidating the influences of size, surface chemistry, and dynamic flow on cellular association of nanoparticles made by polymerization-induced self-assembly. Small 14(34):1801702
61. Wang W, Gaus K, Tilley RD, Gooding JJ (2019) The impact of nanoparticle shape on cellular internalisation and transport: what do the different analysis methods tell us? Mater Horiz 6(8):1538–1547
62. Xie X, Liao J, Shao X, Li Q, Lin Y (2017) The effect of shape on cellular uptake of gold nanoparticles in the forms of stars, rods, and triangles. Sci Rep 7(1):3827
63. Garapaty A, Champion JA (2019) Shape of ligand immobilized particles dominates and amplifies the macrophage cytokine response to ligands. PLoS ONE 14(5):e0217022
64. Lamson NG, Berger A, Fein KC, Whitehead KA (2020) Anionic nanoparticles enable the oral delivery of proteins by enhancing intestinal permeability. Nat Biomed Eng 4(1):84–96
65. Banerjee A, Qi J, Gogoi R, Wong J, Mitragotri S (2016) Role of nanoparticle size, shape and surface chemistry in oral drug delivery. J Control Release 238:176–185
66. Le Z, Chen Y, Han H, Tian H, Zhao P, Yang C, He Z, Liu L, Leong KW, Mao H-Q (2018) Hydrogen-bonded tannic acid-based anticancer nanoparticle for enhancement of oral chemotherapy. ACS Appl Mater Interfaces 10(49):42186–42197
67. Tian H, He Z, Sun C, Yang C, Zhao P, Liu L, Leong KW, Mao H-Q, Liu Z, Chen Y (2018) Uniform core–shell nanoparticles with thiolated hyaluronic acid coating to enhance oral delivery of insulin. Adv Healthcare Mater 7(17):1800285
68. Yong JM, Mantaj J, Cheng Y, Vllasaliu D (2019) Delivery of nanoparticles across the intestinal epithelium via the transferrin transport pathway. Pharmaceutics 11(7):298
69. Zhang S, Asghar S, Yu F, Chen Z, Hu Z, Ping Q, Shao F, Xiao Y (2019) BSA nanoparticles modified with N-acetylcysteine for improving the stability and mucoadhesion of curcumin in the gastrointestinal tract. J Agric Food Chem 67(33):9371–9381

70. Li D, Zhuang J, He H, Jiang S, Banerjee A, Lu Y, Wu W, Mitragotri S, Li, Gan, Qi J (2017) Influence of particle geometry on gastrointestinal transit and absorption following oral administration. ACS Appl Mater Interfaces 9(49):42492–42502
71. Zheng N, Li J, Xu C, Xu L, Li S, Xu L (2018) Mesoporous silica nanorods for improved oral drug absorption. Artif Cells Nanomed Biotechnol 46(6):1132–1140
72. Zhuang J, Wang D, Li D, Yang Y, Lu Y, Wu W, Qi J (2018) The influence of nanoparticle shape on bilateral exocytosis from Caco-2 cells. Chin Chem Lett 29(12):1815–1818
73. Bantz C, Koshkina O, Lang T, Galla H-J, Kirkpatrick CJ, Stauber RH, Maskos M (2014) The surface properties of nanoparticles determine the agglomeration state and the size of the particles under physiological conditions. Beilstein J Nanotechnol 5(1):1774–1786
74. Brown SB, Wang L, Jungels RR, Sharma B (2020) Effects of cartilage-targeting moieties on nanoparticle biodistribution in healthy and osteoarthritic joints. Acta Biomater 101:469–483
75. Khanbabaie R, Jahanshahi M (2012) Revolutionary impact of nanodrug delivery on neuroscience. Curr Neuropharmacol 10(4):370–392
76. Kou L, Sun J, Zhai Y, He Z (2013) The endocytosis and intracellular fate of nanomedicines: implication for rational design. Asian J Pharm Sci 8(1):1–10
77. Araujo L, Löbenberg R, Kreuter J (1999) Influence of the surfactant concentration on the body distribution of nanoparticles. J Drug Target 6(5):373–385
78. Labhasetwar V, Song C, Humphrey W, Shebuski R, Levy RJ (1998) Arterial uptake of biodegradable nanoparticles: effect of surface modifications. J Pharm Sci 87(10):1229–1234
79. Angra PK, Rizvi SAA, Oettinger CW, D'Souza MJ (2011) Novel approach for preparing nontoxic stealth microspheres for drug delivery. Eur J Chem 2(2):125–129
80. Li S-D, Huang L (2010) Stealth nanoparticles: high density but sheddable PEG is a key for tumor targeting. J Control Release Off J Control Release Soc 145(3):178
81. McSweeney MD, Wessler T, Price LSL, Ciociola EC, Herity LB, Piscitelli JA, Zamboni WC, Forest MG, Cao Y, Lai SK (2018) A minimal physiologically based pharmacokinetic model that predicts anti-PEG IgG-mediated clearance of PEGylated drugs in human and mouse. J Control Release 284:171–178
82. Wang XinYu, Ishida T, Kiwada H (2007) Anti-PEG IgM elicited by injection of liposomes is involved in the enhanced blood clearance of a subsequent dose of PEGylated liposomes. J Control Release 119(2):236–244
83. Chen B-M, Su Y-C, Chang C-J, Burnouf P-A, Chuang K-H, Chen C-H, Cheng T-L, Chen Y-T, Wu J-Y, Roffler SR (2016) Measurement of pre-existing IgG and IgM antibodies against polyethylene glycol in healthy individuals. Anal Chem 88(21):10661–10666
84. Yang Q, Jacobs TM, McCallen JD, Moore DT, Huckaby JT, Edelstein JN, Lai SK (2016) Analysis of pre-existing IgG and IgM antibodies against polyethylene glycol (PEG) in the general population. Anal Chem 88(23):11804–11812
85. Ganson NJ, Povsic TJ, Sullenger BA, Alexander JH, Zelenkofske SL, Sailstad JM, Rusconi CP, Hershfield MS (2016) Pre-existing anti–polyethylene glycol antibody linked to first-exposure allergic reactions to pegnivacogin, a PEGylated RNA aptamer. J Allergy Clin Immunol 137(5):1610–1613, e1617
86. Povsic TJ, Lawrence MG, Lincoff AM, Mehran R, Rusconi CP, Zelenkofske SL, Huang Z, Sailstad J, Armstrong PW, Steg PG (2016) Pre-existing anti-PEG antibodies are associated with severe immediate allergic reactions to pegnivacogin, a PEGylated aptamer. J Allergy Clin Immunol 138(6):1712–1715
87. Dölen Y, Valente M, Tagit O, Jäger E, Van Dinther EAW, van Riessen NK, Hruby M, Gileadi U, Cerundolo V, Figdor CG (2020) Nanovaccine administration route is critical to obtain pertinent iNKt cell help for robust anti-tumor T and B cell responses. Oncoimmunology 9(1):1738813
88. McLennan DN, Porter CJH, Charman SA (2005) Subcutaneous drug delivery and the role of the lymphatics. Drug Discov Today Technol 2(1):89–96
89. Ding J, Chen J, Gao L, Jiang Z, Zhang Y, Li M, Xiao Q, Seong LS, Chen X (2019) Engineered nanomedicines with enhanced tumor penetration. Nano Today 29:100800

90. Hui Y, Yi X, Hou F, Wibowo D, Zhang F, Zhao D, Gao H, Zhao C-X (2019) Role of nanoparticle mechanical properties in cancer drug delivery. ACS Nano 13(7):7410–7424
91. Key J, Palange AL, Gentile F, Aryal S, Stigliano C, Di Mascolo D, De Rosa E, Cho M, Lee Y, Singh J (2015) Soft discoidal polymeric nanoconstructs resist macrophage uptake and enhance vascular targeting in tumors. ACS Nano 9(12):11628–11641
92. Cox A, Andreozzi P, Dal Magro R, Fiordaliso F, Corbelli A, Talamini L, Chinello C, Raimondo F, Magni F, Tringali M (2018) Evolution of nanoparticle protein corona across the blood–brain barrier. ACS Nano 12(7):7292–7300
93. Tenzer S, Docter D, Kuharev J, Musyanovych A, Fetz V, Hecht R, Schlenk F, Fischer D, Kiouptsi K, Reinhardt C (2013) Rapid formation of plasma protein corona critically affects nanoparticle pathophysiology. Nat Nanotechnol 8(10):772–781
94. Friedman AD, Claypool SE, Liu R (2013) The smart targeting of nanoparticles. Current Pharm Design 19(35):6315–6329
95. Jose S, Cinu TA, Sebastian R, Shoja MH, Aleykutty NA, Durazzo A, Lucarini M, Santini A, Souto EB (2019) Transferrin-conjugated docetaxel–PLGA nanoparticles for tumor targeting: influence on MCF-7 cell cycle. Polymers 11(11):1905
96. Liu R, Kay BK, Jiang S, Chen S (2009) Nanoparticle delivery: targeting and nonspecific binding. MRS Bull 34(6):432–440
97. Hong S-T, Lin H, Wang C-S, Chang C-H, Lin A-Y, Yang J-H, Lo Y-L (2019) Improving the anticancer effect of afatinib and microRNA by using lipid polymeric nanoparticles conjugated with dual pH-responsive and targeting peptides. J Nanobiotechnol 17(1):1–20
98. Berardi A, Baldelli Bombelli F (2019) Oral delivery of nanoparticles-let's not forget about the protein corona. Expert Opin Drug Deliv 16(6):563–566
99. Durán-Lobato M, Niu Z, Alonso MJ (2020) Oral delivery of biologics for precision medicine. Adv Mater 32(13):1901935
100. Hu C-M, Fang RH, Wang K-C, Luk BT, Thamphiwatana S, Dehaini D, Nguyen P, Angsantikul P, Wen CH, Kroll AV (2015) Nanoparticle biointerfacing by platelet membrane cloaking. Nature 526(7571):118–121
101. Wibroe PP, Anselmo AC, Nilsson PH, Sarode A, Gupta V, Urbanics R, Szebeni J, Hunter AC, Mitragotri S, Mollnes TE (2017) Bypassing adverse injection reactions to nanoparticles through shape modification and attachment to erythrocytes. Nat Nanotechnol 12(6):589–594
102. Anselmo AC, Modery-Pawlowski CL, Menegatti S, Kumar S, Vogus DR, Tian LL, Chen M, Squires TM, Sen Gupta A, Mitragotri S (2014) Platelet-like nanoparticles: mimicking shape, flexibility, and surface biology of platelets to target vascular injuries. ACS Nano 8(11):11243–11253
103. Cheng X, Lee RJ (2016) The role of helper lipids in lipid nanoparticles (LNPs) designed for oligonucleotide delivery. Adv Drug Deliv Rev 99:129–137
104. Kulkarni JA, Witzigmann D, Leung J, Tam YYC, Cullis PR (2019) On the role of helper lipids in lipid nanoparticle formulations of siRNA. Nanoscale 11(45):21733–21739
105. Palanikumar L, Al-Hosani S, Kalmouni M, Nguyen VP, Ali L, Pasricha R, Barrera FN, Magzoub M (2020) PH-responsive high stability polymeric nanoparticles for targeted delivery of anticancer therapeutics. Commun Biol 3(1):95
106. Tanaka R, Arai K, Matsuno J, Soejima M, Lee JH, Takahashi R, Sakurai K, Fujii S (2020) Furry nanoparticles: synthesis and characterization of nanoemulsion-mediated core crosslinked nanoparticles and their robust stability in vivo. Polym Chem 11(27):4408–4416
107. Mura S, Nicolas J, Couvreur P (2013) Stimuli-responsive nanocarriers for drug delivery. Nat Mater 12(11):991–1003
108. Son G-H, Lee B-J, Cho C-W (2017) Mechanisms of drug release from advanced drug formulations such as polymeric-based drug-delivery systems and lipid nanoparticles. J Pharm Investig 47:287–296
109. Calvo P, Remuñan-López C, Vila-Jato JL, Alonso MJ (1997) Chitosan and chitosan/ethylene oxide-propylene oxide block copolymer nanoparticles as novel carriers for proteins and vaccines. Pharm Res 14:1431–1436

110. Mora-Huertas CE, Fessi H, Elaissari A (2010) Polymer-based nanocapsules for drug delivery. Int J Pharm 385(1–2):113–142
111. Lee JH, Yeo Y (2015) Controlled drug release from pharmaceutical nanocarriers. Chem Eng Sci 125:75–84

Inorganic, Organic and Polymer-Based Nanomaterials

Prayas Singh, Samta Manori, Kuldeep Kumar Raina, and Ravi K. Shukla

Abstract Nanomaterials have found enormous applications in distinct fields owing to their unique properties viz. large and functional surfaces, ease of functionalization, high surface area to volume ratio, stability, optical, electrooptical, magnetic and dynamic behaviors. The nanomaterials are characterized in various categories based on morphological structures like nanosheets, nanotubes, nanocapsules, dendrimers, quantum dots, and fullerenes etc. Diverse applications of the nanomaterials depend upon their shape& size anisotropy, surface properties and transport mechanism of charge carriers. This chapter is dedicated to the scientific phenomenon, processing and characterization and applications perspective of inorganic, organic, and polymer nanomaterials to provide useful insights to aid the future development of efficient and commercially viable technology for large-scale production. In these aspects, inorganic nanomaterials are non-toxic, hydrophilic, biocompatible, and more stable while organic nanomaterials are compared to inorganic highly toxic but due to their good solubility in various solvents these can be used in the application of life and material science. On the other hand, polymer nanomaterials are colloidal particles within the range of size 1–1000 nm. The unique properties of polymer nanoparticles like large synthetic flexibility, biocompatibility, biodegradation, and absorbance to macromolecular substances properties make it a very impressive nanostructure in the field of pharmaceutical and biomedical science.

Keywords Inorganic nanoparticles · Organic nanoparticles · Polymer nanoparticles · High surface area · Drug delivery applications · Biomedical applications

---

P. Singh · S. Manori · R. K. Shukla (✉)
Advanced Functional Smart Materials Laboratory, School of Physical Sciences, Department of Physics, DIT University, Dehradun, UK 248009, India
e-mail: ravi.shukla@dituniversity.edu.in

K. K. Raina
M.S. Ramaiah University of Applied Sciences, Bangalore 560054, India

S. K. Rath et al. (eds.), *Nanomaterials for Drug Delivery and Neurological Diseases Management*, Smart Nanomaterials Technology,
https://doi.org/10.1007/978-981-97-0308-1_2

1 Introduction

The massive and interdisciplinary area of nanocrystalline technology and science has seen an enormous increase in research and development over the past few years [1]. The methods used to create materials and goods, as well as the range and kind of features and functionality that may be available, have the potential to be fundamentally altered [2–4]. Nanomaterials are a class of substances with at least one dimension falling between 1 and 100 nm [5]. They adhere to the fundamental principles of nanoscience and nanotechnology, whose applications span a wide range of interdisciplinary research and development that is expanding rapidly across the globe [6]. Nanomaterials can change into functionalized substitutes that can be accessed again and again. Quantum dots (QDs), fullerenes, nanotubes, and dendrimers are examples of typical nanomaterials [7]. Due to their distinctive optical qualities, nanomaterials are becoming more and more popular in a wide range of industries, including medicine, electronics, pharmaceuticals, nanocolloids, polymers etc. [3, 8, 9].

Nanoscale materials, used in cosmetics [10–12], sunscreen [13–16], and self-cleaning windows or sensors [17], as well as nano coatings and nanocomposites for windows [18], sports equipment [19], and automobiles [20], as well as other products like wrinkle- and stain-free textiles [21], electronics [22], printing [23, 24], water purification [25–27] and varnishes [28], are commercial uses for nanomaterials. The schematic representation of various application of nanomaterials are given in Fig. 1.

Nanotechnology provides an interdisciplinary platform to combine biological and physical sciences considering the ordering and surface properties of nanomaterials analogous to orientational ordering of biological entities [29]. The plausible results of such collaborative technologies are nanomedicines, nano-based drug delivery systems and nanomotors etc. [30] biosensors [31], antibacterial agents [32–34], microfluidics [35], and tissue engineering [36, 37]. Nanoparticles are typically small nanospheres because they are made of materials that are created at the atomic or molecular level. As a result, they can travel within the human body with greater freedom than bulkier materials [38].

The objective chapter is to syndicate scientific considerations and technological aspects of inorganic and organic nanomaterials, with a focus on methods of preparation & processing, characterization and applications that offer a fresh perspective nanomaterial science in the field of biological arena.

2 Organic Nanomaterials

Organic nanoparticles are defined as solid particles with an average diameter of 10 nm to 1 μm that are made up primarily of lipids or other organic substances [39]. Compared to inorganic materials, which have seen significant investment in both research and industry, they have gotten relatively little attention. There is no doubt about the potential future benefits of inorganic nanoparticles like quantum dots,

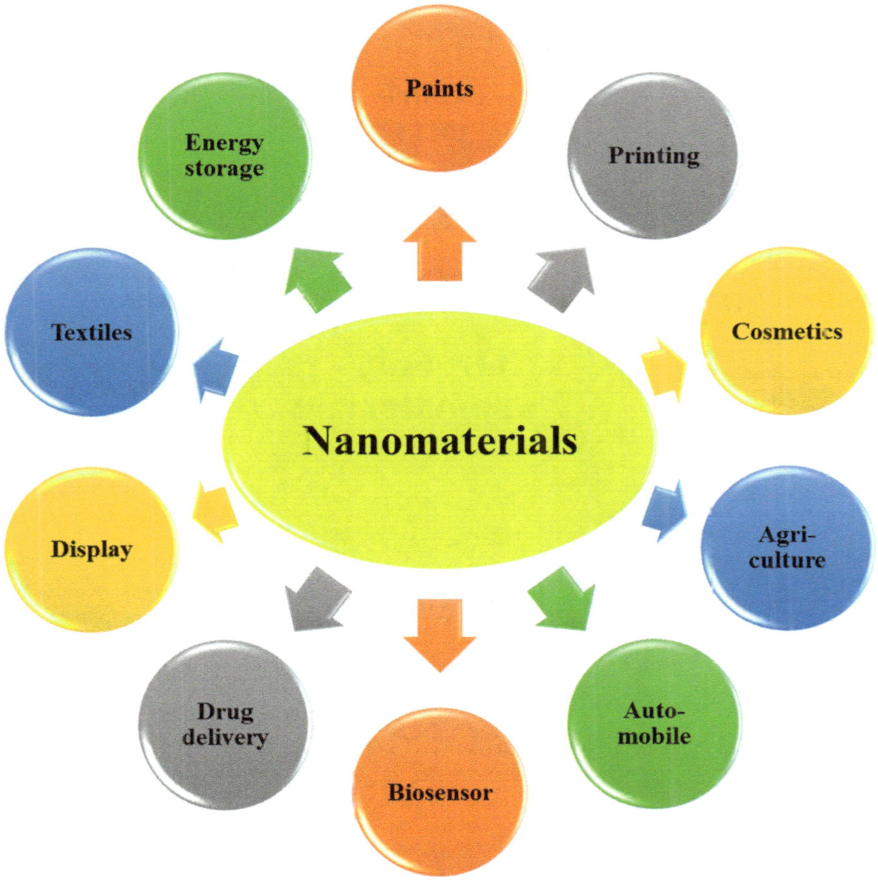

Fig. 1 Applications of nanomaterials

silicas, gold nanoparticles, titania, and various catalysts, but grain nano solutions believes that there is a much greater commercial opportunity in the thousands of insoluble or poorly soluble organic compounds that are used in both high-tech and commodity product fields. In recent years, the study into organic nanoparticles has been driven by the pharmaceutical industry. New materials have been created and tried-and-true methods have been improved as a result of the search for nanomedicine [40].

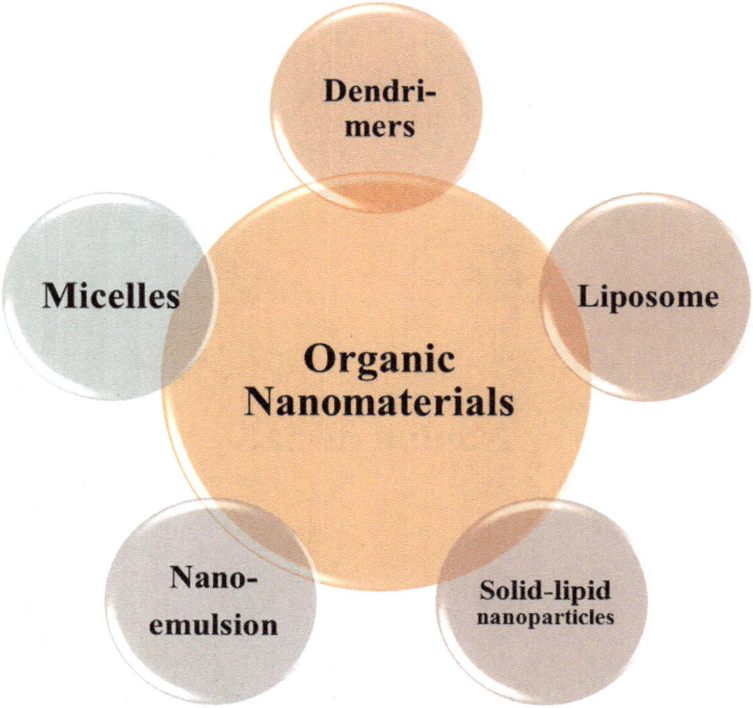

Fig. 2 Classification of organic nanomaterials

2.1 Biomimetics

Biomimetic nano capsules are a different strategy that has been developed. They have a polyglyceryl-6 dioleate and triglyceride-based oily core that is encased in a polyethylene glycol (PEG) and HS-PEG shell. To increase the resistance to quick clearance, they have been used to encapsulate DNA. Complexes with positive charges are concealed by the PEG coating, preventing immune proteins from opsonizing them. DNA nano capsules outperform lipoplexes because PEG causes the lipid endosomal membrane to become unstable [41]. The ability of the nanospheres to biodegrade after passing through the required specific sites is another crucial factor. Initially, synthetic polymers that are non-biodegradable like polyacrylamide and polyethylene were the primary materials used in biopolymer NP design. Soon, it was thought that it is difficult to supervise the systematic introduction of poly(methylacrylate) and polyacrylamide NPs in human body and their chronic toxicity brought on by tissue overload with non-degradable polymers. Owing to this, the emphasis on biodegradable polymers like poly(lactic-co-glycolic acid) and polyanhydride has been shifted [42]. Another restriction applies to administer hydrophilic molecules, such as nucleic acids (oligonucleotides and genes), using bio nanoparticles [43]. This restriction is primarily caused by the hydrophobic nature of the polymers that make up these NPs, as opposed to the hydrophilic nature of biomolecules like nucleic acids. This causes problems with effective encapsulation and enzymatic degradation protection and lead to the investigation about preparing the NPs by using naturally occurring materials and show hydrophilic properties.

2.2 Nucleic Acid Transport

Systems for delivering genes safely and effectively are essential for treating various cardiovascular disorders, genetic diseases, and viral infections. To discontinue the function of the target genes and cause silencing, antisense oligonucleotides or else small interfering RNA can also be delivered as part of gene therapy [44]. For a variety of cells and tissues, numerous techniques for delivering genes have been developed in recent years. Along with these therapeutic uses, delivery of gene is frequently employed in-vitro to examine how gene's role and are regulated in the context of cellular and physiological processes. Through the potential to have a significant impact on fundamental research and technological aspects of biotech and diagnostic the first gene delivery schemes have been developed. In order to release the nucleic acid, gene delivery systems should be able to assemble stable nucleic acid complexes with minimal cytotoxicity [45]. Functional groups are added to the vector to control environmental interactions. These functionalities can target a particular cell type or tissue, stabilize the vector in the extracellular milieu, or keep the vector inside the delivery site. Bioactive assemblies may be fused to help with endosomal escape because intracellular trafficking takes care of the need to have the plasmid to the nucleus for expression. Viral and nonviral vectors are both used in gene delivery systems. Although viral vectors are the most efficient, but they have certain limitations which restrict their therapeutic applications due to their oncogenicity and immunogenicity as well as by their DNA loading capacity [46]. Nonviral vectors are less dangerous and more affordable than viral vectors. Cationic peptides, cationic polymers, or cationic lipids make up the majority of nonviral transfection systems, though combinations of these substances are also possible. Receptor ligands might be used to the NP to enhance the binding to cell-surface receptors and enable cellular internalization, enabling the particular cell types targeting. Before reaching the nucleus, the DNA must navigate a number of dangers to the cell after being introduced. In order to prevent this, intensive research is being done to identify the ideal carrier which enable cell transportation to the DNA's nucleus. The carrier must have flexible tropism, be small enough to pass through nuclear pores and allow cellular internalization, and enable to elude the lysosome- endosome process that occurs after endocytosis [47]. Furthermore, it must not trigger an immune reaction or be cytotoxic. While numerous conditions and readout systems have been used for testing the transfection efficiency and toxicity with gene delivery in various cell types, the absence of a standards types it challenging to directly evaluate various methods. As a result, rather than providing a thorough comparison of the various approaches used over time.

2.3 Solid-Lipid Nanoparticles in Biomedical

When the liquid lipid in emulsions is swapped out for a solid lipid, they solidify at body and room temperature, which results into reduction in the particle size [48]. It has been proven that SLN:DNA vectors can cause the expression of an alien protein when administer intravenously. DNA molecules that are shielded from protons' acidic attack remain intact inside the cell by neutralization of the acidic pH of endosome's. The main distinction with liposomes is that they use a lipophilic core matrix rather than an aqueous one to release and deliver bioactive substances [49].

3 Inorganic Nanomaterials

Inorganic materials are frequently used to create nanomaterials due to their ability to be altered in terms of crystallinity, size, shape, surface area, and ease of functionalization. Unique optical, catalytic, thermodynamic, magnetic and electrochemical properties as well as additional bioactivities are present in inorganic particles [50]. Metallic and non-metallic nanoparticles are two types of inorganic particles. Nanoparticles with surface plasmonic resonance (SPR) likely silver and gold (Ag or Au) are used commonly owing to their strong plasma absorption with improved Rayleigh and surface Raman scattering [51]. With different surface modifications and as hybrids, metal oxides like iron oxide (Fe_2O_3, Fe_3O_4) and silica (SiO_2) are also being used. Inorganic nanomaterials are classified in different types of nanoparticles such as magnetic, metallic, carbon based, silica, etc. (Fig. 3).

3.1 Gold and Silver Nanomaterials

Gold nanoparticles (AuNPs) and their colloidal solutions gold or can be easily produced and employed for wide range of applications. AuNPs strongly absorb and scatter visible light which makes them prominent candidates for bioimaging [52]. Free electrons exists in the gold particles are excited to collective oscillations, or surface plasmons, upon light absorption. For gold, silver, and copper, this absorption is visible, and the SPR of AuNPs is visible till 3 nm. The size of the absorption and scattering produced by AuNPs is dependent on the size of the AuNPs [52]. Particles whose size is less than 20 nm essentially absorb, but particles with size of around 80 nm raise the scattering/absorption ratio. Conversely, silver nanoparticles (AgNPs),

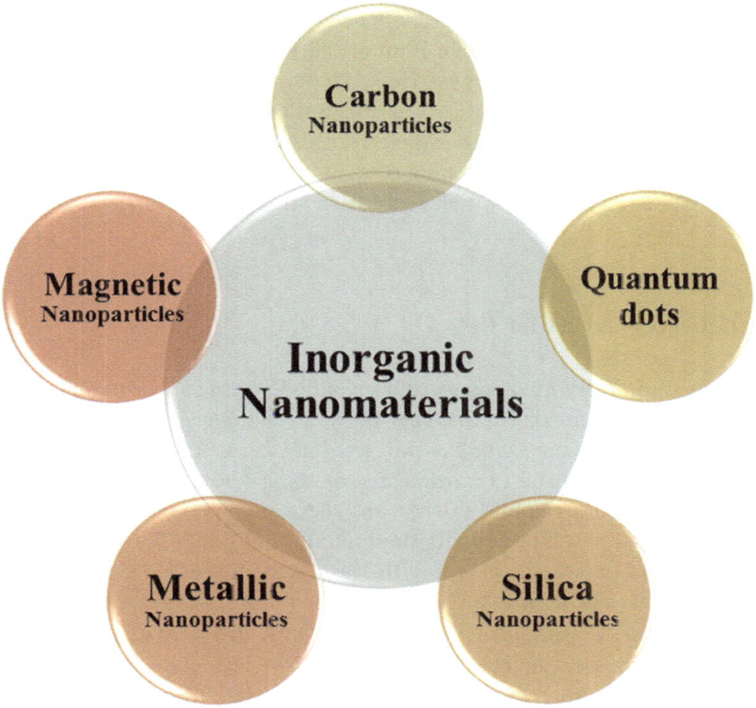

Fig. 3 Classification of inorganic nanomaterials

show outstanding antimicrobic activity against bacteria, viruses, and other microorganisms. AgNPs are therefore widely used in a variety of products, including dental materials [53], clothing [54], coatings for stainless steel [55, 56], water treatment [57, 58], and burn treatments [59].

3.1.1 Biosensor

Plasmon resonance frequency, which can be seen by scattered light, can directly change when molecules bind to the surface of the particle. In similar fashion, the inter nanoparticles distance's in Au affect the plasmon resonance, which play a vital role for sensor applications [60]. When the NPs are linked to a biological analyte, a colour change occurs that forms the foundation of sensing. Colorimetric nucleic acid sensing was the report published on the gold-based biosensor [61]. AuNPs with interparticle distance of 0.34 nm joined to DNA, changing their colour from red to purple depending on whether they were free (red) or bound to the DNA (blue-violet) [62]. Temperature changes can be reversed without losing colour. As a result, even a minor sequence inconsistency will cause the sample to melt at a different temperature than it should, which will alter its colour when heated. AuNPs exhibit antiphotobleaching behaviour when illuminated by bright light and have excellent fluorescent properties. When exposed to relatively high excitation power, AuNPs exhibit robust native fluorescence. As an illustration, fluorescence of AuNP can be captured for imaging of cell if cells stained with AuNPs are exposed to bright light. Another phenomenon is the quenching of many fluorophores' fluorescence when it comes into contact with gold, which can be used in a number of sensing techniques [63].

3.1.2 Delivery Vehicles for Cells

The majority of delivery methods, such as using NPs with cancer-targeting moieties attached to deliver them into the cancer tissue as similar to MNs and others. The delivery of molecules into cells has, in fact, long been accomplished using gold. Cellular uptake can be used to introduce something into cells or it can be forced, as with gene guns, for example. When using the gene gun method, DNA is applied to AuNPs, which are then principally fired into the cells [64]. Usually, gas pressure or electric discharge is used to supply the necessary force. However, in plant cell biology, the use of gene guns to break through the plant cell wall was more common. For delivering DNA into animal cells, gene guns have also been used. AuNP can also be delivered through specific or nonspecific endocytosis of cells. Passive nonspecific uptake is much less efficient than active specific uptake, for instance, transferrin adsorbed onto the AuNPs to trigger cellular uptake. Efforts has been made to prevent endosomal uptake and subsequent vesicle storage. Nucleoplasmin-coated AuNPs (10–35 nm), a Xenopus oocyte protein, were translocated into the nucleus using microinjection on chemically altered cells [65]. Excellent cellular uptake levels can also be achieved by conjugating t-t peptide to AuNPs which enabled direct plasma membrane translocation [66].

3.1.3 Au and AgNPs for Biological Imaging

In terms of bioimaging, immunostaining is arguably where AuNPs are used most frequently. In order to improve contrast, a surplus of gold is typically used to label nearly all entities. Targets inside and outside of cells can both be labelled as the cells are fixed and permeabilized. Gold can be used to immunostain thick/thin sections before embedding or to immunostain ultrathin sections after embedding in order to detect proteins, peptides, or amino acids [67]. Gold serves as an immunolabel, and its particulate nature makes it possible to semi-quantitatively analyze antigen densities on ultrathin sections. AuNPs are more stable than fluorescence microscopy because they are not photobleached, and they typically provide excellent lateral resolution and high contrast in TEM imaging.

3.2 *Magnetic Nanomaterials (MNs)*

Magnetic nanomaterials (MNs) are one of the most useful nanomaterials for the application in field of material science, nanoengineering and biomedical science [68–70]. It is usually decorated by magnetic core such as magnetite (Fe_3O_4) and maghemite (g-Fe_2O_3) [71, 72]. On the other hand, other metals like as nickel and cobalt are less useful because of the toxicity and vulnerability to oxidation [73, 74]. Iron nanoparticles are very prominent for the biomedical applications because of the primary presence of iron in the human body [68, 75–77]. These cationic MNs are present and remain localized in the endosomes for a long time. After that, substances that are being metabolized or expended by hydrolytic enzymes during post-cellular uptake in the lysosomes and endosomes are added to the body's storage. Examples of these compounds include iron and oxygen. Adsorption, excretion, and storage all play important roles in maintaining and postulating the iron level in the human body, which is well controlled by homeostasis. The body processes any excess iron through the use of iron oxide nanoparticles [78]. Although iron is essential to almost all living tissues, its bioavailability is only moderate. When it is not bound to hemoglobin or in the form of free iron, it can occasionally be toxic to cells. Superparamagnetic iron oxide NPs have a special property of superparamagnetic that makes them ideal for use in advanced biomedical materials [79, 80]. Under physiological conditions, the inorganic iron core exhibits a stable behavior, thanks to the application of a biocompatible surface coating (i.e. inhibits aggregation). Synthetic and natural polymers, fatty acids based amphiphilic molecules can be utilized as materials for coating [81]. Findings about MNs are being used more and more as effective delivery vectors, opening up possibilities for targeted therapies, mediators of cancer treatment with hyperthermia, and MRI contrast enhancement [82].

3.2.1 Magnetofection

Application of the magnetic field on the nucleic acid vectors which are coupled to MNs includes the process is referred to as "magnetic transfection," which affects how nucleic acids are delivered. Small constructs and "large" nucleic acids can both be transfected using the magnetic transfection technique [83]. Negatively charged DNAs are bound to MNs via electrostatic interactions, whereupon they are released after cell internalization [84]. In comparison to traditional transfection techniques, magnetic transfection offers a number of benefits, including a quicker turnaround time and higher transfection efficiency at lower vector doses. Lack targeted-specificity in these therapies results in poor diffusion across the cell membrane, which leads to deprived megnetofection efficacies. To overcome these issues, MNs are prescribed for better results and efficiency. It is possible to take advantage of RNA interference, a naturally occurring cellular process that is used to silence gene expression [85]. To use therapeutic RNA silencing on a large scale, a suitable transfection technique must be created which can deliver siRNA molecules to human cells in vivo. Because of their versatility, NPs are desirable siRNA delivery agents, which enables them to circumvent many issues. According to a study, NPs can stop the kidney from rapidly excreting siRNA [86]. The naked siRNA molecules suffer this fate. The half-life of unmodified siRNA in the circulation is prolonged as a result of the pulling of MNs by magnetic force toward target cell which are attached to NPs and thus cause negligible renal filtration [87]. A 2007 study that reported the uptake of MNs into tumors showed that cancer cells could be transfected by NP-delivered siRNA [88]. In this instance, a myristoyl-coupled polyarginine peptide that was attached made membrane translocation easier. Near-IR in vivo optical imaging and MRI both are used for the imaging [89, 90]. Imaging results revealed the staggering of NPs in tumors, which is almost certainly passive because of the leaky tumor vasculature's improved permeability and retention effect. According to the study, NPs with additional tumor-targeting functionalities would improve tumor localization so as to deliver siRNA therapy.

3.2.2 Magnetic Resonance Imaging (MRI)

MRI is a dynamic imaging instrument that provides the benefit of three-dimensional fine spatial resolution of contrast distinction among organs and tissues of body. Contrast agent based on MNs give better image enhancement in comparison to the conformist gadolinium chelates owing to their strong magnetic moments, enhanced cellular internalization, and sluggish clearance from the target site [91]. Iron oxide MNs are used to the reduction of T2 relaxation time due to their unique capacity. So, iron oxide MNs are frequently utilized as a T2 contrast controller agent in MRI applications. Such materials are characterized as a superparamagnetic iron oxide MNs which have the diameter greater than 50 nm or ultrasmall superparamagnetic MNs having diameters < 50 nm and these MNs typically have plasma half-lives of 14 to 30 h [92, 93]. For clinical applications like bowel and liver there are currently a number of formulations available [94]. The research efforts are being paid on the new next generation of active contrast agents and promising to open up exciting new avenues for treatment, diagnostic imaging. In the study of solid tumor, MNs are used as MRI agents to improve the diagnosis study [82].

3.2.3 Hyperthermia

Comparing to the normal healthy cells, temperature-sensitive cells, tumor cells are grown fast. A technique created with the aid of MNs, in particular superparamagnetic iron oxide, has the potential to be used to treat cancer [95]. In order to heat up the cell and cause necrosis, this treatment uses a delivery agent that also serves as a nanoscale heater [96, 97]. Application of the alternating MF to the nanoscale heater causes electromagnetic energy to be converted into heat energy that can be released into the surrounding atmosphere. Magnetic materials whose temperature lies in a range of 42 °C–60 °C offer a successful treatment by serving as an in-vivo switch that can control the temperature to prevent nearby healthy tissue from overheating

[98]. NPs can accumulate in tumor tissue due to its propensity for having “leaky” vasculature, which makes it a passive target for biodistribution. Instead, MNs can be directly injected to the solid tumors imperiled to an additional alternating magnetic field to cause tumor regression. The effectiveness of heating the MNs in human breast cancer has been reported [99]. To get the best performance out of it, however, it is necessary to investigate the optimum conditions for controlling the heat distribution. For instance, a hyperthermia study uses tumor-targeted MNs to assess how well the drug payload is enhanced [100]. Targeting chimeric L6 monoclonal antibody has a high likelihood of success when dextrancoated MNs are used. However, hyperthermia research has also focused on reducing tumor gene expression [101]. Controlling and assessing these gene expressions in tumors is fundamentally important [102–106].

3.3 *Carbon Nanotubes (CNTs)*

The signal and sensitivity can be increased by loading NPs that are hollow and porous. Graphene sheets shaped like tubes make up carbon nanotubes. Owing to the electronic and physical properties, CNTs are primly studied for microelectronic devices. However, they have also proven as potential candidate for use in biomedicine [107]. Both single-walled carbon nanotubes (SWCNTs) and multiwalled CNTs (MWCNTs) have been explored by researchers for various bio applications. SWCNTs shows predominant optical absorbance in the NIR region, where biological systems are known to be highly transparent [108].

3.3.1 Cancer Treatment

SWCNTs are used in the thermal necrosis of cancerous cells in a manner similar to MNs and AuNPs. After treatment, there were few side effects that lasted up to six months, and three months later, the tumor cells were eliminated through urine. In a similar manner, MWCNTs were used in thermal cancer therapy on mice carrying kidney tumors, and the tumors completely disappeared with no sign of recurrence after three months. In order to target tumors, both folate receptors and antibodies have been employed [109]. In targeted applications, CNTs have also been explored as a possible method of therapeutic drug delivery to tumors. The growth of the tumor was almost 60% inhibited by the evenly dispersed particles [110]. Other inorganic NP types exist, including silica, nanorods, nanoshells, and various hybrid nanoparticles, but the four mentioned above are the most frequently used when thinking about bio-applications. Although each of the described particles demonstrates some unique characteristics, many of the bio applications share functionalities and target populations. Each particle type is intended to increase cellular uptake efficiency, enhance images or signals, deliver cargo, or target particular tissues or cells [111].

3.4 *Quantum Dots (QDs)*

Colloidal sub-nanometer sized crystals derived mostly from groups II–VI elements of the periodic table (such as Cd, Zn, Se, and Te) or III to V (such as In, P, and As) are called QDs [112]. The most frequently used QDs in bio-applications were made of CdSe and protected from the highly toxic cadmium by a ZnS shell. Bandgap energy allows for the tuning of the corresponding emission wavelengths from the UV to near-infrared (NIR) region by enclosing the electrons in a range of sizes [113]. With wavelengths between 380 and 440 nm, smaller QDs exhibit blue fluorescence emission, while bigger particles exhibit red emission (within 605–630 nm). In addition to their adjustable fluorescence, QDs have other merits over organic dye molecules. Because they are inorganic, they emit stable and stronger light and are less photosensitive than organic dye molecules. They are very helpful for monitoring cells over longer time periods because of their photostability.

3.4.1 Single-Cell Imaging

Transmembrane proteins, mobility kinetics of receptors and synapses have recently been carried out by using QDs [114]. The method for detecting and monitoring conventional organic dyes can also be used for QDs. Tracking QDs in a cellular environment is technically challenging. First, precision is reduced by background noise brought on by surrounding QDs and cell autofluorescence. This noise is reduced by using QDs that emit in the red wavelength range in which the autofluorescence of cell vanishes [115]. A number of techniques have been established in recent past to acquire image stacks by reconstructing the 3-D structure of the cell [116].

3.4.2 Biomedical Imaging from QDs

QDs are considered as favorable candidates to design probe for long-term experiments in living cells because of their unique properties like high photostability and minimal cytotoxicity, provided a number of issues are addressed. The ability to dissolve in water is a crucial prerequisite for in vivo and in vitro imaging. Hydrophilicity of QDs can be enhanced via thiol functionalization, typically fixed to the ZnS shell with carboxyl (COOH) group at terminal [117]. The cell uptake is typically improved through functionalization of particle surface, just like with magnetic and gold NPs. To get QDs into the cytoplasm of the cell, several approaches have been suggested. The QDs' prolonged entrapment in the endosomes is the main problem in this situation. Pinocytosis is a different route that can be used. A second osmotic shock may then cause pinosomes to rupture, liberating the QDs into the cell cytoplasm [118].

4 Polymer Nanomaterials (PNs)

Over the past few years, polymeric nanoparticles (PNs) are being used for different applications of technological branches. They have been identified as colloidal nanoparticles induced from polymers. Due to their nano size, nanoparticles made of polymers typically have novel properties. Numerous new and exciting properties can be added without altering the makeup of the material by reducing them to nano dimensions. PNs' smaller molecule size is one of the main factors that gives them moderately novel properties compared to bulk polymers [119–124]. The classification of polymer nanoparticles is given in Fig. 4.

As a result of its numerous applications in fields like photonics, sensors, medicine, environmental and purification applications, the study of PNs is quickly growing and becoming a crucial area of study in the field of chemistry. PNs have long been used

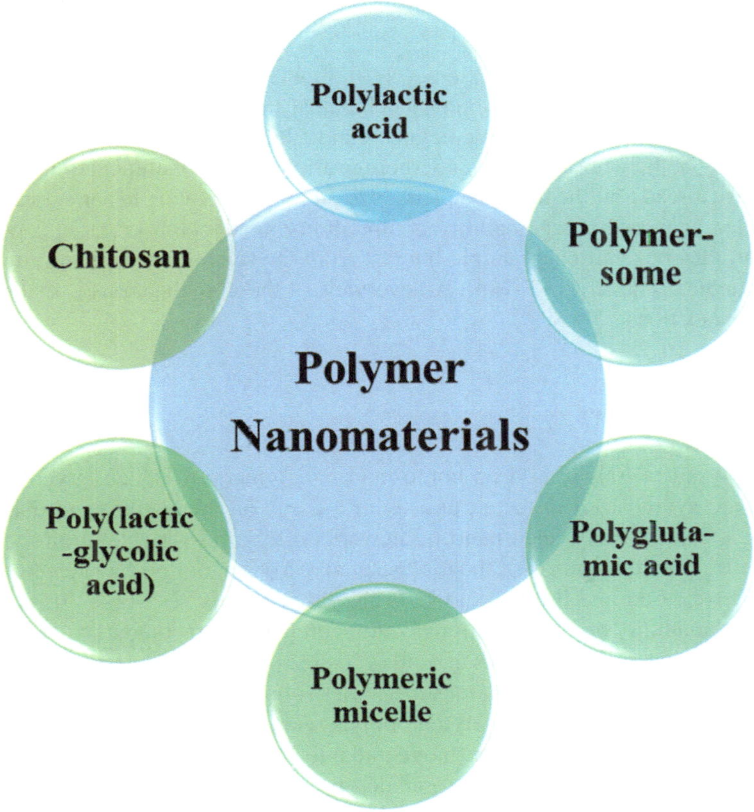

Fig. 4 Classification of polymeric nanomaterials

in the production of numerous essential and practical compounds, including coatings, paints, glues, and many others. Recently, they have been found to have uses in biomedical fields like diagnostics, drug delivery, and bio-imaging [125–128]. Several polymerization techniques, such as surfactant emulsion, miniaturized scale emulsion, and interfacial polymerization, can be used to directly polymerize monomers. Using methods like salting in and out, dialysis, dissipation, fluid nature, PNs arrangements from pre-framed polymers can be crafted. Surfactant PNs can be put together using strategies such as surfactant emulsion polymerization, rapid supercritical fluid expansion, and fast extension of super-critical liquid into liquid. While using any of these techniques, it's important to keep in mind a number of factors, including the application area, particle sizes, particle sizes distribution, surface morphologies, and elasticity [126–135].

4.1 Medical Applications

Nanoparticles have been used extensively in biomedical science over the past few decades because of their superior physicochemical characteristics than that of micromaterials. They are being used for diagnosis and other biomedical applications [136–142]. Many of them are currently undergoing various stages of clinical trials, many of them have already hit the market and are offered for sale. Owing to some fascinating properties, such as bio-degradability, compatibility, small cytotoxicity, etc., polymer nanoparticles have attracted ample interest from the scientific community for their use in medical science [143–146]. An overview of those applications is given in the following sections.

4.1.1 Drug Delivery

Distinct types of PNs (based on homo- and copolymers of lactate, glycolate, and PHAs) are synthesized in recent past, with a focus on therapeutic and diagnostic purposes. Undoubtedly, such nano frameworks offer a possible solution for better drug delivery and diagnosis of the disease at an early stage. PNs have changed how drugs are released and brought closer to the disease cells [2, 147–149]. Based on the cell adaptability built on functionalization, preparation methods, polymers are of interest for remedial applications as well [150–153]. When polymeric nanoparticles (NPs) were first used for applications in a variety of scientific fields, they were based on polymers like PMMA, polystyrene polyacrylamide and polyacrylates. Frameworks should be designed for non-biodegradable particles so that they either exhibit quick release from the body in a stipulated time [151–157]. In medicine PNs are mainly used to create stimuli responsive drug delivery systems [158–161]. Utilizing stimuli-responsive biodegradable PNs for controlled medication delivery has proven substantial therapeutic potential. A targeted delivery of drugs to the site of the disease is simultaneously becoming more and more important, thanks to advances in directed conveyance. Targeted PNs can be used in malignant growth to more effectively deliver chemotherapy to tumor cells while reducing cytotoxicity on surrounding healthy tissues. If only a small amount of water-soluble medications are present, the medication may be released directly from NPs through dispersion, or it may occur concurrently with the breakdown of the NPs into monomeric atoms [162–165]. Altering external stimuli (especially pH or temperature) or external boosts can cause the degradation of polymers to occur (e.g., radiation or ultrasound). In this way, the stacked polymer NPs can degrade in a controlled manner to release the drugs in specific cell compartments as needed by the disease cells, and then they can be easily removed from the living thing. However, there are many stimuli that can be used, including pH, ultrasound, temperature, IR-radiation, magnetic fields, etc. [166–170].

4.1.2 Bioimaging Applications

Bioimaging is a significant use of polymer NP in biomedicine. Various techniques have been developed over the past few decades viz. positron emission tomography (PET), computerized tomography (CT), ultrasound imaging, and magnetic resonance imaging (MRI) etc. [171, 172]. The majority of techniques had a number of drawbacks, including time and health related issues. Therefore, novel techniques those are cheap and safe to use are needs to be developed. Although many different kinds of nanomaterials have been developed for bioimaging, polymer nanoparticles and conjugated polymer nanoparticles have a particularly prominent place in the field [173–176]. Conjugated Polymer Nanoparticles (CPNs), which have made significant contributions to bioimaging, are typically created by mixing various semiconducting nanoparticles with polymer nanoparticles and have shown promising results in clinical imaging. CPNs have low cytotoxicity and are quickly absorbed by cells because they are hydrophobic. Semiconducting conjugated particles exhibit strong fluorescence due to their pi-conjugated electron structure, and the discharge shading can be adjusted to cover the entire visible spectrum into the near infrared (NIR) by simply changing the comonomer composition. CPNs also demonstrate excellent performance for image-guided photodynamic and photothermal treatment. CPNs can also have their surfaces functionalized with a variety of organic and biological molecules. The delivery of CPNs can be accomplished using a range of techniques, such as polymerization scattering conventions, post-polymerization mini-emulsification, and nano-precipitation techniques [138, 156, 174, 177–180]. Hydrophobic conjugated polymers are combined to form conjugated polymer nanoparticles, also known as semiconducting polymer nanospheres (SPNs). Due to their increased brightness and improved biocompatibility, these nanoparticles could be used in applications where QDs are used, and they might even outperform QDs in some cases. Conjugated polymer use in bimodal frameworks was previously explained by the covalent attachment of gadolinium-containing particles to frameworks coming from watery conjugated polymers. CPN is a developing photoacoustic impact-based crossover imaging material that has demonstrated its benefits for high tenacity molecular imaging with remarkable infiltration depth. As a result of numerous studies and experiments, it is now evident that CPN-based multi-modal imaging and treatment that depends on these multi-functional CPNs can pave the way for future advancements in malignant growth theranostics [181–185].

5 Conclusions

Nanomaterials, distinguished by their incredibly small feature sizes, have several industrial, biological, and electronic uses in the future. Substantial large surface area and strong reactivity, make excellent materials for adsorption, catalysis and biosensors. NPs are crucial to many biotechnological applications and have potential for many upcoming and novel applications. Future innovations in this discipline include fields like purification of water, disinfection, production of food and packaging along with medicinal applications (drug delivery to tumor cells and use for regenerative medicine. Finding a straightforward, effective, and manageable method to mass manufacture nanomaterials and connect their optoelectronic applications will be appealing.

References

1. Baig N, Kammakakam I, Falath W, Kammakakam I (2021) Nanomaterials: a review of synthesis methods, properties, recent progress, and challenges. Mater Adv 2(6):1821–1871. https://doi.org/10.1039/d0ma00807a
2. Salata OV (2004) Applications of nanoparticles in biology and medicine. J Nanobiotechnol 2:1–6. https://doi.org/10.1186/1477-3155-2-3
3. Stark WJ, Stoessel PR, Wohlleben W, Hafner A (2015) Industrial applications of nanoparticles. Chem Soc Rev 44(16):5793–5805. https://doi.org/10.1039/c4cs00362d
4. Shafiq M, Anjum S, Hano C, Anjum I, Abbasi BH (2020) An overview of the applications of nanomaterials and nanodevices in the food industry. Foods 9(2):1–27. https://doi.org/10.3390/foods9020148
5. Andrievskii RA (2009) Size-Dependent effects in properties of nanostructured materials. Rev Adv Mater Sci 21:107–133
6. Nanomaterials for medical applications. Elsevier (2013). https://doi.org/10.1016/C2010-0-65569-6
7. Barad HN, Kwon H, Alarcón-Correa M, Fischer P (2021) Large area patterning of nanoparticles and nanostructures: current status and future prospects. ACS Nano 15(4):5861–5875. https://doi.org/10.1021/acsnano.0c09999
8. Aliofkhazraei M (2015) Handbook of nanoparticles. https://doi.org/10.1007/978-3-319-15338-4
9. Subhan M, Choudhury K, Neogi N (2021) Advances with molecular nanomaterials in industrial manufacturing applications. Nanomanufacturing 1(2):75–97. https://doi.org/10.3390/nanomanufacturing1020008
10. Dréno B, Alexis A, Chuberre B, Marinovich M (2019) Safety of titanium dioxide nanoparticles in cosmetics. J Eur Acad Dermatol Venereol 33(S7):34–46. https://doi.org/10.1111/jdv.15943

11. Salvioni L, Morelli L, Ochoa E, Labra M, Fiandra L, Palugan L, Prosperi D, Colombo M (2021) The emerging role of nanotechnology in skincare. Adv Colloid Interfa Sci 293:102437. https://doi.org/10.1016/j.cis.2021.102437
12. Aziz ZAA, Mohd-Nasir H, Ahmad A, Siti SH, Peng WL, Chuo SC, Khatoon A, Umar K, Yaqoob AA, Mohamad Ibrahim MN (2019) Role of nanotechnology for design and development of cosmeceutical: application in makeup and skin care. Front Chem 7(Nov):1–15. https://doi.org/10.3389/fchem.2019.00739
13. Dalla Colletta A, Pelin M, Sosa S, Fusco L, Prato M, Tubaro A (2022) CARBON-BASED nanomaterials and SKIN: an overview. Carbon N Y 196:683–698. https://doi.org/10.1016/j.carbon.2022.05.036
14. Widsten P, Tamminen T, Liitiä T (2020) Natural sunscreens based on nanoparticles of modified Kraft Lignin (CatLignin). ACS Omega 5(22):13438–13446. https://doi.org/10.1021/acsomega.0c01742
15. Nasir A, Wang S, Friedman A (2011) The emerging role of nanotechnology in sunscreens: an update. Expert Rev Dermatol 6(5):437–439. https://doi.org/10.1586/edm.11.49
16. Morsella M, D'Alessandro N, Lanterna AE, Scaiano JC (2016) Improving the sunscreen properties of TiO_2 through an understanding of its catalytic properties. ACS Omega 1(3):464–469. https://doi.org/10.1021/acsomega.6b00177
17. Cedillo-González EI, Riccò R, Montorsi M, Montorsi M, Falcaro P, Siligardi C (2014) Self-Cleaning glass prepared from a commercial TiO_2 Nano-Dispersion and its photocatalytic performance under common anthropogenic and atmospheric factors. Build Environ 71:7–14. https://doi.org/10.1016/j.buildenv.2013.09.007
18. Al-Qahtani SD, Binyaseen AM, Aljuhani E, Aljohani M, Alzahrani HK, Shah R, El-Metwaly NM (2022) Production of smart nanocomposite for glass coating toward photochromic and long-persistent photoluminescent smart windows. Ceram Int 48(1):903–912. https://doi.org/10.1016/j.ceramint.2021.09.174
19. Feng Q, Wang L (2022) The effect of polymer composite materials on the comfort of sports and fitness facilities. J Nanomater 2022(2). https://doi.org/10.1155/2022/9108458
20. Garcés JM, Moll DJ, Bicerano J, Fibiger R, McLeod DG (2000) Polymeric nanocomposites for automotive applications. Adv Mater 12(23):1835–1839. https://doi.org/10.1002/1521-4095(200012)12:23%3c1835::AID-ADMA1835%3e3.0.CO;2-T
21. Gowri S, Almeida L, Amorim T, Carneiro N, Pedro Souto A, Fátima M (2010) Polymer nanocomposites for multifunctional finishing of textiles—a review. Text Res J 80(13):1290–1306. https://doi.org/10.1177/0040517509357652
22. Gong M, Zhang L, Wan P (2020) Polymer nanocomposite meshes for flexible electronic devices. Prog Polym Sci 107:101279. https://doi.org/10.1016/j.progpolymsci.2020.101279
23. Singh P, Chamoli P, Sachdev S, Raina KK, Shukla RK (2020) Structural, optical and rheological behavior investigations of graphene oxide/glycerol based lyotropic liquid crystalline phases. Appl Surf Sci 2020:509. https://doi.org/10.1016/j.apsusc.2019.144710
24. Pajor-Świerzy A, Szczepanowicz K, Kamyshny A, Magdassi S (2021) Metallic core-shell nanoparticles for conductive coatings and printing. Adv Colloid Interf Sci 2022:299. https://doi.org/10.1016/j.cis.2021.102578
25. Nagar A, Pradeep T (2020) Clean water through nanotechnology: needs, gaps, and fulfillment. ACS Nano 14(6):6420–6435. https://doi.org/10.1021/acsnano.9b01730
26. Chamoli P, Shukla RK, Bezbaruah AN, Kar KK, Raina KK (2021) Microwave-Assisted rapid synthesis of Honeycomb Core-ZnO tetrapods nanocomposites for excellent photocatalytic activity against different organic dyes. Appl Surf Sci 2021:555 (January). https://doi.org/10.1016/j.apsusc.2021.149663
27. Singh P, Sachdev S, Chamoli P, Raina KK, Shukla RK (2022) Highly stable GO/Formamide based GOLLCs for free standing film fabrication and their photodegradation applications against organic dyes colloids surfaces a physicochem. Eng Asp 652(July):129840. https://doi.org/10.1016/j.colsurfa.2022.129840
28. Amin KF, Asrafuzzaman NAM, Hoque ME (2022) Polymer nanocomposites for adhesives and coatings. In: Advanced polymer nanocomposites, pp 235–265. Elsevier. https://doi.org/10.1016/B978-0-12-824492-0.00014-3

29. Abdel-Mageed HM, AbuelEzz NZ, Radwan RA, Mohamed SA (2021) Nanoparticles in nanomedicine: a comprehensive updated review on current status, challenges and emerging opportunities. J Microencapsul 38(6):414–436. https://doi.org/10.1080/02652048.2021.1942275
30. Mitchell MJ, Billingsley MM, Haley RM, Wechsler ME, Peppas NA, Langer R (2021) Engineering precision nanoparticles for drug delivery. Nat Rev Drug Discov 20(2):101–124. https://doi.org/10.1038/s41573-020-0090-8
31. Holzinger M, Goff AL, Cosnier S (2014) Nanomaterials for biosensing applications: a review. Front Chem 2(AUG):1–10. https://doi.org/10.3389/fchem.2014.00063
32. Sharmin S, Rahaman MM, Sarkar C, Atolani O, Islam MT, Adeyemi OS (2021) Nanoparticles as antimicrobial and antiviral agents: a literature-based perspective study. Heliyon 7(3):e06456. https://doi.org/10.1016/j.heliyon.2021.e06456
33. Wang L, Hu C, Shao L (2017) The-Antimicrobial-Activity-of-Nanoparticles–Present-Situati. Int J Nanomed 12:1227–1249
34. Singh P, Farheen SS, Chamoli P, Kumar K, Shukla RK (2022) Rheological behaviour and antibacterial activities of MWCNTs/Lyotropic liquid crystals based nanocolloids. Liq Cryst 00(00):1–19. https://doi.org/10.1080/02678292.2022.2070782
35. Liu Y, Yang G, Hui Y, Ranaweera S, Zhao CX (2022) Microfluidic nanoparticles for drug delivery. Small 18(36). https://doi.org/10.1002/smll.202106580
36. Zhao Y, Zhang Z, Pan Z, Liu Y (2021) Advanced bioactive nanomaterials for biomedical applications. Exploration 1(3):20210089. https://doi.org/10.1002/exp.20210089
37. Fathi-Achachelouei M, Knopf-Marques H, Ribeiro da Silva CE, Barthès J, Bat E, Tezcaner A, Vrana NE (2019) Use of nanoparticles in tissue engineering and regenerative medicine. Front Bioeng Biotechnol 7(May):1–22. https://doi.org/10.3389/fbioe.2019.00113
38. Christian P, Von Der Kammer F, Baalousha M, Hofmann T (2008) Nanoparticles: structure, properties, preparation and behaviour in environmental media. Ecotoxicology 17(5):326–343. https://doi.org/10.1007/s10646-008-0213-1
39. Grillo R, Rosa AH, Fraceto LF (2015) Engineered nanoparticles and organic matter: a review of the state-of-the-art. Chemosphere 119:608–619. https://doi.org/10.1016/j.chemosphere.2014.07.049
40. Shatrohan Lal RK (2014) Synthesis of organic nanoparticles and their applications in drug delivery and food nanotechnology: a review. J Nanomater Mol Nanotechnol 03(04). https://doi.org/10.4172/2324-8777.1000150.
41. Vonarbourg A, Passirani C, Desigaux L, Allard E, Saulnier P, Lambert O, Benoit JP, Pitard B (2009) The encapsulation of DNA molecules within biomimetic lipid nanocapsules. Biomaterials 30(18):3197–3204. https://doi.org/10.1016/j.biomaterials.2009.03.009
42. Zahr AS, Davis CA, Pishko MV (2006) Macrophage uptake of core-shell nanoparticles surface modified with poly(Ethylene Glycol). Langmuir 22(19):8178–8185. https://doi.org/10.1021/la060951b
43. Sundar S, Kundu J, Kundu SC (2010) Biopolymeric nanoparticles. Sci Technol Adv Mater 11(1):014104. https://doi.org/10.1088/1468-6996/11/1/014104
44. Lares MR, Rossi JJ, Ouellet DL (2011) Applications. East 28(11):570–579. https://doi.org/10.1016/j.tibtech.2010.07.009.RNAi
45. De Laporte L, Cruz Rea J, Shea LD (2006) Design of modular non-viral gene therapy vectors. Biomaterials 27(7):947–954. https://doi.org/10.1016/j.biomaterials.2005.09.036
46. Kim MH, Na HK, Kim YK, Ryoo SR, Cho HS, Lee KE, Jeon H, Ryoo R, Min DH (2011) Facile synthesis of monodispersed mesoporous silica nanoparticles with ultralarge pores and their application in gene delivery. ACS Nano 5(5):3568–3576. https://doi.org/10.1021/nn103130q
47. Kobiler O, Drayman N, Butin-Israeli V, Oppenheim A (2012) Virus strategies for passing the nuclear envelope barrier. Nucl (USA) 3(6). https://doi.org/10.4161/nucl.21979
48. Gómez-Aguado I; Rodríguez-Castejón J, Vicente-Pascual M, Rodríguez-Gascón A, Pozo-Rodríguez AD; Aspiazu, MÁS (2020) Nucleic Acid delivery by solid lipid nanoparticles containing switchable lipids: plasmid DNA versus messenger RNA. Molecules 25(24). https://doi.org/10.3390/MOLECULES25245995

49. Park TG, Jeong JH, Kim SW (2006) Current status of polymeric gene delivery systems. Adv Drug Deliv Rev 58(4):467–486. https://doi.org/10.1016/j.addr.2006.03.007
50. Auffan M, Rose J, Bottero JY, Lowry GV, Jolivet JP, Wiesner MR (2009) Towards a definition of inorganic nanoparticles from an environmental health and safety perspective. Nat Nanotechnol 4(10):634–641. https://doi.org/10.1038/nnano.2009.242
51. Noah N (2018) Green synthesis: characterization and application of silver and gold nanoparticles. Elsevier Inc. https://doi.org/10.1016/B978-0-08-102579-6.00006-X
52. Jiang K, Smith DA, Pinchuk A (2013) Size-Dependent photothermal conversion efficiencies of plasmonically heated gold nanoparticles. J Phys Chem C 117(51):27073–27080. https://doi.org/10.1021/jp409067h
53. Bapat RA, Chaubal TV, Joshi CP, Bapat PR, Choudhury H, Pandey M, Gorain B, Kesharwani P (2018) An overview of application of silver nanoparticles for biomaterials in dentistry. Mater Sci Eng C 91(May):881–898. https://doi.org/10.1016/j.msec.2018.05.069
54. Montes-Hernandez G, Di Girolamo M, Sarret G, Bureau S, Fernandez-Martinez A, Lelong C, Eymard Vernain E (2021) In Situ formation of silver nanoparticles (Ag–NPs) onto textile fibers. ACS Omega 6(2):1316–1327. https://doi.org/10.1021/acsomega.0c04814
55. Soloviev M, Gedanken A (2011) Coating a stainless steel plate with silver nanoparticles by the sonochemical method. Ultrason Sonochem 18(1):356–362. https://doi.org/10.1016/j.ultsonch.2010.06.015
56. Fahmy HM, Mosleh AM, Elghany AA, Shams-Eldin E, Abu Serea ES, Ali SA, Shalan AE (2019) Coated silver nanoparticles: synthesis, cytotoxicity, and optical properties. RSC Adv 9(35):20118–20136. https://doi.org/10.1039/c9ra02907a
57. Yu Y, Zhou Z, Huang G, Cheng H, Han L, Zhao S, Chen Y, Meng F (2022) Purifying water with silver nanoparticles (AgNPs)-Incorporated membranes: recent advancements and critical challenges. Water Res 222:118901. https://doi.org/10.1016/j.watres.2022.118901
58. Che W, Xiao Z, Wang Z, Li J, Wang H, Wang Y, Xie Y (2019) Wood-Based mesoporous filter decorated with silver nanoparticles for water purification. ACS Sustain Chem Eng 7(5):5134–5141. https://doi.org/10.1021/acssuschemeng.8b06001
59. Zhang K, Lui VCH, Chen Y, Lok CN, Wong KKY (2020) Delayed application of silver nanoparticles reveals the role of early inflammation in burn wound healing. Sci Rep 10(1):1–12. https://doi.org/10.1038/s41598-020-63464-z
60. Lu M, Hong L, Liang Y, Charron B, Zhu H, Peng W, Masson JF (2018) Enhancement of gold nanoparticle coupling with a 2D plasmonic crystal at high incidence angles. Anal Chem 90(11):6683–6692. https://doi.org/10.1021/acs.analchem.8b00496
61. Zhao W, Brook MA, Li Y (2008) Design of gold nanoparticle-based colorimetric biosensing assays. ChemBioChem 9(15):2363–2371. https://doi.org/10.1002/cbic.200800282
62. Boisselier E, Astruc D (2009) Gold nanoparticles in nanomedicine preparations, imaging, diagnostics therapies and toxicity. Chem Soc Rev 38(6):1759–1782. https://doi.org/10.1039/b806051g
63. De Silva AP, Gunaratne HQN, Gunnlaugsson T, Huxley AJM, McCoy CP, Rademacher JT, Rice TE (1997) Signaling recognition events with fluorescent sensors and switches. Chem Rev 97(5):1515–1566. https://doi.org/10.1021/cr960386p
64. Cho EC, Xie J, Wurm PA, Xia Y (2009) Understanding the role of surface charges in cellular adsorption versus internalization by selectively removing gold nanoparticles on the cell surface with a I 2/KI etchant. Nano Lett 9(3):1080–1084. https://doi.org/10.1021/nl803487r
65. Brewer SH, Glomm WR, Johnson MC, Knag MK, Franzen S (2005) Probing BSA binding to citrate-coated gold nanoparticles and surfaces. Langmuir 21(20):9303–9307. https://doi.org/10.1021/la050588t
66. Oh E, Delehanty JB, Sapsford KE, Susumu K, Goswami R, Blanco-Canosa JB, Dawson PE, Granek J, Shoff M, Zhang Q, Goering PL, Huston A, Medintz IL (2011) Cellular uptake and fate of PEGylated gold nanoparticles is dependent on both cell-penetration peptides and particle size. ACS Nano 5(8):6434–6448. https://doi.org/10.1021/nn201624c
67. Chan J, Aoki C, Pickel VM (1990) Optimization of differential immunogold-silver and peroxidase labeling with maintenance of ultrastructure in brain sections before plastic embedding. J Neurosci Methods 33(2–3):113–127. https://doi.org/10.1016/0165-0270(90)90015-8

68. Jiang K, Zhang L, Bao G (2021) Magnetic iron oxide nanoparticles for biomedical applications. Curr Opin Biomed Eng 20:100330. https://doi.org/10.1016/j.cobme.2021.100330
69. Manori S, Singh P, Yadav P, Kumar A, Chandra R, Raina KK, Shukla RK (2022) Magnetically tunable rheological properties of PVDF doped with superparamagnetic Fe3O4 nanoparticles synthesized by rapid microwave method. J Phys Chem Solids 2023(174):111137. https://doi.org/10.1016/j.jpcs.2022.111137
70. Martins PM, Lima AC, Ribeiro S, Lanceros-Mendez S, Martins P (2021) Magnetic nanoparticles for biomedical applications: from the soul of the earth to the deep history of ourselves. ACS Appl Bio Mater 4(8):5839–5870. https://doi.org/10.1021/acsabm.1c00440
71. Pantic I (2010) Magnetic nanoparticles in cancer diagnosis and treatment: novel approaches. Rev Adv Mater Sci 26(1–2):67–73
72. Farzin A, Etesami SA, Quint J, Memic A, Tamayol A (2020) Magnetic nanoparticles in cancer therapy and diagnosis. Adv Healthc Mater 9(9):1901058. https://doi.org/10.1002/adhm.201901058
73. Valko M, Morris H, Cronin M (2005) Metals, toxicity and oxidative stress. Curr Med Chem 12(10):1161–1208. https://doi.org/10.2174/0929867053764635
74. Malhotra N, Lee JS, Liman RAD, Ruallo JMS, Villaflore OB, Ger TR, Der HC (2020) Potential toxicity of iron oxide magnetic nanoparticles: a review. Molecules 25(14):1–26. https://doi.org/10.3390/molecules25143159
75. Sangaiya P, Jayaprakash R (2018) A review on iron oxide nanoparticles and their biomedical applications. J Supercond Nov Magn 31(11):3397–3413. https://doi.org/10.1007/s10948-018-4841-2
76. Hou Z, Liu Y, Xu J, Zhu J (2020) Surface engineering of magnetic iron oxide nanoparticles by polymer grafting: synthesis progress and biomedical applications. Nanoscale 12(28):14957–14975. https://doi.org/10.1039/d0nr03346d
77. Pourmadadi M, Rahmani E, Shamsabadipour A, Mahtabian S, Ahmadi M, Rahdar A, Díez-Pascual AM (2022) Role of Iron Oxide (Fe2O3) nanocomposites in advanced biomedical applications: a state-of-the-art review. Nanomaterials 12(21):3873. https://doi.org/10.3390/nano12213873
78. Berry CC (2005) Possible exploitation of magnetic nanoparticle-cell interaction for biomedical applications. J Mater Chem 15(5):543–547. https://doi.org/10.1039/b409715g
79. Fang C, Zhang M (2009) Multifunctional magnetic nanoparticles for medical imaging applications. J Mater Chem 19(35):6258–6266. https://doi.org/10.1039/b902182e
80. Kim BH, Lee N, Kim H, An K, Park YIl, Choi Y, Shin K, Lee Y, Kwon SG, Na H, Bin Park J, Ahn T, Kim Y, Moon WK, Choi SH, Hyeon T (2011) Large-Scale synthesis of uniform and extremely small-sized iron oxide nanoparticles for high-resolution T 1 magnetic resonance imaging contrast agents. J Am Chem Soc 133(32):12624–12631. https://doi.org/10.1021/ja203340u
81. Mahmoudi M, Sant S, Wang B, Laurent S, Sen T (2011) Superparamagnetic iron oxide nanoparticles (SPIONs): development, surface modification and applications in chemotherapy. Adv Drug Deliv Rev 63(1–2):24–46. https://doi.org/10.1016/j.addr.2010.05.006
82. Sun C, Lee JSH, Zhang M (2008) Magnetic nanoparticles in MR imaging and drug delivery. Adv Drug Deliv Rev 60(11):1252–1265. https://doi.org/10.1016/j.addr.2008.03.018
83. Dietz HC (1998) Delivery construct for antisense nucleic acids and methods of use. US5814500A
84. Arsianti M, Lim M, Marquis CP, Amal R (2010) Assembly of polyethylenimine-based magnetic iron oxide vectors: insights into gene delivery. Langmuir 26(10):7314–7326. https://doi.org/10.1021/la9041919
85. Davidson BL, McCray PB (2011) Current prospects for RNA interference-based therapies. Nat Rev Genet 12(5):329–340. https://doi.org/10.1038/nrg2968
86. Zuckerman JE, Choi CHJ, Han H, Davis ME (2012) Polycation-SiRNA nanoparticles can disassemble at the kidney glomerular basement membrane. Proc Natl Acad Sci USA 109(8):3137–3142. https://doi.org/10.1073/pnas.1200718109

87. Min KA, Shin MC, Yu F, Yang M, David AE, Yang VC, Rosania GR (2013) Pulsed magnetic field improves the transport of iron oxide nanoparticles through cell barriers. ACS Nano 7(3):2161–2171. https://doi.org/10.1021/nn3057565
88. Draz MS, Fang BA, Zhang P, Hu Z, Gu S, Weng KC, Gray JW, Chen FF (2014) Nanoparticle-Mediated systemic delivery of SiRNA for treatment of cancers and viral infections. Theranostics 4(9):872–892. https://doi.org/10.7150/thno.9404
89. Zhang NN, Lu CY, Chen, MJ, Xu XL, Shu, GF; Du YZ, Ji, JS (2021) Recent advances in near-infrared II imaging technology for biological detection. J Nanobiotechnol 19(1):1–14. https://doi.org/10.1186/s12951-021-00870-z
90. Grabska J, Huck CW (2020) Near-Infrared spectroscopy in bio-applications
91. Cheng W, Haedicke IE, Nofiele J, Martinez F, Beera K, Scholl TJ, Cheng HLM, Zhang XA (2014) Complementary strategies for developing Gd-Free High-Field T1 MRI contrast agents based on MnIII porphyrins. J Med Chem 57(2):516–520. https://doi.org/10.1021/jm401124b
92. Daldrup-Link HE, Rudelius M, Oostendorp RAJ, Settles M, Piontek G, Metz S, Rosenbrock H, Keller U, Heinzmann U, Rummeny EJ, Schlegel J, Link TM (2003) Targeting of hematopoietic progenitor cells with MR contrast agents. Radiology 228(3):760–767. https://doi.org/10.1148/radiol.2283020322
93. Gallo J, Long NJ, Aboagye EO (2013) Magnetic nanoparticles as contrast agents in the diagnosis and treatment of cancer. Chem Soc Rev 42(19):7816–7833. https://doi.org/10.1039/c3cs60149h
94. Thanh, NTK, El Sayed MA (eds) (2018) Clinical applications of magnetic nanoparticles. CRC Press: Boca Raton: Taylor & Francis. https://doi.org/10.1201/9781315168258
95. Skitzki JJ, Repasky EA, Evans SS (2009) Hyperthermia as an immunotherapy strategy for cancer. Curr Opin Investig Drugs 10(6):550–558
96. Kalambur VS, Longmire EK, Bischof JC (2007) Cellular level loading and heating of superparamagnetic iron oxide nanoparticles. Langmuir 23(24):12329–12336. https://doi.org/10.1021/la701100r
97. Tay ZW, Chandrasekharan P, Chiu-Lam A, Hensley DW, Dhavalikar R, Zhou XY, Yu EY, Goodwill PW, Zheng B, Rinaldi C, Conolly SM (2018) Magnetic particle imaging-guided heating in vivo using gradient fields for arbitrary localization of magnetic hyperthermia therapy. ACS Nano 12(4):3699–3713. https://doi.org/10.1021/acsnano.8b00893
98. Berry CC (2009) Progress in functionalization of magnetic nanoparticles for applications in biomedicine. J Phys D Appl Phys 42(22). https://doi.org/10.1088/0022-3727/42/22/224003
99. Medeiros SF, Santos AM, Fessi H, Elaissari A (2011) Stimuli-Responsive magnetic particles for biomedical applications. Int J Pharm 403(1–2):139–161. https://doi.org/10.1016/j.ijpharm.2010.10.011
100. Huang J, Li Y, Orza A, Lu Q, Guo P, Wang L, Yang L, Mao H (2016) Magnetic nanoparticle facilitated drug delivery for cancer therapy with targeted and image-guided approaches. Adv Funct Mater 26(22):3818–3836. https://doi.org/10.1002/adfm.201504185
101. Williams MJ, Corr SA (2013) Magnetic nanoparticles for targeted cancer diagnosis and therapy. Front Nanosci 5(5):29–63. https://doi.org/10.1016/B978-0-08-098338-7.00002-9
102. Vekris A, Maurange C, Moonen C, Mazurier F, De Verneuil H, Canioni P, Voisin P (2000) Control of transgene expression using local hyperthermia in combination with a heat-sensitive promoter. J Gene Med 2(2):89–96. https://doi.org/10.1002/(SICI)1521-2254(200003/04)2:2%3c89::AID-JGM90%3e3.0.CO;2-J
103. Angelakeris M (2017) Magnetic nanoparticles: a multifunctional vehicle for modern theranostics. Biochim Biophys Acta-Gen Subj 1861(6):1642–1651. https://doi.org/10.1016/j.bbagen.2017.02.022
104. Lunnoo T, Puangmali T (2015) Capture efficiency of biocompatible magnetic nanoparticles in arterial flow: a computer simulation for magnetic drug targeting. Nanoscale Res Lett 10(1). https://doi.org/10.1186/s11671-015-1127-5
105. Lübbe AS, Bergemann C, Brock J, McClure DG (1999) Physiological aspects in magnetic drug-targeting. J Magn Magn Mater 194(1):149–155. https://doi.org/10.1016/S0304-8853(98)00574-5

106. Parveen S, Misra R, Sahoo SKN (2012) A boon to drug delivery, therapeutics, diagnostics and imaging. Nanomed Nanotechnol Biol Med 8(2): 147–166. https://doi.org/10.1016/j.nano.2011.05.016.
107. Tasis D, Tagmatarchis N, Bianco A, Prato M (2006) Chemistry of carbon nanotubes. Chem Rev 106(3):1105–1136. https://doi.org/10.1021/cr050569o
108. Li H, He X, Liu Y, Huang H, Lian S, Lee ST, Kang Z (2011) One-Step ultrasonic synthesis of water-soluble carbon nanoparticles with excellent photoluminescent properties. Carbon N Y 49(2):605–609. https://doi.org/10.1016/j.carbon.2010.10.004
109. Sheikhpour M, Golbabaie A, Kasaeian A (2017) Carbon nanotubes: a review of novel strategies for cancer diagnosis and treatment. Mater Sci Eng C 76:1289–1304. https://doi.org/10.1016/j.msec.2017.02.132
110. Razak M, Prasad Boggupalli S, Viswanath B (2015) Drug-Loaded nanocarriers in tumor targeted drug delivery. Curr Biotechnol 4(3):319–344. https://doi.org/10.2174/2211550104666150525221950
111. Torchilin VP (2014) Multifunctional, stimuli-sensitive nanoparticulate systems for drug delivery. Nat Rev Drug Discov 13(11):813–827. https://doi.org/10.1038/nrd4333
112. Kargozar S, Hoseini SJ, Milan PB, Hooshmand S, Kim HW, Mozafari M (2020) Quantum dots: a review from concept to clinic. Biotechnol J 15(12):1–18. https://doi.org/10.1002/biot.202000117
113. Near- SS, Ruddy DA, Johnson JC, Smith ER, Neale NR (2010) Size and bandgap control in the. ACS Nano 4(12):7459–7466
114. Renner M, Lacor PN, Velasco PT, Xu J, Contractor A, Klein WL, Triller A (2010) Deleterious effects of amyloid β oligomers acting as an extracellular scaffold for MGluR5. Neuron 66(5):739–754. https://doi.org/10.1016/j.neuron.2010.04.029
115. Rurack K, Spieles M (2011) Fluorescence quantum yields of a series of red and near-infrared dyes emitting at 600–1000 Nm. Anal Chem 83(4):1232–1242. https://doi.org/10.1021/ac101329h
116. Yildiz A, Vale RD (2015) Total internal reflection fluorescence microscopy. Cold Spring Harb Protoc 2015(9):801–810. https://doi.org/10.1101/pdb.top086348
117. Yildiz I, Deniz E, McCaughan B, Cruickshank SF, Callan JF, Raymo FM (2010) Hydrophilic CdSe-ZnS Core-Shell quantum dots with reactive functional groups on their surface. Langmuir 26(13):11503–11511. https://doi.org/10.1021/la1010488
118. Breger J, Delehanty JB, Medintz IL (2015) Continuing progress toward controlled intracellular delivery of semiconductor quantum dots. Wiley Interdiscip Rev Nanomed Nanobiotechnol 7(2):131–151. https://doi.org/10.1002/wnan.1281
119. Hejtmancik JF, Nickerson JM (2015) Preface. In: Molecular Biology of Eye Disease, pp xix–xx. https://doi.org/10.1016/S1877-1173(15)00179-9
120. Srikanth H, Hajndl R, Chirinos C, Sanders J, Sampath A, Sudarshan TS (2001) Magnetic studies of polymer-coated Fe nanoparticles synthesized by microwave plasma polymerization. Appl Phys Lett 79(21):3503–3505. https://doi.org/10.1063/1.1419237
121. Matsumura S, Hlil AR, Lepiller C, Gaudet J, Guay D, Shi Z, Holdcroft S, Hay AS (2008) Stability and utility of pyridyl disulfide functionality in RAFT and conventional radical polymerizations. J Polym Sci Part A Polym Chem 46(April): 7207–7224. https://doi.org/10.1002/pola
122. Schmidt AM (2005) The synthesis of magnetic core-shell nanoparticles by surface-initiated ring-opening polymerization of ε-Caprolactone. Macromol Rapid Commun 26(2):93–97. https://doi.org/10.1002/marc.200400426
123. Shi D, He P, Lian J, Wang L, Van Ooij WJ (2002) Plasma deposition and characterization of acrylic acid thin film on ZnO nanoparticles. J Mater Res 17(10):2555–2560. https://doi.org/10.1557/JMR.2002.0371
124. Schadler LS, Kumar SK, Benicewicz BC, Lewis SL, Harton SE (2007) Designed interfaces in polymer nanocomposites: a fundamental viewpoint. MRS Bull 32(4):335–340. https://doi.org/10.1557/mrs2007.232

125. Wang YJ, Larsson M, Huang WT, Chiou SH, Nicholls SJ, Chao JI, Liu DM (2016) The use of polymer-based nanoparticles and nanostructured materials in treatment and diagnosis of cardiovascular diseases: recent advances and emerging designs. Prog Polym Sci 57:153–178. https://doi.org/10.1016/j.progpolymsci.2016.01.002
126. Caro E, Marcé RM, Borrull F, Cormack PAG, Sherrington DC (2006) Application of molecularly imprinted polymers to solid-phase extraction of compounds from environmental and biological samples. TrAC—Trends Anal Chem 25(2):143–154. https://doi.org/10.1016/j.trac.2005.05.008
127. Adliene D, Urbonavicius BG, Laurikaitiene J, Puiso J (2020) New application of polymer gels in medical radiation dosimetry: plasmonic sensors. Radiat Phys Chem 168:108609. https://doi.org/10.1016/j.radphyschem.2019.108609
128. Shi Y, Zhang JH, Shi D, Jiang M, Zhu YX, Mei SR, Zhou YK, Dai K, Lu B (2006) Selective solid-phase extraction of cholesterol using molecularly imprinted polymers and its application in different biological samples. J Pharm Biomed Anal 42(5):549–555. https://doi.org/10.1016/j.jpba.2006.05.022
129. Marvel CS, Casey DJ (1959) Preparation of polymers containing pyridine units from polyvinyl ketones. J Org Chem 24(7):957–963. https://doi.org/10.1021/jo01089a018
130. Sugimoto M, Morimoto M, Sashiwa H, Saimoto H, Shigemasa Y (1998) Preparation and characterization of water-soluble chitin and chitosan derivatives. Carbohydr Polym 36(1):49–59. https://doi.org/10.1016/S0144-8617(97)00235-X
131. Ting TH (2019) Synthesis, characterization of fe3o4/polymer composites with stealth capabilities. Res Phys 2020(16):102975. https://doi.org/10.1016/j.rinp.2020.102975
132. Qi XD, Wang Y (2020) Novel techniques for the preparation of shape-memory polymers, polymer blends and composites at micro and nanoscales, vol 115. Springer Singapore. https://doi.org/10.1007/978-981-13-8574-2_3
133. Messina MS, Messina KMM, Bhattacharya A, Montgomery HR, Maynard HD (2020) Preparation of biomolecule-polymer conjugates by grafting-from using ATRP, RAFT, or ROMP. Prog Polym Sci 100:101186. https://doi.org/10.1016/j.progpolymsci.2019.101186
134. Harada A, Furue M, Nozakura SI (1976) Cyclodextrin-Containing polymers. 1. Preparation of polymers. Macromolecules 9(5): 701–704. https://doi.org/10.1021/ma60053a003
135. Hawker CJ, Fréchet JMJ (1990) Preparation of polymers with controlled molecular architecture. A new convergent approach to dendritic macromolecules. J Am Chem Soc 112(21): 7638–7647. https://doi.org/10.1021/ja00177a027
136. Chen R, Huang D (2011) Preparation of polymer nanoparticles, and the effect of nanoconfinement on glass transition, structural relaxation and crystallization. Front Chem China 6(4):332–340. https://doi.org/10.1007/s11458-011-0262-5
137. Zhou D, Li L, Li Y, Zhang J, Xue G (2003) Metastable isotactic polystyrene prepared by freeze-extracting concentrated solutions in solvents of middle molecular size. Macromolecules 36(12):4609–4613. https://doi.org/10.1021/ma034230k
138. Feng L, Zhu C, Yuan H, Liu L, Lv F, Wang S (2013) Conjugated polymer nanoparticles: preparation, properties, functionalization and biological applications. Chem Soc Rev 42(16):6620–6633. https://doi.org/10.1039/c3cs60036j
139. Taylor-Pashow KML, Della Rocca J, Huxford RC, Lin W (2010) Hybrid nanomaterials for biomedical applications. Chem Commun 46(32):5832–5849. https://doi.org/10.1039/c002073g
140. Blum AP, Kammeyer JK, Rush AM, Callmann CE, Hahn ME, Gianneschi NC (2015) Stimuli-Responsive nanomaterials for biomedical applications. J Am Chem Soc 137(6):2140–2154. https://doi.org/10.1021/ja510147n
141. Chimene D, Alge DL, Gaharwar AK (2015) Two-Dimensional nanomaterials for biomedical applications: emerging trends and future prospects. Adv Mater 27(45):7261–7284. https://doi.org/10.1002/adma.201502422
142. Fang RH, Jiang Y, Fang JC, Zhang L (2017) Cell membrane-derived nanomaterials for biomedical applications. Biomaterials 128:69–83. https://doi.org/10.1016/j.biomaterials.2017.02.041

143. Duan C, Liang L, Li L, Zhang R, Xu ZP (2018) Recent progress in upconversion luminescence nanomaterials for biomedical applications. J Mater Chem B 6(2):192–209. https://doi.org/10.1039/c7tb02527k
144. Sun L, Zheng C, Webster TJ (2017) Self-Assembled peptide nanomaterials for biomedical applications: promises and pitfalls. Int J Nanomed 12:73–86. https://doi.org/10.2147/IJN.S117501
145. Erol O, Uyan I, Hatip M, Yilmaz C, Tekinay AB, Guler MO (2018) Recent advances in bioactive 1D and 2D carbon nanomaterials for biomedical applications. Nanomed Nanotechnol Biol Med 14 (7): 2433–2454. https://doi.org/10.1016/j.nano.2017.03.021
146. Bhardwaj V, Kaushik A (2017) Biomedical applications of nanotechnology and nanomaterials. Micromachines 8(10):298. https://doi.org/10.3390/mi8100298
147. Wackerlig J, Schirhagl R (2016) Applications of molecularly imprinted polymer nanoparticles and their advances toward industrial use: a review. Anal Chem 88(1):250–261. https://doi.org/10.1021/acs.analchem.5b03804
148. Repenko T, Rix A, Ludwanowski S, Go D, Kiessling F, Lederle W, Kuehne AJC (2017) Bio-Degradable highly fluorescent conjugated polymer nanoparticles for bio-medical imaging applications. Nat Commun 8(1):8–15. https://doi.org/10.1038/s41467-017-00545-0
149. Kumar B, Das A, Alagirusamy R (2014) Introduction to compression therapy. Sci Comp Bandages 1–19. https://doi.org/10.1533/9781782422723.1
150. Moreno-Vega AI, Gómez-Quintero T, Nuñez-Anita RE, Acosta-Torres LS, Castaño V (2012) Polymeric and ceramic nanoparticles in biomedical applications. J Nanotechnol. https://doi.org/10.1155/2012/936041
151. Boyer C, Whittaker MR, Bulmus V, Liu J, Davis TP (2010) The design and utility of polymer-stabilized iron-oxide nanoparticles for nanomedicine applications. NPG Asia Mater 2(1):23–30. https://doi.org/10.1038/asiamat.2010.6
152. Moscatelli D, Sponchioni M (2017) Bioresorbable polymer nanoparticles in the medical and pharmaceutical fields: a promising field. Bioresorbable Polym Biomed Appl Fundam Transl Med 265–283. https://doi.org/10.1016/B978-0-08-100262-9.00012-4
153. Moghimi SM, Hunter AC (2000) Poloxamers and poloxamines in nanoparticle engineering and experimental medicine. Trends Biotechnol 18(10):412–420. https://doi.org/10.1016/S0167-7799(00)01485-2
154. Novio F, Simmchen J, Vázquez-Mera N, Amorín-Ferré L, Ruiz-Molina D (2013) Coordination polymer nanoparticles in medicine. Coord Chem Rev 257(19–20):2839–2847. https://doi.org/10.1016/j.ccr.2013.04.022
155. Hamad K, Kaseem M, Yang HW, Deri F, Ko YG (2015) Properties and medical applications of polylactic acid: a review. Exp Polym Lett 9(5):435–455. https://doi.org/10.3144/expresspolymlett.2015.42
156. Tuncel D, Demir HV (2010) Conjugated polymer nanoparticles. Nanoscale 2(4):484–494. https://doi.org/10.1039/b9nr00374f
157. Francis R, Joy N, Aparna EP, Vijayan R (2014) Polymer grafted inorganic nanoparticles, preparation, properties, and applications: a review. Polym Rev 54(2):268–347. https://doi.org/10.1080/15583724.2013.870573
158. Quinn MT, Deleo FR (eds) (2020) Nanoparticles in biology and medicine. Methods and Protocols, 2nd ed.
159. Koseva NS, Rydz J, Stoyanova EV, Mitova VA (2015) Hybrid protein–synthetic polymer nanoparticles for drug delivery, vol 98, 1st ed. Elsevier Inc. https://doi.org/10.1016/bs.apcsb.2014.12.003
160. Rempel GL (2015) Introduction of polymer nanoparticles for drug delivery applications. Nanotechnol Nanomed Nanobiotechnol 2(3): 1–6. https://doi.org/10.24966/ntmb-2044/100008
161. Deirram N, Zhang C, Kermaniyan SS, Johnston APR, Such GK (2019) PH-Responsive polymer nanoparticles for drug delivery. Macromol Rapid Commun 40(10):1–23. https://doi.org/10.1002/marc.201800917

162. Zheng M, Gong P, Zheng C, Zhao P, Luo Z, Ma Y, Cai L (2015) Lipid-Polymer nanoparticles for folate-receptor targeting delivery of doxorubicin. J Nanosci Nanotechnol 15(7):4792–4798. https://doi.org/10.1166/jnn.2015.9604
163. Lane DD, Chiu DY, Su FY, Srinivasan S, Kern HB, Press OW, Stayton PS, Convertine AJ (2015) Well-Defined single polymer nanoparticles for the antibody-targeted delivery of chemotherapeutic agents. Polym Chem 6(8):1286–1299. https://doi.org/10.1039/c4py01250j
164. Modrejewski J, Walter JG, Kretschmer I, Kemal E, Green M, Belhadj H, Blume C, Scheper T (2016) Aptamer-Modified polymer nanoparticles for targeted drug delivery. BioNanoMaterials 17(1–2):43–51. https://doi.org/10.1515/bnm-2015-0027
165. Masood F (2016) Polymeric nanoparticles for targeted drug delivery system for cancer therapy. Mater Sci Eng C 60:569–578. https://doi.org/10.1016/j.msec.2015.11.067
166. Zhou J, Horev B, Hwang G, Klein MI, Koo H, Benoit DSW (2016) Characterization and optimization of PH-Responsive polymer nanoparticles for drug delivery to oral biofilms. J Mater Chem B 4(18):3075–3085. https://doi.org/10.1039/c5tb02054a
167. Dararatana N, Seidi F, Hamel J, Crespy D (2020) Controlling release kinetics of Ph-Responsive polymer nanoparticles. Polym Chem 11(10):1752–1762. https://doi.org/10.1039/c9py01946d
168. Wang H, Rempel GL (2013) PH-Responsive polymer core-shell nanospheres for drug delivery. J Polym Sci Part A Polym Chem 51(20): 4440–4450. https://doi.org/10.1002/pola.26860
169. Schmaljohann D (2006) Thermo- and PH-Responsive polymers in drug delivery. Adv Drug Deliv Rev 58(15):1655–1670. https://doi.org/10.1016/j.addr.2006.09.020
170. Zhu J, Tang J, Chang SS (2018) Strong convergence theorems for a class of split feasibility problems and fixed point problem in hilbert spaces. J Inequal Appl 1–15. https://doi.org/10.1186/s13660-018-1881-x
171. Kasban H, El-Bendary MAM, Salama DH (2015) A comparative study of medical imaging techniques. Int J Inf Sci Intell Syst 4(2):37–58
172. Kwee TC, Zaidi H (2013) Evolving medical imaging techniques. PET Clin 8(3):xi–xii. https://doi.org/10.1016/j.cpet.2013.04.005
173. Braeken Y, Cheruku S, Seneca S, Smisdom N, Berden L, Kruyfhooft L, Penxten H, Lutsen L, Fron E, Vanderzande D, Ameloot M, Maes W, Ethirajan A (2019) Effect of branching on the optical properties of poly(p-Phenylene Ethynylene) conjugated polymer nanoparticles for bioimaging. ACS Biomater Sci Eng 5(4):1967–1977. https://doi.org/10.1021/acsbiomaterials.8b01416
174. Braeken Y, Cheruku S, Ethirajan A, Maes W (2017) Conjugated polymer nanoparticles for bioimaging. Materials (Basel) 10(12):1–23. https://doi.org/10.3390/ma10121420
175. Peters M, Seneca S, Hellings N, Junkers T, Ethirajan A (2018) Size-Dependent properties of functional PPV-Based conjugated polymer nanoparticles for bioimaging. Colloids Surfaces B Biointerfaces 169(May):494–501. https://doi.org/10.1016/j.colsurfb.2018.05.055
176. Li K, Liu B (2012) Polymer encapsulated conjugated polymer nanoparticles for fluorescence bioimaging. J Mater Chem 22(4):1257–1264. https://doi.org/10.1039/c1jm14397b
177. Wang X, Groff LC, McNeill JD (2013) Photoactivation and saturated emission in blended conjugated polymer nanoparticles. Langmuir 29(45):13925–13931. https://doi.org/10.1021/la402767j
178. Ray SK (2019) Nonradioactive and radioactive telomerase assays for detecting diminished telomerase activity in cancer cells after treatment with retinoid. Methods Mol Biol 2019 257–273. https://doi.org/10.1007/978-1-4939-9585-1_18
179. Li M, Nie C, Feng L, Yuan H, Liu L, Lv F, Wang S (2014) Conjugated polymer nanoparticles for cell membrane imaging. Chem—An Asian J 9(11):3121–3124. https://doi.org/10.1002/asia.201402711
180. Li Y, Liu J, Liu B, Tomczak N (2012) Highly emissive PEG-Encapsulated conjugated polymer nanoparticles. Nanoscale 4(13):5694–5702. https://doi.org/10.1039/c2nr31267k
181. Zhao P, Wu Y, Feng C, Wang L, Ding Y, Hu A (2018) Conjugated polymer nanoparticles based fluorescent electronic nose for the identification of volatile compounds. Anal Chem 90(7):4815–4822. https://doi.org/10.1021/acs.analchem.8b00273

182. Hashim Z, Green M, Chung PH, Suhling K, Protti A, Phinikaridou A, Botnar R, Khanbeigi RA, Thanou M, Dailey LA, Commander NJ, Rowland C, Scott J, Jenner D (2014) Gd-Containing conjugated polymer nanoparticles: bimodal nanoparticles for fluorescence and MRI imaging. Nanoscale 6(14):8376–8386. https://doi.org/10.1039/c4nr01491j
183. Liu Y, Wang YM, Zhu WY, Zhang CH, Tang H, Jiang JH (2018) Conjugated polymer nanoparticles-based fluorescent biosensor for ultrasensitive detection of hydroquinone. Anal Chim Acta 1012:60–65. https://doi.org/10.1016/j.aca.2018.01.027
184. Peters R, Sandiford L, Owen DM, Kemal E, Bourke S, Dailey LA, Green M (2016) Red-Emitting protein-coated conjugated polymer nanoparticles. Photochem Photobiol Sci 15(11):1448–1452. https://doi.org/10.1039/c6pp00160b
185. Zhang YL, Ren JT, Gao HY, Liu JW, Xia WJ, Qiao WQ, Wang ZY (2020) Characterizations and photothermal properties of narrow bandgap conjugated polymer nanoparticles. Chinese J Polym Sci English ed. 38(8): 814–818. https://doi.org/10.1007/s10118-020-2420-z

Fundamentals of Drug Delivery

Shubham Kumar, Nidhi, Babita Thakur, Vagish Dwibedi, and Jasdeep Singh

Abstract Drug delivery systems have the potential of deciding the efficiency of a therapeutic agent. The potential of a drug is often limited by the lack of effective delivery systems and therefore, past few years have seen tremendous upsurge in the research oriented towards development of different systems for the drug delivery systems. From the development of orally administered pills to nanoparticles-based delivery systems, the technologies for drug deliveries have come a long way. The first big success is the development of biological, chemical and physical means that are adopted to alter the pharmacokinetic properties of the drug to exhibit the desired pharmacological effect and remove undesirable physiochemical properties. Development in drug delivery systems can be described through different phases which are described as different generations of the drug delivery system. Sustained gradual release is the first generation of control drug release practice in which a drug is packed in a capsule or in the form of a capsule that releases drug with it when mixed with water in the stomach. On the other hand, targeted drug delivery system is a special system of drug delivery in which the drug is selectively targeted only to the site of action/absorption and not to the non-target tissues, cells or organ. This chapter provides a glimpse of various physiochemical and biological barriers that restrict effective drug delivery and the techniques adopted to overcome these barriers for effective drug delivery.

Keywords Drug delivery system · Pharmacokinetic · Sustained gradual release · Targeted delivery · Drug release

S. Kumar · Nidhi · B. Thakur · V. Dwibedi · J. Singh (✉)
University Institute of Biotechnology, Chandigarh University, Gharuan, Mohali, Punjab 140413, India
e-mail: jasdeep.e9434@cumail.in

S. K. Rath et al. (eds.), *Nanomaterials for Drug Delivery and Neurological Diseases Management*, Smart Nanomaterials Technology,
https://doi.org/10.1007/978-981-97-0308-1_3

1 Introduction

Drug delivery refers to the approaches or a system developed to administer a particular drug to its site of action. The treatment of various diseases is often limited due to the lack an efficient drug delivery system. Drug delivery technology face major challenges of delivering drug to its physiologically relevant site of action in a certain concentration. The history of the drug delivery system traces back to the usage of pills to administrate a particular drug. It involves mixing of a particular drug with excipients such as sugar, starch and filler material to protect the formulation. The basic principle behind using pills to administer the drug is that on swallowing the pill will dissolve in the stomach, the drug will be subsequently absorbed in the intestine which will then enter the blood stream. However, this method is not applicable to the drugs that are liable to the acid present in the stomach and degrade to sub-products. For example, insulin must be injected into the adipose tissues because it cannot survive in the stomach. Injection of insulin into the fatty tissues helps it to get absorbed to the systemic circulation of the body [1]. The earliest drug delivery system traces back to 1932 when the enteric coated tablet was patented. In 1952, first oral Spansules technology tablets, Spansules, Dexedrine was introduced. Following the success, Spansules technology, Christenson in 1962 patented the first sustained release matrix tablet with hydrophilic polymer. In later years, matrix tablets with swelling and gelling controllable hydrogels were developed.

In 1980, the first patent for transdermal patches was awarded to Zaffaroni. It allows transdermal delivery of drug at a controlled rate. Scopoderm was introduced in the market in 1979 against sea sickness (26). Nitroglycerine patch for the treatment of angina, fentayl patch for pain relief, hormone containing patches and vitamin B12 patches were subsequently introduced in the market. Apart from oral delivery, other non-invasive routes for drug delivery were also considered. For instance, pulmonary administration of insulin in the form of dry powder inhaler was approved in 2014. For treatment of neurodegenerative disorders, nasal drug delivery route for administration of peptide drugs has been introduced in the market. It provides benefit of direct carriage of drug to the brain through the olfactory passage. This chapter is an update on some of the existing drug delivery technologies for oral controlled release, oral disintegrating dosage forms, test-masking formulations, liposomes, and targeting drug delivery and transdermal drug delivery. The fundamental principles, applications, advanced methodologies, and technologies employed by pharmaceutical scientists, researchers, and pharmaceutical industries to transform a drug candidate or new chemical entity into a final administrable drug delivery system is discussed. In addition, it also provides up-to-date information on translating the physicochemical properties of drugs into drug delivery systems. The past background and future direction of drug delivery research and development are also discussed.

2 Transformation of Drug to Final Administrable Drug

For any drug to exhibit the desired pharmacological effect and remove undesirable physiochemical and biological properties, its therapeutic efficiency needs to be enhanced. Various biological, chemical and physical means are adopted to alter the pharmacokinetic properties of the drug. The biological approaches alter the route of administration. Physical approaches modify the design of the drug dosage, whereas chemical approaches enhance the drug selectivity while minimising the toxicity. There are three basic objectives of drug transformation including the pharmacokinetic, pharmacodynamic and pharmaceutical objective (Fig. 1). Firstly, the aim is to enhance the solubility, chemical stability and organoleptic properties of the drug. Certain drugs induced pain on injection and cause gastrointestinal irritation which needs to be reduced. Secondly, the absorption of the drug through various oral and non-oral routes should be increased. Improving the time profile and increasing organ selective delivery of the active agent should be considered. Thirdly, decreased toxicity and improved therapeutic index of the drug should be considered for designing the drug.

Rate of passage drug transportation is decided by lipophilicity and hydrophilicity. The increase in lipophilic nature causes decrease in water solubility and decreases the diffusion of the drug across the membrane. Therefore, the drug needs to be prepared keeping in mind a balance between water solubility and lipophilic nature. It has been recommended that the drug should have a molecular weight ≤500 for good membrane permeability. It has also been proved that the drug should be neutral, unionised and lipophilic for efficient absorption. In many drugs, hydrophobic groups have been added in order to increase the lipophilicity of the drug for better gastrointestinal absorption. Oral bioavailability of ampicillin in horses can be increased by addition of lipophilic esters. For instance, alampicillin, pivampicillin and bacampicillin, the lipophilic esters of the drug ampicillin, are 25–40% more soluble than ampicillin salt [2].

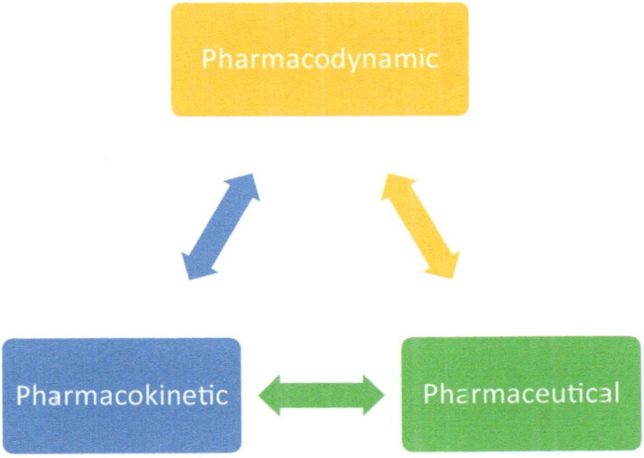

Fig. 1 Basic three objective of drug transformation research

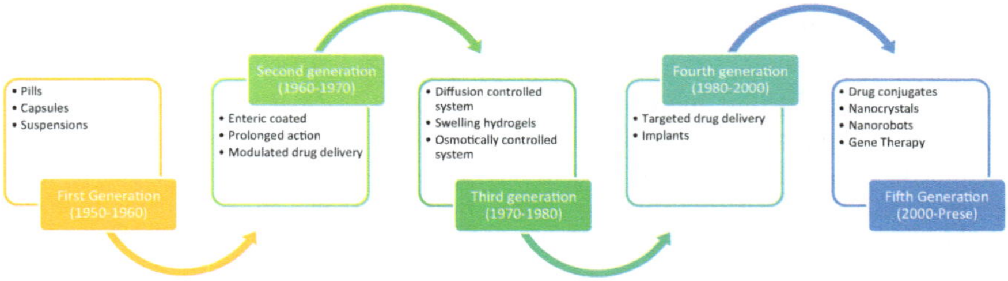

Fig. 2 Development in drug delivery systems as described through different phases

Another technique of transformation of the parent drug to its clinical form is improving the gastrointestinal tolerance of the drug by masking the carboxylic acid present in anti-inflammatory drugs. For instance, masking the carboxylic acid group in naproxen and indomethacin enhances the oral availability of the drug by 30–36% and reduced the irritation in gastric mucosa. Oral drugs are also modified to enhance the taste to enhance the patience compliance. Chloramphenicol has been modified to chloramphenicol palmitate which does not give any taste in the mouth because it does not get dissolved in the mouth [3].

3 Different Approaches of Drug Delivery

Ever since the discovery of pills to administer a particular drug into the body, drug delivery systems have come a long way. The history of drug delivery systems can be broadly divided into five phases which are known as five generations of drug delivery (Fig. 2). The different phases in the drug delivery systems are described below.

4 Sustained Gradual Drug Release

This is the first generation of controlled drug release practice in which a drug is packed in a capsule or in the form of a capsule that releases drug with it is mixed with water in the stomach. Spansules® developed by SmithKline Beecham in 1952 were the first sustained release drug. The pill of Spansules® released dextroamphetamine sulphate from the capsule for a longer time thus prolonging the medicine release. Sustained drug release generally does not attain zero order release kinetics and usually does not contain mechanisms to promote localization of the drug at the active site [4]. This sustained drug delivery system is a type of controlled drug delivery in which sustained level of drug concentration is released in blood over a period time of time [5]. However, sustained drug release is different from controlled drug release in various ways. Controlled drug release delivers the drug at a pre-determined rate for a specific period of time. It is perfectly zero-order release that is the drug release is constant. The basic goal of sustained gradual drug release is to achieve a steady state blood level that is therapeutically effective and non-toxic for an extended period of time. However, the following disadvantages are associated with sustained drug release:

- Non-Targeted delivery
- Drug dissolution and release process is similar to food digestion and takes longer period over 5–7 h
- Difficulty in attaining steady state drug concentration which may arise due to patient incompliance
- Retrieval of drug is difficult in case of toxicity or poisoning
- Less flexibility in designing drug dose
- Therapeutic index of the drug designed for sustained drug release should be high
- The drug should not show any cumulative action

5 Targeted Drug Delivery

Targeted drug delivery system is a special system of drug delivery in which the drug is selectively targeted only to the site of action/absorption and not to the non-target tissues, cells or organ. It involves the delivering of the drug to the patient in a way that increases the concentration of the drug to the targeted site compared to other body parts. It means the concentration of the drug in the cell of interest is high while the relative concentration in the non-targeted tissues is minimal which reduces any side effect and increases the efficiency of the treatment. The primary objective of the targeted drug delivery is to achieve the desired pharmacological response at the selective site without any unwanted interaction at the non-target site. It is an excellent way of enhancing the therapeutic index of the drug and minimising side effects. It allows efficient delivery of the drug in appropriate dosage and time [6]. Targeted drug delivery is the fourth generation of the drug delivery systems and offers the following benefits:

- Requirement of less dosage compared to conventional drug delivery systems
- Drug delivery protocols are simple
- Less toxicity and reduced side effects
- Small dosage can be applied to produce desired effect
- No peak and valley plasma concentration
- Selective target to the target tissues
- The system combines pharmacology, chemistry and molecular biology to control pharmacokinetics and pharmacodynamics of the drug

Targeted drug delivery can be achieved by using a carrier or marker system which includes the use of special molecules that can load the drug and deliver it to the target site [7]. Carriers are usually engineered vectors which have the capability to retain the drug inside it via the process of encapsulation or spacer moiety and transporting it to the target tissue. Pharmaceutical carriers include microcapsules, microparticles, lipoproteins, liposomes, micelles and polymers. Targeted drug delivery can be achieved through different types of systems that are explained below:

- Nanotubes
- Nanowires
- Nano shells
- Quantam dots
- Nanopores
- Gold Nano
- Dendrimers
- Liposomes
- Niosomes
- Ufasomes
- Nanocrystals.

6 Physiochemical and Biochemical Barriers to Drug Delivery

Drug delivery to the target site is often limited by physiological, biological, biochemical and physiochemical barriers. The first barrier that any drug has to pass before reaching the target site is the physiological barrier. Upon ingestion, when the drug reaches the intestine, it has to pass the mucus layer on the luminal side of the gastrointestinal tract that varies from 100 to 150 μm. This mucus layer is composed of glycoproteins and water which must be passed by the drug before reaching its second barrier, a layer of different epithelial cells including goblet cells, endocrine cells, Paneth cells and enterocytes [8]. For any drug to pass through this physiological pathway, various methods can be employed. A drug can passively pass through the cell membrane through the transcellular route. This method is used in case of hydrophobic drugs [9]. Hydrophilic drugs can use paracellular pathways to cross the physiological barriers [10]. Active transport with the help of receptor mediated transporters is acheived. For instance, dipeptide-based drugs are often transported across intestinal mucosal membrane through the use of transporters.

Another, major barrier that leads to interindividual variations in drug response is the presence of metabolizing enzymes. Peptide drugs are subjected to acidic hydrolysis and gastric proteolysis while the smaller size peptides are unaffected by the enzymes. Pancreatic proteases are also responsible for degradation of smaller peptidic drugs. Trypsin, chymotrypsin, carboxypeptidase A and B and elastase are present in the duodenum. These enzymes are responsible for degradation of upto 30–40% peptidic drugs [11]. Peptidase present in lower part of ileum and cytosolic proteases are responsible for degradation of dipeptides [12]. Conjugating enzymes including 'Phase II metabolizers' are present in the intestine and can metabolise various drugs.

The chemical structure and composition of the drugs decides its permeability and solubility profile. Also, the permeation of the drugs in the mucosal membrane of the intestine is responsible for the extent and rate of absorption [13]. The presence of hydrogen bonding is responsible for the permeation of peptides. For the drug to dissolve and enter into the cell membrane, the polar amide bonds in the proteins need to be disintegrated.

7 Pathways of Drug Delivery to Central Nervous System

There are certain blood brain barriers that inhibit easy delivery of the drug to the brain. The first barrier that restricts the drug entry is the brain capillary endothelial cells. Pores and channels that are usually present in the plasma membrane are absent in the brain capillary endothelial cells and therefore, the pinocytic activity is very low. The brain capillary endothelial cells are connected to each other by well-developed tight junctional complexes, which slow down the passive diffusion of the drugs between the endothelial cells [14]. This highlights the fact that the paracellular pathway is highly restricted. The second barrier is the blood-cerebrospinal fluid barrier which involves choroid plexuses and arachnoid membranes [15].

There are generally three basic routes for the delivery of the drugs into the brain which are given below:

- Direct administration of drug.
- Blood–brain barrier disruption.
- Transcellular delivery routes.

7.1 Direct Administration of Drug

Direct administration of drug to the brain can be acheived through intracerebral, intrathecal and nasal routes. These methods involve the strategy of delivering drug to the brain by circumventing the problem of the drug penetrating the blood brain barrier through direct injection into the brain. This method is based upon drilling a small hole into the intracerebroventricular or intracerebral portion for the direct injection to the brain. Therapeutic drugs of various sizes either in single formulation or polymer formulation can be delivered for sustained disease. However, there are certain disadvantages related to the direct administration of the drug to the brain which are given below:

- It involves craniotomy procedure which is invasive.
- The direct implant of the drug causes limited distribution of the drug to the brain.

For the delivery of macro molecular drugs to the brain intrathecal administration is used. It involves injection of the drug to the cerebrospinal fluid surrounding the spinal cord. This method is used for the delivery of the small lipophilic molecules to the brain for pain management. Molecules administered to the intrathecal route are slowly cleared from the cerebrospinal fluid [16]. There are several studies that report the intrathecal delivery of the protein and peptides to the brain. McCarthy et al. reported that leptin can be transferred to the hypothalamus region of the brain within 4 h of injection into the lumbar region [17]. In another study, [18] reported that leptin could be infused intrathecal to the brain for reduction of body weight in the rats.

Third method of direct drug administration is the intranasal drug delivery. It is a non-invasive means in which the connection between the brain and the nose (olfactory neural pathway) is used for the delivery of the drug to the brain. It is used for the delivery of proteins, small molecular weight compounds such as cephalexin, cocaine, insulin and neurotrophic factors [19]. Intranasal drug delivery system offers advantage of direct drug administration eliminating the requirement of systemic delivery and reduced side effects. Also, the drug does not need to be coupled with any carrier molecule and can be inhaled without any modification. There are certain disadvantages associated with the intranasal administration of the drug which are given below:

- Many drugs do not get absorbed to the olfactory nasal pathway and therefore do not produce the desired therapeutic effect [20].
- It requires a smaller dosage of drug because the excess will be drained into the pharynx [21].

7.2 Blood–Brain Barrier Disruption

Due to the presence of tight junctions in the brain capillary endothelial cells, paracellular diffusion of molecules into the brain is highly restricted. Therefore, slight modification in these tight junctions can indirectly control the permeability of the brain capillaries. Different routes including use of an osmotic agent, vasoactive compounds and alkylglycerols can be undertaken to disrupt these tight junctions to deliver drug to the brain. First, the strategy in disrupting the blood brain barrier is useful via osmotic agents that can physically pull apart the tight junction due to the shrinkage of cerebral endothelial tissues. Generally, a hypertonic solution of mannitol sugar of concentration of 1.4–2 M is administered into the brain which causes the expansion of the blood volume [22]. On changing the osmolarity, tight cellular junctions in the capillary endothelial cells got disrupted which can cause increased delivery of the drug. Cerebral endothelial cells can resume their normal barrier function after returning to the normal osmolarity of the blood [23]. This technique has been used to deliver chemotherapeutic drugs to the brain for the treatment of brain tumours [24]. Use of osmotic regulators have been achieved for the delivery of genes and protein therapy to the central nervous system [25]. Antibodies have been delivered to the brain in rats through osmotic blood brain barrier disruption.

Certain pharmacological active agents such as histamine, bradykinin and nitric oxides are known to enhance the cerebral endothelial cell permeability. These agents worked in a dose limited and time dependent manner and have proved for safe supply of drugs to the central nervous system. For instance, bradykinin increases the cell permeability through the opening of tight junctions between the capillary endothelial cells via B2 receptors (53 54). The injection of the short chain alkylglycerols through the intra-arterial route opens up the blood brain barriers in the brain, thereby increasing the delivery of therapeutic drugs to the brain. Concentration dependent delivery of alkylglycerol to the brain has been used as antibiotic and anticancer agents. The effect of 2-*O*-hexyldiglycerol and 1-*O*-pentylglycerol have been examined for the in-vitro effect on paracellular and tight junctions. The study reports that alkylglycerol enhanced the endothelial paracellular permeability by altering the shape of cells and redistribution of junctional proteins [26]. The study has showed that the destruction of blood brain barrier with the help of alkylglycerol does not have any long-term side effects or toxicity in animal models suggesting that these compounds can be used for delivery of drugs to the brain. However, human clinical trials have not initiated yet.

7.3 Transcellular Delivery Routes

The delivery of therapeutic agents to the brain can be increased by enhancing the transcellular migration systems. The transcellular delivery routes include different mechanisms like transporters, passive diffusion and transcytosis. This method is more promising because it utilizes the regular biological route and do not disrupt the integrity and functioning of the blood brain barrier.

Passive diffusion is the primary transcellular route that can be used to deliver drugs with certain physiochemical characteristics and hydrophobicity. The delivery of the drug through the transcellular route can be increased by reducing the molecular size of the drug and increasing the hydrophilicity. Therefore, modifications in the functional group present in the drug can alternatively be used to improve the passive diffusion of the drug across the blood brain barrier. The development of a pro-drug to increase the lipophilicity is generally applied to enhance the passive diffusion. Polar functional groups including acids and amides are chemically modified to increase the lipophilicity. Therefore, the drugs are conjugated with asters containing hydroxyl, carboxyl and thiol groups [27]. Peptides usually have lower rate of diffusion across the biological membranes [28], the permeability of peptides across the membrane can be increased by converting them into cyclic confirmation by the process called as cyclization [29].

Another approach for the efficient drug delivery to the brain can be achieved through the use of a carrier or transport system that is present in the luminal side of the membrane. For meeting the metabolic requirements of the brain several amino acids, glucose, peptide, nucleoside transporters are present for delivering the required nutrients from the blood to the brain [30]. The drugs can be designed in such a way that it structurally resembles natural substrates present in the body or can be linked to endogenous compounds that can be transported into the brain by carriers or transporters [31]. For instance, GLUT are specific transporters present for the transport of glucose. It has special affinity for the transport of glucose. Therefore, glucose-based analogues /glycosylated analogues of various drugs have been developed that can be penetrated through the blood brain barrier using the GLUT transporters [32].

8 Oral Drug Delivery Systems

Oral route has been the most popular and successful route for controlled delivery of the drug because of convenience, ease of examination, greater flexibility in dosage and ease of production. Around 60% of the smaller molecular weight drugs are consumed orally. This is due to high compliance of the patient compared to parenteral routes [33]. Although, highly acceptable, the oral drug delivery system is one of the most problematic delivery systems. This is mainly because delivery of the drug through gastrointestinal tract is due to the lengthy exposure of the drug to various enzymes. There are numerous factors including physiochemical, physiological and formulation factors that restrict the absorption of the drug in the gastrointestinal tract. Firstly, the absorption of the drug requires that the drug should pass through multiple barriers including pericellular matrix, mucous layer, gastric juices, epithelial layer and blood capillaries [34]. pH of the gastrointestinal tract also influences the absorption of drug into the tract. The drugs that do not with stand acidic pH need to be formulated for protection against low pH. As the drug travels further, the mucosal layers present in the duodenum, ileum, jejunum and colon also restricts the movement and absorption of the drug. Solubility of the drug and the permeability through epithelial cells are critical determinants for drug absorption in the gastrointestinal tract. There are several strategies involved to enhance the solubility of the drug administrated through oral route. These strategies are given below:

1. **Salt formation**—This technique is used to enhance oral absorption of weakly basic and weakly acidic drugs. The principle behind this technique is that the salts of the weakly acidic or basic drugs have high solubility compared to pure form of the drug. pH can be used to enhance the solubility profile of the drug. The drug is designed such that its dissolution is independent of the environmental pH of the gastrointestinal tract. Sufficient amount of the buffering agent is used for the formulations.
2. **Chemical modifications**—The properties of the drug molecule like aqueous solubility, stability, permeability, lipophilicity and therapeutic index can be improved by conjugation of the drug to amides, esters, carbonates, or polyethylene glycol [35]. For instance, oral absorption of Paclitaxel is increased by polyethylene glycolation [36]. The solubility of the poor soluble drug can be improved by using various solubilizing materials. Polyethylene glycol 400 is used for increasing the solubility of hydrochlorothiazide 85.

3. **Drug complexation**—There are many oral drug formulations that are developed using the complexation technique [37]. Complexation is the reversible association between two or more molecules to form a non-bonded entity with a well-defined stoichiometry. The bonding between two molecules is based on relatively weak forces such as van der Waal forces, hydrogen bonding and hydrophobic interactions. It involves insertion of the nonpolar molecule or the nonpolar region of one molecule into the cavity of another molecule. The most commonly used molecule for drug complexation is cyclodextrins. Cyclodextrins are chains of glucopyranose structures arranged in donut shape with a hydrophobic cavity which can provide the microenvironment for small sized non-polar molecules. This process can be helpful to enhance the solubility of oral drugs that are water-insoluble or slightly soluble.
4. **Absorption enhancers**—Many molecules such as cholesterol, surfactants, bile salts, salicylates and glycerides are used as absorption enhancers which enhance the transport of hydrophilic drugs through alteration of paracellular permeability [38]. For instance, ethylene diamine is used to enhance the permeability of tight junctions by depleting calcium and magnesium [39].
5. **Physical modifications**—The crystal habit of the drug is modified to polymorphic, amorphous or pseudopolymorps form to enhance the oral solubility. For instance, polymorphic form III of riboflavin has 20 times more water solubility compared to I form. Similarly, amorphous forms have a greater aqueous solubility than the crystalline form because the energy required to transfer the molecule from the crystal lattice is greater than that required for amorphous solid. Amorphous form of Novobiocin is 10 times more soluble than the crystalline form. The anhydrous nature for the drug has greater aqueous solubility than the hydrates, because the hydrates are already in interaction with the water and therefore have lss energy for the crystal breakup in comparison to the anhydrous form for further interaction with water. For example, anhydrous form of theophylline has higher solubility in comparison to the monohydrate form.
6. **Nanocarriers**—Natural or synthetic carriers such as polycaprolactone, polylactide-coglycolide, polylactide, chitosan, gelatin, polyaziridine, dextran and alginate are used for the preparation of polymeric nanocarriers for drug delivery. Development of nanosized drug particles, effectively enhance the surface area which enhances the solubility and the dissolution of the drug molecules [40]. Nanosuspension based technology is used for the efficient delivery of hydrophobic drugs. This technique has been used for the enhanced dissolution and absorption of drugs such as tarazepide, amphotericin B and paclitaxel.

9 Receptor Mediated Drug Delivery

For the specific dispersion of the drug to the targeted cell in order to minimise or cause negligible side effects to the healthy cells, receptor mediated drug delivery system can be used as an effective way to deliver drugs to the targeted sites. Receptor mediated delivery of the drug is also a potential way to carry drugs to the targeted site. Receptor is the specific chemical constituent of the cell with which a drug interacts to produce its pharmacological effect. Some receptors sites have been identified with some specific parts of the proteins and nucleic acid. In most cases, the chemical nature of the receptor sites remained obscure. Receptors largely determined the quantitative relations between concentrations or dose of drug and pharmacological effect. They are responsible for selectivity of the drug action, molecular size, shape and electrical charge of a drug. Receptors mediate the actions of both pharmacological agonists and antagonists.

The ability of the receptor to bind is mediated by the chemical structure of the drug that allows it to interact with the complimentary surfaces on the receptors [41]. Once bound to the receptor the agonists activate the cellular activity. For instance, drugs that binds to the β-receptors in the heart to increase the force of myocardial contraction or drugs that bind to α- receptors present on blood vessels to enhance the blood pressure. The binding of the agonists triggers a series of biochemical events that ultimately leads to alterations in functions. The receptor is believed to have following characteristics:

- Ability to recognise specific molecular shapes..
- Binding of ligand is only temporary.
- Ligand binding produces physical changes in protein conformation, initiating intracellular changes that ultimately generate behavioural effects.
- Receptors have a life cycle and can be upregulated and downregulated.

10 Lipid Based Vesicular Drug Delivery Systems

With developing novel systems of drug delivery different types of pharmaceutical drug delivery systems such as microparticles, nanoparticles, nanospheres, micelles and vesicular systems have been developed to deliver the drug at a constant rate and to the targeted cells. Vesicles are colloidal molecules consisting of an amphiphilic concentric bilayer surrounding an aqueous compartment [42, 43]. Vesicles are an useful tool for the delivery of both hydrophobic drugs and hydrophilic drugs. Lipid based vesicular systems were first introduced by Bingham in 1965. Due to targeted drug delivery and improvement in drug bioavailability vesicular systems are potential candidates in the field of drug delivery. Vesicles can be made up of either natural or synthetic phospholipids which are called as liposomes. Non-ionic surfactants and cholesterol consisting vesicular system are called niosomes. The vesicular drug delivery is widely accepted and offers following advantages:

- Hydrophilic and hydrophobic drugs can be encapsulated easily
- It offers targeted drug delivery
- Quick metabolization of drugs can be delayed
- Stability of liable drugs can be enhanced
- Drugs encapsulated in vesicles are less toxic and offer minimal side effects
- Circulation time of drugs in the body can be prolonged.

Liposomes are minute spherical sac of phospholipid molecules of size 10-300 μm that enclose a water droplet, especially as formed artificially to carry drugs of other substances into the tissues. Liposomes may consist of either many, few or one phospholipid by layer. Weiner et al. described liposomes as a microstructure that consists of a concentric lipid by layers separated by aqueous buffer compartments [44]. Structurally, liposomes constitute of two components, cholesterol and phospholipids, in which cholesterol not does not form the bi-layered structure and acts as a fluidity buffer only [45]. It can be incorporated in liposomes in high concentrations of 1:1 or 2:1. On the other hand, phospholipids form the major components of the liposomes. Different phospholipids used for drug delivery constitute of phosphoglycerides and sphingolipids. Phosphatidylcholine is the most commonly used phospholipids which is an amphipathic molecule in which a glycerol bridge links a pair of hydrophobic acyl hydrocarbon chains with a hydrophilic polar head group, phosphatidylcholine [46]. Phosphatidylcholine is in soluble in water and it aligns itself closely in planar bilayer sheets to reduce unfavourable action between the aqueous phase and long fatty acid chains.

If the permeability of liposomes structure needs to be reduced, cholesterol is added to the bilayer structure. Similarly, lipids with a special affinity for target cells is added to the bilayer. Lactosylceramide is a special ligand which has affinity for hepatocytes. For the targeted delivery to hepatocytes, lactosylceramide is added in the liposomes [47].

Liposomal drug delivery has been extensively used for the treatment of cancer. Cytotoxic drugs are generally administered to body in a non-targeted fashion which leads to unnecessary death of normal cells. Entrapment of anti-cancerous drugs into liposomes increased circulation life time, enhanced deposition in the malignant cells, enhanced targeted delivery. Doxorubicin, daunorubicin and vincristine are the drugs which are usually entrapped in liposomes for targeted delivery. Doxil, an anticancerous drug market by Sequus Pharmaceuticals is designed as polyethylene glycol doxorubicin liposomes [48]. LipoDox is another polyethylene glycol based liposomal formulation marketed by Sun Pharma [49].

Ambisome and Fungisome are liposome based antifungal drugs which have more targeted drug delivery and less side effects. These are lipids formulations in which the amino group of amphotericin B forms an ionic complex with disteareoylphosphatidyl glycerol to form the liposomal bilayer. Cholesterol is added to the structure for the retention of amphotericin B within the liposomal bilayer. The outer layer is formed by phosphatidylcholine which is composed of a major lipid bilayer [50].

Dubey et al. developed liposomes for the delivery of melatonin across the human cadaver skin [51]. The developed liposomes were spherical in shape with 70.71%

entrapment efficiency of the drug. It was reported that ethosomal carrier provided enhanced transdermal delivery of melatonin to the skin. Glavas-Dodov et al. (2003) fabricated 5-fluouracil loaded liposomes for topical use [52]. The rate of drug release was found to be dependent on bilayer composition and offers continuous delivery of the drug.

11 Conclusion and Future Prospective

The delivery of micro and macro molecules to the targeted organ in an integrated manner is a challenge for many emerging drugs. There are numerous ways that have been studied and approved for therapeutic use. 'One of the efficient ways common to all the drug delivery methods is increasing the drug solubility, permeability and bioavailability. Although, a lot of study has been carried out, critical in vitro–in vivo *correlation* models need to be given more consideration for the development of better formulations. Human models-based drug testing needs to be taken into account while designing new formulations. It is expected that the future medicines will be a blend of different drug delivery systems in order to shorten the drug dosage and effective response. One of the challenging tasks in the drug delivery system is the reduction of toxicity related to the drugs which needs to be studied in a more realistic way from laboratories of commercial scale.

References

1. Vogel WH, Berke A (2009) Brief history of vision and ocular medicine. Kugler, Amsterdam
2. Jones KH (1977) Bioavailability of talampicillin. BMJ 2(6081):232
3. Hu L (2005) Prodrug approaches to drug delivery. Drug Deliv: Princ Appl:125–165
4. Zhang W, Zhao Q, Deng J, Hu Y, Wang Y, Ouyang D (2017) Big data analysis of global advances in pharmaceutics and drug delivery 1980–2014. Drug Discov Today 22:1201–1208
5. Hillery AM, Park K (2017) Drug delivery: fundamentals & applications, 2nd edn. CRC Press
6. Thakur A, Roy A, Chatterjee S, Chakraborty P, Bhattacharya K, Mahata PP (2015) Recent trends in targeted drug delivery. SMGroup
7. Prato M, Kostarelos K, Bianco A (2008) Functionalized carbon nanotubes in drug design and discovery. Acc Chem Res 41:60–68
8. Hochman J, Artursson P (1994) Mechanisms of absorption enhancement and tight junction regulation. J Control Release 29(3):253–267
9. Martinez MN, Amidon GL (2002) A mechanistic approach to understanding the factors affecting drug absorption: a review of fundamentals. J Clin Pharmacol 42(6):620–643
10. Yap AS, Mullin JM, Stevenson BR (1998) Molecular analyses of tight junction physiology: insights and paradoxes. J Membr Biol 163(3):159–167
11. Fricker G, Drewe J (1996) Current concepts in intestinal peptide absorption. J Pept Sci: Off Publ Eur Pept Soc 2(4):195–211
12. Lipka E, Crison J, Amidon GL (1996) Transmembrane transport of peptide type compounds: prospects for oral delivery. J Control Release 39(2–3):121–129

13. Goodwin JT, Conradi RA, Ho NF, Burton PS (2001) Physicochemical determinants of passive membrane permeability: role of solute hydrogen-bonding potential and volume. J Med Chem 44(22):3721–3729
14. Kadry H, Noorani B, Cucullo L (2020) A blood–brain barrier overview on structure, function, impairment, and biomarkers of integrity. *Fluids and Barriers of the CNS*, *17*(1),
15. Solár P, Zamani A, Kubíčková L, Dubový P, Joukal M (2020) Choroid plexus and the blood–cerebrospinal fluid barrier in disease. Fluids Barriers CNS 17(1):1–29
16. Verma A, Hesterman JY, Chazen JL, Holt R, Connolly P, Horky L, … Mozley PD (2020) Intrathecal 99mTc-DTPA imaging of molecular passage from lumbar cerebrospinal fluid to brain and periphery in humans. Alzheimer's & Dement: Diagn, Assess & Dis Monit 12(1):e12030
17. McCarthy TJ, Banks WA, Farrell CL, Adamu S, Derdeyn CP, Snyder AZ, Laforest R, Litzinger DC, Martin D, LeBel CP, Welch MJ (2002) Positron emission tomography shows that intrathecal leptin reaches the hypothalamus in baboons. J Pharmacol Exp Ther 301(3):878–883. https://doi.org/10.1124/jpet.301.3.878
18. Yaksh TL, Scott B, LeBel CL (2002) Effects of continuous lumbar intrathecal infusion of leptin in rats on weight regulation. Neuroscience 110(4):703–710
19. Talegaonkar S, Mishra PR (2004) Intranasal delivery: an approach to bypass the blood brain barrier. Indian journal of pharmacology 36(3):140
20. Erdő F, Bors LA, Farkas D, Bajza Á, Gizurarson S (2018) Evaluation of intranasal delivery route of drug administration for brain targeting. Brain Res Bull 143:155–170
21. Appasaheb PS, Manohar SD, Bhanudas SR, Anjaneri N (2013) A review on intranasal drug delivery system. J Adv Pharm Educ Res 3(4)
22. Wacher VJ, Salphati L, Benet LZ (2001) Active secretion and enterocytic drug metabolism barriers to drug absorption. Adv Drug Deliv Rev 46(1–3):89–102
23. Ndemazie NB, Inkoom A, Morfaw EF, Smith T, Aghimien M, Ebesoh D, Agyare E (2022) Multi-disciplinary approach for drug and gene delivery systems to the brain. AAPS Pharm Sci Tech 23(1):1–21
24. Han HK, Amidon GL (2000) Targeted prodrug design to optimize drug delivery. AAPS PharmSci 2(1):48–58
25. Hashimoto Y, Tachibana K, Kondoh M (2020) Tight junction modulators for drug delivery to the central nervous system. Drug Discovery Today 25(8):1477–1486
26. Hülper P, Veszelka S, Walter FR, Wolburg H, Fallier-Becker P, Piontek J … Deli MA (2013) Acute effects of short-chain alkylglycerols on blood-brain barrier properties of cultured brain endothelial cells. Br J Pharmacol 169(7):1561–1573
27. Singh S, Aggarwal A, Bhupathiraju NDK, Arianna G, Tiwari K, Drain CM (2015) Glycosylated porphyrins, phthalocyanines, and other porphyrinoids for diagnostics and therapeutics. Chem Rev 115(18):10261–10306
28. Sanderson JM (2012) Resolving the kinetics of lipid, protein and peptide diffusion in membranes. Mol Membr Biol 29(5):118–143
29. Cardona VMF, Hartley O, Botti P (2003) Synthesis of cyclic peptides from unprotected precursors using removable Nα-(1-(4-methoxyphenyl)-2-mercaptoethyl) auxiliary. J Pept Res 61(3):152–157
30. Alam MI, Beg S, Samad A, Baboota S, Kohli K, Ali J … Akbar M (2010) Strategy for effective brain drug delivery. Eur J Pharm Sci 40(5) 385–403
31. Denora N, Trapani A, Laquintana V, Lopedota A, Trapani G (2009) Recent advances in medicinal chemistry and pharmaceutical technology-strategies for drug delivery to the brain. Curr Top Med Chem 9(2):182–196
32. Fu J, Yang J, Seeberger PH, Yin J (2020) Glycoconjugates for glucose transporter-mediated cancer-specific targeting and treatment. Carbohyd Res 498:108195
33. Ingersoll KS, Cohen J (2008) The impact of medication regimen factors on adherence to chronic treatment: a review of literature. J Behav Med 31(3):213–224. https://doi.org/10.1007/s10865-007-9147-y

34. Zhu L, Lu L, Wang S, Wu J, Shi J, Yan L, Liu Z (2017) Oral absorption basics: pathways and physicochemical and biological factors affecting absorption. Elsevier, Developing solid oral dosage forms. Amsterdam, pp 297–329
35. Greenwald RB, Conover CD, Choe YH (2000) Poly(ethylene glycol) conjugated drugs and prodrugs: a comprehensive review. Crit Rev Ther Drug Carrier Syst 17(2):101–161. https://doi.org/10.1615/critrevtherdrugcarriersyst.v17.i2.20
36. Hussain Z, Wang S, Imran M, Sohail M, Shah SWA, de Matas M (2019) PEGylation: a promising strategy to overcome challenges to cancertargeted nanomedicines: a review of challenges to clinical transition and promising resolution. Drug Deliv Transl Res 9(3):721–734. https://doi.org/10.1007/s13346-019-00631-4
37. Choudhury H, Gorain B, Madheswaran T, Pandey M, Kesharwani P, Tekade BW (2018) Drug complexation implications in drug solubilization and oral bioavailability enhancement. Elsevier, Dosage form design considerations. Amsterdam, pp 473–512
38. Aungst BJ (2012) Absorption enhancers: applications and advances. Aaps J 14(1):10–18. https://doi.org/10.1208/s12248-011-9307-4
39. Lemmer HJ, Hamman JH (2013) Paracellular drug absorption enhancement through tight junction modulation. Expert Opin Drug Deliv 10(1):103–114. https://doi.org/10.1517/17425247.2013.745509
40. Mei L, Zhang Z, Zhao L, Huang L, Yang XL, Tang J, Feng SS (2013) Pharmaceutical nanotechnology for oral delivery of anticancer drugs. Adv Drug Deliv Rev 65(6):880–890. https://doi.org/10.1016/j.addr.2012.11.005
41. Salahudeen MS, Nishtala PS (2017) An overview of pharmacodynamic modelling, ligand-binding approach and its application in clinical practice. Saudi Pharm J 25(2):165–175
42. Negi LM, Garg AK, Chauhan M (2009) Ultradeformable vesicles: concept and execution. Pharma Times 41(9):11–14
43. Sankar V, Ruckmani K, Jailani S, Siva Ganesan K, Sharavanan SP (2010) Niosome drug delivery system. Indian Pharm 9(92):16–18
44. Weiner N, Martin F, Riaz M (1989) Liposomes as a drug delivery system. Drug Dev Indust Phar 15(10):1523–1554. https://doi.org/10.3109/03639048909052502
45. Nsairat H, Khater D, Sayed U, Odeh F, Al Bawab A, Alshaer W (2022) Liposomes: structure, composition, types, and clinical applications. Heliyon 8(5):e09394
46. Li J, Wang X, Zhang T, Wang C, Huang Z, Luo X, Deng Y (2015) A review on phospholipids and their main applications in drug delivery systems. Asian J Pharm Sci 10(2):81–98
47. Harashima H, Kiwada H (1996) Liposomal targeting and drug delivery: kinetic consideration. Adv Drug Deliv Rev 19(3):425–444
48. Cabanes A, Even-Chen S, Zimberoff J, Barenholz Y, Kedar E, Gabizon A (1999) Enhancement of antitumor activity of polyethylene glycol-coated liposomal doxorubicin with soluble and liposomal interleukin 2, Clinical cancer research. Off J Am Assoc Canc Res 5:687–693
49. Chou H, Lin H, Liu JM (2015) A tale of the two PEGylated liposomal doxorubicins. Onco Targets Ther 8:1719–1720
50. Wasan EK, Gershkovich P, Zhao J, Zhu X, Werbovetz K, Tidwell RR et al (2010) A novel tropically stable oral amphotericin B formulation (iCo-010) exhibits efficacy against visceral Leishmaniasis in a murine model. PLoS Negl Trop Dis 4(12):e913
51. Dubey V, Mishra D, Jain NK (2007) Melatonin loaded ethanolic liposomes: Physicochemical characterization and enhanced transdermal delivery. Eur J Pharm Biopharm 67(2):398–405. https://doi.org/10.1016/j.ejpb.2007.03.007
52. de Oliveira BE, Junqueira Amorim OH, Lauro Lima L, Rezende RA, Mestnik NC, Bagatin E, Leonardi GR (2021) 5-Fluorouracil innovative drug delivery systems to enhance bioavailability for topical use. J Drug Deliv Sci Technol 61102155-10. https://doi.org/1016/j.jddst.2020.102155

Smart Development of Nano Materials and Nanomedicine Formulations

Ravi Parashar, Shilpi Prasad, Narayan Hemnani, and Preeti K. Suresh

Abstract The field of nanotechnology has brought in a giant revolution and nanomedicine has emerged as a key player in offering cross-sectoral and cross-technological solutions for various treatment modalities. The domain of nanomedicine includes the nanocarriers and the nanomaterials themselves. The new generation of nanomaterials with their unique properties (acoustic, electrical, mechanical, optical) has unique interactions in the biological milieu. This has undoubtedly opened up new clinical perspectives for better management of various diseases and disorders. Over 50 formulations based on nanotechnology have reached the market and are approved as anesthetics, anti-cancer therapies, anti-fungal, and iron-replacement therapies among others. But, the development of nanomedicine that has the desired and reproducible functionalities, and can successfully transit from bench to bedside is a tedious, rigorous, and arduous pursuit. The Fourth Paradigm of scientific research including rational design, high throughput experimental techniques, process automatization, artificial intelligence technology, and machine learning has immense potential to be integrated with nanomedicine/ nanomaterial research to achieve smart products having the desirable features. The chapter would cover the concepts, historical evolution, and application of these smart nanomaterials, implementation of AI in healthcare, biosensors/smart sensors in neurodegenerative diseases, telemedicine, and its fine-tuning to generate nano pharmaceuticals with requisite profiles to enable their successful clinical translation.

Keywords Nanotechnology · Smart nanomaterials · Nanorobot · Artificial intelligence · Telemonitoring · Cloud computing · e-health · Remote neuronal stimulation

R. Parashar · N. Hemnani · P. K. Suresh (✉)
University Institute of Pharmacy, Faculty of Technology, Pt. Ravishankar Shukla University, Raipur, Chhattisgarh 492010, India
e-mail: sureshpreeti@gmail.com

S. Prasad
Siddhi Vinayaka Institute of Technology and Sciences, Bilaspur, Chhattisgarh 495001, India

S. K. Rath et al. (eds.), *Nanomaterials for Drug Delivery and Neurological Diseases Management*, Smart Nanomaterials Technology,
https://doi.org/10.1007/978-981-97-0308-1_4

1 Introduction

1.1 Smart Nanomaterials

Nanotechnology brings materials, equipment, and engineering together at the nanoscale. Lately, the human life has been revolutionized by the application of materials at the nanoscale in almost every walk of life [1]. The past decade has witnessed a boom in the synthesis and progress of "smart" nanomaterials. The term "smart materials" are alternatively utilized for active, stimuli-responsive, or adaptive materials. These materials alter certain critical properties during use and respond to any external stimuli upon exposure [2]. They mark their presence in various forms such as carbon–metal nanohybrids, lightweight graphene structures, shape-controlled inorganic nanoparticles, stimuli-responsive polymeric materials, and biohybrid self-assembling nanoscale architectures, etc. Some key innovations in the field of drug delivery, catalysis, flexible electronics, environmental remediation, etc. have been catalysed by these "smart nanomaterials" [3].

1.2 Responsive Polymers

In the past decades, tremendous progress has been made towards characterising and developing stimuli-responsive polymeric systems [4, 5]. By definition, these polymers upon exposure to an external stimulus undergo a physical or chemical transformation. The range of stimuli is vast and may include redox reaction, pH change, magnetic field, enzymatic activity, light and temperature change [6–11] (see Fig. 1).

A. ***PH-Responsive Polymers***

This class of polymers witness altered surface activity, chain conformation, and solubility profile upon any induced change in the pH of the solution. They are categorized as polyacids and polybases. At high pH, weak acidic groups in polymers release protons, whereas, at low pH, weak basic groups accept protons. Based on their specific pKa values, they behave as polyelectrolytes in particular acidic or basic conditions [12]. Most common examples of acidic groups include sulfonic, phosphonic, carboxylic and boronic acid, whereas pyrrolidine, pyridine, imidazole, morpholino, piperazine, and the tertiary amines constitute widely used functional groups for responsive polybases [13].

B. ***Thermo-Responsive Polymers***

Sudden change in solvation state leads to a phase transition in the thermo-responsive polymers within a specific temperature range. These polymers have a distinctive critical solution temperature, which induces changes in the hydrophobic/hydrophilic interactions between a polymer chain and an aqueous medium. Chain collapse or

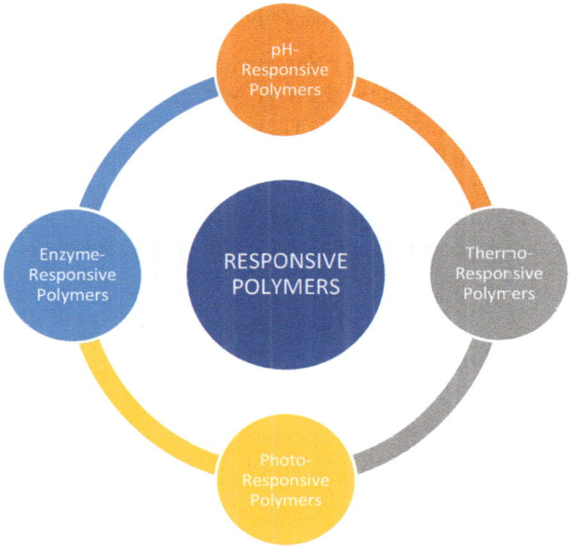

Fig. 1 Classification of responsive polymers

swelling are observed as a result of induced changes. Critical solution temperature can be categorized as lower critical solution temperature (LCST) and upper critical solution temperature (UCST) on the basis of behaviour of mixture at different temperatures. The changeover of polymer–solvent mixture at low temperature from a single phase to a biphasic system at high temperature is referred to as LCST, while a shift from a biphasic system at low temperature to a single phase at high temperature is referred to as UCST [14]. Most common examples of thermo-responsive polymers exhibiting LCST includes Poly(N-isopropylacrylamide) (PNIPAM), poly(N-ethyl oxazoline), poly(N,N-diethylacrylamide), and poly(N-vinyl caprolactam) [15–17].

C. ***Photo-Responsive Polymers***

The polymers that on exposure to light radiation such as ultraviolet (UV), near-infrared (NIR) or visible, undergo changes in physical properties and chemical constitution are referred to as photo-responsive polymers. Polymer chains containing functional groups that are capable of triggering either isomerization, self-annihilation or dimerization can result in systems that are responsive, that on interaction with light induce physical changes or morphological conversions, in terms of shape change, dissociation or crosslinking [18, 19]. Poly(ethylene glycol)-block-poly(dimethylamino-azobenzene) (PEGb-PMDA-Azo) and poly(N-acryloylmorpholine)-o-nitrobenzyl–poly(N-acryloylmorpholine) (PNAM-ONB PNAM) are examples of photo-responsive polymers having azobenzene and benzyl ester moieties, respectively [20, 21].

D. ***Enzyme-Responsive Polymers***

Compounds such as oligopeptide, dipeptide, or tripeptide act as enzyme-sensitive groups, undergoing physical or chemical changes when activated by the catalytic action of enzymes [22]. They function in mild environments (such as aqueous solutions with pH levels between 5 and 8 and temperatures about 37 °C), are highly selective and have a significant impact on healthy and diseased biological pathways. Examples include cleavage of copolymers of PEG and acrylamide at pre-programmed sites using tripeptides as enzymatically cleavable linkers [23].

1.3 Smart Nano-vehicle in Neurodegenerative Diseases

Globally, the median human lifespan has increased and the driving factors have been primarily the improved living conditions and better healthcare facilities. By 2050, Europe's median age is projected to rise by nearly 5 years while population over the age of 65 years in the US is also expected to increase by 88 million in 2050 [24]. Increase in the life expectancy, has been marked with a corresponding increase in the diseases associated with old people. Neurodegenerative diseases (NDDs) mostly affect elderly persons, and these include Alzheimer's disease (AD), Huntington's disease (HD), Parkinson's disease (PD), and amyotrophic lateral sclerosis (ALS). In the advanced stages of certain diseases, such as multiple sclerosis (MS), neuronal degeneration occurs. Initially, multiple sclerosis is characterized by demyelination but it progresses to neuronal death. For improving patient's quality of life, an early diagnosis, prediction of disease progression or the treatment response is required. Early-stage therapeutic effectiveness can avert the permanent damage linked to MS and NDDs, for instance, the neuronal loss.

The majority of NDDs and demyelinating illnesses are identified conventionally by CSF analysis, cognitive evaluations, genetic testing, or imaging. These methods are although accepted at wide level, but have inherent drawbacks like high costs, difficult protocols as well as invasive procedures.

Pathological alterations in the cerebral vasculature, such as the buildup of amyloid β-protein (Aβ), are a predominant pathological characteristic of Alzheimer's disease (AD) and cerebral amyloid angiopathy (CAA) [25, 26]. These pathological changes may result in stroke, brain haemorrhage, or dementia [27, 28]. Several studies have confirmed that cerebral haemorrhages occurring in non-hypertensive individuals may be caused by the cerebral microvascular amyloid deposits [26, 29]. Targeting of novel agents for detecting and treating amyloid deposits is obstructed by cerebrovascular endothelium, where well-formed paracellular tight junctions constitute the blood–brain barrier (BBB).

Polymeric nanoparticles if efficiently designed to traverse the BBB and deliver large drug payloads, can be viable candidates for both diagnostics and treatment. However, the challenges encountered by these nanoparticles to selectively target cerebrovascular amyloid are addressed by designing smart nano-vehicles (SNVs). The SNVs have drug entrapped within their biocompatible polymeric core with requisite size and surface properties, and/or diagnostic agent is coated on the surface. An additional biosensor coating can be included on the surface of the polymeric core to determine amyloid deposits. This additional coating makes it easier for SNVs to target diseased tissue that has amyloid deposits [30].

1.4 Biosensors/Smart Sensors in Neurodegenerative Diseases

Biosensors are a type of chemical sensor that convert biological data into an analytical signal for monitoring chemical and physiological analytes [31]. Through particular bioreceptors, the biosensor can target analytes of various types and sizes. A physicochemical transducer then converts the biochemical event into a useful, quantifiable signal. These signals are transformed and sent to a secondary device for data processing and analysis.

Advantages of biosensors over traditional screening procedure include:

1. quick response
2. easy handling
3. economical
4. minimal power requirements
5. portability
6. permit patient proximity with point-of-care (POC) devices
7. biomarkers can be screened using incredibly sensitive and selective biosensors in low concentration and complex biomatrices (e.g. blood, urine, tears, sweat, saliva).

Nanobiosensors

With the development of nanotechnology, various nanomaterials are being fabricated that have found wide application in the healthcare industry. The nanobiosensors, with improved sensitivity have brought in a giant revolution. Smart biosensors take advantage of microtechnology and wireless technology in combination with actuators. Nanomaterials that are used or are being investigated for their application in biosensors include gold nanoparticles, carbon nanotubes, magnetic nanoparticles, and quantum dots. Some biomarkers like GABA (Gamma-aminobutyric acid)/ glutamate, purine, ATP, and adenosine have been detected using nanostructures mixed with biopolymers such as chitosan, polyethylene glycol, etc. [32]. The biopolymers exhibit high permeation, good adhesive properties, and display reduced or negligible toxicity. These biopolymers can be reused following few simple processes. By effective diagnosis of sensory and motor changes, neurogenerative diseases can be detected nearly 10–15 years earlier.

The advantages of nanobiosensors include [33]:

1. detection of biomolecule that is facilitated with higher specificity and sensitivity.
2. capability of detection of molecules and atoms.
3. biomolecular recognition, detection of pathogens, environment monitoring.
4. Usage of nanaodevices, rendering these products cost-effective with commercial value, e.g., carbon nanotubes.
5. Usage in recognizing various body fluids-based biomarkers (CSF, blood, plasma, urine, tears, sweat, and saliva) and are not limited to only enzymes, proteins, and antibodies.
6. influencing enzymatic immobilisation and considerably enhancing the transducer's responsive surface.
7. possessing increased catalytic activity, better magnetic characteristics, and high electrical conductivity

Carbon-based nanobiosensors

In the field of biosensor research and development, nanostructures based on carbon, such as two-dimensional graphene and one-dimensional carbon nanotubes, are already in use and are undergoing further development [32]. They are able to translate chemical responses in living things into electrical impulses. They are reusable, and the functionalization of their surfaces can improve the biorecognition, specificity, and sensitivity of the assay. They can be utilised in challenging environments while keeping their specificity in a range of temperatures. Since graphene is naturally hydrophobic, its application as a possible biosensor is restricted. Graphene oxide offers higher electrical conductivity qualities as well as increased hydrophilicity and thus, graphene oxide has found application as optical biosensors, particularly in the development of label-free optical biosensors and photoluminescence.

Gold-based nanobiosensors

Gold possesses unique characteristics at the nanoscale, such as increased reactivity, good electrical conductivity, a large surface ratio, the ability to have its surface functionalized, and the ability to incorporate other composite elements, such as chitosan, graphene oxide, and other chemicals, in order to improve the specificity, sensitivity, and stability of nanoscale gold biosensors. In addition, by adding electrodes, they can be transformed into microchips that have a better level of durability and can be utilised in the domains of medicine as well as electronics. Miniaturizing the devices and combining them with multichip and fluid systems are two of the most pressing difficulties in this industry at the moment.

The various types of nanobiosensors along with their uses and advantages are presented in Table 1.

Nano-enabled sensing systems are being investigated for periodic study of neurological diseases/disorders, cardiovascular and motor functioning impairments. These

Table 1 Types of nanobiosensors and their uses

S. no.	Types of nanobiosensor	Uses	Advantages	References
1	Gold nanorods	Alpha-Synuclein (a PD biomarker) detection	Apart from serum, these biosensors can also be used for saliva	Adam et al. [34]
2	Thioflavin-T (ThT)-modified 20 nm multi-branched nanopillared (MNS) polymeric films	Detection of beta-amyloid peptide (Aβ1–42) detection, a biomarker linked with the emergence of Alzheimer's disease (AD)	Apart from serum these biosensors can also be used for saliva	Altuntas and Buyukserin [35]
3	Nanocomposite biosensor	Detection of DJ-1 protein	Used in earlier detection of Parkinson's disease from saliva	Karaboğa and Sezgintürk [36]
4	Nanoparticles of titanium dioxide (TiO_2)	Detection of multiple sclerosis	Employed for the construction of immunosensors owing to their high surface area and characteristics that encourage electron transfer rates	Kim et al. [37]
5	Platinum nanoparticles (PtNPs) with glutmate oxidase immobilized on top of them	Biomarker of neurodegenerative conditions like PD and AD	Enhanced nanocomposite's electro-catalytic activity	Nguyen [38]
6	Modified nanocomposite, carbon-coated mesoporous SiO_2 nanoparticles	Detection of DA, a biomarker for AD, PD, and schizophrenia	Increased nanocomposite's electrochemical performance	Liu et al. [12]
7	Carbon nanotubes-altered Au electrodes on a porous polyester track etched Trans well membrane	Dynamic, quantitative detection of serotonin (5-HT), a neurotransmitter responsible for neuronal synaptic communication in the brain and peripheral nervous systems	Resulted in enhanced electroactive surface area, 5-HT sensitivity, specificity, and saturation time	Chapin et al. [39]

(continued)

Table 1 (continued)

S. no.	Types of nanobiosensor	Uses	Advantages	References
8	Carbon nanotube-based microelectrode system	Used for the identification of brain disorders like epilepsy	Improved resolution in comparison to conventional neurochemical sensing systems	Hu and Hu [40]
9	Transistor based on graphene	Used for the in depth neural activity as well as surface alterations	High flexibility, mechanical strength, conductance and chemical stability in comparison to other reported metal or silicon-based probes	Kujawska et al. [41]
10	Graphene ink-based, ultrasensitive electrochemical sensor	Utilized in detection of dopamine for PD	Sensor's high selectivity, and sensitivity	Butler et al. [42]
11	Nanocomposites of zinc oxide and reduced graphene oxide (ZnO-rGO)	Employed as a transducer matrix for the accurate detection of dopamine	Exhibit better electron transport	Verma et al. [43]
12	Surface enhanced Raman scattering (SERS) technique and SERS biosensor platform utilizing Raman dye coated Poly A aptamer-AuNPs (PAapt-AuNPs)	Aβ42 oligomers and tau protein detection with a wide linear detection range	The sensor demonstrated a very low limit of detection for the Aβ42 peptide	Phan et al. [44]

systems include wireless e-bra, e-band, various integrated electronics, headwear, shoes, among others. Technological improvements have not only aided in the detection or diagnosis of neurodegenerative disorders, but also in their treatment of diseases using aptamers, polymersomes, nanodendrimers, nanoparticles, nanocomposites, and nanobots. The advantages of these nanosized sensors include the lack of invasive procedures, active monitoring, mobile tracking, infection-free database acquisition, for monitoring response, and advising the concerned about potential remedies [45].

Nanomaterial-based graphene electrodes, like reduced graphene oxide (rGO) and graphene oxide (GO), have garnered considerable attention for electrochemical biosensing applications [41]. Graphene has excellent electrical conductivity and have large surface area which is used in electrochemical measurement systems.

Remote Neuronal Stimulation

Neuronal stimulations have been employed to study brain functions and neurological illnesses. Remote neural circuit stimulation have also been explored for brain-machine interfaces [46]. It allows for the direct linkage of neuronal events (e.g., membrane hyperpolarization/depolarization, action potential firing, neurotransmitter release) or activation of a specific receptor and second messenger-induced signalling pathway and a behavioural outcome [47]. Researchers in the field of neuroscience have created a wide range of instruments and methods that may remotely translate chemical and electrical signals into behaviours that provide geographical, temporal, and directional control. These methods use light, tiny chemicals, peptides, toxins, and other substances to change neuronal activity at the levels of neurotransmitter release, membrane potential and electrical excitability, post-synaptic receptors, and second messenger pathways [46, 48].

Some of the technologies which are being utilized for remote management of neural networks are:

1. Magnetic nanoparticles: They can produce heat or apply mechanical forces to regulate brain circuits from a distance [49].
2. Light, peptides, and tiny molecules to activate ion channels and G protein-coupled receptors (GPCRs) and, in turn, induce or retard neuronal firing.
3. Opsins, the microbial light-gated receptors found in mammalian tissue, modify cell membrane potential in response to light and may either hyperpolarize or depolarize neurons.
4. Numerous peptide receptors have been successful in controlling neuronal activity, including the *Drosophila melanogaster* allatostatin receptor (AlstR) and the transient receptor potential vanilloid 1 (TRPV1) ligand-gated ion channel [46].

There are three types of controls for remote neuronal stimulation, i.e., spatial, temporal and directional [46]. In spatial control, expression of some protein, receptors or light is required whose position is controlled or presence of their associated ligands (i.e., small molecules or photons) gives the data to modulate neuronal signals. A receptor's or pathway's duration, which can range from milliseconds to hours, is determined by the temporal control. The term "directional control" describes how the instrument affects neural activity overall (activation versus inhibition). This provides details on the function of that cell in neuronal depolarization, hyperpolarization, firing, and silencing.

Smart Insole Dataset

Currently several wearable devices are in use for monitoring the wearer's condition continuously with newly developed devices. Since each gait event (the way the person walks) can be characterised by a pressure pattern, sensor insoles for monitoring foot pressure are one of cutting-edge technology currently being utilized for gait analysis. This allows for the analysis of phases and gait patterns [50]. Human gait pattern may also divulge possible illness and ingrained healthcare practises. Gait is a rhythmic, periodic movement governed primarily by coordination, balance, and synchronisation, and is activated by the appropriate functioning of the central and peripheral (musculoskeletal) nerve systems. A loose, thin strip called an insole is inserted inside a pair of shoes for comfort or warmth. Developments in the medical field of diagnostics has led to the invention of Smart Insole which uses pressure sensors in addition to shoe products. A Smart Insole is supposed to replace the huge medical devices and costs. These insoles can predict motor dysfunction at an early stage and thus predict the onset of neurodegenerative diseases especially in elderly patients [51]. Several insoles have been invented, e.g., Flexinfit, Samsung Smart Insole, Triboelectric nanogenerator, etc. [50, 52, 51].

FlexinFit is the evolution in the smart insole dataset which analyses biomechanics and posture. It has got more than 400 sensors and it takes around 4 h to analyse the data. It is tied to the baropodometric platforms that is inserted in the shoes. One of the major drawbacks is the slipping on the foot while walking, as it is made using the printing method [52].

With a variety of sensors attached, **Samsung's smart insole** is a wearable Internet of Things (IoT) gadget that monitors a variety of activities, including walking style, activity level, movement data, and calorie computation. As it is a separate accessory designed to wear on shoes, it is more comfortable.

For real-time gait analysis, a smart insole powered by a **Triboelectric Nanogenerator** (TENG) is being developed. Its revolutionary air-pressure-driven structural architecture boasts interesting qualities including easy fabrication, quick response times, great durability, and exceptional mechanical resilience for the sensors. The mechanical activities of these TENG-based sensors may be simply converted into electrical output and they can be conveniently integrated into the traditional insole. Simply by examining the electrical data, the smart insole was able to accurately track and distinguish different gait patterns such as leap, step, walk, and run in real time. Thus, it can also monitor the abnormality of the gait, and play an important role in healthcare applications. It can also be used as a fall-alert system for the elderly [51]. It offers a fresh perspective on the practical uses of remote clinical biomotion analysis.

Some advancements were also done in Smart Insole. Recently an insole, composed of two electrode layers and elastomeric layers have been reported, which has a common top electrode flooded in the insole [52]. The upper non-conductive layer is made up of poly-dimethyl-siloxane (PDMS) and the lower layer is constituted by carbon nanotube (CNT)-dispersed PDMS for detection of pressure. The 16 electrodes present under the lower sensing layer serve as pressure sensors. The smart insole is cost-effective as there is no need of sewing and manufacturing is easy.

1.5 Telemedicine

Telemedicine, the practice of providing healthcare services remotely by using communication devices and AI software allows patients to consult healthcare professionals, receive medical advice, get diagnosed and even receive treatment without physically visiting a healthcare facility. Three separate layers make up the hierarchical tier structure used by telemedicine systems viz., remote or rural area, city or district hospital and specialty centre. The system enables in-home patients to engage with nurses, doctors, and occasionally a multidisciplinary team in real-time, high-quality voice and video. Levodopa-carbidopa intestinal gel (LCIG) home titration, optimization, and healthcare provider and patient satisfaction were evaluated in a study by Willows et al. [53]. The time between the introduction of the pump and the choice to either have a permanent percutaneous endoscopic trans gastric jejunostomy (PEG-J) procedure or quit receiving LCIG treatment was referred to as the telemedicine-assisted LCIG home management phase. From 4 clinics, a total of 15 patients with advanced stages of Parkinson's disease (PD) were enrolled. All technical incidents were documented and further examined in order to evaluate technical feasibility as well as procedural restrictions. The technique was shown to be very effective, technically practicable, and widely accepted. Patients, neurologists, and nurses thought the approach worked well and took lesser time than a patient being admitted to the hospital for LCIG care. The technical issues with this unique home-based telemedicine system included infrequency and connection with internet outages, that were quickly fixed. Except for one occurrence of a tube occlusion, there were no significant adverse effects. By reducing in-ward bed occupancy as well as hospitalisation and travel costs, the home-based telemedicine system for administering LCIG may reduce healthcare spending [53]. A pilot study on 61 patients of Parkinson's disease (PD) was based on examination of a novel idea i.e., the PD virtual clinic in an effort to create a productive system that combined digital wearable technologies and home-based telemedicine. Clinicians employed the Parkinson's Kineti Graph, a wrist-worn device that provides objective movement evaluation, to manage and optimise treatment [54].

However, telehealth demands a number of considerations and reflections:

(1) Legal issues: It is required to protect data integrity, accessibility, and security tracking and reporting (as with in-person and outpatient appointments). Till date, no global legislation is in place, but there are various restrictions in many jurisdictions: First and foremost, in many nations, telemedicine visits are not looked upon as official, and is still thought as an experimental study. Another issue is related to the usage of this data is informed consent for data collection in order to protect the privacy and manage sensitive data. Virtual private network tunnels must be used for the internet connection while telemedicine technologies must create encryption between the connected devices [55]. The European Union expanded the use of telemedicine as a standard medical service in Europe in 2015, although there is still a lack of clear European regulations and different national approaches to telemedicine [56].

(2) Personal barriers: Telemedicine implementation may be slowed down by scepticism of patient and healthcare provider. Nevertheless, numerous studies, patients, caretakers, and doctors all demonstrated a high level of acceptability. Barriers for patients include personal complexity in using technology owing to motor impairments, as well as the lack of devoted caretakers and a suitable environment. In some cases, the requirement for a caregiver can prevent the use of telemedicine. This is valid for both ALS patients with motor limits and dementia patients due to cognitive deficits. Additionally, some patients—particularly those who are elderly and reside in rural areas—limited access to smart electronic devices (such as a personal computer, tablet, or smartphone) and a subpar internet connectivity, which may prevent them from having satisfactory televisits with substantial anxiety. The practice of telemedicine can be greatly facilitated by advances in technology, more specifically in preserving technological resources and connectivity.

(3) Differences from in-person evaluation: There are significant differences between in-person examinations and tele-neurological consultations despite their similarities. It may be challenging to assess certain aspects of the examination only by visual inspection, like tone and coordination, because information from the virtual visit can only be obtained by monitoring the patient. Additionally, it can be more challenging for telemedicine to identify inconsistent responses brought on by poor hearing or slight cognitive and behavioural impairment. Therefore, neurologists who take part in telehealth should be trained on methods for enhancing telemedicine interactions and tools [57].

(4) Research and clinical trials: Telemedicine can be applied in research for various operations, such as patient recruitment and screening (to prevent taxing travel to the nearest recruiting facility), signing informed consent, and monitoring patients [58]. Telemedicine could, in fact, ease the strain of participation by lowering the number of outpatient visits. However, a fresh approach to clinical trials is required. To acquire an objective score directly from the patients (rather than through the provider's video interpretation), the virtual patient's evaluation must be built, validated, and collected self-reported outcome measures that are properly integrated with the physician measures.

1.6 Cloud Computing

The term "cloud computing" refers to an on-demand network system that provides users with efficient and suitable access to massive amounts of computing resources that are accessible from anywhere and easy to manage. The cloud model has several distinct features, such as on-demand self-service, broad network access, resource pooling, rapid elasticity, measured service, and so on. Cloud computing encompasses both internet-based services and the infrastructure and software that support them. The cloud provides Software as a Service (SaaS), Platform as a Service (PaaS), and Infrastructure as a Service (IaaS).

Cloud Computing in Healthcare

Nowadays, there is an increasing need for patient's remote monitoring of various disorders and especially patients with different neurological conditions require close observation, in particular. But it is generally observed that mostly, the patients neglect visits to hospitals/clinics for a routine checkup and it is impossible for medical professionals to personally visit each patient.

However, a remote monitoring system has a number of challenges, including sensing biological data and handling data collection, storage, computation, analysis, and transmission. If a remote system is to be created, massive computational and storage resources are needed to store, access, and analyse patient files. Almost all the smartphones in use today have various sensors that can detect and store biomedical data (such as speech/voice, image, video, etc.). Because of the elasticity, on-demand self-service, ubiquity, resource pooling, and scalability of clouds in terms of data collecting, data storage, data analysis, and data transfer, a cloud-based healthcare system accessed by smartphones may be a realistic solution for both patients and clinicians [59]. The following section discusses a practical implementation of a cloud computing-based technique for Parkinson's disease identification.

1.7 Fog-Assisted Intelligent Detection of Parkinson's Disease (Fog-IDPD)

This system offers fast storage, efficient data processing, precise measurement of critical parameters, and genuine report for the user. The physical space that makes up the proposed system is accountable for gathering data and exchanging it with the end users, whereas the internet itself includes a layer of fog and clouds. The information obtained from the physical area is sent to the Parkinson patient processing and detection fog layer. In order to lessen the severity of symptoms, the study intends to create a smart system to identify and monitor the health condition of patients with Parkinson's disease. The suggested system offers a detailed evaluation of voice data to assess the degree of severity. Simultaneously, the patient's medical history and health record are backed up to the cloud and kept for future use. The Fog-IDPD framework consists of these components:

1. Smart devices: Users looking to determine if they have Parkinson's disease or not may use smartphones that are web applications and sensor-equipped. Voice signals from the user are detected, recorded, and sent to the fog server using Bluetooth, Wi-Fi, or ZigBee communications. For gathering gait-related symptoms, additional wearable sensors are also used, such as a 3D accelerometer.
2. Fog Layer: After the information has been gathered, it is transferred to the individual's smartphone for local data analysis, categorization, and anomaly detection. It offers data dimensionality reduction, aggregation, and filtering services. Data that has undergone pre-processing is sent to a cloud server for centralized storage and in-depth analytics. In the instance of an alarming condition, an

immediate alert is sent to the patient or their family to acquaint them with the condition.

3. Cloud computing platform: This layer provides services such as central storage, data analytics, and graphical user interfaces for visualisation of report, prescription, and recommendations. To use a healthcare service, a user must first send a request to the cloud over an internet connection. The cloud administrator will then authenticate the user and register them by creating a special identifier for use in subsequent communications. The cloud administrator maintains each user's profile and preserves their personal data in a database [60].

Artificial Intelligence and Internet of Things for Diagnosis and Management of Parkinson's Disease

Artificial intelligence (AI) is focussed on creating intelligent agents/machines capable of perceiving their surroundings and take actions to achieve specific goals. They are designed to mimic human-like cognitive abilities like learning from experience, problem-solving and decision-making. Traditionally, AI is rule-based i.e. they rely on the explicit sets of rules created by human experts. expertise of human specialists. But, with the advent of machine learning and data-driven approaches, AI are now capable of learning from data and adapt without sole reliance on explicit rules. The Internet of Things (IoT) is a network of physical objects or "things" embedded with sensors, software and connectivity, that enable them to collect and exchange data over the internet or other communication networks and unique identifiers to exchange data across a network [61].

AI and IoT technologies can contribute to both the early diagnosis of Parkinson's disease (PD) and the monitoring of PD patients, with the goal of enabling improved individualized treatments and evaluating those that have been offered, supplementing the existing conventional approaches [62].

References

1. Choi S, Tripathi A, Singh D (2014) Smart nanomaterials for biomedics. J Biomed Nanotechnol 10:3162–3188
2. Gottardo S, Mech A, Drbohlavova J, Malyska A, Bowadt S, Riego Sintes J, Rauscher H (2021) Towards safe and sustainable innovation in nanotechnology: state-of-play for smart nanomaterials. NanoImpact 21:100297
3. Palchoudhury S, Aich N, Zhou Z (2020) Advances in smart nanomaterials: environmental perspective. J Nanomater 2020
4. Schmaljohann D (2006) Thermo- and pH-responsive polymers in drug delivery. Adv Drug Deliv Rev 58:1655–1670
5. Stuart MA, Huck WT, Genzer J, Müller M, Ober C, Stamm M, Sukhorukov GB, Szleifer I, Tsukruk VV, Urban M, Winnik F (2010) Emerging applications of stimuli-responsive polymer materials. Nat Mater 9:101–113
6. Cabane E, Zhang X, Langowska K, Palivan CG, Meier W (2012) Stimuli-responsive polymers and their applications in nanomedicine. Biointerphases 7:9

7. Chung JW, Lee KA, Neikirk C, Nelson CM, Priestley RD (2012) Photoresponsive coumarin-stabilized polymeric nanoparticles as a detectable drug carrier. Small 8:1693–700
8. Filipcsei G, Csetneki I, Szilágyi A, Zrínyi M (2007) Magnetic field-responsive smart polymer composites. In: Oligomers-polymer composites-molecular imprinting, pp 137–89
9. Huo M, Yuan J, Tao L, Wei Y (2014) Redox-responsive polymers for drug delivery: from molecular design to applications. Polym Chem 5:1519–1528
10. Kocak G, Tuncer C, Bütün V (2017) pH-responsive polymers. Polym Chem 8:144–76
11. Zelzer M, Todd SJ, Hirst AR, McDonald TO, Ulijn RV (2013) Enzyme responsive materials: design strategies and future developments. Biomater Sci 1:11–39
12. Liu X, Yang Y, Urban MW (2017) Stimuli-responsive polymeric nanoparticles. Macromol Rapid Commun 38:1700030
13. Zhao J, Lee VE, Liu R, Priestley RD (2019) Responsive polymers as smart nanomaterials enable diverse applications. Annu Rev Chem Biomol Eng 10:361–382
14. Manikandan M, Nisha Francis P, Dhanuskodi S, Maheswari N, Muralidharan G (2018) High performance supercapacitor behavior of hydrothermally synthesized CdTe nanorods. J Mater Sci: Mater Electron 29:17397–17404
15. Aoki T, Kawashima M, Katono H, Sanui K, Ogata N, Okano T, Sakurai Y (1994) Temperature-responsive interpenetrating polymer networks constructed with poly (acrylic acid) and poly (N,N-dimethylacrylamide). Macromolecules 27:947–952
16. Idziak I, Avoce D, Lessard D, Gravel D, Zhu XX (1999) Thermosensitivity of aqueous solutions of poly (N,N-diethylacrylamide). Macromolecules 32:1260–1263
17. Van Durme K, Verbrugghe S, Prez FED, Mele BV (2004) Influence of poly (ethylene oxide) grafts on kinetics of LCST behavior in aqueous poly (N-vinylcaprolactam) solutions and networks studied by modulated temperature DSC. Macromolecules 37:1054–1061
18. Gohy JF, Zhao Y (2013) Photo-responsive block copolymer micelles: design and behavior. Chem Soc Rev 42:7117–7129
19. Yang L, Tang H, Sun H (2018) Progress in photo-responsive polypeptide derived nano-assemblies. Micromachines 9:296
20. Dong R, Zhu B, Zhou Y, Yan D, Zhu X (2012) "Breathing" vesicles with jellyfish-like on–off switchable fluorescence behavior. Angew Chem Int Ed 51:11633–11637
21. Ercole F, Thissen H, Tsang K, Evans RA, Forsythe JS (2012) Photodegradable hydrogels made via RAFT. Macromolecules 45:8387–8400
22. Ulijn RV (2006) Enzyme-responsive materials: a new class of smart biomaterials. J Mater Chem 16:2217–2225
23. Thornton PD, McConnell G, Ulijn RV (2005) Enzyme responsive polymer hydrogel beads. Chem Commun, 5913–5915
24. Goldoni R, Dolci C, Boccalari E, Inchingolo F, Paghi A, Strambini L, Galimberti D, Tartaglia GM (2022) Salivary biomarkers of neurodegenerative and demyelinating diseases and biosensors for their detection. Ageing Res Rev, 101587
25. Jellinger KA (2002) Alzheimer disease and cerebrovascular pathology: an update. J Neural Transm 109:813–836
26. Vinters HV, Farag ES (2003) Amyloidosis of cerebral arteries. Adv Neurol 92:105–112
27. Brierley AS, Fernandes PG, Brandon MA, Armstrong F, Millard NW, McPhail SD, Stevenson P, Pebody M, Perrett J, Squires M (2002) Antarctic krill under sea ice: elevated abundance in a narrow band just south of ice edge. Science 295:1890–1892
28. Schwerd T, Twigg SRF, Aschenbrenner D, Manrique S, Miller KA, Taylor IB, Capitani M, McGowan SJ, Sweeney E, Weber A, Chen L, Bowness P, Riordan A, Cant A, Freeman AF, Milner JD, Holland SM, Frede N, Muller M, Schmidt-Arras D, Grimbacher B, Wall SA, Jones EY, Wilkie AOM, Uhlig HH (2017) A biallelic mutation in IL6ST encoding the GP130 co-receptor causes immunodeficiency and craniosynostosis. J Exp Med 214:2547–2562
29. Wisniewski HM, Vorbrodt AW, Wegiel J (1997) Amyloid angiopathy and blood-brain barrier changes in Alzheimer's disease a, b. Ann N Y Acad Sci 826:161–172
30. Agyare EK, Curran GL, Ramakrishnan M, Yu CC, Poduslo JF, Kandimalla KK (2008) Development of a smart nano-vehicle to target cerebrovascular amyloid deposits and brain

parenchymal plaques observed in Alzheimer's disease and cerebral amyloid angiopathy. Pharm Res 25:2674–2684
31. Duocastella M, Fernández-Pradas JM, Morenza JL, Zafra D, Serra P (2010) Novel laser printing technique for miniaturized biosensors preparation. Sens Actuators B: Chem 145:596–600
32. Pandit S, Dasgupta D, Dewan N, Prince A (2016) Nanotechnology based biosensors and its application. Pharma Innov 5:18
33. Zhang X, Guo Q, Cui D (2009) Recent advances in nanotechnology applied to biosensors. Sensors 9:1033–1053
34. Adam H, Gopinath SCB, Arshad MKM, Parmin NA, Hashim U (2021) Distinguishing normal and aggregated alpha-synuclein interaction on gold nanorod incorporated zinc oxide nanocomposite by electrochemical technique. Int J Biol Macromol 171:217–224
35. Altuntas S, Buyukserin F (2018) Fabrication of thioflavin-T-modified nanopillared SERS substrates for ultrasensitive beta-amyloid peptide detection. J Raman Spectrosc 49:1247–1256
36. Karaboğa MNS, Sezgintürk MK (2021) A nano-composite based regenerative neuro biosensor sensitive to Parkinsonism-associated protein DJ-1/Park7 in cerebrospinal fluid and saliva. Bioelectrochemistry 138:107734
37. Kim JH, Suh YJ, Park D, Yim H, Kim H, Kim HJ, Yoon DS, Hwang KS (2021) Technological advances in electrochemical biosensors for the detection of disease biomarkers. Biomed Eng Lett 11:309–334
38. Nguyen TNH (2020) Printable electrochemical biosensors for the detection of neurotransmitter and other biological molecule. Purdue University Graduate School
39. Chapin AA, Rajasekaran PR, Quan DN, Hu L, Herberholz J, Bentley WE, Ghodssi R (2020) Electrochemical measurement of serotonin by Au-CNT electrodes fabricated on microporous cell culture membranes. Microsyst Nanoeng 6:90
40. Hu C, Hu S (2009) Carbon nanotube-based electrochemical sensors: principles and applications in biomedical systems. J Sens 2009
41. Kujawska M, Bhardwaj SK, Mishra YK, Kaushik A (2021) Using graphene-based biosensors to detect dopamine for efficient parkinson's disease diagnostics. Biosensors 11:433
42. Butler D, Moore D, Glavin NR, Robinson JA, Ebrahimi A (2021) Facile post-deposition annealing of graphene ink enables ultrasensitive electrochemical detection of dopamine. ACS Appl Mater Interfaces 13:11185–11194
43. Verma S, Arya P, Singh A, Kaswan J, Shukla A, Kushwaha HR, Gupta S, Singh SP (2020) ZnO-rGO nanocomposite based bioelectrode for sensitive and ultrafast detection of dopamine in human serum. Biosens Bioelectron 165:112347
44. Phan LM, Tu TX, Hoang TA, Vo T, Pham HL, Ngoc HT, Le SR, Chinnadayyala JY, Kim S-M, Cho WW, Kim YH (2021) Nanomaterial-based optical and electrochemical biosensors for amyloid beta and tau: potential for early diagnosis of Alzheimer's disease. Expert Rev Mol Diagn 21:175–193
45. Tiwari S, Sharma V, Mujawar M, Mishra YK, Kaushik A, Ghosal A (2019) Biosensors for epilepsy management: state-of-art and future aspects. Sensors 19:1525
46. Rogan SC, Roth BL (2011) Remote control of neuronal signaling. Pharmacol Rev 63:291–315
47. Battaglini M, Marino A, Carmignani A, Tapeinos C, Cauda V, Ancona A, Garino N, Vighetto V, La Rosa G, Sinibaldi E (2020) Polydopamine nanoparticles as an organic and biodegradable multitasking tool for neuroprotection and remote neuronal stimulation. ACS Appl Mater Interfaces 12:35782–35798
48. Yuan M, Harnett MC, Yan TH, Georgas E, Qin YX, Zhou HC, Wang Y (2022) Progress, opportunities, and challenges of magneto-plasmonic nanoparticles under remote magnetic and light stimulation for brain-tissue and cellular regeneration. Nanomaterials (Basel) 12:2242
49. Tay A, Di Carlo D (2017) Remote neural stimulation using magnetic nanoparticles. Curr Med Chem 24:537–548
50. Chatzaki C, Skaramagkas V, Tachos N, Christodoulakis G, Maniadi E, Kefalopoulou Z, Fotiadis DI, Tsiknakis M (2021) The smart-insole dataset: gait analysis using wearable sensors with a focus on elderly and Parkinson's patients. Sensors 21:2821

51. Lin Z, Wu Z, Zhang B, Wang Y-C, Guo H, Liu G, Chen C, Chen Y, Yang J, Wang ZL (2019) A triboelectric nanogenerator-based smart insole for multifunctional gait monitoring. Adv Mater Technol 4:1800360
52. Lee W, Hong S-H, Oh H-W (2018) Characterization of elastic polymer-based smart insole and a simple foot plantar pressure visualization method using 16 electrodes. Sensors 19:44
53. Willows T, Dizdar N, Nyholm D, Widner H, Grenholm P, Schmiauke U, Urbom A, Groth K, Larsson J, Permert J (2017) Initiation of levodopa-carbidopa intestinal gel infusion using telemedicine (video communication system) facilitates efficient and well-accepted home titration in patients with advanced Parkinson's disease. J Parkinsons Dis 7:719–728
54. Evans L, Mohamed B, Thomas EC (2020) Using telemedicine and wearable technology to establish a virtual clinic for people with Parkinson's disease. BMJ Open Qual 9:e001000
55. Bassan S (2020) Data privacy considerations for telehealth consumers amid COVID-19. J Law Biosci 7:lsaa075
56. Raposo VL (2016) Telemedicine: the legal framework (or the lack of it) in Europe. GMS Health Technol Assess 12
57. Grossman SN, Han SC, Balcer LJ, Kurzweil A, Weinberg H, Galetta SL, Busis NA (2020) Rapid implementation of virtual neurology in response to the COVID-19 pandemic. Neurology 94:1077–1087
58. Govindarajan R, Berry JD, Paganoni S, Pulley MT, Simmons Z (2020) Optimizing telemedicine to facilitate amyotrophic lateral sclerosis clinical trials. Muscle Nerve 62:321–326
59. Mell P, Grance T (2011) The NIST definition of cloud computing
60. Devarajan M, Ravi L (2019) Intelligent cyber-physical system for an efficient detection of Parkinson disease using fog computing. Multimed Tools Appl 78:32695–32719
61. Norvig PR, Rani M, Nayak R, Vyas OP (2002) A modern approach. Prentice Hall Up Saddle River, NJ, USA 90:33–48
62. Giannakopoulou K-M, Roussaki I, Demestichas K (2022) Internet of things technologies and machine learning methods for parkinson's disease diagnosis, monitoring and management: a systematic review. Sensors 22:1799

Nanomaterials and Neurological Disorders Management

Sibasankar Sahu, Debasis Gantayat, Sipu Kumar Sahu, Gursharan Kaur, Vagish Dwibedi, and Santosh Kumar Rath

Abstract Neurodegenerative diseases (NDs) is the most common illnesses that affect majorly our healthcare systems including dementia, Alzheimer's disease, Parkinson's disease, frontotemporal dementia, and amyotrophic lateral sclerosis. As no specific treatments are available to pass the blood–brain barrier (BBB) and significantly reach the brain for the pharmacological impact, these ailments are regarded as incurable diseases. It is still difficult to create diagnostic and therapeutic tools for the surveillance and treatment of these disorders. The recent use of specialized nanomaterials (nanocarriers and nanoparticles) has improved diagnosis and therapies for neurodegenerative illnesses. The immense potential of nanopharmaceuticals as carriers for the spatial and temporal distribution of bioactive and diagnostics in drug delivery has recently come to light. Numerous pharmaceutical nanotechnology-based systems, also known as nanopharmaceuticals, have revolutionized both drug delivery and the entire medical system. These include polymeric nanoparticles, magnetic nanoparticles, liposomes, carbon nanotubes, quantum dots, dendrimers, metallic nanoparticles, polymeric nanoparticles, etc. These nanoparticles are employed recurrently for imaging studies and the treatment of neurological illnesses because of their distinctive properties, which include sensitivity, selectivity, and the capacity to cross the BBB when used in nano-sized particles.

Keywords Liposomes · Carbon nanotubes · Quantum dots · Dendrimers · Polymeric nanoparticles · Metalic nanoparticles · Micelles

Sibasankar Sahu and Debasis Gantayat authors are contributed equally.

S. Sahu · D. Gantayat · S. K. Sahu · S. K. Rath (✉)
School of Pharmaceuticals and Population Health Informatics, Faculty of Pharmacy, DIT University, Dehradun 248009, Uttarakhand, India
e-mail: skrath1985@gmail.com; santoshk.rath@dituniversity.edu.in

G. Kaur
University Institute of Biotechnology, Chandigarh University, Mohali 140413, India

V. Dwibedi
Institute of Soil, Water and Environmental Sciences, Volcani Research Center, Agricultural Research Organization, Rishon Lezion 7528809, Israel

S. K. Rath et al. (eds.), *Nanomaterials for Drug Delivery and Neurological Diseases Management*, Smart Nanomaterials Technology,
https://doi.org/10.1007/978-981-97-0308-1_5

1 Introduction

Generally, our nervous system is broadly divided into two main parts: the central and peripheral nervous systems. The diseases that are coming into the part of this particular central nervous system are called neurodegenerative disorders (NDs). As the name suggests, neurodegenerative disorders mainly involve our brain and spinal cord which contain various types of neurons. The loss of structure and function of neurons are called neurodegenerative disorders and as per WHO they are the most challenging as well as devastating to our society because their mechanism is associated with the brain. There are different types of NDs including Alzheimer's disease, Parkinson′s disease, Huntington′s disease, Amyotrophic lateral sclerosis, Frontotemporal dementia, Prion disease, Brain tumor, Spinal cord injury, and Stroke [1]. Although the mechanisms of all these diseases are different from each other, they involve quite similar forms of mechanism for achieving desired therapeutic response by the crossing of the blood–brain barrier (BBB).

The BBB is located in the central nervous system and mainly has the criteria to prevent neurotoxic plasms components, blood cells, and pathogens from entering the brain. The BBB has the power in terms of controlling influx and efflux of various biologically active substances which are very useful for the brain's metabolic activity as well as various neuronal functions. In the case of all NDs, the foremost challenge is to cross the BBB as BBB is considering those therapeutic agents in the same way [2]. So these NDs are considered incurable, as there are no particular therapies invented nowadays to provide such therapeutic efficacy as much is particularly required. As a result, approximately 15% of the worldwide population is barely affected by neurogenerative disorders [3]. As per WHO and the United Kingdom National Health Services data for the treatment of any kind of neurological disease the available resources are insufficient in most countries of the world and redesign must be needed [4]. Among all the challenges, molecular size is the biggest challenge to cross the BBB as only lipophilic drugs having a molecular size of less than 500 daltons can certainly cross while other traditional drugs fail. So there are different strategies are being developed and from there the role of nanoparticles emerges in a gigantic way to overcome these challenges as a result there are various nanoformulations are being developed previously and a lot of research work is continuing to fulfill the required criteria as an accountable dosage form. This nanotechnology involves the particle size range between 1 and 100 nm and contains various types of engineered nanomaterials in a single dimension and they can interact in a molecular level [5]. These nanomaterials particularly open new opportunities in the case of biomedical science and mainly play an impact role in the case of brain studies. Various formulations are recently trending like metal chelators, gold nanoparticles, micelles, quantum dots, polymeric nanoparticles, liposomes, solid lipid nanoparticles, microparticles, carbon nanotubes, etc. These are mainly composite-based formulations where a combination of two different types of nanoparticles are present. In the case of dendrimer-based formulations, there is presence of branching system of nanoparticles. The carbon-based formulations mainly involve nanotubes and fullerenes, and metal-based formulations that which comprise the formulation of nanoparticles with the help of various metals e.g. gold, silver, metal oxides, etc. [6, 7]. Many reported formulations are also significantly able to produce desired pharmacological responses in various neurodegenerative disorders that's why the use of nanomaterial is increased commercially as well as industrially.

2 Nanotechnology

Nanotechnology, a technology used at the nanoscale, is described as the manipulation or reorganisation of matter at the atomic and molecular levels in the 1 to 100 nm size range. It includes creating nanostructures at a nanoscales ranging from a single atom or molecule to submicron dimensions and applying them to physical, chemical, and biological systems. It also includes integrating the resulting nanostructures into greater systems. Nanotechnology has had a significant impact on medical devices such diagnostic biosensors, drug delivery systems, and imaging probes in the pharmaceutical communities of practice [8]. The limited anatomical access makes diagnosis and treatment more challenging. As a result, systemic administration of drugs for the treatment of CNS diseases is frequently ineffective. The most significant successes of nanotechnology claims in neuroscience from a biological standpoint will be those that value a thorough understanding of neurobiology and make use of the known (and undiscovered) molecular details. The creation of tactics that can increase medicine efficacy and get around BBB is necessary. The usage of various nano-scale materials is one of the potential strategies to overcome BBB, for which the desired therapeutic effect can be expected. These nano-based medications or drugs that have undergone nanoscale transformations have good stability, targeted delivery, drug loading capacity, the capability to boost therapeutic efficacy, sustained circulation, improve drug localization, and reduced toxicity [6, 9]. Numerous engineering techniques based on nanoparticles have been created and are being researched to prevent or treat nerve damage. As previously discussed nanotechnology is the most appropriate drug delivery approach in the future to treat all neurodegenerative disorders which are mainly categorized into various types (Fig. 1), among them Quantum dots, Metallic nanoparticles, Dendrimers, Carbon nanotubes, Polymeric nanoparticles, Liposomes, Micelles are most widely researched worldwide [10, 11, 6, 12].

3 Polymeric Nanoparticles

Neurological disorders that affect the brain and spinal cord are a significant health challenge worldwide, leading to high rates of morbidity and disability. Among these disorders, stroke stands as the second most common cause of death [13]. However, it

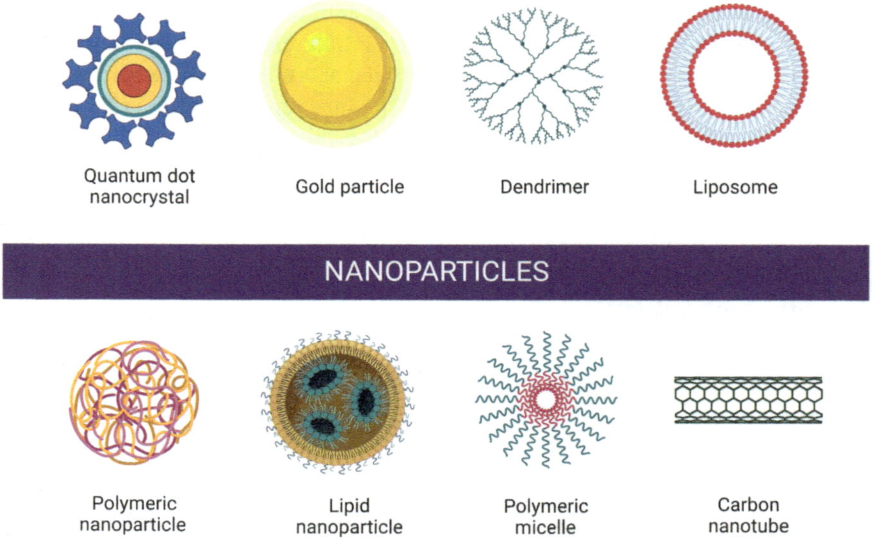

Fig. 1 Types of nanomaterials used for the treatment of NDs

is not the only the condition of the plagues individuals as there are several other prevalent neurological disorders including Alzheimer's disease, Parkinson's disease, Huntington's disease, motor neuron disease, multiple sclerosis, traumatic brain injury, stroke, and brain cancers. The impact of these disorders is substantial, with a comprehensive study conducted in 2016 estimating that approximately 276 million people suffer from a neurological disability, while approximately 9 million deaths occur annually due to neurological disorders [14].

The central nervous system (CNS), comprising the brain and spinal cord, plays a vital role in regulating the body's functions. It is protected by three barriers: the blood–brain barrier (BBB), the blood-cerebrospinal fluid barrier (formed by the choroid plexus epithelium), and the cerebrospinal fluid-blood barrier (established by the avascular arachnoid epithelium). These natural barriers pose significant challenges when it comes to delivering pharmaceutical treatments to the CNS [15]. Among these barriers, the BBB is particularly formidable, as it restricts the entry of many therapeutic agents into the brain. This limited permeability makes it difficult to develop effective treatments for neurological disorders [16, 17]. Neurons, the fundamental units of the CNS responsible for transmitting information and coordinating bodily functions, are highly sensitive and vulnerable to various factors. They are exquisitely sensitive to temperature fluctuations, pathogens, and toxins, which can cause severe damage or cell death. Consequently, neurodegenerative diseases, such as Parkinson's, Huntington's, and Alzheimer's disease, are commonly observed. These disorders involve the irreversible degeneration and death of neurons, leading to progressive deterioration of cognitive and motor functions [16, 18]. The consequences for individuals suffering from neurodegenerative diseases are profound, often resulting in a significant decline in quality of life.

The process of neurodegeneration can also be triggered by ischemic or hypoxic conditions, such as those experienced during a stroke, birth asphyxia, or traumatic brain injuries. These events can lead to a slow and progressive loss of neuronal functions over time [19]. The brain's vulnerability to these insults is due to its high metabolic demands and limited ability to regenerate damaged tissue. Consequently, individuals who experience stroke or traumatic brain injuries often face long-term consequences and require comprehensive management and rehabilitation to optimize their recovery [20, 21]. Solid hypoxic cancer cells oxidise glucose and the byproduct of the same process resulted lactate that builds up in the tumour microenvironment. Glioma stem cells (GSC) when they lack glucose utilize lactate as a fuel in the Krebs cycle and generate GTP. After consuming lactate, cancer cells become more aggressive and start to spread. HIF-1a that has been triggered by hypoxia aids hypoxic cancer cells in overcoming energy stress by promoting angiogenesis [22, 23]. Brain cancers, such as glioblastoma, pose another significant challenge in the realm of neurological disorders. These cancers arise from the abnormal transformation of genetic and cellular factors within neurons and glial cells. Glioblastoma is an aggressive and invasive form of brain cancer with limited treatment options and poor prognosis. Additionally, secondary brain tumours, known as brain metastases, can occur in adults with cancer, further exacerbating the burden of neurological disorders [24, 25]. Neurological disorders affecting the brain and spinal cord, such as stroke, Alzheimer's, Parkinson's, and brain cancers, have a significant impact on global health. The blood–brain barrier poses challenges for drug delivery, while neurodegenerative diseases, ischemic conditions, traumatic injuries, and brain tumours cause irreversible neuronal damage. With an ageing population, effective management and treatment options are in high demand. Overcoming barriers and addressing neuronal sensitivity is crucial for advancing therapies and improving outcomes in neurological disorders. In addition to being reasonably simple to modify with targeting ligands to improve BBB transport or route the loading medication to particular CNS areas, polymers can be created to be intrinsically multipurpose. Polymers have the potential to be biologically active, which makes them useful for controlling the body's endogenous transport systems and enhancing medication targeting [26]. The ideal polymer for transport to the brain is stable in blood, biodegradable, biocompatible, nontoxic, nonthrombogenic, nonimmunogenic, and noninflammatory. Additionally, polymeric NPs must be scalable and economical to make, and they must be able to resist aggregation.

4 Metal Chelators

Metal chelators, also known as chelates or chelating agents, or else we can say sequestering agents are the agents or compounds that form a stable water-soluble complex by reacting with metal ions. The ring-like structure of these chelates forms two or more bonds with the metal ions, allowing them to excrete easily. As the imbalance of the metal ions in our body is harmful, the regulation of metal ion concentrations in our tissue level is mandatory for normal body functioning [27]. These chelators are having a large advancement in our medical fields. In certain cases of heavy metal poisoning, chelation therapy is used, which can be done either orally or intravenously, where by using the chelating agents, heavy metals can be retarded out from our body, no matter if it is in simpler form or it is combined with a complex. Once the heavy metal is bound with the chelating agent, it forms another complex with it and can be easily excreted out from our body [28].

4.1 Metal Chelators in Various Brain Diseases

Alzheimer's disease is a brain disorder caused by the deposition of a certain type of proteins in the brain, which distorts brain cells. It is a common cause of dementia, in which a person loses the ability to think and memory loss occurs.

As Alzheimer's disease has no modified treatments available, Chand et al. [29]. Conducted an experiment in which they developed a drug combination of tacrine, which is an anti-Alzheimer's disease drug used previously with a metal chelator drug called deferiprone to target the disease poly pharmacologically. The enzyme called acetylcholinesterase, which plays a primary role in the pathology of Alzheimer's disease can be inhibited successfully with low concentrations along with can inhibit certain attributes of Alzheimer's disease [29]. In an another study, researchers have reported the use of redox of copper ions in the case of Alzheimer's disease, in which the copper homeostasis is regulated by a specific copper chelator known as TDMQs. The oral administration of the specific chelator can fully recover the cognitive and behavioural impairments in the models that are taken for the experiment [30]. The scientists have taken three models of Alzheimer's disease, where two non-transgenic models which indicate the initial stage of Alzheimer's disease and a model that shows an advanced form of that disease. So it was concluded that the oral administration of that copper chelator TDMQs is fully effective in all three models administered orally over 16 days [30, 31].

Parkinson's disease is characterized by a neurodegenerative disorder that affects the motor neurons, causing involuntarily shaking of limbs, face, and jaw and it makes simple tasks very difficult to do. It can be caused by the loss of dopamine-generating cells in a specific part of the brain which involves the regulation of motions of different parts of our body. As the increase in iron concentration is marked on different regions of the brain. In the case of Parkinson's disease, Zucca et al. [32]

suggested neuromelanins can take part in neuroprotective or harmful processes in Parkinson's disease depending on the cellular environment. Their manufacture is a protective process because it inhibits the accumulation of reactive chemicals formed from catechols, which depends on the concentration of cytosolic catechols. Synthetic neuromelanins that closely resemble the natural brain pigment in terms of melanin, protein structure, and metal concentration have been created, and these models can activate microglia [32]. Few experiments also demonstrated the use of chelation therapy is one of the best strategy to treat Parkinson's disease. As the presence of microgliosis and neuroinflammation can hamper the iron extraction from the targeted areas by chelating therapy, they demonstrated an approach in which they used an anti-inflammatory drug along with chelation therapy. This combination therapy is proven as the best strategy in the case of Parkinson's disease [33, 34, 32].

5 Micelles

Micelles are polymeric formulations consisting of both hydrophilic and lipophilic particles, with size, ranging from 10 to 1000 nm, draws the attention of researchers due to certain characteristics, such as biocompatibility, ease of use, a large variety of drug loading capacity of both hydrophilic and lipophilic drugs etc. Because of their small molecular size and both hydrophilic and lipophilic nature, they can easily cross the blood–brain barrier which makes them a potential drug-targeting strategy for numerous brain diseases. Due to the reduced size, extended circulation time in blood and stability, micelles are used to treat various brain-related diseases such as Parkinson's disease, Alzheimer's disease, glioblastoma, migraine etc. As they are formed by polymers, we can modify their shapes according to the requirements and sizes as we need to target them potentially to our desired site [35]. In 2022, a study conducted by Heng [36] in which they developed a dual-targeted drug delivery system with paclitaxel and lapatinib, where paclitaxel is an anti-neoplastic agent which is used to treat a certain types of cancers such as breast cancer and lapatinib is having an effect against human epidermal growth factor receptor-2 (HER-2) which is a prime cause of human breast cancers. As breast cancer cells can be metastasized to the brain, the targeting of drugs to the brain is very critical due to the blood–brain barrier. As the combination of these two drugs shows a synergic effect against the cancer tissues, they can be given by micelles for easily targeting the therapeutic agents in the brain [36]. Meng et al. [37] conducted an experiment in which they primarily focused on an electro-responsive polymer to target the therapeutic particles in the brain. He gave the theory that the nanoparticles such as micelles are formed by these electro-responsive or stimuli-responsive polymers, which can undergo structural changes under certain circumferences and can load a wide range of both hydrophilic and lipophilic drugs that can easily cross the BBB due to smaller size as discussed before [37]. Ferrocene, an electrosensitive group is considered should be incorporated in the polymeric micelle. It is a hydrophobic state generally, which upon activation by an oxidation potential or by an electric current, converts from a hydrophobic to a hydrophilic stage, followed by the swelling of the polymer and release of the drug [38, 39, 37]. The loaded poorly water-soluble drug lamotrigine, which is a potential drug for epilepsy, into the F127/TPGS- Ferrocene mixed micelles, which upon activation by electric potential releases the drug by undergoing alteration in particle size and then they access the potential of the system to target the drug to brain along with its in-vivo characteristics [37].

6 Gold Nanoparticles (AuNP)

In the field of nanoparticles, gold nanoparticles have drawn the attention of researchers due to the ease of preparation and flexibility of altering their shape, size and charge according to the need. Besides drug delivery, these gold nanoparticles can be utilized in certain fields such as gene delivery, photothermal and photon radiation therapy and X-ray radiation therapy etc. [40]. For the better utilization of these nanoparticles, we have to develop certain treatment and preventive strategies. Raji et al. [41] conducted research where they demonstrate various future perspectives of these gold nanoparticles in case of brain targeting [41]. The glioblastoma is a dangerous form of brain cancer which is caused by disfunction of miRNAs, which is a prime cause for tumor growth and initiation. One strategy to target these miRNAs is RNA interference, where RNA nucleotides are used to target these misfunctioning miRNAs. In this strategy there are a large number of limitations such as the poor stability of the RNAs and they can cause certain side effects by interfering with certain cellular processes, besides the crossing of these particles through BBB is another hurdle. Grafals et al. [42] stated that gold nanoparticles in the form of neosomes can be utilized for brain targeting, as they can easily cross BBB and they can hold up these RNAs and release them at the sight of action [42]. As gold nanoparticles are having antioxidant and anti-inflammatory properties, they can be used as a treatment for Alzheimer's disease. Santos Tramontin et al., in 2020 conducted an experiment in which they used gold nanoparticles to reverse the brain cell damage by Alzheimer's disease. Here they used the Alzheimer's disease model that was caused by okadaic acid. The rat models group used are Male Wistar rats, which include gold nanoparticles, okadaic acid, and gold nanoparticles + okadaic acid. Here the AuNP prevents the effects caused by okadaic acids, such as increased tau phosphorylation and spatial memory impairment [43]. Neurotrophic factors (BDNF and NGF-β) in the cortex and hippocampus were reduced by OA, but AuNPs helped maintain their normal levels. Both OA and OA + AuNP groups exhibited increased interleukin (IL)-1β levels in the hippocampus and cortex, while the AuNP group showed increased IL-1β only in the hippocampus. S100 protein levels in the cortex and hippocampus were elevated by OA, and IL-4 levels were increased in the OA + AuNP group. AuNPs mitigated oxidative stress induced by OA, as evidenced by the restoration of sulfhydryl and nitrite levels [43].

7 Quantum Dots

Quantum dots are nano-sized particles that are applied in neurodegenerative diseases as theragnostic agents. They are also called semiconductor nanocrystals having both optical and electronic properties that mainly differ from those of larger particles which mainly give the advantages like high sensitivity, stability, and selectivity when used as a nanoparticle. Also, Quantum dots have photoluminescent properties due to the dimensional quantization effect and a discrete spectrum of excitons, making them different from other bulk materials [44]. The emission band of QDs can cover a wide range of the light spectrum, from ultraviolet (UV) to infrared, allowing for optical coding and investigation of biological cell structures. They mainly stand out due to their long fluorescence lifetime and excellent anti-photobleaching performances [45]. Nowadays graphene quantum dots are coming into the spotlight because they are reported useful in Parkinson's and Alzheimer's diseases. They have the property to bypass the BBB and easily getting targeted at the interested site makes them most useful. Somehow QDs have not had any broad applications in the treatment of neurodegenerative disorders but they are the future of nanoparticles [46, 47, 48].

8 Various Nanoformulation for the Treatment of Alzheimer Disease

Alzheimer's disease (AD) is the most common cause of mental dwindling. It grows progressively year after year as the percentage of persons above the age of 60 rises. The most typical symptom in neurodegenerative diseases is difficulty in remembering, and additional symptoms include behavioural changes, problems with self-care, and bewilderment. However, no actually causes are identified. Its increase risk for the diabetes, hypertension and cardiovascular disease, there is no sufficient treatment for this disease [48]. The marketed drug only shows suggestive relief but currently many FDA approved marketed products are present to prevent symptoms of AD. These are donepezil, memantine, rivastigmine and galantamine. Alzheimer disease is marked by the presence of β-amyloid plaques and neurofibrillary tangles relaxed of hyper phosphorylated proteins [49]. It is also related with oxidative nitrative stress, mitochondrial dysfunction, endoplasmic reticulum stress, disbalance in neurotransmitter levels and neuroinflammation. Symptoms of Alzheimer was contributed by the above pathological attributes. Neuronal communication disrupts by the β-amyloid plaques and internal structure of neurons diminish by neurofibrillary tangles. Dysfunction and cellular damage lead by the endoplasmic reticulum and mitochondrial dysfunction [50].

The cause of Alzheimer disease is partially understood and blood brain barrier restrict the drug due to its efficacy, low bioavailability, poor solubility, low stability and large particle size these two are the main reason to create difficulty in the design formulation and carrying research in the recent study we discover a new therapy

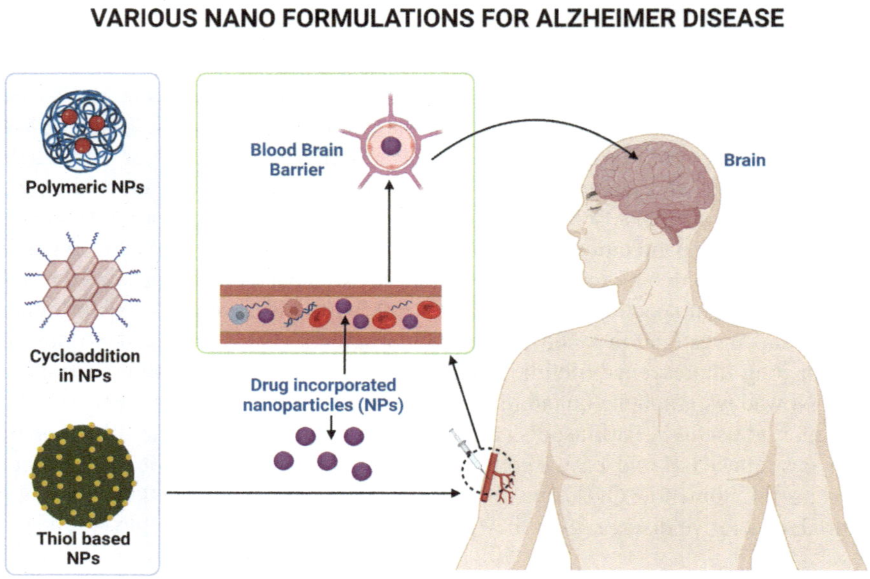

Fig. 2 Types of nanoformulations in Alzheimer disease

for the treatment of Alzheimer disease [51]. Stem cell based therapy was perceived secure, effective and creative therapeutic solution to overcome Alzheimer disease because of its several functional nature and insufficient care [52]. Present day developments in nanotechnology frequently offer chance for the delivery of active drug candidates with some limitations. Most used nanoparticle against Alzheimer are polymeric nanoparticles, lipid based and inorganic nanoparticles. Nano drug delivery are optimistic vehicle for targeting various therapeutic moieties for penetration by the CNS and improving its bioavailability and increases lipophilicity (Fig. 2).

9 Polymeric Strategies

Polymeric nanoparticles (NPs) have emerged as a promising and cutting-edge strategy for delivering therapeutic drugs to the brains of Alzheimer's disease (AD) patients. These NPs provide a novel and safe tool to enhance the efficacy of pharmaceuticals by improving their pharmacokinetics and bio distribution. They are composed of block co-polymers, which can be derived from natural sources like albumin and polysaccharides, as well as synthetic materials that are biocompatible, biodegradable, and easily excretable [53, 54]. The selection of polymers plays a crucial role in the synthesis of NPs. Common choices include chitosan, albumin, PLGA, and others. The internal structures of these macromolecules can form three-dimensional nano networks through covalent crosslinking or by reacting with other polymers, resulting in either one-polymer-based NPs or heterogeneous NPs. Additionally, the chemical groups within the polymers can be modified to incorporate diverse functional groups or allow for targeted drug release [53].

Polymeric NPs offer versatility in drug delivery. They can entrap drug payloads through chemical reactions or steric hindrance, enabling the controlled release of therapeutics. By functionalizing the NPs with targeting biomolecules, such as proteins or nucleic acids, specific brain areas or cell types can be selectively reached. This targeted delivery approach holds great potential for improving the effectiveness of AD treatments [55, 56]. In addition, polymeric nanoparticles (NPs) can be further modified by conjugating various ligands to their surface, aiming to facilitate their entry through the blood–brain barrier (BBB) [57].

Macromolecular drug-encapsulating nanoparticles (NPs) can be efficiently delivered to the AD brain by conjugating them with cationic oligoes, proteins, or cell-penetrating peptides. This surface modification allows electrostatic interaction with the negatively charged endothelial cells of the brain's capillaries [53]. Orthogonal chemistry, which enables selective conjugation between complementary functional groups, is widely used in NP design to achieve controlled drug delivery. Various techniques, such as cycloaddition reactions, thiol-based chemistry, coupling reactions, and imine chemistry, are employed for polymer functionalization and chemo selective grafting [58]. Additionally, the polymer backbone itself can serve as a therapeutic agent in AD [59]. For example, sialic acid-modified selenium nanoparticles (SeNPs) conjugated with B6 peptide demonstrated high blood–brain barrier permeability and the ability to inhibit amyloid-beta (Aβ) aggregation. Selenium is known for its antioxidant properties and has shown protection against cognitive decline in animal models. Other examples include the use of nanoparticles functionalized with biphenyl ethers for amyloid fibril disruption and polyphenol-based nanostructures for stimuli-responsive drug delivery. These advancements in NP technology hold promise for targeted and effective drug delivery in AD treatment [60, 53, 61].

10 Cycloaddition Reaction

Copper-catalyzed azide-alkyne cycloaddition (CuAAC), strain-promoted azide-alkyne cycloaddition (SPAAC), and nitrile oxide-alkyne cycloaddition (NOAC) are widely used click chemistry approaches for the synthesis of bio hybrid scaffolds and functionalized polymer nanoparticles. These reactions offer several advantages, including simple reaction conditions, high yields, and compatibility with various functional groups. CuAAC and SPAAC are commonly employed for functionalization with azide and alkyne groups, resulting in the formation of stable triazole linkages [62]. CuAAC utilizes copper catalysts to enhance reaction rates and regioselectivity, while SPAAC is a metal-free alternative with slower kinetics. NOAC, on the other hand, forms hydrolytically stable is oxazole linkages through interactions between reactive dipoles and alkyne motifs. These click chemistry methods enable the conjugation of biomolecules such as proteins, peptides, carbohydrates, and fatty acids to generate bio hybrid scaffolds with improved properties [63, 62, 64].

In the context of neurological disorders, click chemistry has been applied to develop neuroactive candidates for the central nervous system (CNS). For instance, polyglutamic acid (PGA) has been functionalized with azide and alkyne units, leading to the formation of a neuroprotective nanostructure through CuAAC-mediated crosslinking. Similarly, CuAAC has been used to decorate nanoparticles with specific ligands for targeting proteins associated with pathological conditions in the brain. The functionalization of nanocarriers with anti-Aβ1–42 antibody via CuAAC has shown promising results in inhibiting aggregation and rescuing toxicity in therapies against Alzheimer's disease. Furthermore, click chemistry has been utilized to functionalize polymer nanoparticles with sialic acid mimetics, which exhibit a high affinity for counteracting amyloid-beta protein deposition and plaque formation, potentially slowing down the progression of Alzheimer's disease [65, 53].

Overall, click chemistry provides a versatile and efficient tool for the synthesis of biohybrid scaffolds and functionalized nanoparticles, enabling targeted drug delivery and therapeutic interventions in neurological disorders [66].

11 Thiol Based Chemistry

Thiol groups provide another functional moiety essential for polymer-biomolecule pairing. Thiols reactivity with carbon–carbon double bonds by radical and light-mediated mechanisms enables NP functionalization, combining the benefits of click chemistry with the control given by photoinitiated reactions [67]. Thiol-based chemistry has high reaction rates, quantitative yields, good reaction conditions (such as room temperature and aqueous solutions), and simple purification methods. Free radical thiol-alkene and thiol-alkyne effects, nucleophilic Michael addition, and isulphide transfer are all important reactions [68, 67].

Crosslinking between thiol groups found in peptides and proteins as well as maleimide-modified polymers is a typical synthetic technique used in controlled drug delivery and selective targeting. For example, to facilitate nose-to-brain drug administration of neuroprotective peptides, researchers grafted thiolated lactoferrin, a natural iron-binding protein, onto PEG-PCL copolymers bearing maleimide units [69]. In a further study, the thiol-maleimide reaction was used to conjugate the peptide cRGDfK and the Nanobody 11A4, both of which contain a free thiol group, to maleimide-functionalized PLGA NPs [53]. This enabled the tailoring of NP cellular internalisation by cell surface receptor targeting. For intracellular delivery of curcumin, PLGA nanocarriers containing PEG and GSH are proposed, improving neuronal absorption and changing the NP internalisation route, increasing therapeutic possibilities for Alzheimer's disease therapy [53, 69].

Overall, thiol-based chemistry provides a versatile strategy for NP functionalization, enabling targeted drug delivery and enhancing the therapeutic efficacy of nanoparticles in various biomedical applications.

12 Parkinson Disease

Parkinson's disease (PD) is characterized by the progressive loss of dopaminergic neurons, leading to neurodegeneration. Researchers have explored the use of nanoparticles (NPs) to restore dopamine levels and protect against further damage. Chitosan NPs encapsulating dopamine and conducted in vitro and in vivo experiments. The NPs efficiently loaded and released dopamine, resulting in increased dopamine concentrations in the striatum and successful transport across the blood–brain barrier (BBB) in rat models [70]. Notably, the chitosan NPs exhibited a prompt and pulsatile release profile, which was considered more advantageous than the sustained release observed with cellulose acetate phthalate (CAP) NPs. Moreover, chitosan demonstrated the ability to improve the uptake of hydrophilic drugs into the brain by opening tight junctions in BBB endothelial cells. These findings highlight the potential of chitosan NPs as promising carriers for dopamine delivery, offering neuroprotection and enhanced drug penetration in PD treatment [71, 72, 70].

Polymers are highly versatile materials that surpass metals and ceramics in terms of versatility. However, non-degradable particles such as fullerenes, metal particles, quantum dots, carbon nanotubes, and silica nanoparticles have been less utilized in various applications. The materials commonly employed in the production of nanoparticles (NPs) include: [73–79].

(i) Poly (lactic-co-glycolic acid) (PLGA): NPs made from PLGA can have different compositions, which determine their biodegradation rate.
(ii) Poly (lactic acid): This polymer is also used for NP fabrication.
(iii) Poly n-butyl cyanoacrylate (PBCA): PBCA is known for its high degradation rate among polymers.
(iv) Poly (ε-caprolactone): Although not extensively used, this low-cost polymer is easy to handle.
(v) Human serum albumin: NPs made from this protein offer certain advantages.
(vi) Chitosan: Chitosan can be used in NP production through the ionic gelation method, which does not require organic solvents. This is particularly advantageous when incorporating peptides or proteins.

13 Protein Nanoparticles

Anand K Kondapi et al., Proteins are important in biological systems for signalling, transport, and stimulation. Bovine serum albumin (BSA) has been used as a delivery vehicle, and protein denaturation/folding techniques have been employed for preparing nano/microparticles for drug delivery [80]. Maintaining the native conformation of proteins is crucial for their biological activities. The hydrophobic environment provided by oils can protect proteins and induce multimerization, leading to the formation of nanosized particles when controlled by sonication and freezing. Proteins have complex surfaces with hydrophobic, hydrophilic, and charged groups. Bioactive molecules can interact with proteins at their surfaces, forming weak complexes, which, when exposed to oils, can result in the encapsulation of the bioactive molecules within protein particles. The size of these particles can be controlled through sonication and freezing techniques [80, 81]. To avoid the BBB's different transport protein's efflux mechanism, trans-activating transcriptor (TAT) conjugation made sure that BBB absorption was mediated by transport mechanisms other than transcytosis. Protein-based nanoparticles have been successfully formed using techniques, including salt precipitation (salting out), emulsion solvent extraction, coacervation or desolvation, polyelectrolyte complexation, and electrospraying. These techniques typically produce protein nanoparticles between the diameters of 100 and 1000 nm, while techniques that produce particles smaller than 100 nm are far less prevalent [82]. It is frequently necessary to chemically alter protein nanoparticles during or after synthesis to increase the stability and slower down the rate of degradation that can be accomplished by adding a natural or synthetic crosslinkers [83].

14 Lactoferin Based Targeted Delivery System

Lactoferrin receptors are highly expressed in gliomas (a type of brain tumour), and lactoferrin itself has an affinity for capillary endothelial cells in the blood–brain barrier (BBB). These characteristics enable lactoferrin to localize in the brain through a process called transcytosis. Due to these properties, lactoferrin is considered an appealing target-specific ligand for conjugation in brain cancer research studies [84].

Bioconjugated lactoferrin and iron oxide nanoparticles have shown considerable effects on glioma cells. Iron oxide nanoparticles were prepared by paralyzing an iron oleate precursor in the presence of an oleic acid surfactant. This pyrolysis process resulted in the formation of iron oxide nanoparticles. To facilitate the conjugation of lactoferrin, the iron oxide nanoparticles were activated using N-(3-dimethyl aminopropyl)-N-ethyl carbodiimide hydrochloride (EDC) and N-hydroxysulfosuccinimide. These reagents are commonly used to activate nanoparticles for subsequent bioconjugation. Lactoferrin, a protein with high affinity for lactoferrin receptors found in gliomas and capillary endothelial cells in the blood–brain barrier (BBB), was conjugated to the activated iron oxide nanoparticles. In C6 glioma cells, the Lf-coupled iron oxide nanoparticles displayed substantial localisation. The significant localization observed indicates that the nanoparticles successfully targeted and interacted with the glioma cells. This conjugation process involves the specific binding of lactoferrin to the surface of the nanoparticles [85, 86]. Lactoferrin and Lower Generation PAMAM Dendrimers conjugation was investigated and assessed in vitro and in vivo in the disease-induced mice model for the effect on behavioural responses. The result have shown the behavioural responses in the in vivo investigation of $AlCl_3$-induced Alzheimer's (AD) mice were significantly improved [87]. Oral administration of Lactoferrin-heparin (Lf-Hp) conjugated formulation to glioblastoma multiforme orthotopic mice observed better interaction with the lactoferrin receptor (Lf-R) expressed on the intestine. After being orally supplied, Lf-Hp was precisely delivered to the brain tumour by receptor Lf-R that resulted a good oral therapy in the treatment of glioblastoma [84].

15 Liposomes

15.1 Film Hydration Techniques

The passage outlines a technique known as film hydration, which is employed for the preparation of liposomes. Liposomes are lipid-based vesicles that can encapsulate various substances and have applications in drug delivery systems. In this specific method, liposomes are prepared using a combination of lipids, including DOPE, DOTAP, CPP-conjugated PEGylated DSPE, MAN-conjugated PEGylated DSPE, and cholesterol, in a precise molar ratio [88]. The process begins by dissolving these lipids in a solution of methanol and chloroform, followed by evaporation using a rotary evaporator, resulting in the formation of a uniform lipid film. Chitosan and ApoE2 pDNA are then complexed electrostatically and added to a hydration buffer containing HEPES at a specific pH. This complex is subsequently added to the lipid film, and the mixture is sonicated using a bath sonicator to create small unilamellar vesicles [88, 89]. The size and surface charge of the liposomes can be measured using dynamic light scattering, which provides information about their distribution and properties. The entrapment efficiency of pApoE2, a plasmid DNA, is determined using Hoechst 33,342 fluorescent dye. Additionally, the surface morphology of the liposomes is examined using atomic force microscopy, which allows for high-resolution imaging of the liposome surface [88, 89].

15.2 Liposomal Approaches for Alzheimer Disease

Sureshbabu Ram Kumar Pandian et al., Alzheimer's disease (AD) is a debilitating and progressive neurological disorder that is expected to impact a staggering 115 million people worldwide by 2050. It is characterized by the accumulation of misfolded proteins, particularly β-amyloid and tau, resulting in the formation of plaques in the brain. Despite being discovered a century ago, currently approved drugs for AD only provide temporary relief for symptoms, with no available preventive or long-term solutions [90].

Researchers have been striving to develop more effective treatments by targeting the underlying mechanisms of AD. Studies have indicated that reducing the levels of Aβ protein, which plays a significant role in the progression of AD, could be beneficial. Another crucial factor associated with AD is apolipoprotein E (ApoE), which influences Aβ levels and amyloid burden [91]. To deliver therapeutic agents with precision, liposomes have emerged as a promising tool. Liposomes are tiny vesicles capable of encapsulating drugs or genetic material. Chitosan, a biocompatible polysaccharide, is utilized to protect the genetic material, such as plasmid-encoded ApoE2 (pApoE2), from degradation. Furthermore, the surface of liposomes can be modified with molecules like mannose and rabies virus peptide to facilitate their passage across the blood–brain barrier (BBB) and target specific receptors [92, 90].

Exciting advancements have been made with bi-functionalized liposomes, demonstrating their potential to reduce amyloid burden and enhance memory in animal models of AD. Other strategies involve utilizing liposomes loaded with glutathione or imatinib mesylate for targeted delivery to the brain. These approaches aim to improve the delivery and retention of therapeutic agents specifically in affected brain regions [93, 94].

15.3 Liposomal Approaches for Parkinson Disease

Parkinson's disease (PD) is characterized by the aggregation of α-Synuclein protein and the formation of irregular protein clusters in the brain [95]. Key features of PD include the selective loss of dopaminergic neurons and neuroinflammation in the substantia nigra. Existing treatments for PD do not effectively slow down disease progression, although levodopa (L-dopa) is commonly used to restore dopamine levels in the brain. Research suggests that nanomaterials can interact with α-Synuclein to inhibit fibril formation [95, 96].

A novel approach for central nervous system (CNS) gene delivery involves the use of a microbubble (MB) liposomal complex combined with ultrasound-targeted microbubble destruction (UTMD) to trigger blood–brain barrier (BBB) opening. This complex, consisting of clinically approved MB formulations and neurotrophic factor (NF)-loaded PEGylated liposomes, enables the delivery of various genes across the BBB. NFs, such as glia cell-derived neurotrophic factors (GDNF) and brain-derived neurotrophic factors (BDNF), have shown potential in reducing neuronal loss and protecting dopaminergic neurons. Studies have demonstrated that GDNF or BDNF gene carriers can improve behavioral symptoms and provide neuroprotection in animal models of PD [97, 98].

15.4 Dual Targeting Liposomal Drug Delivery

Dual-targeted liposomes, which have ligands on their surface, offer advantages in targeted drug delivery. They can simultaneously target multiple receptors, transport multiple drugs, and provide synergistic effects while reducing toxicity. Ligands improve liposome delivery to specific cells or structures for active targeting. Immunoliposomes, a type of dual-targeted liposomes, incorporate ligands or antibodies that bind to rapidly internalizing receptors. This allows efficient internalization and intra-cellular drug release [99]. Immunoliposomes have demonstrated reduced cellular cytotoxicity compared to traditional liposomes. They hold promise for enhancing drug delivery and therapeutic outcomes. The use of dual-targeted liposomes has led to the approval of liposomal medicines for autoimmune diseases and malignancies. By incorporating ligands, liposomes can actively target tumor cells or other structures. Additionally, stimuli-responsive liposomes, such as pH-sensitive liposomes, can enhance the internalization and release of drugs. The field of dual-targeted liposomes and immunoliposomes shows great potential for targeted and safer drug delivery in various diseases [100, 101].

16 Lipid Nanoparticles

16.1 Nanostructure Lipid Carrier

Yoon et al., solid lipid nanoparticles (SLNs) and nanostructured lipid carriers (NLCs), in particular, have been created as revolutionary drug delivery platforms using lipid-based Nanoparticulate systems. Lipids are the main component used in these systems to encapsulate and distribute medications to specific organ targets [102]. Solid lipid inclusion in SLNs and NLCs offers stability, regulated drug release, and enhanced therapeutic effect due to stable nanoparticles and solid state at body temperature. SLNs, created by substituting solid lipids in oil-in-water emulsions, maintain their solid state at body temperature. NLCs, a mixture of solid and liquid lipids, are the second generation of lipid nanoparticles, maintaining their solid form despite the presence of liquid lipids [103]. Particularly, NLCs show considerable advantages. The mixture of solid and liquid lipids in NLCs lowers the melting point of the core substance, enabling the inclusion of a wider variety of drugs. When compared to SLNs and other Nanocarrier systems, this characteristic improves the encapsulation efficiency of NLCs. Higher drug loading efficiency in NLCs is also a result of the solid lipid's incorrect arrangement inside the liquid lipid. NLCs' features depend on lipid blend and production technique, with liquid and solid lipids like olive oil, sesame oil, and soy lecithin and Surfactants, like Poloxamer 188, Tween® 80, and SDS, aiding in nanoparticle synthesis and stabilization [104, 105].

17 Limitations

Due to difficulties in technique development and scale-up, the clinical use of nanostructured lipid carriers as targeted drug carriers is restricted. Wide-range replication of effective outcomes is still challenging. Delivery of delicate biomolecules needs careful optimisation. There may be issues with sensitivity, irritability, or cytotoxicity depending on the kind and quantity of surfactants employed [106, 107].

18 Different Method

18.1 Fabrication Method

Unique lipid nanocarrier systems called nanostructured lipid carriers are made up of a combination of solid and liquid lipids that are stabilised by an appropriate surfactant and used excipients and the ratio of solid to liquid lipids in NLCs can range from 30:70 to 0.1:99.90 for the types of lipids, respectively [108, 109]. In general, the quantity of surfactant depends on the kind of lipid desired NLC qualities, and medication load. For NLC development, multiple types of fabrication methods are used, with high-pressure homogenization being the most well-known and widely used. It is common to use this method to create solid lipid nanoparticles, microemulsions, and other lipid drug carriers in the pharmaceutical industry. In addition, several different techniques are used to fabricate NLC [110, 111].

18.2 Hot Pressure Homogenization

To create lipid nanocarrier systems, high-pressure homogenization (HPH) is a frequently used technique. The drug, lipid, and aqueous phases must be homogenised by applying high shear and pressure. Due to its cheap production costs, simplicity in handling, and appropriateness for mass manufacturing of different lipid Nanocarrier systems, HPH is preferred [111]. Additionally, HPH is an environmentally non-cancerous process since it can be carried out without the use of organic solvents. To decrease particle size to the submicron or nanoregion, HPH uses high pressures of 100 to 2000 bars coupled with significant shear stress. HPH may be divided into two categories based on the temperature used during the nanoparticle formation process [112, 113].

18.3 Hot Homogenization

In this method, the process temperature is kept above the lipid's melting point. A hot pre-emulsion is created when the drug and lipid mixture is homogenised with the aqueous surfactant phase while being subjected to high shear stress and extreme temperature. A Nanoemulsion is then created by further homogenising the pre-emulsion at high pressure and temperature. Then goes through recrystallization to create nanostructured lipid carriers (NLCs), which are then used in various applications [111]. Although this procedure is simple and inexpensive, the high temperature used in the process may restrict its compatibility with thermosensitive active or bioactive substances. However, some heat-sensitive chemicals may degrade or lose their therapeutic action [114, 111].

18.4 *Cold Homogenization*

A drug and lipid combination is milled and solidified using liquid nitrogen (−196 °C) or dry ice and liquid helium before being homogenised using the cold high-pressure homogenization process. After that, the frozen mix is blended with a cold surfactant phase. The drug-lipid combination is next dispersed in the cold surfactant and subjected to high-pressure homogenization at low temperatures. This method produces nanostructured lipid carriers [115, 111]. Because of the low-temperature settings used, this approach is particularly beneficial for delivering heat-sensitive active molecules, proteins, and peptides.

19 Microemulsification

A lipid phase is formed in this process by combining active substance, fused solid lipid, and liquid lipid. At the same temperature and with steady stirring, this lipid phase is mixed with an aqueous phase containing surfactant and co-surfactant. This method produces a transparent and thermodynamically stable microemulsion [116]. To make a Nanoemulsion, a heated microemulsion is continually stirred with a cool aqueous phase. This causes the mixture to recrystallize, resulting in the creation of nanostructured lipid carriers (NLC). Although the micro emulsification technology allows for large-scale production, the greater surfactant concentration may restrict its commercial applicability [116].

19.1 *Solvent Emulsification Evaporation*

Initial solubilisation of the lipid content and lipophilic compound dissolved in an organic solvent like ethanol, methanol, etc. This organic phase is then emulsified with an aqueous phase that contains surfactant and co-surfactant using a homogenizer [117]. Furthermore, the organic solvent is evaporated at room temperature and leaving the solid by-product behind. This approach uses a microfluidizer to reduce the particle size without using heat. As a result, Using organic solvents for thermolabile compounds may cause unfavourable effects [118].

19.2 Solvent Diffusion

To distribute the active compound and lipid components, a water-immiscible or slightly miscible organic solvent is used and saturated with the aqueous phase to maintain thermodynamic equilibrium. The resultant oil-in-water emulsion is then injected into a unit of water while mixing continuously, causing the dispersed phase to solidify then nanoparticles are collected and dried. This method enables the creation of stable lipid nanoparticles [119, 120]. It is crucial to note, however, this approach is dependent on the selection of an adequate organic solvent and careful removal to minimise any potential residual solvent effects.

19.3 Emulsification Sonication

The emulsification sonication method is similar to the HPH approach, which uses high shear pressures to produce Nanoemulsions. The main distinction is the use of ultrasonication to transform the pre-emulsion into nanostructured lipid carriers (NLC) [121]. However, it is critical to use caution while using a probe sonicator to avoid metallic contamination. To secure the desired outputs and avoid any unfavourable impacts, proper care and attention should be given during the preparation phase [122, 123].

20 Conclusion

In the complex realm, the neurodegenerative disorders, such as Alzheimer's, Parkinson's, and brain cancers, healthcare confronts formidable challenges. A significant barrier to effective treatment lies in the blood–brain barrier (BBB). Overcoming this obstacle demands innovative solutions, and nanotechnology has emerged as a beacon of hope, offering novel strategies to counter these challenges and revolutionize neurological disease management.

Among diverse nanoparticles under investigation, including polymeric nanoparticles, micelles, and gold nanoparticles, a promising avenue emerges for circumventing the BBB and precisely delivering treatments to affected brain regions. These nanoparticles serve as carriers, encapsulating drugs and genes with precision and efficiency. The small size and versatile properties of nanotechnology hold transformative potential in reshaping our approach to brain diseases. Metal imbalances play a pivotal role in neurodegenerative disorders, and metal chelators offer a potential therapeutic strategy for conditions like Alzheimer's and Parkinson's. Chelation therapy, employing these agents, presents a viable approach to mitigate disease progression by targeting root causes. The interplay between metal homeostasis and neurodegeneration provides a compelling avenue for intervention, instilling new optimism among patients and healthcare practitioners.

Collaboration stands as a linchpin of progress in this domain. The convergence of expertise from researchers, clinicians, and engineers is paramount to refining and ushering these innovative approaches into reality. With the ageing global population intensifying the burden of neurological diseases, the urgency to find effective solutions has never been more pronounced. With its remarkable capacity to navigate barriers and precisely deliver therapies, nanotechnology assumes heightened significance. The ongoing research endeavours hold substantial promise. Quantum dots (QDs), semiconductor nanocrystals with unique properties, offer neuroimaging and drug delivery avenues. Their distinct photoluminescence properties span applications from optical coding to cellular exploration, showcasing the multifaceted contributions of nanotechnology to neuroscience.

As focus sharpens on Alzheimer's disease, the urgency for breakthroughs becomes palpable. Polymeric nanoparticles, with their versatility and biocompatibility, emerge as prominent contenders for brain drug delivery. Functionalization of these nanoparticles with ligands like proteins, peptides, and nucleic acids enhances their BBB-crossing ability and targeted drug release. Click chemistry techniques, including copper-catalyzed azide-alkyne cycloaddition (CuAAC) and thiol-based chemistry, play pivotal roles in nanoparticle functionalization, enabling controlled drug delivery and tailored therapeutic interventions. Parkinson's disease, marked by dopamine deficiency, finds a potential ally in chitosan nanoparticles, offering avenues for neuroprotection and enhanced drug penetration through the BBB. Additionally, protein-based nanoparticles, leveraging ligands such as lactoferrin, exhibit promise for precise brain cancer interventions, capitalizing on their affinity for glioma cells and BBB endothelial cells.

While scientific strides are inspiring, a crucial bridge must connect laboratory discoveries to clinical applications. The translation of these innovative nano formulations into effective neurodegenerative disorder treatments hinges on collaborative efforts spanning nanotechnology, neuroscience, and medicine. This convergence holds the power to propel breakthroughs from concept to tangible improvements, paving the way for a transformed landscape of neurological disease management, enriched outcomes, and renewed quality of life for individuals grappling with these daunting conditions.

References

1. Waris A, Ali A, Khan AU, Asim M, Zamel D, Fatima K, Raziq A, Khan MA, Akbar N, Baset A, Abourehab MA (2022) Applications of various types of nanomaterials for the treatment of neurological disorders. Nanomaterials 12(13):2140
2. Kadry H, Noorani B, Cucullo L (2020) A blood–brain barrier overview on structure, function, impairment, and biomarkers of integrity. Fluids Barriers CNS 17(1):1–24

3. Feigin VL, Vos T, Nichols E, Owolabi MO, Carroll WM, Dichgans M, Deuschl G, Parmar P, Brainin M, Murray C (2020) The global burden of neurological disorders: translating evidence into policy. The Lancet Neurol 19(3):255–265
4. Dorsey ER, Glidden AM, Holloway MR, Birbeck GL, Schwamm LH (2018) Teleneurology and mobile technologies: the future of neurological care. Nat Rev Neurol 14(5):285–297
5. Guidance D (2011) Guidance for industry considering whether an FDA-regulated product involves the application of nanotechnology. Biotechnol Law Rep 30(5):613–616
6. Nguyen TT, Nguyen-Thi PT, Nguyen TH, Ho TT, Tran NM, Van Vo T, Van Vo G (2023) Recent advancements in nanomaterials: a promising way to manage neurodegenerative disorders. Mol Diagn Ther:1–17
7. Siddiqi KS, Husen A, Sohrab SS, Yassin MO (2018) Recent status of nanomaterial fabrication and their potential applications in neurological disease management. Nanoscale Res Lett 13:1–17
8. Bhushan B (2017) Introduction to nanotechnology. Springer Handbook of Nanotechnology, pp 1–19
9. Silva GA (2006) Neuroscience nanotechnology: progress, opportunities and challenges. Nat Rev Neurosci 7(1):65–74
10. Bhatia S, Bhatia S (2016) Nanoparticles types, classification, characterization, fabrication methods and drug delivery applications. Nat Polymer Drug Deliv Syst Nanopart Plants Algae:33–93
11. Kumar R, Aadil KR, Ranjan S, Kumar VB (2020) Advances in nanotechnology and nanomaterials based strategies for neural tissue engineering. J Drug Deliv Sci Technol 57:101617
12. Shete MB, Patil TS, Deshpande AS, Saraogi G, Vasdev N, Deshpande M, Rajpoot K, Tekade RK (2022) Current trends in theranostic nanomedicines. J Drug Deliv Sci Technol 71:103280
13. Kaiafa G, Savopoulos C, Kanellos I, Mylonas KS, Tsikalakis G, Tegos T, Kakaletsis N, Hatzitolios AI (2017) Anemia and stroke: where do we stand? Acta Neurol Scand 135(6):596–602
14. Dumurgier J, Tzourio C (2020) Epidemiology of neurological diseases in older adults. Revue Neurol 176(9):642–648
15. Abbott NJ (2013) Blood–brain barrier structure and function and the challenges for CNS drug delivery. J Inherit Metab Dis 36:437–449
16. Golpich M, Amini E, Mohamed Z, Azman Ali R, Mohamed Ibrahim N, Ahmadiani A (2017) Mitochondrial dysfunction and biogenesis in neurodegenerative diseases: pathogenesis and treatment. CNS Neurosci Ther 23(1):5–22
17. Stanimirovic DB, Sandhu JK, Costain WJ (2018) Emerging technologies for delivery of biotherapeutics and gene therapy across the blood–brain barrier. BioDrugs 32(6):547–559
18. Lo Furno D, Mannino G, Giuffrida R (2018) Functional role of mesenchymal stem cells in the treatment of chronic neurodegenerative diseases. J Cell Physiol 233(5):3982–3999
19. Galluzzi L, Bravo-San Pedro JM, Blomgren K, Kroemer G (2016) Autophagy in acute brain injury. Nat Rev Neurosci 17(8):467–484
20. Marklund N, Bellander BM, Godbolt AK, Levin H, McCrory P, Thelin EP (2019) Treatments and rehabilitation in the acute and chronic state of traumatic brain injury. J Intern Med 285(6):608–623
21. Vannucci SJ, Hagberg H (2004) Hypoxia–ischemia in the immature brain. J Exp Biol 207(18):3149–3154
22. Chipurupalli S, Ganesan R, Martini G, Mele L, Reggio A, Esposito M, Kannan E, Namasivayam V, Grumati P, Desiderio V, Robinson N (2022) Cancer cells adapt FAM134B/BiP mediated ER-phagy to survive hypoxic stress. Cell Death Dis 13(4):357
23. Singh L, Nair L, Kumar D, Arora MK, Bajaj S, Gadewar M, Mishra SS, Rath SK, Dubey AK, Kaithwas G, Choudhary M (2023) Hypoxia induced lactate acidosis modulates tumor microenvironment and lipid reprogramming to sustain the cancer cell survival. Front Oncol 13:1034205

24. Booth TC, Thompson G, Bulbeck H, Boele F, Buckley C, Cardoso J, Dos Santos Canas L, Jenkinson D, Ashkan K, Kreindler J, Huskens N (2021) A position statement on the utility of interval imaging in standard of care brain tumour management: defining the evidence gap and opportunities for future research. Front Oncol 11:620070
25. D'Asti E, Chennakrishnaiah S, Lee TH, Rak J (2016) Extracellular vesicles in brain tumor progression. Cell Mol Neurobiol 36:383–407
26. Manek E, Petroianu GA (2021) Brain delivery of antidotes by polymeric nanoparticles. J Appl Toxicol 41(1):20–32
27. Kontoghiorghes GJ (2020) Advances on chelation and chelator metal complexes in medicine. Int J Mol Sci (MDPI)21:2499
28. Crichton RR, Ward RJ, Hider RC (2016) Metal chelation in medicine. Royal Society of Chemistry
29. Chand K, Candeias E, Cardoso SM, Chaves S, Santos MA (2018) Tacrine–deferiprone hybrids as multi-target-directed metal chelators against Alzheimer's disease: a two-in-one drug. Metallomics 10(10):1460–1475
30. Huang L, Zeng Y, Li Y, Zhu Y, He Y, Liu Y, Robert A, Meunier B (2022) Distribution in rat blood and brain of TDMQ20, a copper chelator designed as a drug-candidate for Alzheimer's Disease. Pharmaceutics 14(12):2691
31. Zhao J, Shi Q, Tian H, Li Y, Liu Y, Xu Z, Robert A, Liu Q, Meunier B (2020) TDMQ20, a specific copper chelator, reduces memory impairments in Alzheimer's disease mouse models. ACS ChemNeurosci 12(1):140–149
32. Zucca FA, Capucciati A, Bellei C, Sarna M, Sarna T, Monzani E, Casella L, Zecca L (2023) Neuromelanins in brain aging and Parkinson's disease: synthesis, structure, neuroinflammatory, and neurodegenerative role. IUBMB Life 75(1):55–65
33. Andersen HH, Johnsen KB, Moos T (2014) Iron deposits in the chronically inflamed central nervous system and contributes to neurodegeneration. Cell Mol Life Sci 71:1607–1622
34. Ward RJ, Dexter DT, Martin-Bastida A, Crichton RR (2021) Is chelation therapy a potential treatment for Parkinson's disease? Int J Mol Sci 22(7):3338
35. Kanoujia J, Kishore A, Parashar P (2023) Progress in polymeric micelles as viable wagons for brain targeting. Curr Pharm Des 29(2):116–125
36. Lu H, Chen T, Wang Y, He Y, Pang Z, Wang Y (2022) Dual targeting micelles loaded with paclitaxel and lapatinib for combinational therapy of brain metastases from breast cancer. Sci Rep 12(1):2610
37. Meng XY, Li JJ, Ni TJ, Xiao-tong L, He T, Men ZN, Liu JS, Shen T (2020) Electro-responsive brain-targeting mixed micelles based on Pluronic F127 and d-α-tocopherol polyethylene glycol succinate–ferrocene. Colloids Surf A: Physicochem Eng Aspects 601:124986
38. Kondapaneni LP, Bobde Y, Ghosh B (2022) Exogenous stimuli–responsive polymeric micelles for drug delivery. In: Polymeric micelles for drug delivery. Elsevier, pp 409–428
39. Li JJ, Meng XY, Men ZN, Chen X, Shen T, Liu JS (2022) Electric and reactive oxygen species dual-responsive polymeric micelles improve the therapeutic efficacy of lamotrigine in pentylenetetrazole kindling rats. Colloids Surf A Physicochem Eng Aspects 642:128628
40. Hu X, Zhang Y, Ding T, Liu J, Zhao H (2020) Multifunctional gold nanoparticles: a novel nanomaterial for various medical applications and biological activities. Front Bioeng Biotechnol 8:990
41. Raji V, Pal K, Zaheer T, Kalarikkal N, Sabu T, de Souza FG, Asiya SI (2020) Gold nanoparticles against respiratory diseases: oncogenic and viral pathogens review. Ther Deliv 11(8): 521
42. Grafals-Ruiz N, Rios-Vicil CI, Lozada-Delgado EL, Quiñones-Díaz BI, Noriega-Rivera RA, Martínez-Zayas G, Santana-Rivera Y, Santiago-Sánchez GS, Valiyeva F, Vivas-Mejía PE (2020) Brain targeted gold liposomes improve rnai delivery for glioblastoma. Int J Nanomed:2809–2828
43. dos Santos Tramontin N, da Silva S, Arruda R, Ugioni KS, Canteiro PB, de Bem Silveira G, Mendes C, Silveira PC, Muller AP (2020) Gold nanoparticles treatment reverses brain damage in Alzheimer's disease model. Mol Neurobiol 57:926–936

44. Singh A, Mallika TN, Gorain B, Yadav AK, Tiwari S, Flora SJ, Shukla R, Kesharwani P (2021) Quantum dot: Heralding a brighter future in neurodegenerative disorders. J Drug Deliv Sci Technol 65:102700
45. Pleskova S, Mikheeva E, Gornostaeva E (2018) Using of quantum dots in biology and medicine. Cell Mol Toxicol Nanopart:323–334
46. Duwa R, Jeong JH, Yook S (2021) Development of immunotherapy and nanoparticles-based strategies for the treatment of Parkinson's disease. J Pharm Investig 51:465–481
47. Kumar A, Sudevan ST, Nair AS, Singh AK, Kumar S, Jose J, Behl T, Mangalathillam S, Mathew B, Kim H (2023) Current and future nano-carrier-based approaches in the treatment of Alzheimer's disease. Brain Sci 13(2):213
48. Pool J (2018) Reducing the symptoms of Alzheimer's Disease and other dementias: a guide to personal cognitive rehabilitation techniques. Jessica Kingsley Publishers
49. Hansen RA, Gartlehner G, Webb AP, Morgan LC, Moore CG, Jonas DE (2008) Efficacy and safety of donepezil, galantamine, and rivastigmine for the treatment of Alzheimer's disease: a systematic review and meta-analysis. ClinInterv Aging 3(2):211–225
50. Bhatt S, Puli L, Patil CR (2021) Role of reactive oxygen species in the progression of Alzheimer's disease. Drug Discov Today 26(3):794–803
51. Martinelli C, Pucci C, Battaglini M, Marino A, Ciofani G (2020) Antioxidants and nanotechnology: promises and limits of potentially disruptive approaches in the treatment of central nervous system diseases. Adv Healthcare Mater 9(3):1901589
52. Agrawal M, Prathyusha E, Ahmed H, Dubey SK, Kesharwani P, Singhvi G, Naidu VG, Alexander A (2021) Biomaterials in treatment of Alzheimer's disease. Neurochem Int 145:105008
53. La Barbera L, Mauri E, D'Amelio M, Gori M (2022) Functionalization strategies of polymeric nanoparticles for drug delivery in Alzheimer's disease: current trends and future perspectives. Front Neurosci 16:939855
54. Sharma M, Dube T, Chibh S, Kour A, Mishra J, Panda JJ (2019) Nanotheranostics, a future remedy of neurological disorders. Expert Opin Drug Deliv 16(2):113–128
55. Ekladious I, Colson YL, Grinstaff MW (2019) Polymer–drug conjugate therapeutics: advances, insights and prospects. Nat Rev Drug Discov 18(4):273–294
56. Elsabahy M, Wooley KL (2012) Design of polymeric nanoparticles for biomedical delivery applications. Chem Soc Rev 41(7):2545–2561
57. Tosi G, Bortot B, Ruozi B, Dolcetta D, Vandelli MA, Forni F, Severini GM (2013) Potential use of polymeric nanoparticles for drug delivery across the blood-brain barrier. Curr Med Chem20(17):2212–2225
58. Das A, Theato P (2016) Activated ester containing polymers: opportunities and challenges for the design of functional macromolecules. Chem Rev 116(3):1434–1495
59. Machtakova M, Thérien-Aubin H, Landfester K (2022) Polymer nano-systems for the encapsulation and delivery of active biomacromolecular therapeutic agents. Chem Soc Rev 51(1):128–152
60. Gallardo-Toledo E, Velasco-Aguirre C, Kogan MJ (2021) Inorganic nanoparticles and their strategies to enhance brain drug delivery. Nanomed Brain Drug Deliv:149–172
61. Mehta TA, Shah N, Parekh K, Dhas N, Patel JK (2019) Surface-modified PLGA nanoparticles for targeted drug delivery to neurons. Surf Modif Nanopart Target Drug Deliv:33–71
62. Li S, Zhu H, Wang J, Wang X, Li X, Ma C, Wen L, Yu B, Wang Y, Li J, Wang PG (2016) Comparative analysis of Cu (I)-catalyzed alkyne–azide cycloaddition (CuAAC) and strain-promoted alkyne–azide cycloaddition (SPAAC) in O-GlcNAc proteomics. Electrophoresis 37(11):1431–1436
63. Anderton GI, Bangerter AS, Davis TC, Feng Z, Furtak AJ, Larsen JO, Scroggin TL, Heemstra JM (2015) Accelerating strain-promoted azide–alkyne cycloaddition using micellar catalysis. Bioconjugate Chem 26(8):1687–1691
64. Singh S, Dubinsky-Davidchik IS, Kluger R (2016) Strain-promoted azide–alkyne cycloaddition for protein–protein coupling in the formation of a bis-hemoglobin as a copper-free oxygen carrier. Org Biomol Chem 14(42):10011–10017

65. Gupta J, Fatima MT, Islam Z, Khan RH, Uversky VN, Salahuddin P (2019) Nanoparticle formulations in the diagnosis and therapy of Alzheimer's disease. Int J Biol Macromolecules 130:515–526
66. Kobeissy F, Kobaisi A, Peng W, Barsa C, Goli M, Sibahi A, El Hayek S, Abdelhady S, Ali Haidar M, Sabra M, Orešič M (2022) Glycomic and glycoproteomic techniques in neurodegenerative disorders and neurotrauma: towards personalized markers. Cells 11(3):581
67. He P, He L (2009) Synthesis of surface-anchored DNA-polymer bioconjugates using reversible addition-fragmentation chain transfer polymerization. Biomacromolecules 10(7):1804–1809
68. Escorihuela J, Marcelis AT, Zuilhof H (2015) Metal-free click chemistry reactions on surfaces. Adv Mater Interfaces 2(13):1500135
69. Nicolas J, Mura S, Brambilla D, Mackiewicz N, Couvreur P (2013) Design, functionalization strategies and biomedical applications of targeted biodegradable/biocompatible polymer-based nanocarriers for drug delivery. ChemSoc Rev 42(3):1147–1235
70. Trapani A, De Giglio E, Cafagna D, Denora N, Agrimi G, Cassano T, Gaetani S, Cuomo V, Trapani G (2011) Characterization and evaluation of chitosan nanoparticles for dopamine brain delivery. Int J Pharm 419(1–2):296–307
71. Chatzitaki AT, Jesus S, Karavasili C, Andreadis D, Fatouros DG, Borges O (2020) Chitosan-coated PLGA nanoparticles for the nasal delivery of ropinirole hydrochloride: in vitro and ex vivo evaluation of efficacy and safety. Int J Pharm 589:119776
72. Di Gioia S, Trapani A, Mandracchia D, De Giglio E, Cometa S, Mangini V, Arnesano F, Belgiovine G, Castellani S, Pace L, Lavecchia MA (2015) Intranasal delivery of dopamine to the striatum using glycol chitosan/sulfobutylether-β-cyclodextrin based nanoparticles. Eur J Pharm Biopharm94:180–193
73. Aillon KL, Xie Y, El-Gendy N, Berkland CJ, Forrest ML (2009) Effects of nanomaterial physicochemical properties on in vivo toxicity. Adv Drug Deliv Rev 61(6):457–466
74. Elmowafy EM, Tiboni M, Soliman ME (2019) Biocompatibility, biodegradation and biomedical applications of poly (lactic acid)/poly (lactic-co-glycolic acid) micro and nanoparticles. J Pharm Investig 49:347–380
75. Huang CY, Chen CM, Lee YD (2007) Synthesis of high loading and encapsulation efficient paclitaxel-loaded poly (n-butyl cyanoacrylate) nanoparticles via miniemulsion. Int J Pharm 338(1–2):267–275
76. Lai P, Daear W, Löbenberg R, Prenner EJ (2014) Overview of the preparation of organic polymeric nanoparticles for drug delivery based on gelatine, chitosan, poly (d, l-lactide-co-glycolic acid) and polyalkylcyanoacrylate. Colloids Surf B Biointerfaces 118:154–163
77. Liu X, Jin J, Chen Y, Lu B, Sun Q, Wang J, Chen JF, Le Y (2020) Controllable polymerization of n-butyl cyanoacrylate using a high-gravity rotating packed bed. Chem Eng J 379:122400
78. Mi HY, Salick MR, Jing X, Jacques BR, Crone WC, Peng XF, Turng LS (2013) Characterization of thermoplastic polyurethane/polylactic acid (TPU/PLA) tissue engineering scaffolds fabricated by microcellular injection molding. Mater Sci Eng C 33(8):4767–4776
79. Wahit MU, Akos NI, Laftah WA (2012) Influence of natural fibers on the mechanical properties and biodegradation of poly (lactic acid) and poly (∈-caprolactone) composites: a review. Polym Compos 33(7):1045–1053
80. Kondapi AK (2020) Targeting cancer with lactoferrin nanoparticles: recent advances. Nanomedicine 15(21):2071–2083
81. Wang W, Nema S, Teagarden D (2010) Protein aggregation—pathways and influencing factors. Int J Pharm 390(2):89–99
82. Jain A, Singh SK, Arya SK, Kundu SC, Kapoor S (2018) Protein nanoparticles: promising platforms for drug delivery applications. ACS Biomater Sci Eng 4(12):3939–3961
83. Khanbabaie R, Jahanshahi M (2012) Revolutionary impact of nanodrug delivery on neuroscience. Curr Neuropharmacol 10(4), 370–392
84. Hwang HH, Kim HS, Lee DY (2023) Gastrointestinally absorbable lactoferrin-heparin conjugate with anti-angiogenic activity for treatment of brain tumor. J Control Release 355:730–744

85. Mofidian R, Barati A, Jahanshahi M, Shahavi MH (2019) Optimization on thermal treatment synthesis of lactoferrin nanoparticles via Taguchi design method. SN Appl Sci 1:1–9
86. Zhi D, Yang T, Yang J, Fu S, Zhang S (2020) Targeting strategies for superparamagnetic iron oxide nanoparticles in cancer therapy. Acta Biomaterialia 102:13–34
87. Gothwal A, Kumar H, Nakhate KT, Ajazuddin, Dutta A, Borah A, Gupta U (2019) Lactoferrin coupled lower generation PAMAM dendrimers for brain targeted delivery of memantine in aluminum-chloride-induced Alzheimer's disease in mice. Bioconjug Chem 30(10):2573–2583
88. Arora S, Layek B, Singh J (2020) Design and validation of liposomal ApoE2 gene delivery system to evade blood–brain barrier for effective treatment of Alzheimer's disease. Mol Pharm 18(2):714–725
89. dos Santos Rodrigues B, Kanekiyo T, Singh J (2019) ApoE-2 brain-targeted gene therapy through transferrin and penetratin tagged liposomal nanoparticles. Pharm Res 36:1–11
90. Pandian SR, Vijayakumar KK, Murugesan S, Kunjiappan S (2022) Liposomes: an emerging carrier for targeting Alzheimer's and Parkinson's diseases. Heliyon
91. Williams T, Borchelt DR, Chakrabarty P (2020) Therapeutic approaches targeting Apolipoprotein E function in Alzheimer's disease. Mol Neurodegener 15:1–19
92. Choi C, Nam JP, Nah JW (2016) Application of chitosan and chitosan derivatives as biomaterials. J Ind Eng Chem 33:1–10
93. Balducci C, Mancini S, Minniti S, La Vitola P, Zotti M, Sancini G, Mauri M, Cagnotto A, Colombo L, Fiordaliso F, Grigoli E (2014) Multifunctional liposomes reduce brain β-amyloid burden and ameliorate memory impairment in Alzheimer's disease mouse models. J Neurosci 34(42):14022–14031
94. Mancini S, Balducci C, Micotti E, Tolomeo D, Forloni G, Masserini M, Re F (2017) Multifunctional liposomes delay phenotype progression and prevent memory impairment in a presymptomatic stage mouse model of Alzheimer disease. J Control Release 258:121–129
95. Lee SJ (2008) Origins and effects of extracellular α-synuclein: implications in Parkinson's disease. J Mol Neurosci 34:17–22
96. Zecca L, Wilms H, Geick S, Claasen JH, Brandenburg LO, Holzknecht C, Panizza ML, Zucca FA, Deuschl G, Sievers J, Lucius R (2008) Human neuromelanin induces neuroinflammation and neurodegeneration in the rat substantia nigra: implications for Parkinson's disease. Acta Neuropathol 116:47–55
97. Kaushik A, Jayant RD, Bhardwaj V, Nair M (2018) Personalized nanomedicine for CNS diseases. Drug Discov Today 23(5):1007–1015
98. Lin CY, Lin YC, Huang CY, Wu SR, Chen CM, Liu HL (2020) Ultrasound-responsive neurotrophic factor-loaded microbubble-liposome complex: preclinical investigation for Parkinson's disease treatment. J Control Release 321:519–528
99. Zhang P, Zhang L, Qin Z, Hua S, Guo Z, Chu C, Lin H, Zhang Y, Li W, Zhang X, Chen X (2018) Genetically engineered liposome—like nanovesicles as active targeted transport platform. Adv Mater 30(7):1705350
100. Belfiore L, Saunders DN, Ranson M, Thurecht KJ, Storm G, Vine KL (2018) Towards clinical translation of ligand-functionalized liposomes in targeted cancer therapy: challenges and opportunities. J Control Release 277:1–13
101. Mojarad-Jabali S, Farshbaf M, Walker PR, Hemmati S, Fatahi Y, Zakeri-Milani P, Sarfraz M, Valizadeh H (2021) An update on actively targeted liposomes in advanced drug delivery to glioma. Int J Pharm 602:120645
102. Yoon G, Park JW, Yoon IS (2013) Solid lipid nanoparticles (SLNs) and nanostructured lipid carriers (NLCs): recent advances in drug delivery. J Pharm Investig 43:353–362
103. Elbahwy IA, Ibrahim HM, Ismael HR, Kasem AA (2017) Enhancing bioavailability and controlling the release of glibenclamide from optimized solid lipid nanoparticles. J Drug Deliv Sci Technol 38:78–89
104. Ashkar A, Sosnik A, Davidovich-Pinhas M (2022) Structured edible lipid-based particle systems for oral drug-delivery. Biotechnol Adv 54:107789

105. Neves AR, Lúcio M, Martins S, Lima JL, Reis S (2013) Novel resveratrol nanodelivery systems based on lipid nanoparticles to enhance its oral bioavailability. Int J Nanomed:177–187
106. Garg J, Pathania K, Sah SP, Pawar SV (2022) Nanostructured lipid carriers: a promising drug carrier for targeting brain tumours. Fut J Pharm Sci 8(1):25
107. Ghasemiyeh P, Mohammadi-Samani S (2018) Solid lipid nanoparticles and nanostructured lipid carriers as novel drug delivery systems: applications, advantages and disadvantages. Res Pharm Sci 13(4):288
108. Agrawal M, Saraf S, Saraf S, Dubey SK, Puri A, Patel RJ, Ravichandiran V, Murty US, Alexander A (2020) Recent strategies and advances in the fabrication of nano lipid carriers and their application towards brain targeting. J Control Release 321:372–415
109. Müller RH, Alexiev U, Sinambela P, Keck CM (2016) Nanostructured lipid carriers (NLC): the second generation of solid lipid nanoparticles. Percutaneous Penetr Enhanc Chem Methods Penetr Enhanc Nanocarriers:161–185
110. Souto EB, Müller RH (2006) Investigation of the factors influencing the incorporation of clotrimazole in SLN and NLC prepared by hot high-pressure homogenization. J Microencapsul 23(4):377–388
111. Vinchhi P, Patel JK, Patel MM (2021) High-pressure homogenization techniques for nanoparticles. In: Emerging technologies for nanoparticle manufacturing. Springer, pp 263–285
112. Duan Y, Dhar A, Patel C, Khimani M, Neogi S, Sharma P, Kumar NS, Vekariya RL (2020) A brief review on solid lipid nanoparticles: part and parcel of contemporary drug delivery systems. RSC Adv 10(45): 26777–26791
113. Hussein HA, Abdullah MA (2022) Novel drug delivery systems based on silver nanoparticles, hyaluronic acid, lipid nanoparticles and liposomes for cancer treatment. Appl Nanosci 12(11):3071–3096
114. Baspinar Y, Keck CM, Borchert HH (2010) Development of a positively charged prednicarbate nanoemulsion. Int J Pharm 383(1–2):201–208
115. Katouzian I, Esfanjani AF, Jafari SM, Akhavan S (2017) Formulation and application of a new generation of lipid nano-carriers for the food bioactive ingredients. Trends Food Sci Technol 68:14–25
116. Ganesan P, Narayanasamy D (2017) Lipid nanoparticles: different preparation techniques, characterization, hurdles, and strategies for the production of solid lipid nanoparticles and nanostructured lipid carriers for oral drug delivery. Sustain Chem Pharm 6:37–56
117. Sahbaz Y, Williams HD, Nguyen TH, Saunders J, Ford L, Charman SA, Scammells PJ, Porter CJ (2015) Transformation of poorly water-soluble drugs into lipophilic ionic liquids enhances oral drug exposure from lipid based formulations. Mol Pharm 12(6):1980–1991
118. Đorđević V, Balanč B, Belščak-Cvitanović A, Lević S, Trifković K, Kalušević A, Kostić I, Komes D, Bugarski B, Nedović V (2015) Trends in encapsulation technologies for delivery of food bioactive compounds. Food Eng Rev 7:452–490
119. Shchukina EM, Shchukin DG (2011) LbL coated microcapsules for delivering lipid-based drugs. Adv Drug Deliv Rev 63(9):837–846
120. Tamjidi F, Shahedi M, Varshosaz J, Nasirpour A (2013) Nanostructured lipid carriers (NLC): a potential delivery system for bioactive food molecules. Innov Food Sci Emerg Technol 19:29–43
121. Sakellari GI, Zafeiri I, Batchelor H, Spyropoulos F (2021) Formulation design, production and characterisation of solid lipid nanoparticles (SLN) and nanostructured lipid carriers (NLC) for the encapsulation of a model hydrophobic active. Food Hydrocolloids Health 1:100024
122. Hidajat MJ, Jo W, Kim H, Noh J (2020) Effective droplet size reduction and excellent stability of limonene nanoemulsion formed by high-pressure homogenizer. Colloids Interfaces 4(1):5
123. Kentish S, Wooster TJ, Ashokkumar M, Balachandran S, Mawson R, Simons L (2008) The use of ultrasonics for nanoemulsion preparation. Innov Food SciEmerg Technol 9(2):170–175

Going Nano for Neuro: Nanoparticle-Based Treatment of Central Nervous System Diseases

Palak Singhal, Shweta Kumari, Rudhvi Jain, Aman Bhushan, and Sahil Jain

Abstract Central nervous system (CNS) disorders effect more than 1 billion people (~50% of these are children) globally and account for nearly 9 million deaths annually. Therefore, CNS disorders have received due attention in the past few decades, with a lot of research focused on formulating novel strategies to treat them. However, overcoming the blood–brain barrier (BBB) challenge has posed a major challenge in drug and therapeutic development efforts. Usage of nanoparticles to deliver drugs specifically to target cells across the BBB presents a way forward. In this chapter, we focus on various studies conducted in the last decade to address the BBB penetration conundrum by utilizing nanoplatforms, including solid lipid nanoparticles (SLNs), nanoemulsions, liposomes, nanostructured lipid carriers (NLCs), and transfersomal nanoparticles, against brain tumor, epilepsy, meningitis, and multiple sclerosis. We hope that this chapter will encourage the scientific community to formulate novel nanoplatforms, as well as validate the current nanoparticle-based therapeutic systems for treatment of various CNS diseases.

Palak Singhal and Shweta Kumari are co-first authors, having contributed to the content equally.

P. Singhal
Department of Human Genetics, Inselspital, Bern University Hospital, University of Bern, Bern, Switzerland

Department of Biomedical Research, University of Bern, Bern, Switzerland

S. Kumari
University Institute of Biotechnology (UIBT), Chandigarh University, Mohali, Punjab 140413, India

R. Jain
Department of Biotechnology, Thapar Institute of Engineering and Technology, Patiala, Punjab 147004, India

R. Jain · S. Jain (✉)
Department of Biochemistry and Molecular Biology, Faculty of Life Sciences, Tel-Aviv University, Tel-Aviv, Israel
e-mail: sahilj@tauex.tau.ac.il

A. Bhushan
University Institute of Engineering and Technology (UIET), Panjab University, Chandigarh, India

S. K. Rath et al. (eds.), *Nanomaterials for Drug Delivery and Neurological Diseases Management*, Smart Nanomaterials Technology,
https://doi.org/10.1007/978-981-97-0308-1_6

Keywords Brain tumor · Epilepsy · Meningitis · Multiple sclerosis · Nanoparticles · Blood–brain barrier

1 Introduction

The central nervous system (CNS) disorders present a significant challenge to the healthcare industry, evident from the steadily increasing number of patients [1]. Globally, 1.5 billion people suffer from CNS disorders, which accounts for 1% of fatalities [2]. This makes CNS disorders the second leading cause of global deaths, with 9 million deaths per year [2]. CNS disorders are also the leading cause of disability-adjusted life-years (DALYs), which is calculated by adding the years of life lost to premature mortality and the years spent with a disability as a result of the disease's high prevalence in a population [3, 4]. Also, CNS diseases seem to effect both, men and women, as indicated by a 2019 Pan American Health Organization (PAHO) report that nearly 33 CNS-related deaths per 100,000 US male population and 32 deaths per 100,000 US female population were witnessed [5].

CNS diseases comprise a diverse range of severe neurological disorders, including brain tumor, meningitis, strokes, epilepsy, Alzheimer's disease, Parkinson's disease, Huntington's disease, and multiple sclerosis (MS). As per a WHO 2016 report, stroke (42.2%), migraine (16.3%), dementia (10.4%), meningitis (7.9%), and epilepsy (4.9%) were majorly responsible for DALYs [6]. According to the National Brain Tumor Society (NBTS), nearly 0.7 million US citizens suffer from a primary brain tumor, while approximately 18,000 would lose their life in 2022 [7]. Epilepsy is one of the most common neurological diseases worldwide [8]. Nearly 50 million people suffer from epilepsy worldwide, with 10% of the affected population in developed countries [9]. About 30 million effected people, residing in the low-income countries, do not have access to proper treatment [9]. Meningitis is a major global public-health challenge, particularly in the African Meningitis Belt region in the sub-Sahara Africa [10]. Different types of meningitis are known to majorly affect specific age groups. For example, infants are more vulnerable to Group B streptococcus, while elders are more likely to contract pneumococcal disease [10]. MS is estimated to affect nearly 3 million people globally, with almost 33% of the affected population in the US [11]. Females are twice as likely to contract MS as compared to human males [11]. MS is a global nemesis and was estimated to affect nearly 1 million people within the last decade [11].

Although different therapeutic approaches are being clinically tested currently for treatment of CNS disorders, a validated strategy eludes us, partly due to ignorance about the exact pathology of various conditions. Radiotherapy, chemotherapy, gene therapy, immunotherapy, and surgery are currently used to treat CNS disorders, each with its own benefits and limitations [12]. The therapeutic impact of commonly used drugs is constrained by the characteristic selective transportation of the blood–brain barrier (BBB) [13, 14]. Some other reasons for the low efficacy of such drugs include slow drug action, association or conversion of the drug into non-transporting forms, and lower neuronal absorption [15]. To increase the effectiveness of drug delivery for CNS disorders, it is crucial to develop novel therapeutic systems, such as nanomedicine [16]. Drug administration based on nanotechnology has proven beneficial over conventional drug delivery. Nanocarriers are promising candidates and have drawn widespread attention in the healthcare industry, owing to their desirable (10–100 nm) size, high biocompatibility, and amphiphilicity [17]. Various nanoformulations, including liposomes, dendrimers, gold nanoparticles (Au-NPs), solid lipid nanoparticles (SLNs), exosomes, carbon nanostructure-based vehicles, and polymer-based vehicles, have been used for targeted drug delivery. Various strategies, such as crossing the BBB without functionalization, adsorptive-mediated transcytosis, receptor-mediated transcytosis, retrograde transport, BBB Breakdown, and exploiting monocyte/macrophage infiltration in the CNS, have been developed to improve the drug delivery to the brain using nanoparticles (NPs) [18].

In this chapter we enlist various studies performed to overcome the drug delivery issue against four major CNS disorders viz., brain tumor, epilepsy, meningitis, and multiple sclerosis. We specifically focus on the NP-based studies conducted in the last decade. We hope that this chapter will highlight the enormous potential of NP-based strategies in overcoming the CNS-disorder-treatment hurdles and encourage further experimentation and validation of existing as well as novel nanoformulations.

2 NP-Based Treatment in Various CNS Disorders

2.1 Brain Tumor

Brain tumor is an abnormal growth of brain cells, characterized by poor prognosis and low survival rate of patients [19]. The World Health Organization (WHO) has classified the brain tumor into four grades viz., I, II, III, and IV, based on their manifestations and malignancies [20]. Amongst these grades, grade IV (glioblastoma; GB) is the most aggressive and lethal tumor to humans [20, 21], with a global incidence rate of 0.59–5 per 100,000 people per annum [22]. In 2016, around 3,30,000 cases and 2,27,000 deaths were reported globally due to CNS tumors [23].

Current treatment available for GB is surgical evacuation, followed by radiotherapy and chemotherapy with temozolomide (TMZ), an alkylating agent [24, 25]. However, this treatment may cause severe myelosuppression and may increase the risk of radiotherapy-induced cognitive deficits [24, 25]. Another major obstacle in the treatment process of brain tumor is the blood–brain barrier (BBB), which restricts the transport of drugs to the targeted site [26]. This indicates at a need for an ideal system that can help in controlled and targeted delivery of drugs to brain by crossing the BBB. NPs can play a significant role in the therapeutic treatment of brain tumors in comparison to traditional management methods, as NP-based treatment approaches overcome the hindrance caused by biological barriers while simultaneously enhancing the therapeutic effect of chemotherapy and immunotherapy [27,

28]. Various studies analyzing the efficacy of NP-based brain tumor treatment have been enlisted in Table 1, while some of the recent studies have been discussed here.

In 2014, Cheng et al. employed a transactivator of transcription (TAT) peptide-modified-Au NP system to deliver the anticancer drug, doxorubicin (Dox), across the BBB of mice with intracranial glioma xenografts [29]. They reported a significant increase in BBB penetration by Dox-conjugated TAT-Au NPs, as compared to free Dox [29]. This might be due to the small core size of TAT-Au NPs (5 nm) [29]. Further, the study also reported better delivery of Gd^{3+} chelates when conjugated with the TAT-Au NPs, thus supplementing the brain tumor imaging efforts [29].

In 2017, Richard et al. synthesized non coated maghemite γFe_2O_3 NPs and coated their surface with phosphonate-poly(ethylene glycol) (PO-PEG-COOH) [30]. PO-PEG-COOH helped to improve the stability of the synthesized NPs [30]. Further, they covalently coupled the cRGD (cyclic aspartic acid-glycine-arginine; a model molecule to target integrins) peptide onto γFe_2O_3@PO-PEG-COOH [30]. This nanoplatform was used to target the $\alpha_v\beta_3$ integrin, which is over expressed in brain tumors [30]. The authors observed a high potential of this nanoplatform as a potential MRI contrast agent for glioblastoma diagnosis [30]. In the same year, Kuo and Hsu employed Dox-loaded cationic solid lipid nanoparticles (CSLNs), covalently linked with surface anti-melanotransferrin (AMT) and apolipoprotein (ApoE), to investigate their effect on Dox delivery across BBB [31]. They targeted human brain-microvascular endothelial cells (HBMECs), human astrocytes, and U87MG (a malignant glioma cell line) cells [31]. The researchers observed improved Dox delivery across the BBB and negligible toxic effects of this nanoplatform [31]. Further, they reported that AMT-ApoE-Dox-CSLNs prepared at 10 μg/mL of AMT and at 5–10 μg/mL of ApoE provided optimum results [31].

In 2018, Liu et al. estimated the effectiveness of carbonized polymer dots (CPDs) in early stage visualization of brain tumor [32]. They observed that CPDs exhibited long emission wavelength, high photostability, favorable biocompatibility, and high internalization property to glioma cells in time and dose dependent manner [32]. The study suggested the usage of this nanoplatform for non-invasive visualization of brain tumors, and guiding surgical brain-tumor resection by real-time fluorescence imaging [32].

In 2019, Wahab et al. employed multivarient-sized gold nanoparticles (MVS-GNPs) to investigate their potential in inhibiting tumorigenesis in various cell lines, such as human T98G, U87, and U373 glioblastoma cells, SNU-80 (thyroid cancer cell line), and H460 (lung cancer cell line) [33]. They observed that gold quantum dots (GQDs; size <10 nm) are non-toxic, biocompatible, and markedly reduce the tumorigenic potential of glioma spheroid cells [33]. This might be due to the exploitation of the interaction between E-cadherin and Catenin Beta 1 (CTNNB1) gene by the GQDs, and potentially inhibiting the self-renewal ability of these cells [33]. In the same year, a study performed in Shanghai Jiao Tong University and Nanjing Tech University employed polyethylenimine-entrapped gold nanoparticles (Au PENPs) for glioma theranostics (therapy and diagnostics) in vitro as well as in vivo [34]. Their nanoplatform exhibited high radiochemical purity and stability and may be employed for targeted SPECT/CT imaging [34]. Also, the nanoprobe exhibited remarkable BBB

Table 1 A non-exhaustive summary of various studies analyzing the effects of NP-based treatments for brain tumor

Year	Study type	Nanoplatform	Drug	Result	Reference
2021	In vitro	Graphene quantum dots	Doxorubicin	Downregulation of nanosphere formation	[37]
2020	In vitro, In vivo	Carbon nitride dots	Gemcitabine	Selective targeting and apoptosis of tumor cells	[35]
2020	In vitro	Iron-oxide NPs	Doxorubicin	Inhibited human U251 cell proliferation and induced apoptosis of GB cells	[36]
2019	In vitro, In vivo	Gold NPs	–	Targeted SPECT/CT imaging of glioma cells	[34]
2019	In vitro	Gold quantum dots	–	Inhibition of spheroid cell growth and CTNNB1 signaling	[33]
2018	In vitro, In vivo	Carbonized polymer dots (CPDs)	–	Application in early-stage diagnosis of brain disorders, and real time fluorescence imaging of brain during surgery	[32]
2018	In vitro	Alginate nanogel co-loaded with AuNPs	Cisplatin	Induced apoptosis of U87-MG human glioblastoma cells	[38]

(continued)

Table 1 (continued)

Year	Study type	Nanoplatform	Drug	Result	Reference
2017	In vitro	Cationic SLN	Doxorubicin	Increased BBB permeability and inhibited U87-MG human glioblastoma cells	[31]
2017	In vivo	Iron-oxide nanoparticle	–	Enhanced MRI imaging for better diagnosis of brain tumor	[30]
2016	In vitro, In vivo	SLN and NLC	Vincristine and temozolomide	Dual-drug loaded NLCs displayed enhanced antitumor activity	[39]
2016	In vitro, In vivo	Nanogel	Doxorubicin	Higher drug uptake and acute toxicity against C6 glioma cancerous cell line. Inhibition of tumor growth in glioma rat model	[40]
2016	In vitro, In vivo	Iron oxide core and PEG/PEI/polysorbate 80	Doxorubicin	Suppression of glioma growth via induction of apoptosis through the caspase-3 pathway	[41]
2016	In vitro	Lipid nanocapsules	Lauroyl-gemcitabine	Prolonged drug release, and enhanced cytotoxicity against U-87 MG glioma cells	[42]

(continued)

Table 1 (continued)

Year	Study type	Nanoplatform	Drug	Result	Reference
2016	In vitro	Poly(acrylamide-co-N-(3-aminopropyl)methacrylamide) (PAA) and branched polyethylenimine (PEI)	Cisplatin	Enhanced drug uptake and higher cytotoxicity in 9L glioma cell line	[43]
2015	In vivo	Liposome nanoparticle	–	Enhanced near-infrared (NIR) imaging	[44]
2015	In vivo	Hydrogel	Temozolomide	Sustained drug release, and apoptosis of tumor cells	[45]
2014	In vitro, In vivo	PLA NPs	Temozolomide	Enhanced permeation of drug into brain	[46]
2014	In vitro, In vivo	An-PEG-DOX-AuNPs	Doxorubicin	Enhanced median survival time in mice model	[47]
2014	In vivo	TAT-AuNP	Doxorubicin	Enhanced survival of glioma mice models, and enhanced brain tumor imaging	[29]
2013	In vivo	Cy7-micelles	–	Enhanced permeability and better imaging	[48]
2013	In vivo	Magnetic nanogels	–	Highly specific targeted MR/fluorescence imaging	[49]
2012	In vitro	PEG-iron oxide hydrogel nanocomposites	Paclitaxel	Sustained drug release and cytotoxicity against cancer cell lines	[50]

(continued)

Table 1 (continued)

Year	Study type	Nanoplatform	Drug	Result	Reference
2011	In vivo	Silver nanoparticles	–	Enhanced the apoptosis rate of cancer cells during magnetic nanoparticles hyperthermia (MNPH) treatment	[51]
2011	In vitro, In vivo	Procationic liposomes	Doxorubicin	Enhanced drug uptake observed in cell lines, and inhibited tumor growth in rat models	[52]

NP: Nanoparticle; GB: Glioblastoma; SLN: Solid lipid nanoparticles; NLC: nanostructured lipid carriers; PLA: poly(lactic acid); TAT: Trans-activator of transcription peptide; PEG: poly(ethylene glycol); NIR: Near Infrared permeability and was able to specifically target the glioma cells in rat intracranial glioma models [34].

In 2020, a collaborative in vitro study employed carbon nitride dots (CN-dots or CNDs) for efficient delivery of gemcitabine to treat pediatric glioblastoma [35]. They targeted SJGBM2 glioma cells and observed ~95% selective removal of cancerous cells at 1 μM concentration of the CND-Gemcitabine conjugate [35]. To lower the concentration of the conjugate required for this action, the authors experimented with a CND-Gemcitabine-Transferrin conjugate and observed selective targeting at 1 nM concentration [35]. Thus, delivery of gemcitabine via a nanoplatform was shown to improve the BBB permeability of the drug [35]. Interestingly, before this study, gemcitabine had never been administered successfully to treat brain cancer [35]. Another study reported usage of magnetic iron-oxide NPs (IONPs), stabilized with trimethoxysilylpropyl-ethylenediamine triacetic acid (EDT), to enhance BBB penetration of Dox for glioblastoma treatment in human U251 cells (glioma cell line) [36]. The nanocarrier, DOX-EDT-IONPs, enabled almost threefold BBB penetration by Dox, affecting the glioma cell proliferation, and resulting in apoptotic death of ~90% glioma cells [36]. The plausible causes of this favorable effect may be the downregulation of enzymes involved in DNA repair and replication and upregulation of p53 and MEG3 genes [36].

In a recent study, graphene quantum dots (GQDs) and carboxylated GQDs (COOH-GQDs) were used to deliver Dox to neurospheres (a cluster of glioma cells) [37]. The authors observed a marked reduction in size and population of neurospheres upon administration of the nanoplatform [37]. The mechanism behind these observations was suggested to be an increase in cell membrane fluidity, which consequently reduced the cell-to-cell interaction [37].

2.2 *Epilepsy*

Epilepsy is characterized by abnormal neuronal electrical activity that may lead to repeated seizures, erratic behavior, disturbances in sensations (vision, hearing, and taste), and sometimes loss of consciousness [9]. Around 50 million people worldwide suffer from this disease, with approximately 10 million in high-income countries [9]. Approximately 5 million new cases are discovered globally per annum, with 50 new cases per 0.1 million people in high-income countries [9]. Epilepsy increases the risk of premature death, as well as makes the patient prone to fractures, bruises, anxiety, and depression [9].

Currently, no drug is known to cure epilepsy [53]. Anti-epileptic drugs (AEDs), such as lamotrigine, topiramate, and carbamazepine, are used to control seizures in epilepsy [54]. The disease is difficult to cure as antiepileptic drugs (AEDs) cannot pass the BBB readily [55]. Additionally, despite the availability of promising new AEDs and the potential to use IN administration as a distinct method of delivering medications to the brain, the desirable efficacy of epilepsy treatment hasn't been obtained [56]. Recently, a number of nanostructured drug delivery carriers have been suggested as efficient targeted drug delivery for the treatment of epilepsy by circumventing the barrier of AED elimination at the BBB, facilitating efficient medication bioavailability. Various studies analyzing the efficacy of NP-based epilepsy treatment have been enlisted in Table 2, while some of the recent studies have been discussed here.

In 2018, El-Zaafarany et al. employed emulsomes as nanocarriers for Oxcarbazepine (OX), an AED [57]. Further, the localized the nanoplatform in a poly(lactic acid-co-glycolic acid)-poly(ethylene glycol)-poly(lactic acid-co-glycolic acid) (PLGA-PEG-PLGA) thermogel [57]. This platform reportedly increased the drug residence time in rat model, thus, obtaining sustained drug release [57]. Moreover, the thermogel platform also exhibited a safer toxicology profile as compared to the standard (drug solution) [57]. In the same year, Kaur et al. utilized poly-lactide-co-glycolide (PLGA)-chitosan NPs, in a bid to address the limitations of L-pGlu-(1-benzyl)-L-His-L-ProNH_2 (NP-355) and L-pGlu-(2-propyl)-L-His-L-ProNH_2 (NP-647) as AEDs [58]. The BBB permeability of NP-355 and NP-647 was reportedly increased upon usage of this nanoplatform [58]. Also, sustained drug release was obtained, consequently overcoming the short life limitation of these AEDs [58].

A collaborative study conducted in Italy and Portugal employed PLGA NPs loaded with OX drug to treat epileptic rodent model [59]. This was done with an objective to obtain sustained OX drug release, lower the number of drug doses required, and enhance the brain target efficiency [59]. Upon intranasal (IN) administration, a neuroprotective effect of OX-PLGA-NPs was reported within three weeks of treatment [59]. The findings indicated that OX-PLGA-NPs might be beneficial in the treatment of epileptic seizures by enhancing the release of drug across the BBB and increasing the brain-drug bioavailability [59].

In 2018, a nanostructured lipid carrier, consisting of Compritol® 888, stearic acid, glyceryl monostearate, oleic acid, and glyceryl monooleate, was loaded with superparamagnetic iron oxide NPs, to enhance the brain targeting efficiency of clonazepam [60]. This nanoplatform delayed the onset time for convulsion in chemically induced convulsive Swiss Albino mice models [60]. Moreover, the nanoplatform was able to reduce the mortality rate in Swiss Albino mice, as well as displayed a better pharmacokinetic profile as compared to clonazepam alone [60]. In the same year, Montoto et al. presented a nanoplatform that could be modified for treatment of refractory epilepsy linked to efflux transporters upregulation [61]. They presented a spherical nanoplatform with Carbamazepine (CBZ) entrapped in an amorphous state [61]. In vitro experimentation indicated a 100% release of the drug within 24 h of administration in a controlled manner, while in vivo experiments in a mice model indicated at the protective effects of the nanostructured lipid carrier (NLC) nanoplatform upon intraperitoneal administration [61].

A study conducted in Jamia Hamdard University formulated a letrozole loaded nanoemulsion (LET-NE) administered intranasally and compared it to the intraperitoneal administration of free letrozole (LET) [62]. The study applied status epilepticus (SE) Swiss Albino mice [62]. It was reported that LET-NE administration resulted in delayed SE onset and reduced the incidence rate of SE [62]. Further, LET-NE displayed a more favorable neuroprotective activity of the hippocampus,

Table 2 A non-exhaustive summary of various studies analyzing the effects of NP-based treatments for epilepsy

Year	Study type	Nanoplatform	Drug	Result	Reference
2022	In vitro, In vivo	Polymeric NPs	Phenytoin	Sustained drug release in vitro, and antiseizure effects in rodents	[66]
2022	In vivo	Polymeric NPs	Oxytocin	Enhancement of neurogenesis, and apoptotic reduction in hippocampus	[67]
2021	In vivo	PLGA NPs	Clonazepam	Enhanced clonazepam transport in the brain via intranasal administration	[68]
2021	In vitro, In vivo	e-caprolactone (e-CL) NPs	Carbamazepine	Enhanced uptake and accumulation of drug in brain	[65]
2020	In vivo	AuNPs	Lacosamide	Targeted drug delivery, lowering the required doses	[63]
2020	In vivo	PLGA NPs	Catechin hydrate	Enhanced brain bioavailability, lowering the required doses	[64]
2020	In vitro, In vivo	NLC	Carbamazepine	Enhanced anticonvulsant and anxiolytic activities	[69]
2020	In vitro, In vivo	PLGA NPs	Thymoquinone	Sustained drug release and improved drug bioavailability	[70]
2020	In vitro, In vivo	SLN	Curcumin	Reduced neuronal apoptosis through BCL-2 family and P38 MAPK pathways	[71]
2019	In vitro, In vivo	Nanoemulsion	Letrozole	Prolonged drug release in vitro, and showed anticonvulsant activity in mice models	[62]

(continued)

Table 2 (continued)

Year	Study type	Nanoplatform	Drug	Result	Reference
2018	In vitro	Polymeric NPs	Oxytocin	Rabies virus glycoprotein conjugated bovine serum albumin nanoparticles enhance brain drug delivery	[72]
2018	In vivo	PLGA NPs	L-pGlu-(1-benzyl)-L-His-L-ProNH2 (NP-355) and L-pGlu-(2-propyl)-L-His-L-ProNH2 (NP-647)	Sustained release of TRH analogues via IN administration	[58]
2018	In vivo	PLGA NPs	Oxcarbazepine	Reduction in required doses, helping to control epileptic seizures	[59]
2018	In vitro, In vivo	NLC	Clonazepam	Prolonged convulsion onset time, and reduced mice model death	[60]
2018	In vitro, In vivo	SLN, NLC	Carbamazepine	Controlled drug release in vitro, and protection against seizures in mice models	[61]
2018	In vitro, In vivo	Emulsomes nanocarriers	Oxcarbazepine	Sustained drug release, and higher uptake in brain upon localization of drug loaded emulsomes in a copolymer thermogel	[57]
2018	In vitro, Ex vivo	Nanoliposomes	Lamotrigine	Enhanced drug entrapment, and permeation in goat nasal mucosa	[73]
2018	In vitro, In vivo	PEGylated-PLGA NPs	Epigallocatechin-3-gallate	Sustained drug release, reduction in epileptic episodes, and reduced neuroinflammation	[74]

(continued)

Table 2 (continued)

Year	Study type	Nanoplatform	Drug	Result	Reference
2017	In vitro, In vivo	Carboxymethyl chitosan NPs	Carbamazepine	Enhanced drug bioavailability and brain targeting	[75]
2016	In vitro, In vivo	Emulsomes nanocarriers	Oxcarbazepine	Reduced drug toxicity, and prolonged release time	[76]
2016	In vitro	PLGA NPs	Diazepam	Sustained release of diazepam	[77]
2015	In vitro, In vivo, Ex vivo	PLGA NPs	Diazepam	Desirable drug release in sheep nasal mucosa, and higher uptake in Sprague–Dawley rats via IN administration	[78]
2014	In vitro, In vivo, Ex vivo	PLGA NPs	Lorazepam	Sustained drug release, desirable permeation in sheep nasal mucosa, and sustained brain concentration in Sprague–Dawley rats	[79]
2014	In vitro, In vivo	SLN	Haloperidol	Enhanced drug-targeting, and drug brain concentration	[80]
2012	In vitro, In vivo	SLN	Alprazolam	Enhanced rate and extent of transport of alprazolam, reducing the required doses	[81]

NP: Nanoparticle; PLGA: poly lactic-co-glycolic acid; NLC: nanostructured lipid carrier; SLN: Solid lipid nanoparticles; TRH: Thyrotropin-releasing hormone which may be attributed to decreased 17-β estradiol levels [62]. Moreover, the 5α-Dihydrotestosterone (5α-DHT) and 3α-androstanediol (3α-Diol) levels were markedly increased, stressing on the higher efficacy of LET-NE as compared to LET alone [62].

In 2020, Yilmaz et al. employed glucose-coated gold nanoparticles (GNPs) loaded with lacosamide (LCM) for synthesizing nanocarrier LCM-GNPs [63]. They targeted temporal lobe epilepsy (TLE), one of the most common epilepsies with focal seizures [63]. This resulted in decreased levels of glutathione in the hippocampus region [63]. Also, significant decrease in amplitude and frequency of EEG-waves was observed after intravenous administration of LCM-GNPs [63]. The authors have suggested that glucose-coated NPs might defend the neurons by reducing oxidative damage and decreasing neuronal excitation [63]. The study concluded that LCM-GNPs can efficiently deliver LCM into brain parenchyma by crossing the BBB and eliminating the need for higher dose administration for TLE treatment [63]. In the same year, Ahmad et al. used chitosan-coated-PLGA-nanoparticles (CS-PLGA-NPs) loaded with catechin hydrate (CH) to increase the brain bioavailability of CH for epilepsy treatment [64]. They observed that CS-CH-PLGA-NPs show a sustained release profile over 24 h, with increased nasal permeability and longer retention for nose-to-brain distribution [64]. Also, the nanoplatform effectively avoided hepatic first pass metabolism [64]. Overall, the results indicated at better BBB permeability of CH encapsulated in CS-PLGA-NPs at a reduced dose via IN administration [64].

In a recent study, Parashar et al. employed angiopep-2 (ANG) anchored lipoprotein-coated e-caprolactone (e-CL) NPs loaded with CBZ in a bid to identify a novel delivery system for CBZ across the BBB [65]. It was reported that the cumulative release within the first 48 h was ~80% [65]. Also, ANG is a 19-residue peptide that exhibits high LRP-mediated brain penetration capability [65]. Therefore, ANG enabled higher permeability of the formulation across the BBB [65]. Further, a great improvement in the solubility of CBZ was observed upon using this nanoplatform [65]. The study concluded that CBZ-loaded angiopep-conjugated PEG-PCL NPs exhibit targeting effects through transport of the ANG-NP across the BBB through LRP targeting for better treatment of epilepsy [65].

2.3 *Meningitis*

Meningitis is an inflammation of the meninges, a protective membrane of the brain and spinal cord [82]. Meningitis is primarily caused by bacteria, viruses, fungi, and parasites; amongst these, bacterial meningitis is of major concern [10]. Almost 50% of global deaths from meningitis are due to infection by *Neisseria meningitidis* (meningococcus), *Streptococcus pneumoniae* (pneumococcus), *Haemophilus influenza*, and *Streptococcus agalactiae* (group B streptococcus) [82]. Around 1 in 10 individuals who get bacterial meningitis die, and 1 in 5 are found to have severe complications [82].

Some vaccines are available against different meningitis types, but they suffer from major limitations. For example, protein based vaccines and polysaccharide vaccines against meningococcus cannot prevent transmission of the infection, thus cannot provide herd immunity [82]. Also, most of the available vaccines confer protection only against a specific serotype [82]. Additionally, biofilms are a major problem and pose a great challenge for the treatment of bacterial meningitis, as they are able to respond to any environmental changes and become resistant to multiple drugs [83]. Moreover, various drugs used for treatment of meningitis exhibit low efficacy due to lesser BBB penetration. This can be avoided by encapsulating the drug in a proper carrier system such as lipid or polymeric NP [84]. Various studies analyzing the efficacy of NP-based meningitis treatment have been enlisted in Table 3, while some of the recent studies have been discussed here.

In 2011, Xu et al. used polybutylcyanoacrylate NPs (PBCA NPs) loaded with the antifungal drug amphotericin B deoxycholate (AmB) to address the BBB permeability of AMB during cryptococcal meningitis treatment [85]. The resultant AmB-PBCA-NPs were coated with polysorbate 80 to enhance the CNS uptake of the drug [85]. Experiments in BALB/c mice models indicated a significant reduction in the fungal titers upon administration of AmB-PBCA-NPs [85]. Also, ~80% survival rate was found for these mice, as compared to mice administered AmB alone (0%) [85]. Moreover, the polysorbate 80 coating enhanced the brain targeting, as the drug concentration in the brain was detected after 30 min of administration and increased to its maximum by 3 h [85]. In another study, Shao et al. addressed the same issue (BBB permeability of AmB during cryptococcal meningitis treatment), by designing a brain-targeting delivery system consisting of Angiopep-PEG-PE/AmB polymeric micelles [86]. For target-specific drug delivery, angiopep-2 was selected as it exhibits high BBB penetration ability via interaction with the lipoprotein receptor-related protein (LRP) receptor [86]. This resulted in improved CNS permeability of AmB through LRP-mediated transcytosis and maintaining a higher drug level in brain parenchyma of immunosuppressive murine models [86]. Also, Angiopep-PEG-PE/AmB polymeric micelles minimized the dose requirement and significantly reduced the brain fungal burden [86].

In 2017, Garcia et al. employed tat_{47-57} functionalized liposomes as nanocarriers loaded with vancomycin, methicillin, and ampicillin antibiotics [87]. Tat (YGRKKRRQRRR) is a peptide sequence which shows high BBB penetration capability at 4 $\mu L/(g \times min)$ [87]. The authors targeted three meningitis-causing bacterial strains, including *Streptococcus pneumoniae*, *Staphylococcus aureus* (methicillin-resistant strain), and *Escherichia coli* [87]. This study resulted in improved antibiotic release with liposome-loaded drugs [87]. Moreover, tat-functionalized liposomes loaded with methicillin presented higher penetration capability, with a minimum inhibitory concentration of 1.7 μg/ml against methicillin-resistant *Staphylococcus aureus* [87]. The study concluded that tat-functionalized liposomes improved localized release of drug and enhanced bacteria killing efficiency [87].

In 2018, a study in Shenyang Agricultural University employed PEGylated nano-self-assemblies of bacitracin A (BA) with brain targeting ligands such as RVG_{29} (rabies virus glycopeptide-29) and Pluronic® P85 unimers (P-glycoprotein inhibitor)

Table 3 A non-exhaustive summary of various studies analyzing the effects of NP-based treatments for meningitis

Year	Study type	Nanoplatform	Drug	Result	Reference
2021	In vitro, In vivo	Poly (n-butyl cyanoacrylate) NPs	Propolis	In vitro antifungal activity against *Cryptococcus neoformans*. Reduced fungal titers in infected mice models	[93]
2020	In vitro	Polymeric NPs	Ansamycin	Sustained, progressive release of drug for 36 h	[92]
2020	In vitro, In vivo, Ex vivo	SLN	Levofloxacin and Doxycycline	Prolonged drug release, brain targeting, and direct transport percentage	[91]
2019	In vitro, In vivo	Borneol and poly (ethylene glycol) modified BSA NPs	Itraconazole	Enhanced cellular uptake and biodistribution in brain	[94]
2019	In vitro, In vivo	Transfersomal NPs	Ofloxacin	Enhanced brain bioavailability via IN administration, and delayed drug release	[89]
2019	In vivo	NLC	Ketoconazole	Antifungal activity against *Cryptococcus neoformans*, and prolonged residence in tissues	[90]
2019	In vitro, In vivo	NLC	Oleuropein	Observed brain tissue regeneration, and controlled drug release	[84]
2019	In vitro, In vivo	RDP liposomes	Polypyridyl ruthenium complex RC-7	Enhanced antifungal activity, targeted drug delivery, and prolonged survival in mice models	[95]
2018	In vitro, In vivo	PEGylated nanocarrier	Bacitracin A	Antibacterial activity against *Streptococcus pneumonia*, and enhanced drug uptake	[88]
2018	In vivo	Liposomes	Amphotericin B and VT-1598	A dose-dependent reduction in brain fungal burden	[96]

(continued)

Table 3 (continued)

Year	Study type	Nanoplatform	Drug	Result	Reference
2017	In vivo	Liposomes	Amphotericin B	A dose-dependent decline in fungal burden in mice models	[97]
2017	In vitro	Poly (butyl cyanoacrylate) NPs	Itraconazole	An efficient, targeted itraconazole delivery system	[98]
2017	In vitro	Tat-functionalized Liposomes	Methicillin	100% eradication of bacterial population	[87]
2015	In vivo	PLA-PEG NPs	Amphotericin B	Significant reduction of fungal burden, and increase in survival time of mice models	[99]
2014	In vitro, In vivo	Polymeric micelles	Itraconazole	Targeted drug delivery by penetrating BBB, and increased the drug stability in blood circulation	[100]
2013	In vitro	Polypropylene imine (PPI) dendrimers	Choline and NH_2	Enhanced phagocytosis of pneumococcal long chain by microglia	[101]
2013	In vivo	Liposomes	Amphotericin B and flucytosine	Additive effect of both drugs resulted in near-maximal antifungal activity	[102]
2012	In vivo	Polymeric micelles	Amphotericin B	Enhanced BBB permeability, drug bioavailability, antifungal activity, and median survival time	[86]
2011	In vivo	Liposomes	Amphotericin B and voriconazole	A synergistic effect of drugs on reduction of fungal titers and inflammation	[103]
2011	In vivo	Polybutylcyanoacrylate NPs	Amphotericin B	Enhanced drug bioavailability, and mice survival rate	[85]

(continued)

Table 3 (continued)

Year	Study type	Nanoplatform	Drug	Result	Reference
2010	In vitro, In vivo	Polymeric micelles	Amphotericin B	Enhanced BBB permeability	[104]
2009	In vitro, In vivo	CG(3)R(6)TAT NPs	Amphotericin B and fluconazole	Lowered dosage requirement for most tested samples. Increased BB permeability and better toxicological profile in rabbit models	[105]

NP: Nanoparticle; BSA: Bovine serum albumin; SLN: Solid lipid nanoparticles; NLC: nanostructured lipid carrier; RDP: Rabies virus-derived peptide; TAT: Trans-Activator of Transcription; PLA-PEG: Poly(lactic acid)-Poly(ethylene oxide)

to get a RVG_{29}-Nano-BA_{P85} nanocarrier against *Streptococcus pneumonia* [88]. This nanoplatform was reported to accumulate in the mice brain parenchyma and resulted in enhanced antibacterial activity and higher drug cellular uptake in brain capillary endothelial cells [88]. Additionally, reduced membrane viscosity and exhaustion of ATP also contributed to boosting the BBB permeability [88]. The study concluded that RVG_{29}-Nano-BA_{P85} nanocarriers exhibit very high therapeutic efficiency against both, drug-resistant and drug-sensitive *Streptococcus pneumonia* [88].

Eid et al. (2019) prepared ofloxacin loaded transfersomal nanovesicles (OFLOX-TNVs) against bacterial meningitis [89]. There nanoplatform, ~270 nm in size, was able to release 75–80% of entrapped OFLOX within 24 h of administration [89]. The drug-brain bioavailability was also enhanced, while delayed drug release over a period of 8 h was observed, with enhanced transnasal flux [89]. Based on the encouraging preliminary results, the authors suggested clinical experimentation of the proposed colloidal drug delivery system against bacterial meningitis [89]. In the same year, a study in China was based on development of a nanosystem for the intranasal delivery of ketoconazole (keto), so as to bypass the BBB during treatment of *Cryptococcus neoformans*-mediated meningoencephalitis [90]. A NLC loaded with keto was utilized, and the nanosystem reached the target site via olfactory bulb region, bypassing the BBB [90]. This nanosystem resulted in high antifungal activity due to enhanced tissue colonization and prolonged residual time [90]. The study concluded that keto-NLCs could be an effective nanocarrier system for the successful treatment of cryptococcal meningoencephalitis by crossing the BBB via the olfactory system [90]. Another study reported application of NLCs loaded with oleuropein (a secondary metabolite isolated from olive leaf) [84]. They targeted *Streptococcus pneumonia*, the leading cause of pneumococcal meningitis [84]. This resulted in controlled drug release of $81.15 \pm 2.42\%$ within 12 h of administration, as compared to free oleuropein, which shows immediate drug release (~98%) within 60 min [84]. Moreover, compared to the control group, the hippocampus area of the treated group showed signs of brain tissue regeneration, indicating at the effectiveness of the employed nanosystem [84].

In 2020, Hady et al. employed SLN nanoparticles for the targeted delivery of the combination of levofloxacin/doxycycline (LEVO/DOX) via intranasal route against meningitis [91]. The administration of drugs using this nanoplatform resulted in an enhanced percentage of drug targeting efficiency (DTE%), i.e., 149.815 (LEVO) and 161.969 (DOX), and a better direct transport percentage (DTP%) of 33.285 (LEVO) and 40.236 (DOX) for LEVO and DOX, in comparison to free drug delivery [91]. Also, a decline in the required dosage concentration was observed due to increased brain targeting [91]. The study concluded the intranasal administration of a LEVO/DOX combination loaded onto a SLN has potential for targeting and treating bacterial meningitis [91]. Recently, Nair et al. worked upon optimizing the PLGA based nanoplatform loaded with drug ansamycin [92]. Their response surface methodology resulted in a mean particle size of ~121 nm and an increased encapsulation efficiency of 89% [92]. Moreover, sustained drug release was observed for 36 h upon in vitro experimentation, indicating that the optimized polymeric NPs can be effectively used as drug carriers for the treatment of bacterial meningitis [92].

2.4 *Multiple Sclerosis*

Multiple sclerosis (MS) is a progressive neuroinflammatory and autoimmune disease affecting the brain, optic nerves, and the spinal cord [106]. It is a multifactorial disease encompassing various pathomechanisms, including gliosis, inflammation, and neuronal loss resulting in demyelination of myelinated axons, which further leads to slower signals from nerves [106]. MS therapeutics and medications are expected to be delivered via BBB to eventually reach the lesion sites, but mostly the BBB obstructs the perforation of the delivered drugs [107, 108]. Only traces of drugs make it through the BBB and reach lesion sites, consequently, not delivering the expected response efficacy. Therefore, even though many medications, including Cladribine (Mavenclad) [109], Ocrelizumab (Ocrevus) [110], and Alemtuzumab (Lemtrada) [111], are available for MS treatment, it still remains a challenge to administer drugs effectively to the MS lesion sites.

In the past few years, a wide range of NP-based platforms have been used for early detection, prognosis, and treatment of MS. In general, these NPs enable efficient delivery of target drugs for neuroprotection and anti-inflammation [112, 113]. Researchers have explored various NPs such as exosomes, lipid-based nanoparticles, cerium oxide NPs, aptamers, gold NPs, etc. to deliver therapeutic medications across the BBB more precisely [27, 114–116], which could help in better drug delivery to treat MS. Various studies analyzing the efficacy of NP-based MS treatment have been enlisted in Table 4, while some of the recent studies have been discussed here.

In 2000, Merodio et al. examined the activity of albumin NPs to cross the BBB and their distribution across the brain using experimental autoimmune encephalomyelitis (EAE) rat models [117]. The authors reported the presence of NPs in the lumbar

Table 4 A non-exhaustive summary of various studies analyzing the effects of NP-based treatments for multiple sclerosis

Year	Study type	Nanoplatform	Drug	Result	Reference
2022	In vitro, In vivo	PLGA NPs	$MOG_{35–55}$ peptide analogues	Reduced clinical symptoms and inflammation in EAE mice models	[128]
2022	In vivo	SLN	Dimethyl fumarate	Reduced inflammation, weight loss and pulmonary dysfunction in female C57BL/6J mice models	[124]
2021	In vivo	Nanoformulation	1 methylpseudouridine-modified messenger RNA	Delayed onset and reduced severity in mice models	[129]
2021	In vitro, In vivo	Chitosan/ sulfobutylether-β-cyclodextrin NPs	IFN-β	Sustained drug release, high brain bioavailability, and amelioration of clinical symptom in EAE mice	[123]
2018	In vitro	Nanomicelle	Curcumin	Decreased mRNA expression levels of IFN-γ, IL-1β, IL-6, CCL2, CCL5 and TNF-α in human blood samples	[130]
2017	In vitro	Graphene oxide-Dendrimer NPs	–	Quantification of MBP and Tau proteins	[131]

(continued)

Table 4 (continued)

Year	Study type	Nanoplatform	Drug	Result	Reference
2016	In vitro, In vivo	Immune polyelectrolyte multilayers	Myelin and GpG oligonucleotide	Reduced myelin-triggered inflammatory response, and TLR9 signaling	[132]
2015	In vitro, In vivo	PLGA NPs	Leukaemia inhibitory factor	Activation of activated pSTAT-3 signaling and oligodendrocyte precursor cells differentiation in vitro, and increased myelin repair in vivo	[133]
2015	In vivo	Cerium oxide NPs (nanoceria)	Lenalidomide	Combination therapy ameliorated EAE symptoms and inflammatory responses in mice models	[134]
2012	In vitro, In vivo	Gold NPs	$MOG_{35–55}$ and 2-(1′H-indole-3′-carbonyl)-thiazole-4-carboxylic acid methyl ester (ITE)	Promoted T_{reg} differentiation and suppressed development of EAE in mouse models	[135]
2012	In vivo	Polyamidoamine dendrimers	N-acetyl-L-cysteine (NAC)	Suppression of neuroinflammation, which might benefit MS treatment	[136]

(continued)

Table 4 (continued)

Year	Study type	Nanoplatform	Drug	Result	Reference
2011	In vivo	Magnetic NPs	–	Magnetic NPs are effective tools for gene delivery to rat oligodendrocyte precursor cells derived for transplantation therapies	[137]
2010	In vivo	Polyamidoamine dendrimers	–	Dendrimers can localize in activated microglia and astrocytes	[138]
2009	In vivo	PEGylated liposomes	Tempamine	Better brain targeting and inhibition of EAE in mice models	[139]
2009	In vivo	Cationic liposomes	–	Cationic (but not anionic) liposomes target acute neuroinflammatory sites in EAE rats	[140]
2008	In vitro, In vivo	NMDA receptor antagonist conjugated-ABS-75 compound (fullerene derivative)		Reduced axonal loss, oxidative injury, and disease progression in NOD mice	[118]
2000	In vivo	Albumin NPs	–	Albumin NPs can effectively reach lumbar portion of the spinal cord, the optic chiasma, iris, and Purkinje cells of cerebellum	[117]

PLGA: Poly Lactic-co-Glycolic Acid; NP: Nanoparticle; MOG: Myelin oligodendrocyte glycoprotein; EAE: Experimental autoimmune encephalomyelitis; SLN: Solid lipid nanoparticles; MBP: Myelin basic protein; NMDA: N-methyl-D-aspartate receptor; NOC: Non-obese diabetic region of the spinal cord, optic chiasma, iris, and area of the Purkinje cells of the cerebellum [117]. They also showed that macrophages (ED1) and activated microglial cells (OX42) facilitated the distribution of albumin NPs [117]. The study concluded that usage of NPs might help in optimizing the drug dosage as well as confer better BBB permeability while targeting the brain lesions [117]. A 2008 study conducted in Harvard Medical School worked on myelin-oligodendrocyte glycoprotein (MOG) induced-EAE in non-obese diabetic (NOD) mice, for development of a novel MS treatment [118]. Their strategy consisted of administrating a fullerene derivative (ABS-75) attached to a N-methyl-D-aspartate (NMDA) receptor antagonist [118]. The authors reported reduced disease progression, and an alleviation in axonal loss and demyelination in the spinal cord [118]. ABS-75 acted as an antioxidant and was shown to prevent CD11b+ infiltration in the spinal cord [118]. Moreover, in vitro experimentations suggested that ABS-75 could normalize the expression of glutamine synthetase and glutamate transporter under inflammatory insult [118]. Encouragingly, no disturbance in antigen-specific T cell responses was observed [118].

In 2012, Gaillard et al. employed glutathione pegylated (GSH-PEG) liposomes to improve the therapeutic window of methylprednisolone, a glucocorticoid-based anti-inflammatory drug, during MS treatment in EAE rat models [119]. Glutathione was used as it is a brain targeting ligand and is expected to enhance the permeability of the nanoplatform [119]. The results indicated a significant reduction in clinical signs upon administration of GSH-PEG methylprednisolone upon disease onset, as compared to free methylprednisolone [119]. Also, the finding affirmed the role of glutathione, as PEG liposomes (without GSH) were found to be less effective as compared to GSH-PEG liposomes [119].

In a study in The University of Sydney, immune-modifying particles (IMPs), derived from polystyrene, microdiamonds, or poly(lactic-co-glycolic) acid, were used to modulate inflammatory monocyte-derived effector cells [120]. Monocytes were observed to take up these IMPs via macrophage receptor with collagenous structure (MARCO) [120]. Consequently, no monocyte trafficking to inflammatory sites was observed, while caspase-3-mediated apoptosis was reported [120]. Reduced inflammation and alleviated symptoms were observed in EAE mouse models upon administration of the IMPs [120]. In the same year, Hunter et al. studied the induction of antigen-specific T-cell tolerance in a relapsing–remitting EAE mice model using PLGA NPs [121]. They demonstrated that the conjugate obtained from myelin antigen and NP could efficiently prevent the disease, as well as enervate the disease symptoms [121]. Interestingly, this nanoplatform was able to attenuate disease symptoms in both cases: upon administration at the onset or at the peak of the disease [121]. Moreover, the nanoplatform reportedly minimized epitope spreading when administered during remission phase [121]. The action mechanism was proposed to be a significant reduction in populations of TH1 cells, TH17 cells, inflammatory monocytes, and macrophages [121].

In 2015, Binyamin et al. studied the effects of punicic acid, a strong natural antioxidant and a major constituent of pomegranate seed oil (PSO), on MS treatment

[122]. For this, they compared the effects of administering free PSO and nano-formulated PSO, in an EAE mouse model [122]. They observed that nano-PSO was able to exhibit a more desirable effect at lesser concentrations, as compared to free PSO [122]. The action mechanism was suggested to be a marked decrease in demyelination and lipid oxidation in the brain of EAE mouse models [122].

Recently, Gonzalez et al. prepared a nanoformulation made of IFN-β-loaded NPs [123]. This nanoformulation consisted of IFN-β-loaded chitosan/sulfobutylether-β-cyclodextrin NPs and was prepared with the objective to overcome IFN-β treatment limitations, such as low BBB permeability and short half-life [123]. The intranasal administration of IFN-NPs showed significantly better protection than systemic administration of free cytokine against MS in a preclinical model [123]. In addition to ameliorating clinical symptoms, delivery of IFN-β from NPs also recovered motor impairment and neurological damage, and controlled neuroinflammation by regulating cell activation [123]. In another recent study, Pinto et al. studied the effects of SLN encapsulated dimethyl fumarate (DMF; an FDA approved drug for treatment of MS) on EAE induced female C57BL/6J mice model [124]. Upon administration post disease onset, the mice models reportedly displayed lesser weight loss, attenuated clinical symptoms, and reduced inflammation, as compared to control models [124]. Further, the authors reported a beneficial effect of the nanoplatform on pulmonary dysfunction, based on reversal of characteristic lung inflammatory and dysfunction symptoms [124].

In an interesting recent study, Triantafyllakou et al. addressed the limitations of peptide based therapeutics [125–127] by entrapping myelin peptide analogues, based on mouse/rat (rMOG) epitope 35–55 of MOG, in PLGA nanoparticles [128]. The results indicated at an effective reduction in EAE clinical scores and inflammation of the CNS [128]. This type of treatment could offer an alternative and promising strategy against MS.

3 Future Perspectives

Nanotechnology is a ray of hope for CNS diseases because it has the potential to overcome the limitations of current and conventional therapeutic approaches [141]. Multiple recent studies have focused on targeted drug delivery to the brain using the nanostructures in order to treat CNS disorders like brain tumors, epilepsy, meningitis, and multiple sclerosis. However, despite the aforementioned advantages, there are still some limitations and challenges, including low transfection efficacy, batch-to-batch fluctuation, poor drug loading capacity and entrapment efficiency, low biocompatibility, low biodegradation, low immunogenicity, scale-up difficulties, and particle–particle aggregation [142, 143]. Further, polycationic NPs may trigger osmotic swelling and lysosome rupture, consequently leading to generation of free radicals and mitochondrial dysfunction [143]. Moreover, little is known about the metabolism, clearance, and toxicological profile of various NPs [142].

Additionally, development of an optimized NP platform requires consideration of various physiochemical, topological, and morphological characteristics of NPs, including size, aggregation/agglomeration, shape, surface charge, reactivity, hydrophilicity, surface morphology, and long-term persistence [144]. The need for improvement in fabrication and formulation of NP-based therapeutics is indicated by the low rate of translation from experimental setups to commercial suitability and availability [142].

Therefore, it is prudent to advance current investigations in a step-by-step manner and to further evaluate their outcomes in order to develop more beneficial approaches that can be translated to the clinic for the treatment of various CNS disorders.

Acknowledgements The authors would like to thank the scientific community.

Authors Contributions Writing—original draft preparation, Formal analysis and investigation: **Palak Singhal**, **Shweta Kumari**; Writing—original draft preparation: **Rudhvi Jain**; Writing—original draft preparation: **Aman Bhushan**; Writing - review and editing, Conceptualization, Supervision: **Sahil Jain.**

Funding The authors declare that no funds, grants, or other support were received during the preparation of this manuscript.

Competing Interests The authors have no relevant financial or non-financial interests to disclose.

References

1. Li Q et al (2022) Recent trends in the development of hydrogel therapeutics for the treatment of central nervous system disorders. NPG Asia Mater 14(1):1–14
2. Domínguez A et al (2013) Central nervous system diseases and the role of the blood-brain barrier in their treatment. Neurosci Discov 1(1):3
3. Chin JH, Vora N (2014) The global burden of neurologic diseases. Neurology 83(4):349–351
4. WHO. Disability-adjusted life years (DALYs). [cited 2022 15 Dec]. https://www.who.int/data/gho/indicator-metadata-registry/imr-details/158
5. PAHO (2021) The burden of Neurological conditions in the Region of the Americas, 2000–2019. [cited 2022 15 Dec]. https://www.paho.org/en/enlace/burden-neurological-conditions
6. WHO (2022) Follow-up to the political declaration of the third high-level meeting of the General Assembly on the prevention and control of non-communicable diseases. [cited 2022 15 Dec]; https://apps.who.int/gb/ebwha/pdf_files/WHA75/A75_10Add4-en.pdf
7. Society NBT (2020) Brain tumor facts. [cited 2022 14 Dec]. https://braintumor.org/brain-tumors/about-brain-tumors/brain-tumor-facts/.
8. Spiciarich MC et al (2019) Global health and epilepsy: update and future directions. Curr Neurol Neurosci Rep 19(6):1–8
9. WHO (2022) Epilepsy [cited 2022 7th Nov]. https://www.who.int/news-room/fact-sheets/detail/epilepsy
10. Torpy JM, Lynm C, Glass RM (2007) Meningitis. JAMA 297(1):122–122
11. Walton C et al (2020) Rising prevalence of multiple sclerosis worldwide: insights from the Atlas of MS, third edition. Mult Scler 26(14):1816–1821
12. Palmer AM (2010) The role of the blood–CNS barrier in CNS disorders and their treatment. Neurobiol Dis 37(1):3–12
13. Lochhead JJ et al (2020) Structure, function, and regulation of the blood-brain barrier tight junction in central nervous system disorders. Front Physiol 11:914

14. Archie SR, Al Shoyaib A, Cucullo L (2021) Blood-brain barrier dysfunction in CNS disorders and putative therapeutic targets: an overview. Pharmaceutics 13(11):1779
15. Upadhyay RK (2014) Drug delivery systems, CNS protection, and the blood brain barrier. Biomed Res Int 2014:869269
16. Domínguez A, Suárez-Merino B, Goñi-de-Cerio F (2014) Nanoparticles and blood-brain barrier: the key to central nervous system diseases. J Nanosci Nanotechnol 14(1):766–779
17. Girdhar V et al (2018) Nanocarriers for drug delivery: mini review. Current Nanomed (Formerly: Recent Patents on Nanomedicine) 8(2):88–99
18. Masserini M (2013) Nanoparticles for brain drug delivery. ISRN Biochem 2013:238428
19. Rosenfeld SS, Massey EW (2019) Epidemiology of primary brain tumor. Neuroepidemiology 121–144
20. Louis DN et al (2016) The 2016 world health organization classification of tumors of the central nervous system: a summary. Acta Neuropathol 131(6):803–820
21. Preusser M et al (2011) Current concepts and management of glioblastoma. Ann Neurol 70(1):9–21
22. Grech N et al (2020) Rising incidence of glioblastoma multiforme in a well-defined population. Cureus 12(5):e8195
23. Patel AP et al (2019) Global, regional, and national burden of brain and other CNS cancer, 1990–2016: a systematic analysis for the global burden of disease study 2016. Lancet Neurol 18(4):376–393
24. Stupp R et al (2005) Radiotherapy plus concomitant and adjuvant temozolomide for glioblastoma. N Engl J Med 352(10):987–996
25. Abbruzzese C et al (2022) Molecular biology in glioblastoma multiforme treatment. MDPI 1850
26. Arvanitis CD, Ferraro GB, Jain RK (2020) The blood–brain barrier and blood–tumour barrier in brain tumours and metastases. Nat Rev Cancer 20(1):26–41
27. Saraiva C et al (2016) Nanoparticle-mediated brain drug delivery: overcoming blood–brain barrier to treat neurodegenerative diseases. J Control Release 235:34–47
28. Debele TA, Yeh C-F, Su W-P (2020) Cancer immunotherapy and application of nanoparticles in cancers immunotherapy as the delivery of immunotherapeutic agents and as the immunomodulators. Cancers 12(12):3773
29. Cheng Y et al (2014) Blood-brain barrier permeable gold nanoparticles: an efficient delivery platform for enhanced malignant glioma therapy and imaging. Small 10(24):5137–5150
30. Richard S et al (2017) Iron oxide nanoparticle surface decorated with cRGD peptides for magnetic resonance imaging of brain tumors. Biochim Biophys Acta (BBA)-General Subjects 1861(6):1515–1520
31. Kuo Y-C, Hsu C-C (2017) Anti-melanotransferrin and apolipoprotein E on doxorubicin-loaded cationic solid lipid nanoparticles for pharmacotherapy of glioblastoma multiforme. J Taiwan Inst Chem Eng 77:10–20
32. Liu Y et al (2018) Noninvasive brain tumor imaging using red emissive carbonized polymer dots across the blood–brain barrier. ACS Omega 3(7):7888–7896
33. Wahab R et al (2019) Gold quantum dots impair the tumorigenic potential of glioma stem-like cells via β-catenin downregulation in vitro. Int J Nanomed 14:1131
34. Zhao L et al (2019) Chlorotoxin peptide-functionalized polyethylenimine-entrapped gold nanoparticles for glioma SPECT/CT imaging and radionuclide therapy. J Nanobiotechnol 17(1):1–13
35. Liyanage PY et al (2020) Pediatric glioblastoma target-specific efficient delivery of gemcitabine across the blood–brain barrier via carbon nitride dots. Nanoscale 12(14):7927–7938
36. Norouzi M et al (2020) Doxorubicin-loaded iron oxide nanoparticles for glioblastoma therapy: a combinational approach for enhanced delivery of nanoparticles. Sci Rep 10(1):1–18
37. Perini G et al (2021) Functionalized graphene quantum dots modulate malignancy of glioblastoma multiforme by downregulating neurospheres formation. C 7(1):4
38. Neshastehriz A et al (2018) Investigating the therapeutic effects of alginate nanogel co-loaded with gold nanoparticles and cisplatin on U87-MG human glioblastoma cells. Anti-Cancer Agents Med Chem (Formerly Current Med Chem Anti Cancer Agents) 18(6):882–890

39. Wu M et al (2016) Vincristine and temozolomide combined chemotherapy for the treatment of glioma: a comparison of solid lipid nanoparticles and nanostructured lipid carriers for dual drugs delivery. Drug Deliv 23(8):2720–2725
40. Panja S et al (2016) Metal ion ornamented ultrafast light-sensitive nanogel for potential in vivo cancer therapy. Chem Mater 28(23):8598–8610
41. Xu H-L et al (2016) Glioma-targeted superparamagnetic iron oxide nanoparticles as drug-carrying vehicles for theranostic effects. Nanoscale 8(29):14222–14236
42. Bastiancich C et al (2016) Lauroyl-gemcitabine-loaded lipid nanocapsule hydrogel for the treatment of glioblastoma. J Control Release 225:283–293
43. Shirakura T, Ray A, Kopelman R (2016) Polyethylenimine incorporation into hydrogel nanomatrices for enhancing nanoparticle-assisted chemotherapy. RSC Adv 6(53):48016–48024
44. Suganami A et al (2015) Liposomally formulated phospholipid-conjugated indocyanine green for intra-operative brain tumor detection and resection. Int J Pharm 496(2):401–406
45. Fourniols T et al (2015) Temozolomide-loaded photopolymerizable PEG-DMA-based hydrogel for the treatment of glioblastoma. J Control Release 210:95–104
46. Jain D et al (2016) Surface-coated PLA nanoparticles loaded with temozolomide for improved brain deposition and potential treatment of gliomas: development, characterization and in vivo studies. Drug Deliv 23(3):989–1006
47. Ruan S et al (2015) Tumor microenvironment sensitive doxorubicin delivery and release to glioma using angiopep-2 decorated gold nanoparticles. Biomaterials 37:425–435
48. Chung EJ et al (2014) Fibrin-binding, peptide amphiphile micelles for targeting glioblastoma. Biomaterials 35(4):1249–1256
49. Jiang L et al (2013) pH/temperature sensitive magnetic nanogels conjugated with Cy5. 5-labled lactoferrin for MR and fluorescence imaging of glioma in rats. Biomaterials 34(30):7418–7428
50. Meenach SA et al (2013) Characterization of PEG–iron oxide hydrogel nanocomposites for dual hyperthermia and paclitaxel delivery. J Biomater Sci Polym Ed 24(9):1112–1126
51. Liu L et al (2011) Silver nanocrystals sensitize magnetic-nanoparticle-mediated thermo-induced killing of cancer cells. Acta Biochim Biophys Sin 43(4):316–323
52. Chen H et al (2011) Lactoferrin modified doxorubicin-loaded procationic liposomes for the treatment of gliomas. Eur J Pharm Sci 44(1–2):164–173
53. Knowles JK et al (2022) Precision medicine for genetic epilepsy on the horizon: recent advances, present challenges, and suggestions for continued progress. Epilepsia 63(10):2461–2475
54. French JA, Gazzola DM (2011) New generation antiepileptic drugs: what do they offer in terms of improved tolerability and safety? Ther Adv Drug Saf 2(4):141–158
55. Falcicchia C, Simonato M, Verlengia G (2018) New tools for epilepsy therapy. Front Cell Neurosci 12:147
56. Löscher W, Schmidt D (2011) Modern antiepileptic drug development has failed to deliver: ways out of the current dilemma. Epilepsia 52(4):657–678
57. El-Zaafarany GM et al (2018) A tailored thermosensitive PLGA-PEG-PLGA/emulsomes composite for enhanced oxcarbazepine brain delivery via the nasal route. Pharmaceutics 10(4):217
58. Kaur S et al (2018) Bioengineered PLGA-chitosan nanoparticles for brain targeted intranasal delivery of antiepileptic TRH analogues. Chem Eng J 346:630–639
59. Musumeci T et al (2018) Oxcarbazepine free or loaded PLGA nanoparticles as effective intranasal approach to control epileptic seizures in rodents. Eur J Pharm Biopharm 133:309–320
60. Abbas H, Refai H, El Sayed N (2018) Superparamagnetic iron oxide–loaded lipid nanocarriers incorporated in thermosensitive in situ gel for magnetic brain targeting of clonazepam. J Pharm Sci 107(8):2119–2127
61. Montoto SS et al (2018) Carbamazepine-loaded solid lipid nanoparticles and nanostructured lipid carriers: physicochemical characterization and in vitro/in vivo evaluation. Colloids Surf, B 167:73–81

62. Iqbal R et al (2019) Design and development of letrozole nanoemulsion: a comparative evaluation of brain targeted nanoemulsion with free letrozole against status epilepticus and neurodegeneration in mice. Int J Pharm 565:20–32
63. Yilmaz CU et al (2020) Targeted delivery of lacosamide-conjugated gold nanoparticles into the brain in temporal lobe epilepsy in rats. Life Sci 257:118081
64. Ahmad N et al (2020) Quantification and evaluations of catechin hydrate polymeric nanoparticles used in brain targeting for the treatment of epilepsy. Pharmaceutics 12(3):203
65. Parashar AK, Kurmi B, Patel P (2021) Preparation and characterization of ligand anchored polymeric nanoparticles for the treatment of epilepsy. Pharmaspire 13(1):1–5
66. Wu D et al (2022) Nanoengineered on-demand drug delivery system improves efficacy of pharmacotherapy for epilepsy. Sci Adv 8(2):eabm3381
67. Sahin H et al (2022) Protective effects of intranasally administrated oxytocin-loaded nanoparticles on pentylenetetrazole-kindling epilepsy in terms of seizure severity, memory, neurogenesis, and neuronal damage. ACS Chem Neurosci 13(13):1923–1937
68. Shah P et al (2021) PLGA nanoparticles for nose to brain delivery of clonazepam: formulation, optimization by 32 factorial design, in vitro and in vivo evaluation. Curr Drug Deliv 18(6):805–824
69. Khan N et al (2020) Nanostructured lipid carriers-mediated brain delivery of carbamazepine for improved in vivo anticonvulsant and anxiolytic activity. Int J Pharm 577:119033
70. Ahmad N et al (2020) A bioanalytical UHPLC based method used for the quantification of thymoquinone-loaded-PLGA-nanoparticles in the treatment of epilepsy. BMC Chem 14(1):1–15
71. Huang R et al (2020) Solid lipid nanoparticles enhanced the neuroprotective role of curcumin against epilepsy through activation of Bcl-2 family and P38 MAPK pathways. ACS Chem Neurosci 11(13):1985–1995
72. Zaman RU et al (2018) Nanoparticle formulations that allow for sustained delivery and brain targeting of the neuropeptide oxytocin. Int J Pharm 548(1):698–706
73. Praveen A et al (2019) Lamotrigine encapsulated intra-nasal nanoliposome formulation for epilepsy treatment: Formulation design, characterization and nasal toxicity study. Colloids Surf, B 174:553–562
74. Cano A et al (2018) Epigallocatechin-3-gallate loaded PEGylated-PLGA nanoparticles: a new anti-seizure strategy for temporal lobe epilepsy. Nanomed Nanotechnol Biol Med 14(4):1073–1085
75. Liu S, Yang S, Ho PC (2018) Intranasal administration of carbamazepine-loaded carboxymethyl chitosan nanoparticles for drug delivery to the brain. Asian J Pharm Sci 13(1):72–81
76. El-Zaafarany GM et al (2016) Identifying lipidic emulsomes for improved oxcarbazepine brain targeting: in vitro and rat in vivo studies. Int J Pharm 503(1–2):127–140
77. Bohrey S, Chourasiya V, Pandey A (2016) Polymeric nanoparticles containing diazepam: preparation, optimization, characterization, in-vitro drug release and release kinetic study. Nano Converg 3(1):1–7
78. Sharma D et al (2015) Nose-to-brain delivery of PLGA-diazepam nanoparticles. AAPS PharmSciTech 16(5):1108–1121
79. Sharma D et al (2014) Formulation and optimization of polymeric nanoparticles for intranasal delivery of lorazepam using Box-Behnken design: in vitro and in vivo evaluation. BioMed Res Int 2014
80. Yasir M, Sara UVS (2014) Solid lipid nanoparticles for nose to brain delivery of haloperidol: in vitro drug release and pharmacokinetics evaluation. Acta Pharm Sin B 4(6):454–463
81. Singh AP, Saraf SK, Saraf SA (2012) SLN approach for nose-to-brain delivery of alprazolam. Drug Deliv Transl Res 2(6):498–507
82. WHO (2021) Meningitis. [cited 2022 8th Nov]. https://www.who.int/news-room/fact-sheets/detail/meningitis
83. Arenas J, Tommassen J (2017) Meningococcal biofilm formation: let's stick together. Trends Microbiol 25(2):113–124

84. Reddy KB (2019) In vitro-in vivo characterization of Oleuropein loaded nanostructured lipid carriers in the treatment of streptococcus pneumoniae induced meningitis. Asian J Pharm (AJP) 13(02)
85. Xu N et al (2011) Efficacy of intravenous amphotericin B-polybutylcyanoacrylate nanoparticles against cryptococcal meningitis in mice. Int J Nanomed 6:905
86. Shao K et al (2012) A brain-vectored angiopep-2 based polymeric micelles for the treatment of intracranial fungal infection. Biomaterials 33(28):6898–6907
87. Garcia CB, Shi D, Webster TJ (2017) Tat-functionalized liposomes for the treatment of meningitis: an in vitro study. Int J Nanomed 12:3009
88. Hong W et al (2018) Brain-targeted delivery of PEGylated nano-bacitracin A against Penicillin-sensitive and-resistant Pneumococcal meningitis: formulated with RVG29 and Pluronic® P85 unimers. Drug Delivery 25(1):1886–1897
89. Eid HM et al (2019) Transfersomal nanovesicles for nose-to-brain delivery of ofloxacin for better management of bacterial meningitis: formulation, optimization by Box-Behnken design, characterization and in vivo pharmacokinetic study. J Drug Deliv Sci Technol 54:101304
90. Du W et al (2019) Development of nose-to-brain delivery of ketoconazole by nanostructured lipid carriers against cryptococcal meningoencephalitis in mice. Colloids Surf, B 183:110446
91. Hady MA, Sayed OM, Akl MA (2020) Brain uptake and accumulation of new levofloxacin-doxycycline combination through the use of solid lipid nanoparticles: formulation; optimization and in-vivo evaluation. Colloids Surf, B 193:111076
92. Nair KG, Velmurugan R, Sukumaran SK (2020) Formulation and optimization of ansamycin-loaded polymeric nanoparticles using response surface methodology for bacterial meningitis. BioNanoScience 10(1):279–291
93. Thammasit P et al (2021) Targeted propolis-loaded poly (butyl) cyanoacrylate nanoparticles: an alternative drug delivery tool for the treatment of cryptococcal meningitis. Front Pharmacol 2198
94. Zhang S et al (2020) Borneol and poly (ethylene glycol) dual modified BSA nanoparticles as an itraconazole vehicle for brain targeting. Int J Pharm 575:119002
95. Wang Q et al (2019) Targeted theranostic of cryptococcal encephalitis by a novel polypyridyl ruthenium complex. Mol Pharm 17(1):145–154
96. Garvey E et al (2018) The novel fungal CYP51 inhibitor VT-1598 is efficacious alone and in combination with liposomal amphotericin B in a murine model of cryptococcal meningitis. J Antimicrob Chemother 73(10):2815–2822
97. Lestner J et al (2017) Experimental models of short courses of liposomal amphotericin B for induction therapy for cryptococcal meningitis. Antimicrob Agents Chemother 61(6):e00090-e117
98. Ćurić A, Möschwitzer JP, Fricker G (2017) Development and characterization of novel highly-loaded itraconazole poly (butyl cyanoacrylate) polymeric nanoparticles. Eur J Pharm Biopharm 114:175–185
99. Tang X et al (2015) Anti-transferrin receptor-modified amphotericin B-loaded PLA–PEG nanoparticles cure Candidal meningitis and reduce drug toxicity. Int J Nanomed 10:6227
100. Shao K et al (2015) Functionalized nanoscale micelles with brain targeting ability and intercellular microenvironment biosensitivity for anti-intracranial infection applications. Adv Healthcare Mater 4(2):291–300
101. Ribes S et al (2013) Multivalent choline dendrimers increase phagocytosis of Streptococcus pneumoniae R6 by microglial cells. Chemotherapy 59(2):138–142
102. O'Connor L et al (2013) Pharmacodynamics of liposomal amphotericin B and flucytosine for cryptococcal meningoencephalitis: safe and effective regimens for immunocompromised patients. J Infect Dis 208(2):351–361
103. Gazzoni AF et al (2012) Efficacy of intrathecal administration of liposomal amphotericin B combined with voriconazole in a murine model of cryptococcal meningitis. Int J Antimicrob Agents 39(3):223–227

104. Shao K et al (2010) Angiopep-2 modified PE-PEG based polymeric micelles for amphotericin B delivery targeted to the brain. J Control Release 147(1):118–126
105. Wang H et al (2010) The efficacy of self-assembled cationic antimicrobial peptide nanoparticles against Cryptococcus neoformans for the treatment of meningitis. Biomaterials 31(10):2874–2881
106. Liu R et al (2022) Autoreactive lymphocytes in multiple sclerosis: Pathogenesis and treatment target. Front Immunol 13:996469
107. Spencer JI, Bell JS, DeLuca GC (2018) Vascular pathology in multiple sclerosis: reframing pathogenesis around the blood-brain barrier. J Neurol Neurosurg Psychiatry 89(1):42–52
108. Pinheiro MAL et al (2016) Immune cell trafficking across the barriers of the central nervous system in multiple sclerosis and stroke. Biochim Biophys Acta (BBA)-Mol Basis Dis 1862(3):461–471
109. Buiter HJ, Derijks L, Mulder CJ (2019) Cladribine repurposed in multiple sclerosis: making a fortune out of a generic drug. British Medical Journal Publishing Group, pp 246–247
110. Syed YY (2018) Ocrelizumab: a review in multiple sclerosis. CNS Drugs 32(9):883–890
111. Havrdova E, Horakova D, Kovarova I (2015) Alemtuzumab in the treatment of multiple sclerosis: key clinical trial results and considerations for use. Ther Adv Neurol Disord 8(1):31–45
112. Serra P, Santamaria P (2015) Nanoparticle-based autoimmune disease therapy. Clin Immunol 160(1):3–13
113. Rahiman N et al (2022) Recent advancements in nanoparticle-mediated approaches for restoration of multiple sclerosis. J Control Release 343:620–644
114. Wohlfart S, Gelperina S, Kreuter J (2012) Transport of drugs across the blood–brain barrier by nanoparticles. J Control Release 161(2):264–273
115. Zhou Y et al (2018) Crossing the blood-brain barrier with nanoparticles. J Control Release 270:290–303
116. Tosi G, Duskey J, Kreuter J (2020) Nanoparticles as carriers for drug delivery of macromolecules across the blood-brain barrier. Expert Opin Drug Deliv 17(1):23–32
117. Merodio M et al (2000) Distribution of albumin nanoparticles in animals induced with the experimental allergic encephalomyelitis. J Drug Target 8(5):289–303
118. Basso AS et al (2008) Reversal of axonal loss and disability in a mouse model of progressive multiple sclerosis. J Clin Investig 118(4):1532–1543
119. Gaillard PJ et al (2012) Enhanced brain delivery of liposomal methylprednisolone improved therapeutic efficacy in a model of neuroinflammation. J Control Release 164(3):364–369
120. Getts DR et al (2014) Therapeutic inflammatory monocyte modulation using immune-modifying microparticles. Sci Transl Med 6(219):219ra7–219ra7
121. Hunter Z et al (2014) A biodegradable nanoparticle platform for the induction of antigen-specific immune tolerance for treatment of autoimmune disease. ACS Nano 8(3):2148–2160
122. Binyamin O et al (2015) Treatment of a multiple sclerosis animal model by a novel nanodrop formulation of a natural antioxidant. Int J Nanomed 10:7165
123. González LF et al (2021) Intranasal delivery of interferon-β-loaded nanoparticles induces control of neuroinflammation in a preclinical model of multiple sclerosis: a promising simple, effective, non-invasive, and low-cost therapy. J Control Release 331:443–459
124. Pinto BF et al (2022) Inhalation of dimethyl fumarate-encapsulated solid lipid nanoparticles attenuate clinical signs of experimental autoimmune encephalomyelitis and pulmonary inflammatory dysfunction in mice. Clin Sci 136(1):81–101
125. Jain S, Khaiboullina SF, Baranwal M (2020) Immunological perspective for Ebola virus infection and various treatment measures taken to fight the disease. Pathogens 9(10):850
126. Jain S, Baranwal M (2021) Immunoinformatics aided design of peptide-based vaccines against ebolaviruses. In: Litwack G (ed) Vitamins and hormones. Academic Press, pp 157–187
127. Jain S, Baranwal M (2019) Computational analysis in designing T cell epitopes enriched peptides of Ebola glycoprotein exhibiting strong binding interaction with HLA molecules. J Theor Biol 465:34–44

128. Triantafyllakou I et al (2022) Development of PLGA nanoparticles with a glycosylated myelin oligodendrocyte glycoprotein epitope (MOG35–55) against experimental autoimmune encephalomyelitis (EAE). Mol Pharm
129. Krienke C et al (2021) A noninflammatory mRNA vaccine for treatment of experimental autoimmune encephalomyelitis. Science 371(6525):145–153
130. Dolati S et al (2018) Nanocurcumin is a potential novel therapy for multiple sclerosis by influencing inflammatory mediators. Pharmacol Rep 70(6):1158–1167
131. Derkus B et al (2017) Simultaneous quantification of Myelin basic protein and Tau proteins in cerebrospinal fluid and serum of multiple sclerosis patients using nanoimmunosensor. Biosens Bioelectron 89:781–788
132. Tostanoski LH et al (2016) Design of polyelectrolyte multilayers to promote immunological tolerance. ACS Nano 10(10):9334–9345
133. Rittchen S et al (2015) Myelin repair in vivo is increased by targeting oligodendrocyte precursor cells with nanoparticles encapsulating leukaemia inhibitory factor (LIF). Biomaterials 56:78–85
134. Eitan E et al (2015) Combination therapy with lenalidomide and nanoceria ameliorates CNS autoimmunity. Exp Neurol 273:151–160
135. Yeste A et al (2012) Nanoparticle-mediated codelivery of myelin antigen and a tolerogenic small molecule suppresses experimental autoimmune encephalomyelitis. Proc Natl Acad Sci U S A 109(28):11270–11275
136. Kannan S et al (2012) Dendrimer-based postnatal therapy for neuroinflammation and cerebral palsy in a rabbit model. Sci Transl Med 4(130):130ra46
137. Jenkins SI et al (2011) Magnetic nanoparticle-mediated gene transfer to oligodendrocyte precursor cell transplant populations is enhanced by magnetofection strategies. ACS Nano 5(8):6527–6538
138. Dai H et al (2010) Intrinsic targeting of inflammatory cells in the brain by polyamidoamine dendrimers upon subarachnoid administration. Nanomedicine (Lond) 5(9):1317–1329
139. Kizelsztein P et al (2009) Pegylated nanoliposomes remote-loaded with the antioxidant tempamine ameliorate experimental autoimmune encephalomyelitis. J Neuroimmunol 213(1–2):20–25
140. Cavaletti G et al (2009) Cationic liposomes target sites of acute neuroinflammation in experimental autoimmune encephalomyelitis. Mol Pharm 6(5):1363–1370
141. Zhu FD et al (2021) Nanoparticles: a hope for the treatment of inflammation in CNS. Front Pharmacol 12:683935
142. Yetisgin AA et al (2020) Therapeutic nanoparticles and their targeted delivery applications. Molecules 25(9)
143. Ahlawat J et al (2020) Nanocarriers as potential drug delivery candidates for overcoming the blood-brain barrier: challenges and possibilities. ACS Omega 5(22):12583–12595
144. Joudeh N, Linke D (2022) Nanoparticle classification, physicochemical properties, characterization, and applications: a comprehensive review for biologists. J Nanobiotechnol 20(1):262

Nano Drug Delivery Therapy—A Novel Approach Towards Common Neurological Disorders

Targeted Therapy for Neurological Disorders Using Nanomaterial-Based Drug Delivery Vehicle

Manu Sharma, Tapasvi Gupta, Namita Gupta, Reetika Rawat, Namita Badoniya, Easha Pandey, and Sheelu Sharma

Abstract Globally, neurological disorders possess great impact on human health and social system. The available current medical therapies have increased the survival period. Although insufficient for complete cure of neurological disorders due to biological barriers like blood–brain barrier (BBB), blood-cerebrospinal fluid barrier and efflux proteins. In respect to present context, nanomaterials are receiving amazing recognition due to their unique physicochemical properties. The biocompatible nanomaterial based targeted therapies such as gene, dendritic cell, receptor, protein, molecular targeted etc. have shown promising results for the management of neurological disorders. Engineering of nanomaterials to deliver therapeutic agents across blood–brain barrier and specifically to target cells have intensified the hope of cure of neurological disorders. However, short-term and long-term effects of nanomaterials based targeted therapies in humans need to be studied to ensure their safety and potential in clinics. Henceforth, this chapter discusses the various approaches based on targeted therapies using nanomaterials for effective comprehension of their utility in terms of current prospective.

Keywords Nanomaterials · Targeted therapy · Barriers · Neurological disorders

1 Introduction

Neurological disorders are the illness of central and peripheral nervous system including Alzheimer's, Parkinsonism, dementia, epilepsy, stroke, brain tumor, brain injury, multiple sclerosis and headache. These disorders possess paramount assault on human health and social system worldwide. Neurological diseases are the extremely

M. Sharma (✉) · T. Gupta · N. Gupta · R. Rawat · N. Badoniya · E. Pandey
Department of Pharmacy, Banasthali Vidyapith, Banasthali, Rajasthan 304022, India
e-mail: smanu@banasthali.in

S. Sharma
PDUNIPPD, Delhi University, New Delhi 110002, India

S. K. Rath et al. (eds.), *Nanomaterials for Drug Delivery and Neurological Diseases Management*, Smart Nanomaterials Technology,
https://doi.org/10.1007/978-981-97-0308-1_7

challenging area appealing for attentiveness of researchers. Since neurological disorders are the leading cause contributing to 11.6 -45% of unresolved issue of global disability-adjusted life-years (DALYs) and 16.5% of deaths [1]. Global burden of neurological diseases is also growing continuously with respect to time. Efforts have been made continuously to understand the cause and pathogenesis of these neurological disorders. However, major gaps still exist to find out the solution for effective management of neurological diseases. Available therapeutic treatment and advanced therapies improve the survival duration but are inadequate to accomplish the cure of neurological disorders. The protective mechanisms of central nervous system offer crucial barriers in management of neurological diseases [2]. Furthermore, non-targeted delivery of therapeutic moieties and diagnostic agent can show harmful effects on neuronal cells and glial cells. These are highly sensitive cellular elements of CNS involved in maintenance of homeostasis and brain functioning. So, considering above facts it is a top priority to design and develop novel and targeted delivery system loaded with therapeutic moieties for instant and long-lasting response for management of the neurological disorders [3].

2 Barriers Encountered During Management of Neurological Diseases

The major neurological disorders are related to central nervous system. In previous few decades, broad range of therapeutics with great potential has been discovered to treat various types of neurological disorders, but their productive success is still limited due to complex architecture of central nervous system [4]. Numerous developed drugs had failed in clinical trial due to their limited permeability to the brain parenchyma due to the presence of different peripheral barriers. These barriers include mainly blood–brain barrier (BBB), blood-cerebrospinal fluid barriers (BCSFB) and efflux proteins [5].

2.1 Blood–Brain Barrier (BBB)

Human brain is protected by a membrane called blood brain barrier (BBB) that regulate the proper functioning of brain and control the diffusion of drug from blood across the wall. It is a physical barrier separating the central nervous system from systemic circulation. This border is also well suited to protect brain neurons against toxic and harmful molecules present in blood. BBB is selectively permeable to the substances such as water, lipophilic drugs and nutrients through passive transport mechanism. Additionally, it also maintains the fluid level of the brain as per the requirement and helpful in the limited transport of fluid and salt to the extracellular matrix [6]. BBB is composed of three distinctive cells i.e., endothelial cells, astrocytes and pericytes.

The tight junctions (TJs) formed by joining of astrocytes and endothelial cells regulate the brain permeability. Briefly the main characteristics of these TJs are to restrict the permeation of ions, macromolecules, and polar compounds via paracellular diffusion pathways into the brain. Various proteins present along TJs such as occludins and claudins maintain the integrity and proper functioning of BBB [7].

Astrocytes are also known as astrocytic glial cells, star-shaped, comprise 90–98% of brain microvasculature and found on basal lamina at the parenchymal side having end-feet projection to associate to endothelial cells (ECs). Astrocytic end feet projections are helpful in maintaining the integrity and tightness of BBB by providing biochemical support required for the maintenance of TJs and ECs. It also promotes the formation of tight junction between ECs. Astrocytes also regulate the homeostatic maintenance of neurotransmitter into the brain as well as ensure the appropriate supply of several required nutrients for nerve tissue. These cells also act as a safeguard to the central nervous system by removing out the waste or toxic metabolites [8].

Pericytes are also vital cellular constituents of BBB having important role in formation of blood vessels, maintenance of BBB, regulation of immune cells entry to the central nervous system [9].

2.2 *Blood-Cerebrospinal Fluid Barrier (BCSFB)*

Choroid plexus formed by a group of ependymal cells operate as a barrier in the CNS by isolating the blood from cerebrospinal fluid. The ependymal cells fold themselves on brain surface to form a double layer known as arachnoid membrane which is selectively permeable for hydrophilic molecules. So, combination of choroid plexus and arachnoid membrane forms a barrier between blood and CSF which is called blood-cerebrospinal fluid barrier (BCSFB). This additional barrier increases CNS complexity and hinders the delivery of therapeutic agents to CNS [10].

2.3 *Efflux Protein*

The availability of several types of efflux transporters significantly contributes in the poor permeation of therapeutic substance to the brain. These efflux proteins are mostly found on the luminal membrane of the epithelial cells of BBB and act as a clearance system. Efflux transport at the blood–brain barrier (BBB) limits the brain tissue exposure to a variety of potential therapeutic agents, including compounds that are relatively lipophilic [11]. The most well-investigated brain efflux transmembrane glycoprotein, P-Glycoprotein (Pgp, Mo weight 170 kDa) is a, ATP-dependent efflux transporter conferring multidrug resistance. Although, regulation of Pgp expression and function in CNS is not well-understood till yet [12].

3 Transport Across BBB

Various kind of transport mechanisms regulate delivery of wide variety of nutrients and therapeutic agents across endothelial transport barrier known as blood brain barrier (Fig. 1). The intercellular cleft between endothelial cells called tight junction facilitates very little paracellular transport of substances. Some essential nutrients enter into the brain via transcellular passage through BBB. The basic requirement for passive diffusion, a most common transport mechanism across BBB is that a molecule should have lipophilic nature with molecular weight < 400–500 Da and less than 9 hydrogen bonds. Several nutrients do not meet above criteria so they follow carrier mediated transport mechanism. Some others mechanism i.e. receptor mediated and adsorptive type transporter is also helpful in promoting transport across BBB. All these mechanism require energy to move molecules against concentration gradients into the brain. However, passive diffusion does not require energy to transport molecules. One another mechanism i.e., efflux transport also works to cross BBB. It acts like a clearance system to move various proteins into blood circulation [13].

Besides the beneficial protective roles of these barriers, they also present obstacles for therapeutic agents to reach to the pharmacological targets located inside brain parenchyma during neurological disorders and brain tumors. One of the important reasons in failing to develop new CNS acting drugs is the inability to design

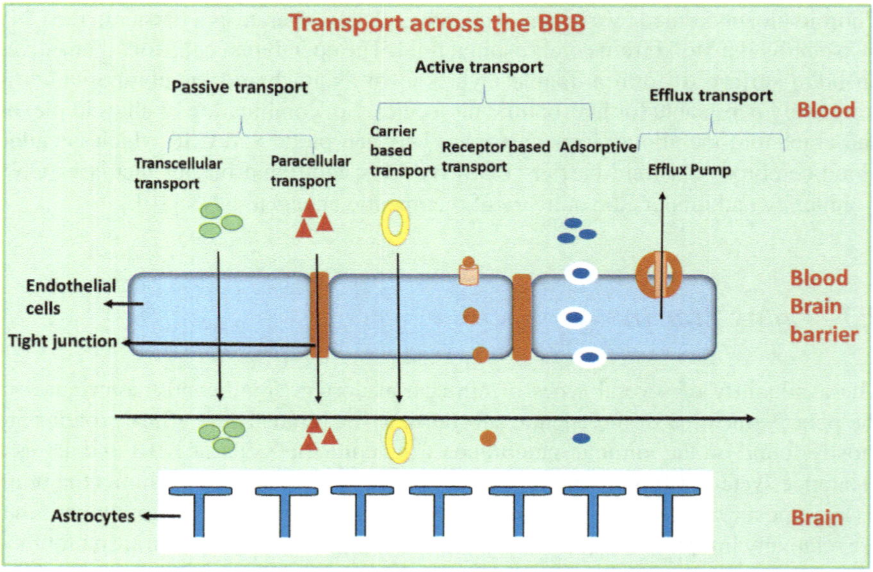

Fig. 1 Various transport mechanisms across blood brain barrier

substances with sufficient capacity to cross BBB and to achieve pharmacologically active concentrations at the respective target sites in brain tissues.

4 Therapies for Neurological Disorders

The development of targeted therapies with safe and accurate amount of active substance to CNS is the prime aim to treat and prevent progression of neurological diseases. The existing therapies cure symptoms but unable to block the advancement of neurological disease. Currently, researchers are working for advancement in therapies employing component of the immune system as therapeutic agents or evolving therapies to target the immune system. Sometimes therapeutic immunomodulation might be beneficial when local immune responses are insufficient or may be damaging [14]. Although, approaches used for managing neurological disorders are to relieve symptoms rather than to regain the quality of life. The application of nanomedicine, a combination of nanotechnology and pharmaceutical science, is a promising approach to selectively enhance permeability across BBB and for targeted drug delivery. A comprehensive range of engineered nanostructures composed of metal, organic or inorganic material like solid lipid nanoparticles (SLNs), liposome, micelles, carbon nanotubes, dendrimers, niosome and nanocapsules are extensively used for controlled and targeted delivery of therapeutic agents. The characteristic features of nanostructures i.e. nano-size, higher surface area to volume ratio, biocompatibility and biodegradability offers various merits in management of chronic disorders by prolonging controlled delivery of drug at target sites [15]. In view of promises of nanomedicine in human diseases management, the present chapter mainly focuses on more efficient targeted therapies for neurological disorders developed utilizing nanomaterial based drug delivery systems [16].

4.1 Immunotherapies

Immunotherapies are widely explored for management of auto-immune, age-associated and non-autoimmune neurodegenerative disorders. A wide category of cells such as immune cells, endothelial cells and fibroblasts are involved in chronic inflammatory disorders reflecting the complexity of neurological conditions. The progression of neurodegenerative disease supports the bloom of immune-based therapies to get rid of cellular immune responses (Fig. 2).

A vivid variety of immunotherapy proposals has been emphasized including:

a. Triggered immune responses, antigen specific via vaccination, gene therapy and cell therapy
b. Alternatively, boosting immune responses, non-antigen specific by cytokine (antibodies) or immunosuppressors [14].

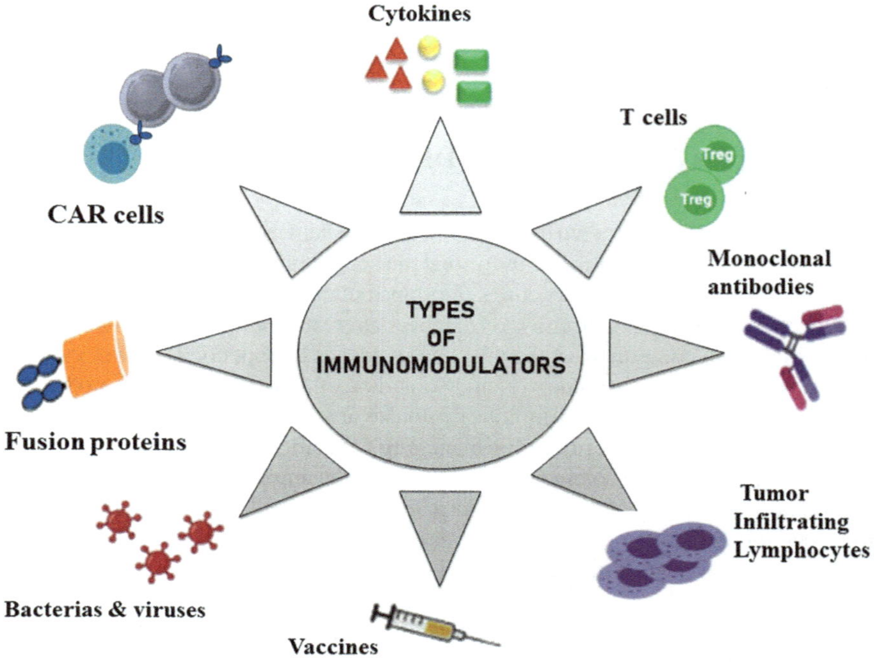

Fig. 2 Types of immunotherapies for various neurological disorders

4.1.1 Vaccine Therapy

Vaccine therapies are the mainstay to instigate robust immune responses via passive or active immunization. Vaccine therapies have flourished for the prevention as well as treatment of neurological disorders associated with auto-immune diseases and cancer of nervous system. Vaccines have likely hindered more diseases than any other medical or public health interventions. The infusion of monoclonal antibodies or specific antigen to promote antibody production or regulate inflammatory responses is the major mechanism of vaccine therapy in neurological disorders management respectively (Fig. 3) [17].

The management of synucleinopathies depends on passive delivery of discrete monoclonal antibodies against distinct areas of α-syn. The intraperitoneal injection of α-syn antibodies which specifically target N-terminal or the central region of α-syn exerted neuroprotective effects by inducing nigral cell death and decreasing activated microglia in the substantia nigra [18]. mAb47 monoclonal antibody has been found effective in reducing intracellular oligomerization of α-syn and levels of α-syn protofibrils in the spinal cord [19, 20]. The active immunization of mice with recombinant human α-syn facilitated production of α-syn antibodies mainly

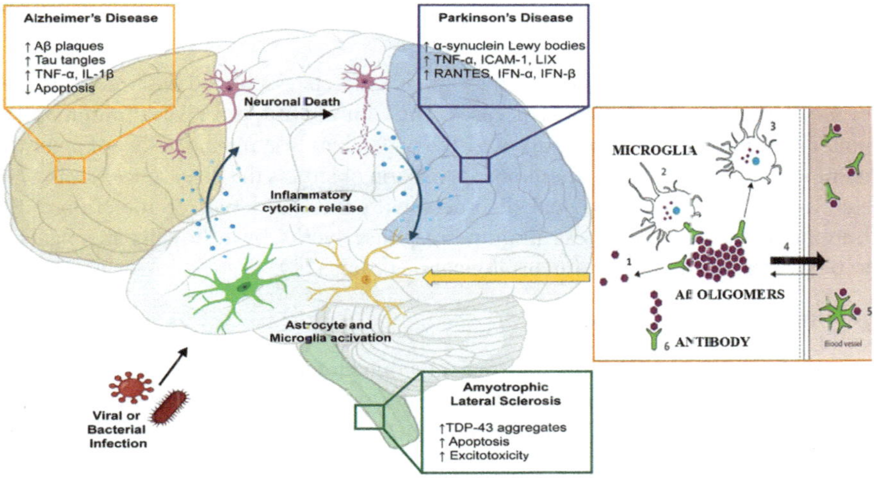

Fig. 3 Various targeting sites of vaccine therapy indicators (Aß antibodies, α-Synuclein, Tau. Amyloid, TNF- α, IFN-ß)

targeting the C-terminus of αsyn with high affinity [21]. AFFITOPE develops anti-α-syn antibodies that infiltered CSF and plasma, target α-syn aggregates and decrease neuronal degeneration of impaired oligomeric α-syn accumulation in neurons [22].

The active phosphorylated tau peptide vaccine activated the generation of anti-tau antibodies responsible for decrement of pathological tau aggregates and Aß depositions. The experimental outcomes revealed the potential use of the tau vaccine against neurodegenerative disorders for clinical application [23]. ACI-35, liposomal-based anti-tau vaccine composed of phosphorylated tau peptide elicited target specific pathological conformers of phosphorylated tau for treatment of neurodegenerative disease. These conformers also evade autoimmune B-cells or T-cells reaction against intracellular protein. [24]. ACI-35 produces 5 times more immunogenicity than its precursors [25].

Anti-Aß antibody targeting the Aß-sequence resulted in the reduction of disease pathology i.e., decreased the level of Aß monomer, oligomer, plaques production, antagonized aggregation & accumulation and increased brain clearance of Aß [26]. ACI-24, a liposome-based anti-amyloid vaccine effectively bound the Aß peptides and prevented induced cell death. Additionally, the vaccine was effectively safe and triggered an immune response [27]. However, evidences of immunogenicity of ACI-24 with pharmacodynamic and target enlargement was observed [28].

4.1.2 Immunosuppressive Therapy

Severe inflammatory conditions, injury or side effects associated with medicaments eventually triggers neurological diseases. Thus, immunosuppressive or immunomodulatory therapies are usually advised by physicians for management of neuroinflammatory disorders [29]. Immunosuppression obstructs the disease worsening and stabilizes neuro-immunological disorders with increased risk of infections [30]. Immunotherapies to suppress immune response works by following mechanisms to target precursor causes of neurological disorders (Fig. 4).

A. Impeding DNA synthesis

Drugs like teriflunomide, mitoxantrone, mycophenolate mofetil and cladribine interfere with DNA synthesis and disrupt the denovo purine synthesis. These drugs chiefly target the proliferation of T and B lymphocytes. Furthermore, reduces the production of lymphocyte-derived proinflammatory cytokines such as IFN-γ and TNF-α [30].

B. Attenuation of immune cells

Monoclonal antibodies (rituximab, ocrelizumab, inebilizumab and alemtuzumab) are often utilized in neurological diseases management. mAbs exhibited pulsed depletion of immune cells and target B cells that are instantaneous cause of neuroinflammation. Mainly, a chimeric anti-CD20 mAb (rituximab) target CD 20 molecules expressed throughout B-cell maturation and on a subset of $CD4^{+}$ T cells [31, 32]. The attack of immune cells on nerve fibres along with insulating membranes surrounding them lead to localized damage in CNS and symptoms of relapsing-remitting multiple sclerosis (RRMS). Humanized anti-CD25 mAb (alemtuzumab) has been approved

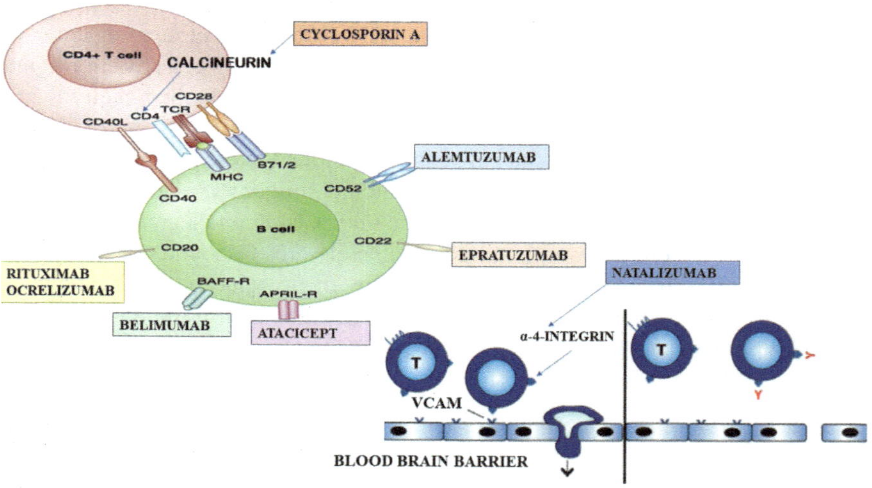

Fig. 4 Pictorial depiction of mechanism of action of various immunosuppressive therapies

for management of RRMS. Alemtuzumab antagonizes CD-52 antigen mostly manifested on the surface of B and T cells and at subsidiary level on monocytes and macrophages [33].

C. Leukocytes sequestration

Natalizumab is a recombinant humanized mAb directed against alpha 4-integrin molecules on leukocytes facilitate transmigration of peripheral immune cells into CNS. In addition, alpha 4-integrin assists the retention of lymphoid progenitor cells in bone marrow. Thus, use of natalizumab (a recombinant humanized mAb) elevates NK cells, T lymphocytes and mainly B cells in the peripheral blood by blocking their passage into CNS [34, 35]. Modulators of sphingosine 1-phosphate receptor in multiple sclerosis exhibited complimentary sequestration of peripheral leukocytes. Fingolimod and siponomid impede the emergence of lymphocytes from secondary lymphoid organs which results in intense curtailment of native and central memory T cells and memory B cells in the periphery [36, 37].

D. Targeting inflammatory mediators

Therapeutic agents manifesting blockage of intracellular signaling pathway plays a vital role in reducing the level of inflammatory mediators. Cyclosporine A ties up to cellular cyclophilins to obstruct the action of calcineurin involved in translocation of nuclear factor of activated T cells from cytosol into the nucleus. This results in reduction of transcription of pro-inflammatory genes [38]. Glucocorticoids are also effective in reducing neuroinflammation. These agents hamper the manufacture of inflammatory markers and emigration of immune cells across BBB [39].

E. Cytokine targeting therapies

Cytokines are diverse group of glycoproteins that synchronize numerous functions such as physiological, immune, inflammation, hematopoiesis and tissue repair. Cytokines modulate debate between the innate and adaptive immune responses for effective immune responses. In various neurological diseases, degranulation of cytokines was noticed. Thus, their involvement in pharmacological therapies proposes an encouraging core for research. Although, certain complications make pharmacological forecast challenging as homeostasis of inflammatory and anti-inflammatory effects are regulated by cytokines via a complex network protocol. Thus, cytokine therapy plays crucial role in offering new strategies for neurological disease modulation and treatment [40].

The wide family of cytokines has similar structure and receptors which authorize super-imposed and supporting actions among cytokines. IFN-ß and secondary progressive cytokine agent switches cytokine production in support of anti-inflammatory cytokines, alters function of dendritic cells and promote anti-inflammatory B-cells function [41, 42]. Likewise, interleukins-6 (IL-6), well known mediators of immune system predominantly associated with production of pro-inflammatory effects in the brain. IL-6 produced in response to infection is also upregulated in chronic autoimmune processes [43]. For example, during stroke and amyotrophic lateral sclerosis, the level of INF-γ and TNF-α is low whereas IL-1,

IL-4 and IL-10 become high. Thus, G-CSF (granulocyte colony-stimulating factor, a hematopoietic factor) was released from neurons to prevent neuron apoptosis and intensify vessel reformation in ischemic tissue. Anti-TNF therapies include mAbs and TNF receptor molecule to prevent TNF interaction with its receptors [40].

Certain clinical trials in neurological diseases management included both neuroprotection and neurodegenerative pathways [44]. Nanomaterials have been visualized as innovative component with distinctive physicochemical properties in diagnosis and management of neurological diseases. Various kinds of nanomaterials including organic (metallic nanoparticles, quantum dots, graphene), organic (polymeric nanoparticles, liposomes, chitosan, exosomes) and their hybrid complexes have been widely used to deliver the therapeutic agents to target site by overcoming the anatomical and physiological barriers (Table 1) [45, 46].

4.1.3 Cell Therapy

Cell therapy is defined as the transfer of allogenic or autologous biological material in a patient for therapeutic purposes. In comparison to conventional therapies, cell therapies can rapidly respond to any biological malignancies or promote regeneration and restoration of impaired tissues or otherwise strengthen the body's own defense mechanism. Now a day's cell therapy is gaining attention of medical professionals as an alternative treatment option for various neurological diseases. Since it works by replacing dead cells or liberate defensive things to the injured cells or altering the microenvironment around the damaged cells in the nervous system [56–58]. With the increasing research, cell therapy has revealed its distinctive potential in treatment of neurological disorders together with brain trauma, stroke, brain tumor, Parkinson's and Alzheimer's disease. Presently variety of cells have been employed in cell therapy studies such as embroyonic stem cell (ESCs), induced pluripotent stem cells (iPSCs), neural stem or progenitor cells (NSPCs), mesenchymal stromal or stem cells (MSCs), dental pulp stem cells (DPSCs), stem cells from human exfoliated deciduous teeth (SHED), multilineage-differentiating stress enduring cells (muse), hematopoietic stem cells (HSC), olfactory unsheathing cells (OECs) and hematopoietic stem cells (HSC). Therapeutic effect of various cell therapies in management of neurological disorders can be achieved by following mechanisms as explained in Fig. 5.

Nanotechnology based cell therapy has unlocked numerous promising opportunities in the field of regenerative medicine to converse and restore injured neural tissues (Fig. 6) [59, 60]. Multidirectional differentiation potential of neural stem cells and their ability to self-renew can urge and amplify functional rehabilitation and constitutional regeneration either directly by replacing for failed cells in the tissues of concern, or indirectly, by restoring the repair operation through paracrine signaling network at damaged sites to actuate endogenous stem cells [61, 62]. Nanomaterials having capability to load drugs and ease of detectability are the preferred candidates for the bio-labeling and bio-imaging of transplanted stem cells in vivo [63]. Moreover, nanomaterials enable the restoration of injured tissues with the aid of the laden drugs. Although nonmaterial's rarely have tissue renovation potential. Thus,

Table 1 Nanomaterials used for development of immunosupressive therapies in treatment of neurological diseases

Active Agent	Delivery system	Neurological disorder	Characteristics	Mechanism	Target site	References
Selenium	Metalloprotein nanoparticle	Alzheimer's disease	Reduce oxidative toxicity in the brain	Inhibit Aß aggregation and cross BBB	Aß-amloyid receptor	[47]
Proto-lipid protein ($PLP_{139-151}$) & ovalbumin protein ($OVA_{323-339}$)	Poly-DL-lactide nanoparticle	Multiple sclerosis	Antigen-specific immunomodulation	Inhibit Th1 and Th17 polarization	Kupffer T-cells	[48]
Melanin	PEG- Nanoparticle	Ischemic stroke	Attenuates the RONS triggered inflammatory responses	Suppressing the expression of inflammatory mediators and cytokines	Neuro 2A cell in the brain	[49]
Interleukine-13	Mesoporous silica Nanoparticle	Encephalomyelitis	Intranasal administration	Induction of chemokines orchestrating immune cell infiltration	Th2 cells	[50]
Atorvastatin	Chitosan oligosaccharide Nanoparticle	Atherosclerosis	Enhance specific payload release and neutralize inflammation	Accumulation of targeted inflammatory tissue	TNFR2, CD36, and CCR2 antigens in macrophages	[51]
Plasmonic Gold	Thiolated polyethylene glycol nanoparticles	Brain tumor ablation	Capable of producing long term survivors for cancer cells	Checkpoint blockage immune-therapy	CT-2A glioma cells	[52]

(continued)

Table 1 (continued)

Active Agent	Delivery system	Neurological disorder	Characteristics	Mechanism	Target site	References
Doxorubicin	Mesoporous silica nanoparticle	Glioblastoma	Effectively inhibit tumor proliferation via permeation through BBB; improve accumulation of drug in orthotopic brain tumors	Immune checkpoint inhibitor	GL261-Tcells	[53]
Doxorubi-cin and Dalargin	Poly-n-butylcyano-acrylate nanoparticle	CNS diseases	Nanoparticles release 12 inflammatory cytokine to neutralize ROS	Nanoparticle stimulates the production of ROS	Cells of BBB	[54]
Methyl-predniso-lone	Chitosan-methylprednisolone nanoparticles	Spinal cord injury	Anti-inflammatory and antiapoptotic effects by terminal deoxynucleotide transferased UTP nick end labeling (TUNEL) and ED1 staining	Regulate gene transcription	Areas of spinal cord injury	[55]

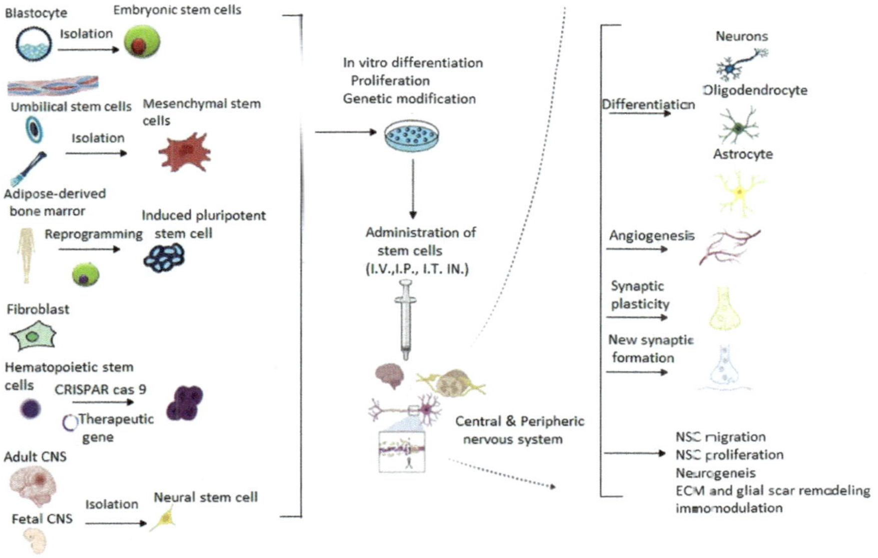

Fig. 5 Therapeutic effect of stem cells in neurological disorders

amalgamation of cell therapy and nanomaterials is mushrooming in development of regenerative medicine.

Researchers have revealed therapeutic benefits of cellular therapy in neurological disorders. However, the major problems associated to cell therapy including their viability, safety, tumorigenicity, unlimited differentiation, metastasis, low survival after transplantation, probable immune actions as well as inadequacy of screening the migration of stem cell to the damaged tissues and real-time imaging-directed

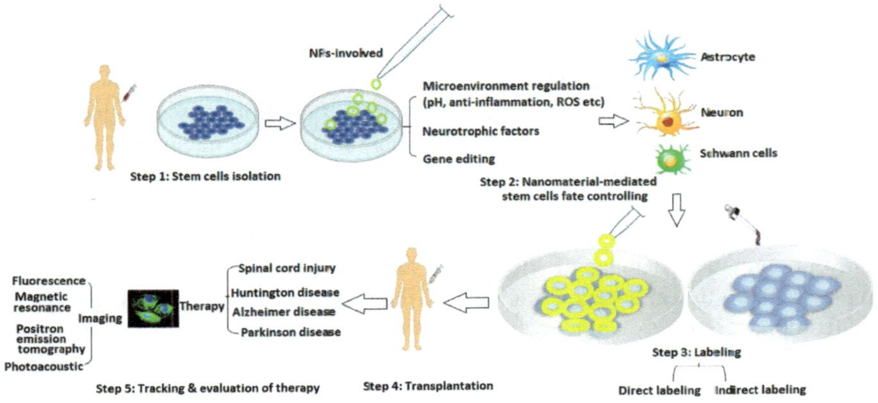

Fig. 6 Applications of nanotechnology based cell therapy in regenerative medicine

therapy in vivo have limited their therapeutic effectiveness in clinical array [64–66]. These limitations are due to the interactions of cell therapy with different inward or outer variables, predominantly surrounding cells, extracellular matrix (ECM), growth factors and inflammation at the injured site. Hence, to make progress in cell mediated therapy approach and to defeat the obstructions of employing stem cells at clinical scale, these issues should be resolved. The distinctive characteristics of nanomaterials such as high surface energy, high surface-to-volume ratio (S/V) and distinctive thermal, electrical, mechanical as well as optical behaviors establish them as suitable carriers to confront the barriers in cell therapy. Presently, a wide variety of nanomaterials have been assessed in neurological disorders such as liposomes, micelles, carbon nanotubes, metallic nanomaterials, quantum dots and micelles. These nanomaterials have the ability of enhancement of cell therapy by offering perfect substrates for huge scale proliferation of cells. These nanomaterials showed improved efficiency by controlling cell adhesion, differentiation and proliferation as well as employed for targeting neural stem cell relocation and delivering it to localized injured sites of neural. Various techniques can be utilized to improve the potential of cell therapy such as directly adding nanomaterials to the culture media, coating of culture container and also conjugation of nanomaterials with definite scaffold for 3D culture systems. Nanomaterials will display diverse features of interaction with intracellular constituents of stem cells. Thus, the internalized nanoparticles will modify the cellular signaling pathways [67–70]. Stem cells have been explored as prospective therapies for neurodegenerative diseases. Neural stem cells and mesenchymal stem cells are multipotent populations that can be united with nanoparticle medication and transplanted into the brain. While embryonic stem cells and induced pluripotent stem cells are pluripotent populations that utilize nanoparticles both for reprogramming and differentiation as well as for drug delivery into the brain (Table 2). The mechanisms involved in delivering of nanomaterials into the brain are shown in Fig. 7.

4.1.4 Gene Therapy

Neurological issues are significantly emphasizing an enormous socioeconomic burden. Neuroinflammation and neurodegeneration are normally seen in different sorts of neurological problems, yet the existing therapeutic strategy has a restricted part in switching and reclamation of lost neuronal capability [89]. Hence, gene therapy has arisen as an intense option in contrast to the current pharmacological intervention and affirms re-establishment of vanished neuronal capability to prevent permanent damage (Table 3) [90, 91]. The general objective of gene treatment in neurological issues is focused on three end points i.e., avoiding neurodegeneration, recovery of injured neurons and replacing defective gene and neurotransmitters [92, 55]. Gene therapy works by augmentation, silencing or editing the genes (Fig. 8). Gene therapy has prosperously served different inherited immune deficiencies including severe combined immune deficiency (SCID) and adenosine deaminase (ADA) deficiency, hereditary blindness [93, 94], blood disorders such as

Table 2 Nanomaterials mediated cell therapies in neurological disorders

Active agent	Nanomaterial	Neurological disorder	Characteristic	Mechanism	References
BMSCs (bone marrow mesenchy-mal stem cells)	Gold NPs	Bone-defect	Stem cells progressively carried to faulty region in cortical bone	Intracellular delivery, cell imaging	[71]
Rat NSCs (neural stem cells)	Silica NPs	Disorder of cell signaling	Deliver silica nanoparticle associated neural stem cells into the cells	Intracellular signaling pathway, cell imaging	[72]
NSCs (neural stem cells)	Mesoporous silica NPs	Intracranial glioma xenograft	Efficient in imaging of stem cell distribution	Intracellular delivery, cell imaging	[73]
NSCs (neural stem cells)	Gd2O3	Injured rat brain	Monitoring NSCs in murine brains	Intracellular delivery, cell imaging	[74]
ESCs (embryonic stem cell)	Graphene oxide GO)	Parkinson's disease	Improve dopamine neural differentiation and axons re-growth	Intracellular delivery	[75]
HNSCs (human neural stem cells)	TiO_2	Neuron regeneration	Attain extremely expedited differentiation	TiO_2 hetero junction film as a biocompatible flash photo stimulator for effective differentiation of HNSCs into neurons	[76]
NSCs (neural stem cells)	TiO_2 NPs	Neural regeneration	Intended for differentiation affinity	TiO_2 NPs lead to differentiational tendency towards neurons from neural stem cells	[77]
HMSCs (Human mesenchymal stem cells)	Carbon dots	Neural regeneration	Lengthen cellular retention in HMSCs	Cell labeling and tracking	[78]

(continued)

Table 2 (continued)

Active agent	Nanomaterial	Neurological disorder	Characteristic	Mechanism	References
NSCs (Neural stem cells)	Carbon tube	Neural regeneration	Advancing neurite elongation and enhancing effects on the differentiation of NSCs into adult neuronal cells	Electrical stimulation of carbon tube may have a synergistic effect neurite elongation	[79]
Hematopoietic and neural progenitor cells	SPIO	Spinal cord injury	Permit in vivo noninvasive tracking and healing stem cells	Monitor the distribution and differentiation of stem cells by high-resolution in vivo imaging techniques	[80]
HNSCs (Human neural stem cells)	19F MRI contrast agent	Stroke	Visualize the operation of denovo tissue formation	19F-MRI contrast agent can adequately monitor the distribution of transplanted cells	[81]
MSCs (mesenchymal stem cells)	CdSe/ZnS QDs	NOD/SCID beta2 M null mice	Invade mesenchymal stem cells effectively	Quantum dots conjugated with Tat peptide, and introduced into living mesenchymal stem cells forcellular labeling and tracking	[82]
C17.2 NSC (neural stem cells)	PFCE/ rhodamine	Neurodegenera-tive diseases in CNS	Stem cells can be proficiently fluorinated with cationic PFCE nanoparticles	Intracellular delivery, cell imaging	[83]
MHP36 cells	PLGA	Stroke	Neuroscaffolds incorporate effectively within host tissue forming a primordial neural tissue	Intracellular delivery	[84]

(continued)

Table 2 (continued)

Active agent	Nanomaterial	Neurological disorder	Characteristic	Mechanism	References
ENSCs (Enteric neural stem/ progenitor cells)	Liposomes	Enteric neuropathies	Enhance neuronal density and proliferation of transplanted cells	Improved cell proliferation and neuronal differentiation	[85]
NSCs/ADSCs (neural stem cells/adipose derived stem cells)	Chitosan	Neural deficit	Provide an ECM-like environment to drive the interaction and morphological assembly	Advance neural different a-tion capacities	[86]
HUVECs (human umbilical vein endothelial cells)/ RT4-D6P2T	Gelatin	Nerve tissue damage	Control release vascular endothelial growth factor to hasten the nerve regeneration course	Intracellular delivery	[87]
MSCs (mesenchymal stromal cells)	Exosomes	Traumatic brain injury	Augment functional recovery and assist neuroplasticity	Intracellular delivery	[88]

hemophilia [95, 96] and beta-thalassemia [97], amyotrophic lateral sclerosis (ALS), spinal muscular atrophy, lysosomal storage diseases and oncologic diseases.

During Parkinson dopaminergic neuron are decreased in substantia nigra (SN) region with impaired GABA concentration [103]. Thus to treat the genetic abnormalities in the biosynthesis of dopamine, equine infectious anemia virus (EIAV) and adeno-associated virus (AAV) as a vector can be used to deliver gene for GTP cyclohydrolase and aromatic L-amino acid decarboxylase (AADC) respectively. GTP cyclohydrolase initiates a cascade of events involved in conversion of guanosine triphosphate (GTP) into tetrahydrobiopterin needed for tyrosine synthesis. Tyrosine hydroxylase (TH) converts tyrosine into L-DOPA which is transformed to dopamine by aromatic L-amino acid decarboxylase (AADC) enzyme (Fig. 9). Another step to manage GABA deficiency in Parkinson's disease is to overcome the deficit of glutamate decarboxylase (GAD) required to concert glutamate to GABA by delivering GAD gene with the aid of AAV vector. Sometimes deficiency of gene involved in production of an important neuropeptide nuerturin (NRTM) also leads to symptoms of Parkinson's disease. Thus, supplement of NRTN gene is required to enhance the genesis of neuropeptide (Fig. 9) [102].

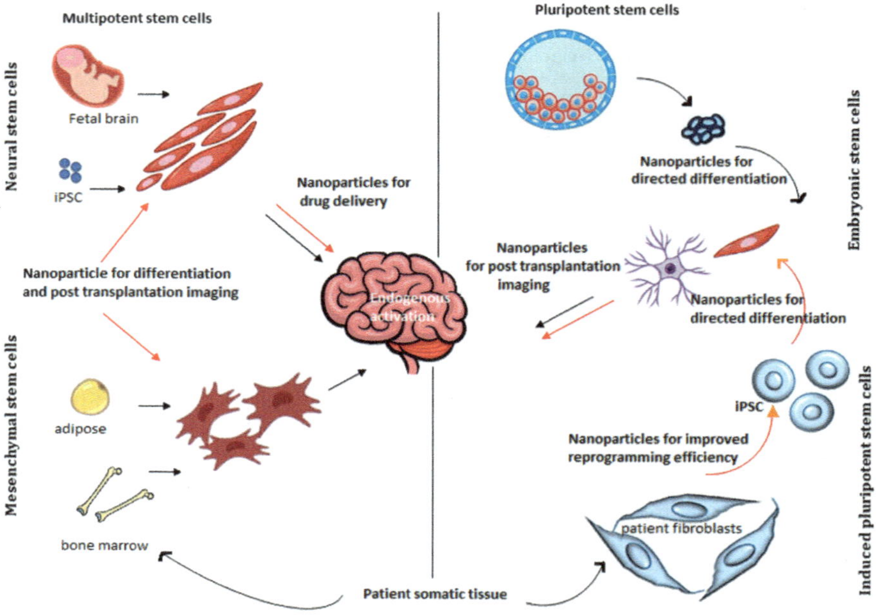

Fig. 7 Potential therapies for neurodegenerative disorders

Similarly, targeted gene therapy utilizing HSV vector is utilized to transport brain-derived neurotrophic factor (BDNF) and fibroblast growth factor (FGF) genes responsible for increasing seizure limit with decrease in event of seizure score. The utilization of lentivirus loaded with gene responsible for overexpression of K^+ channel decreased neuronal excitability and diminished seizure limit [104, 105]. Subsequently, to reduce the overexpression of ADK gene, the lentivirus as vector can be used for gene therapy to obstruct ADK gene and reduce the severity of epilepsy (Fig. 10) [106, 107].

The deficiency of nerve growth factor (NGF), neprilysin (NEP) enzymes and overexpression of CDK5 gene may contribute to increased development of amyloid beta (Aβ) peptides, neuroinflammation and neurodegeneration during Alzheimer's disease. Gene therapy has shown promising results in management and treatment of Alzheimer prognosis and related impacts. Gene therapy has indicated encouraging results in treatment of Alzheimer prognosis and related impacts [108, 109] (Fig. 11).

Table 3 Nanomaterials mediated gene therapies in neurological disorders

Active agent	Delivery system	Neurological disorder	Characteristic	Mechanism	References
Oxidation resistance 1 plasmid (pOXR1)	Vitamin E succinate-grafted ε-polylysine liposomal nanoparticles	Spinal cord injury	Alleviate neuronal apoptosis, attenuates oxidative stress and inhibits inflammation	Augmentation	[98]
Tyrosine hydroxyl-lase (TH) and aromatic L-amino acid decarboxylase (AADC) genes	Plasmid DNA-cationic liposome complex	Parkinson	Improvement of apomorphine-induced rotational behavior	Transfection of TH gene	[99]
Glial fibrillary acidic protein (GFAP) gene promoter	Pegylated immune liposomes (PILs)	Parkinson	Improvement of striatal tyrosine hydroxylase activity	Augmentation	[100]
EGFR antisense gene	Pegylated immuno liposomes (PILs)	Brain cancer	Reduce the growth of epidermal growth factor receptor dependent gliomas	Silencing epidermal growth factor receptor	[101]
Hairpin RNA expression plasmids	Pegylated immune liposomes	Brain cancer	Suppression of epidermal growth factor receptor	Silencing oncogenic genes	[100]
Plasmid DNA and Poly-ethylenimine	plasmid DNA complexed with 25 kDa polyethylenimine	Spinal cord injury	Prolonged transgene expression in spinal cord	Augmenta-tion	[102]

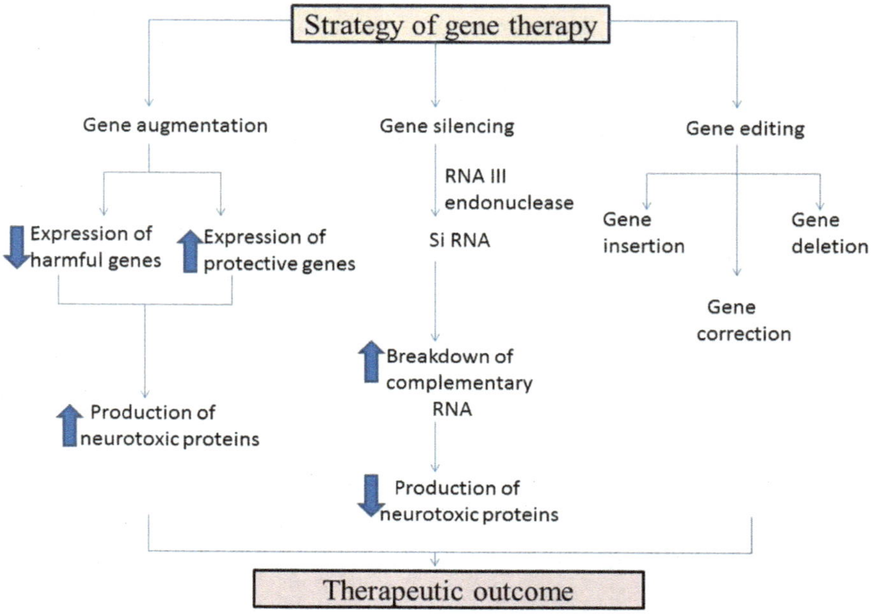

Fig. 8 Different modes of working of gene therapy

5 Future Prospective

The future of neurological disorders management rests in the amalgamation of selective neurological vaccines, immune checkpoint inhibitors, cell therapies or means of alleviating immune suppression associated with neurological disorders. The blockage of inhibitory receptors by nanomaterial-based therapies can possibly lower the threshold for effective anti-neurological immunity. Currently used as well as advanced therapies down-regulate cell signaling at the immune synapse. Common signaling and regulatory pathways of nanomaterial-based therapies could impart additional controlled targets for pharmaceutical intervention. However, the crucial challenge of the succeeding investigations of above-discussed therapies could be to ascertain the accurate time for beginning and suspending treatment.

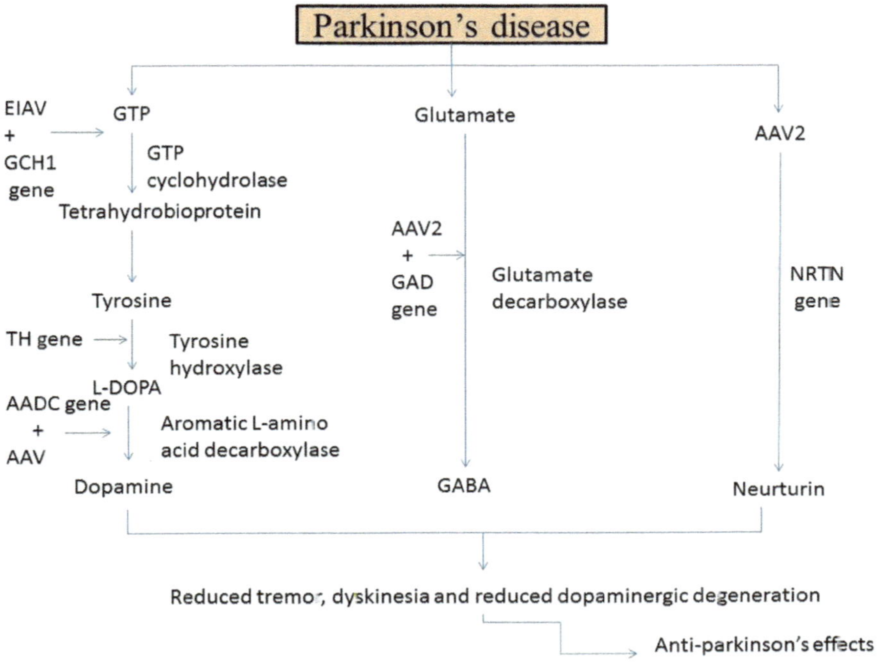

Fig. 9 Diagrammatic representation of various sites targeted by gene therapy in Parkinson's disease

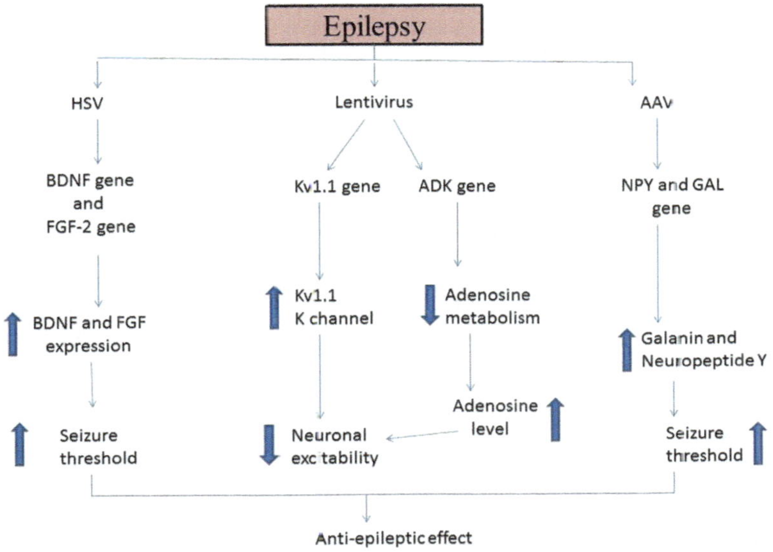

Fig. 10 Gene therapy approaches to manage epilepsy

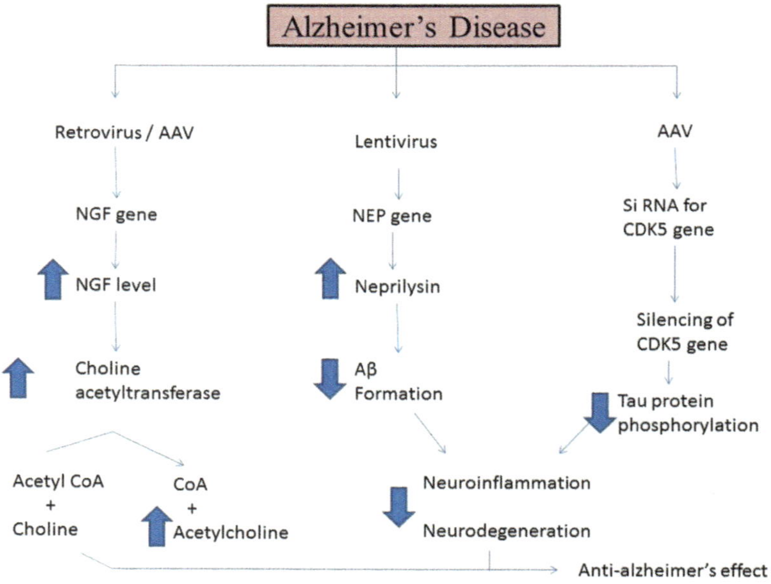

Fig. 11 Gene therapy approaches to prevent prognosis of Alzheimer's disease

References

1. Nguyen TT, Nguyen TT, Vo TK, Nguyen MK, Van Vo T, Van Vo G (2021) Nanotechnology-based drug delivery for central nervous system disorders. BiomedPharmacother143:112117–112130
2. Naqvi S, Panghal A, Flora SJ (2020) Nanotechnology: a promising approach for delivery of neuroprotective drugs. Front Neurosci 14:494–520
3. Kang YJ, Cutler EG, Cho H (2018) Therapeutic nanoplatforms and delivery strategies for neurological disorders. Nano Converg 5(1):1–5
4. Soni S, Ruhela RK, Medhi B (2016) Nanomedicine in central nervous system (CNS) disorders: a present and future prospective. Adv Pharm Bull 6(3):319–336
5. Saeedi M, Eslamifar M, Khezri K, Dizaj SM (2019) Applications of nanotechnology in drug delivery to the central nervous system. Biomed Pharmacother 111:666–675
6. Achar A, Myers R, Ghosh C (2021) Drug delivery challenges in brain disorders across the blood–brain barrier: novel methods and future considerations for improved therapy. Biomed 9(12):1834–1860
7. Anthony DP, Hegde M, Shetty SS, Rafic T, Mutalik S, Rao BS (2021) Targeting receptor-ligand chemistry for drug delivery across blood-brain barrier in brain diseases. Life Sci 274:119326–119341
8. Alajangi HK, Kaur M, Sharma A, Rana S, Thakur S, Chatterjee M, Singla N, Jaiswal PK, Singh G, Barnwal RP (2022) Blood–brain barrier: emerging trends on transport models and new-age strategies for therapeutic intervention against neurological disorders. Mol Brain 15(1):1–28
9. Hirunpattarasilp C, Attwell D, Freitas F (2019) The role of pericytes in brain disorders: from the periphery to the brain. J Neurochem 150(6):648–665
10. McCabe SM, Zhao N (2021) The potential roles of blood–brain barrier and blood–cerebrospinal fluid barrier in maintaining brain manganese homeostasis. Nutrients 13(6):1833–1847

11. Witika BA, Poka MS, Demana PH, Matafwali SK, Melamane S, MalungeloKhamanga SM, Makoni PA (2022) Lipid-based nanocarriers for neurological disorders: a review of the state-of-the-art and therapeutic success to date. Pharmaceutics 14(4):836–880
12. Golden PL, Pollack GM (2003) Blood–brain barrier efflux transport. J Pharm Sci 92(9):1739–1753
13. Furtado D, Björnmalm M, Ayton S, Bush AI, Kempe K, Caruso F (2018) Overcoming the blood–brain barrier: the role of nanomaterials in treating neurological diseases. Adv Mater 30(46):1801362–1801428
14. Hanif S, Pir M, Rose C, Fawad Ur R, Qian R-J, Zheng M, Shi B-Y (2020) Nanomedicine-based immunotherapy for central nervous system disorders. Acta Pharmacol Sin 41(7):936–953
15. Senapati S, Arun KM, Sunil K, Maiti P (2018) Controlled drug delivery vehicles for cancer treatment and their performance. Signal Transduct Target Ther 3(1):7
16. Anthony DP, Hegde M, Shetty SS, Rafic T, Mutalik S, Rao BS (2021) Targeting receptor-ligand chemistry for drug delivery across blood-brain barrier in brain diseases. Life Sci 274:119326
17. Mortada I, Farah R, Nabha S, Ojcius DM, Fares Y, Almawi WY, Sadier NS (2021) Immunotherapies for neurodegenerative diseases. Front Neurol 12:654739
18. Shahaduzzaman Md, Nash K, Hudson C, Sharif M, Grimmig B, Lin X, Bai G, Liu H, Ugen KE, Cao C, Bickford PC (2015) Anti-human a-synuclein N-terminal peptide antibody protects against dopaminergic cell death and ameliorates behavioral deficits in an AAV-α-synuclein rat model of Parkinson's disease. PLoS ONE 10(2): e0116841
19. Gustafsson G, Eriksson F, Möller C, da F TL, Outeiro TF, Lannfelt L, Bergström J, Ingelsson M (2017) Cellular uptake of α-synuclein oligomer-selective antibodies is enhanced by the extracellular presence of α-synuclein and mediated via Fcγ receptors. Cell Mol Neurobiol 37(1):121–131
20. Lindström V, Fagerqvist T, Nordström E, Eriksson F, Lord A, St T, Andersson J, Johannesson M, Schell H, Kahle PJ, Möller C, Gellerfors P, Bergström J, Lannfelt L, Ingelsson M (2014) Immunotherapy targeting α-synuclein protofibrils reduced pathology in (Thy-1)-h[A30P] α-synuclein mice. Neurobiol Dis 69:134–143
21. Valera E, Masliah E (2013) Immunotherapy for neurodegenerative diseases: Focus on α-synucleinopathies. Pharmacol Ther 138(3):311–322
22. McFarthing K, Simuni T (2019) Clinical trial highlights: targetting alpha-synuclein. J Parkinson Dis. 9(1):5–16
23. Rajamohamedsait H, Rasool S, Rajamohamedsait W, Lin Y, Sigurdsson EM (2017) Prophylactic active tau immunization leads to sustained reduction in both tau and amyloid-b pathologies in 3xTg mice. Sci Rep 7(1):17034
24. Shahpasand K, Shamloo AS, Nabavi SM, Zhou XZ, Lu KP (2017) Tau immunotherapy: hopes and hindrances. Hum Vaccin Immunother 14(2):277–284
25. Ayalon G, Lee SH, Adolfsson O, Atkins CF, Atwal JK, Blendstrup M (2021) Antibody semorinemab reduces tau pathology in a transgenic mouse model and engages tau in patients with Alzheimer's disease. Sci Transl Med 13(593):eabb2639
26. Mantile F, Prisco A (2020) Vaccination against ß-Amyloid as a strategy for the prevention of alzheimer's disease. Biology (Basel) 9(12):425
27. Cheng L, Zhang J, Li XY, Yuan L, Pan YF, Chen XR, Gao TM, Qiao JT, Qi JS (2017) A novel antibody targeting sequence 31–35 in amyloid b protein attenuates Alzheimer's disease-related neuronal damage. Hippocampus 27(2):122–133
28. Rafii MS, Sol O, Mobley WC, Delpretti S, Skotko BG, Burke AD, Sabbagh MN, Yuan SH, Rissman RA, Pulsifer M, Evans C, Evans AC, Beth G, Fournier N, Gray AJ, Santos DMA, Hliva V, Vukicevic M, Kosco-Vilbois M, Streffer J, Pfeifer FHH (2022) Safety, tolerability and immunogenicity of the ACI-24 vaccine in adults with down syndrome: a phase 1b randomized clinical trial. JAMA Neurol 79(6):565–574
29. Winkelmann A, Loebermann M, Reisinger EC, Hartung H-P, Zettl UK (2016) Disease-modifying therapies and infectious risks in multiple sclerosis. Nat Rev Neurol 12(4):217–233
30. Pawlitzki M, Zettl UK, Ruck T, Rolfes L, Hartung H-P, Meuth SG (2020) Merits and culprits of immunotherapies for neurological diseases in times of COVID-19. EBioMedicine 56:102822

31. Hauser SL, Bar-Or A, Comi G, Giovannoni G, Hartung H-P, Hemmer B, Leubin F, Montalban X, Rommohan KW, Selmaj K, Traboulsee A, Wolinsky JS, Arnold DL, Klingelschmitt G, Masterman D, Fontoura P, Belachew S, Chin P, Marion N, Garren H, Kappos L (2017) Ocrelizumab versus interferon beta-1a in relapsing multiple sclerosis. N Engl J Med 376(3):221–234
32. Whittam DH, Tallantyre EC, Jolles S, Huda S, Moots RJ, Kim HJ, Robertson NP, Cree BAC, Jacob A (2019) Rituximab in neurological disease: principles, evidence and practice. Pract Neurol 19(1):5–20
33. Ruck T, Bittner S, Wiendl H, Meuth SG (2015) Alemtuzumab in multiple sclerosis: mechanism of action and beyond. Int J Mol Sci 16(7):16414–16439
34. Boing H, Wundes A, Chang KH, Lucas S, Papayannopoulou T (2008) Increased numbers of circulating hematopoietic stem/progenitor cells are chronically maintained in patients treated with the CD49d blocking antibody natalizumab. Blood 111(7):3439–3441
35. Polman CH, O'Connor PW, Havrdova E, Hutchinson M, Kappos L, Miller DH, Phillips JT, Lublin FD, Giovannoni G, Wajgt A, Toal M, Lynn F, Panzara MA, Sandrock AW (2006) A randomized, placebo-controlled trial of natalizumab for relapsing multiple sclerosis. N Engl J Med 354(9):899–910
36. Comi G, Hartung HP, Bakshi R, Williams IM, Wiendl H (2017) Benefit-risk profile of sphingosine-1-phosphate receptor modulators in relapsing and secondary progressive multiple sclerosis. Drugs 77(16):1755–1768
37. Kappos L, Radue E-W, O'Connor P, Polman C, Hohlfeld R, Calabresi P, Selmaj K, Agoropoulou C, Leyk M, Auberson LZ (2010) A placebo-controlled trial of oral fingolimod in relapsing multiple sclerosis. N Engl J Med 362(5):387–401
38. Liddicoat AM, Lavelle C Ed (2019) Modulation of innate immunity by cyclosporine A. Biochem Pharmacol.163:472–480
39. Gold R, Buttgereit F, Toyka KV (2001) Mechanism of action of glucocorticosteroid hormones: possible implications for therapy of neuroimmunological disorders. J Neuroimmunol 117(1–2):1–8
40. Azodi S, Jacobson S (2016) Cytokine therapies in neurological disease. Neurotherapeutics 13(3):555–561
41. Klotz L, Havla J, Schwab N, Hohlfeld R, Barnett M, Reddel S, Wiendl H (2019) Risks and risk management in modern multiple sclerosis immunotherapeutic treatment. Ther Adv Neurol Disord 12:1756286419836571
42. Zettl UK, Hecker M, Aktas O, Wagner T, Rommer PS (2018) Interferon ß-1a and ß-1b for patients with multiple sclerosis: updates to current knowledge. Expert Rev Clin Immunol 14(2):137–153
43. Tanaka T, Narazaki M, Kishimoto T (2014) IL-6 in inflammation, immunity, and disease. Cold Spring Harb Perspect Biol 6(10):a016295
44. Cornelis-Feltz CVF, Brabyn S, Ratcliff J, Varley D, Allgar V, Gilbody S, Clarke C, Dimitris L (2021) Assessment of cytokines, microRNA and patient-related outcome measures in conversion disorder/functional neurological disorder (CD/FND): The CANDO clinical feasibility study. Brain Behav Immun Health 13:100228
45. Bali YH, Kasman GM, Pirzadeh M (2019) Curcumin-loaded nanoparticles: a novel therapeutic strategy in treatment of central nervous system disorders. Int J Nanomedicine 14(4449):4460
46. Zhu D-F, Hu Y-J, Yu L, Zhou X-G, Wu J-M, Tang Y, Qin D-L, Fan Q-Z, Wu A-G (2021) Nanoparticles: a hope for the treatment of inflammation in CNS. Front Pharmacol 12:683935
47. Nazıroglu M, Muhamad S, Pecze L (2017) Nanoparticles as potential clinical therapeutic agents in alzheimer's disease: focus on selenium nanoparticles. Expert Rev Clin Pharmacol 10(7):773–782
48. Saito E, Kuo R, Kramer KR, Gohel N, Giles DA, Moore BB, Miller SD, Shea LD (2019) Design of biodegradable nanoparticles to modulate phenotypes of antigen-presenting cells for antigen-specific treatment of autoimmune disease. Biomaterials 222:119432
49. Yanlan L, Ai K, Ji X, Askhatova D, Du R, Lu L, Shi J (2017) Comprehensive insights into the multi-antioxidative mechanisms of melanin nanoparticles and their application to protect brain from injury in ischemic stroke. J Am Chem Soc 139(2):856–862

50. Park J, Choi SW, Cha BG, Kim J, Kang S-Jo, (2021) Alternative activation of macrophages through interleukin-13-loaded extra-large-pore mesoporous silica nanoparticles suppresses experimental autoimmune encephalomyelitis. ACS Biomater Sci Eng 7(9):4446–4453
51. Gao C, Huang Q, Liu C, Kwong CHT, Yue L, Wan J-Bo, Lee SMY; Wang R, (2020) Treatment of atherosclerosis by macrophage-biomimetic nanoparticles via targeted pharmacotherapy and sequestration of proinflammatory cytokines. Nat Commun 11(1):2622
52. Yang L, Chongsathidkiet P, Crawford BM, Dechant OR, CA, Kemeny HR, Cui X, Maccarini, PF; Lascola CD; Fecci EP; Vo-Dinh Tuan, (2019) Plasmonic gold nanostar-mediated photothermal immunotherapy for brain tumor ablation and immunologic memory. Immunotherapy 11(15):1293–1302
53. Kuang J, Song W, Yin J, Zeng X, Han S, Yi-P Z, Tao J, Liu C-J, He X-H, Zhang X-Z (2018) IRGD Modified Chemo-immunotherapeutic Nanoparticles for Enhanced Immunotherapy against Glioblastoma. Adv Funct Mater 1800025:1–14
54. Kolter M, Ott M, Hauer C, Reimold I, Fricker G (2015) Nanotoxicity of poly(n-butylcyano-acrylate) nanoparticles at the blood–brain barrier, in human whole blood and in vivo. J Control Release 197:165–179
55. Gwak SJ, Koo HY, Yhee Y, Young J, Yeong LH, Yoon DH, Kwangmeyung K, Yoon H (2015) Multifunctional nanoparticles for gene delivery and spinal cord injury. J Biomed Mater Res Part A 103(11):3474–3482
56. Bellak T, Fekecs Z, Torok D, Tancos Z, Nemes C, Tezsla Z, Gal L, Polgari S, Kobolak J, Dinnyes A, Nogradi A, Pajer K (2020) Grafted human induced pluripotent stem cells improve the outcome of spinal cord injury: Modulation of the lesion microenvironment. Sci Rep 10(1):1–33
57. Besusso D, Schellino R, Boido M, Belloli S, Parolisi R, Conforti P, Faedo A, Cernigoj M, Campus I, Laporta A, Bocchi VD, Murtaj V, Parmar M, Spaiardi P, Talpo F, Maniezzi C, Toselli MG, Biella G, Moresco RM, Vercelli A, Buffo A, Cattaneo E (2020) Stem cell-derived human striatal progenitors innervate striatal targets and alleviate sensorimotor deficit in a rat model of huntington disease. Stem Cell Rep 14(5):876–891
58. Marques CR, Marote A, Mendes-Pinheiro B, Teixeira FG, Salgado AJ (2018) Cell secretome based approaches in parkinson's disease regenerative medicine. Expert Opin Biol Ther 18(12):1235–1245
59. Fan C, Li X, Xiao Z, Zhao Y. Liang H, Wang B, Han S, Li X, Xu B, Wang N, Liu S, Xue W, Dai J (2017) A modified collagen scaffold facilitates endogenous neurogenesis for acute spinal cord injury repair. Acta Biomater 51:304–316
60. Gelain F, Cigognini D, Caprini A, Silva D, Colleoni B, Donegá M, Antonini S, Cohen BE, Vescovi A (2012) New bioactive motifs and their use in functionalized self-assembling peptides for NSC differentiation and neural tissue engineering. Nanoscale 4(9):2946–2957
61. Dutta S, Singh G, Sreejith S, Mamidi MK, Husin JM, Datta I, Pal R, Das AK (2013) Cell therapy: the final frontier for treatment of neurological diseases. CNS Neurosci Ther 19(1):5–11
62. Laroni A, Novi G, de Kerlero RN, Uccelli A (2013) Towards clinical application of mesenchymal stem cells for treatment of neurological diseases of the central nervous system. J Neuroimmune Pharmacol 8(5):1062–1076
63. Barreto JA, O'Malley W, Kubeil M, Graham B, Stephan H, Spiccia L (2011) Nanomaterials: applications in cancer imaging and therapy. Adv Mater 23(12):H18–H40
64. Adams C, Israel LL, Ostrovsky S, Taylor A, Poptani H, Lellouche JP, Chari D (2016) Development of multifunctional magnetic nanoparticles for genetic engineering and tracking of neural stem cells. Adv Healthc Mater 5(7):841–849
65. Aswendt M, Henn N, Michalk S, Schneider G, Steiner MS, Bissa U, Dose C, Hoehn M (2015) Novel bimodal iron oxide particles for efficient tracking of human neural stem cells in vivo. Nanomedicine 10(16):2499–2512
66. Qiao S, Liu Y, Han F, Guo M, Hou X, Ye K, Deng S, Shen Y, Zhao Y, Wei H, Song B, Yao L, Tian W (2018) An intelligent neural stem cell delivery system for neurodegenerative diseases treatment. Adv Healthc Mater 7(12):1–10

67. Bannunah AM, Vllasaliu D, Lord J, Stonik S (2014) Mechanisms of nanoparticle internalization and transport across an intestinal epithelial cell model: effect of size and surface charge. Mol Pharm 11(12):4363–4373
68. Dayem A, Lee SB, Cho SG (2018) The impact of metallic nanoparticles on stem cell proliferation and differentiation. Nanomaterials 8(10):761–765
69. Ilie I, Ilie R, Mocan T, Bartos D, Mocan L (2012) Influence of nanomaterials on stem cell differentiation: designing an appropriate nanobiointerface. Int J Nanomed 7:2211–2225
70. Zhao F, Zhao Y, Liu Y, Chang X, Chen C, Zhao Y (2011) Cellular uptake intracellular trafficking and cytotoxicity of nanomaterials. Small 7(10):1322–1337
71. Wan D, Chen D, Li K, Qu Y, Sun K, Tao K, Dai K, Ai S (2016) Gold nanoparticles as a potential cellular probe for tracking of stem cells in bone regeneration using dual-energy computed tomography. ACS Appl Mater Interfaces 8(47):32241–32249
72. Shah DA, Kwon SJ, Bale SS, Banerjee A, Dordick JS, Kane RS (2011) Regulation of stem cell signaling by nanoparticle-mediated intracellular protein delivery. Biomaterials 32(12):3210–3219
73. Cheng SH, Yu D, Tsai HM, Morshed RA, Kanojia D, Lo LW, Leoni L, Govind Y, Zhang L, Aboody KS, Lesniak MS, Chen CT, Balyasnikova IV (2016) Dynamic in vivo SPECT imaging of neural stem cells functionalized with radiolabeled nanoparticles for tracking of glioblastoma. J Nucl Med 57(2):279–284
74. Shen Y, Shao Y, He H, Tan Y, Tian X, Xie F, Li L (2013) Gadolinium(3+)-doped mesoporous silica nanoparticles as a potential magnetic resonance tracer for monitoring the migration of stem cells in vivo. Int J Nanomedicine 8:119–127
75. Yang D, Li T, Xu M, Gao F, Yang J, Yang Z, Le W (2014) Graphene oxide promotes the differentiation of mouse embryonic stem cells to dopamine neurons. Nanomedicine 9(16):2445–2455
76. Akhavan O, Ghaderi E (2013) Flash photo stimulation of human neural stem cells on graphene/ TiO_2 heterojunction for differentiation into neurons. Nanoscale 5(21):10316–10326
77. Liu X, Ren X, Deng X, Huo Y, Xie J, Huang H, Jiao Z, Wu M, Liu Y, Wen T (2010) A protein interaction network for the analysis of the neuronal differentiation of neural stem cells in response to titanium dioxide nanoparticles. Biomaterials 31(11):3063–3070
78. Gao Y, Wang Y, Fu A, Shi W, Yeo D, Luo KQ, Ow H, Xu C (2015) Tracking mesenchymal stem cell tumor-homing using fluorescent silica nanoparticles. J Mater Chem B 3(7):1245–1253
79. Huang YJ, Wu HC, Tai NH, Wang TW (2012) Carbon nanotube rope with electrical stimulation promotes the differentiation and maturity of neural stem cells. Small 8(18):2869–2877
80. Lewin M, Carlesso N, Tung CH, Tang XW, Cory D, Scadden DT, Weissleder R (2000) Tat peptide-derivatized magnetic nanoparticles allow in vivo tracking and recovery of progenitor cells. Nat Biotechnol 18(4):410–414
81. Bible E, Dell'Acqua F, Solanky B, Balducci A, Crapo PM, Badylak SF, Ahrens ET, Modo M (2012) Non-invasive imaging of transplanted human neural stem cells and ECM scaffold remodeling in the stroke-damaged rat brain by (19) F and diffusion MRI. Biomaterials 33(10):2858–2871
82. Lei Y, Tang H, Yao L, Yu R, Feng M, Zou B (2008) Applications of mesenchymal stem cells labeled with Tat peptide conjugated quantum dots to cell tracking in mouse body. Bioconjug Chem 19(2):421–427
83. Ruiz-Cabello J, Walczak P, Kedziorek DA, Chacko VP, Schmieder AH, Wickline SA, Lanza GM, Bulte JW (2008) In vivo "hot spot" MR imaging of neural stem cells using fluorinated nanoparticles. Magn Reson Med 60(6):1506–1511
84. Bible E, Chau DY, Alexander MR, Price J, Shakesheff KM, Modo M (2009) Attachment of stem cells to scaffold particles for intra-cerebral transplantation. Nat Protoc 4(10):1440–1453
85. Hotta R, Cheng L, Graham HK, Nagy N, Belkind-Gerson J, Mattheolabakis G, Amiji MM, Goldstein AM (2016) Delivery of enteric neural progenitors with 5-HT4 agonist-loaded nanoparticles and thermosensitive hydrogel enhances cell proliferation and differentiation following transplantation in vivo. Biomaterials 88:1–11

86. Han HW, Hsu SH (2017) Chitosan derived co-spheroids of neural stem cells and mesenchymal stem cells for neural regeneration. Colloids Surf B Biointerfaces 158:527–538
87. Gnavi S, di Blasio L, Tonda-Turo C, Mancardi A, Primo L, Ciardelli G, Gambarotta G, Geuna S, Perroteau I (2017) Gelatin-based hydrogel for vascular endothelial growth factor release in peripheral nerve tissue engineering. J Tissue Eng Regen Med 11(2):459–470
88. Zhang Y, Chopp M, Meng Y, Katakowski M, Xin H, Mahmood A, Xiong Y (2015) Effect of exosomes derived from multipluripotent mesenchymal stromal cells on functional recovery and neurovascular plasticity in rats after traumatic brain injury. J Neurosurg 122(4):856–867
89. Jeffery ND, McBain SC, Dobson J, Chari DM (2009) Uptake of systemically administered magnetic nanoparticles (MNPs) in areas of experimental spinal cord injury (SCI). J Tissue Eng Regen Med 3:153–157
90. Gribkoff VK, Kaczmarek LK (2017) The need for new approaches in CNS drug discovery: why drugs have failed, and what can be done to improve outcomes. Neuropharmacology 120:11–19
91. Joshi CR, Labhasetwar V, Ghorpade A (2017) Destination brain: the past, present, and future of therapeutic gene delivery. J Neuroimmune Pharmacol 12(1):51–83
92. Choong CJ, Baba K, Mochizuki H (2016) Gene therapy for neurological disorders. Expert Opin Biol Ther 16(2):143–159
93. Cideciyan AV, Jacobson SG, Beltran WA, Sumaroka A, Swider M, Iwabe S, Roman AJ, Olivares MB, Schwartz SB, Komaromy AM, Hauswirth WW, Aguirre GD (2013) Human retinal gene therapy for Leber congenital amaurosis shows advancing retinal degeneration despite enduring visual improvement. PNAS 110(6):E517–E525
94. MacLaren RE, Groppe MB, Alun R, Cottriall CL, Tolmachova T, Seymour L, Clark KRD, Matthew J, Cremers Frans PM, Black Graeme CM, Lotery AJ, Downes SM, Webster AR, Seabra MC (2014) Retinal gene therapy in patients with choroideremia: initial findings from a phase 1/2 clinical trial. Lancet 383(9923):1129–1137
95. Nathwani AC, Tuddenham Edward GD, Rangarajan S, Rosales C, McIntosh J, Linch DC, Chowdary P, Riddell A, Pie AJ, Harrington C, O'Beirne J, Smith K, Pasi J, Glader B, Rustagi PN, Catherine YC, Kay MA, Zhou J, Spence Y, Morton CL, Allay J, Coleman J, Sleep S, Cunningham JM, Srivastava D, Basner-Tschakarjan E, Mingozzi FH, Katherine A, Gray JT, Reiss UM, Nienhuis AW, Davidoff AM (2011) Adenovirus-associated virus vector-mediated gene transfer in haemophilia. N Engl J Med 365(25):2357–2365
96. Nienhuis AW (2013) Development of gene therapy for blood disorders: an update. Blood 122(9):1556–1564
97. Cavazzana-Calvo M, Payen E, Negre O, Wang G, Hehir K, Fusil F, Down J, Denaro M, Brady T, Westerman K (2010) Transfusion independence and HMGA2 activation after gene therapy of human beta-thalassaemia. Nature 467(7313):318–322
98. Zhang J, Li Y, Xiong J, Xu H, Xiang G, Fan M, Zhou K, Lin Y, Chen X, Xie L, Zhang H, Wang J, Xiao J (2021) Delivery of pOXR1 through an injectable liposomal nanoparticle enhances spinal cord injury regeneration by alleviating oxidative stress. Bioact Mater 6(2021):3177–3191
99. Imaoka T, Date I, Ohmoto T, Nagatsu T (1998) Significant behavioral recovery in parkinson's disease model by direct intracerebral gene transfer using continuous injection of a plasmid DNA-liposome complex. Hum Gene ther 1998;9(7):1093–102
100. Zhang Y, Schlachetzki F, Zhang YF, Boado RJ, Pardridge WM (2004) Normalization of striatal tyrosine hydroxylase and reversal of motor impairment in experimental parkinsonism with intravenous nonviral gene therapy and a brain-specific promoter. Hum Gene Ther 15(4):339–350
101. Zhang Y, Lee HJ, Boado RJ, Pardridge WM (2002) Receptor-mediated delivery of an antisense gene to human brain cancer cells. Journal Gene Med 4(2):183–194
102. Shi L, Tang GP, Gao SJ, Ma YX, Liu BH, Li Y, Zeng JM, Ng YK, Leong KW, Wang S (2003) Repeated intrathecal administration of plasmid DNA complexed with polyethylene glycol-grafted polyethylenimine led to prolonged transgene expression in the spinal cord. Gene Ther 10(14):1179–1188

103. Zhang Y (2004) Intravenous RNA interference gene therapy targeting the human epidermal growth factor receptor prolongs survival in intracranial brain cancer. Clin cancer Res 10(11):3667–3677
104. Snowball A, Chabrol E, Wykes RC, Shekh-Ahmad T, Cornford JH, Lieb A, Hughes MP, Massaro G, Rahim AA, Hashemi KS, Kullmann DM, Walker MC, Schorge S (2019) Epilepsy gene therapy using an engineered potassium channel. J Neurosci 39(16):3159–3169
105. Wykes RC, Heeroma JH, Mantoan L, Zheng K, MacDonald DC, Deisseroth K, Hashemi KS, Walker MC, Schorge S, Kullmann DM (2012) Optogenetic and potassium channel gene therapy in a rodent model of focal neocortical epilepsy. Sci Transl Med 4(161):161–171
106. Jack CR (2020) Alzheimer Disease, Biomarkers, and Clinical Symptoms- Quo Vadis? Neurology 77(3):394
107. Wang X, Li T (2020) Role of adenosine kinase inhibitor in adenosine augmentation therapy for epilepsy: a potential novel drug for epilepsy. Curr Drug Targets 21(3):252–257
108. Agnihotri A, Aruoma OI (2020) Alzheimer's disease and parkinson's disease: a nutritional toxicology perspective of the impact of oxidative stress, mitochondrial dysfunction, nutrigenomics and environmental chemicals. J Am Coll Nutr 39(1):16–27
109. Libon DJ, Lamar M, Swenson RA, Heilman KM (2020) Vascular disease, Alzheimer's disease, and mild cognitive impairment: advancing an integrated approach. OUP 9(1):76–92

Nanomaterials for Diagnosis and Treatment of Common Neurological Disorders

Gursharan Kaur, Aleena James Chirayimmel, Palak Rana, Sonia Sharma, Jagadeesh Chandra Bose, Santosh Kumar Rath, and Vagish Dwibedi

Abstract Smart nanomaterials have emerged as a promising approach for drug delivery and the management of neurological diseases. Neurodegenerative disorders pose significant challenges in terms of treatment due to the limited ability of drugs to cross the blood–brain barrier (BBB) and effectively reach the affected regions in the central nervous system (CNS). However, advancements in nanotechnology offer exciting opportunities to overcome these limitations by utilizing smart nanomaterials for targeted drug delivery. Neurodegenerative diseases, such as Parkinson's disease, Alzheimer's disease, and others, are characterized by the gradual deterioration of neuronal structure and function, leading to neuronal death. Despite extensive drug screening efforts, no particular treatment is available that can cure these diseases or effectively reduce their progression. Smart nanomaterials, which possess the ability to respond and adapt to external stimuli, have distinct advantages for neuro-drug delivery. These nanomaterials can be engineered to respond to specific triggers, such as changes in temperature, pH, or enzymatic activity, to release drugs at the desired site within the body. This targeted drug delivery approach enhances therapeutic efficacy, minimizes side effects, and reduces the required dosage, thereby improving patient outcomes. Furthermore, smart nanomaterials can be functionalized to cross the BBB, allowing for the delivery of therapeutic agents directly to the brain. This approach holds great promise for the treatment of neurodegenerative disorders, as it enables higher drug concentrations at the site of action, improving treatment outcomes. Despite these promising advantages, the clinical translation of

G. Kaur · P. Rana · S. Sharma · J. C Bose · V. Dwibedi (✉)
University Institute of Biotechnology, Chandigarh University, Mohali 140413, India
e-mail: vagishdwibedi@gmail.com; vagish.lcc@gmail.com

A. J. Chirayimmel
School of Biosciences and Technology, Vellore Institute of Technology, Vellore 632014, India

S. K. Rath
School of Pharmaceuticals and Population Health Informatics, Faculty of Pharmacy, DIT University, Dehradun, Uttarakhand 248009, India

V. Dwibedi
Institute of Soil, Water and Environmental Sciences, Volcani Research Center, Agricultural Research Organization, 7528809 Rishon Lezion, Israel

S. K. Rath et al. (eds.), *Nanomaterials for Drug Delivery and Neurological Diseases Management*, Smart Nanomaterials Technology,
https://doi.org/10.1007/978-981-97-0308-1_8

smart nanomaterials for neuro-drug delivery also faces challenges and limitations. Ensuring the safety and biocompatibility of these materials is crucial, as they interact with the intricate and sensitive structures of the CNS. A thorough assessment of toxicity, long-term effects, and potential immunological reactions is essential to mitigate any adverse effects on neuronal function or overall health. The journey toward clinical translation of nanomedicines for brain drug delivery is complex and requires careful consideration of regulatory and ethical issues. Adequate in vitro and animal models that accurately represent human physiology are essential for reliable and predictive outcomes in clinical trials.

Keywords Neurological disorders · Smart nanomaterials · Drug delivery · Blood–brain barrier

1 Introduction

In recent years, with an increase in the aging population, the need for developing therapeutic approaches to treat Neurodegenerative disorders (ND) is also increasing. These disorders are characterized by the gradual deterioration of neuronal structure and function, often leading to neuronal death. Despite extensive drug screening efforts, no particular treatment is available that can cure these diseases or effectively reduce their succession. Neurodegenerative disorders such as Parkinson's disease (PD), frontotemporal dementia, amyotrophic lateral sclerosis (ALS), Huntington's disease, Alzheimer's disease (AD), brain tumors, epilepsy, and prion disease affect a significant number of individuals worldwide [1, 2]. Neurodegenerative diseases arise when nerve cells in the brain experience functional impairment or premature cell death [3].

The treatment of neurodegenerative diseases has encountered several challenges, including limitations imposed by the blood-cerebrospinal fluid barrier (BCFB), blood–brain barrier (BBB), and P-glycoproteins [4]. The average molecular weight of the drugs used in treating neurological diseases is greater than 400–500 Dalton, which does not pass through the blood–brain barrier (BBB) in therapeutically significant quantity [5]. However, recent advancements in nanotechnology offer promising opportunities to overcome these limitations by leveraging nanomaterials and designing improved drug delivery systems to transport active drug candidates effectively [6].

Nanotechnology has revolutionized technological advancements by introducing innovative inventions such as nanoparticles (NPs), nanocarriers, microparticles (MPs), polymeric nanomaterials (NMs), nanomedicines, and nanotubes. Nanotechnology has gained significant recognition in the field of biomedical science, as evidenced by the approval of over 100 nanomedicine products by the US FDA. This demonstrates the profound impact of nanotechnology on modern biomedical research. In recognition of its significance, the US federal authorities have allocated more than $1.4 billion in funding for the National Nanotechnology Initiative, underscoring the importance placed on this field. Globally, nanotechnology has garnered substantial attention, and a recent Forbes report highlights it as one of the top five emerging technologies to closely monitor in the upcoming decade [7]. Nano-drug delivery systems offer enhanced control and safety in the release of loaded drugs by providing continuous release. This feature enables a reduction in the dosage requirement and facilitates precise dosage regimen control [8]. These breakthroughs have significantly contributed to the field of managing neurodegenerative diseases by enabling precise drug delivery to specific molecular targets and action sites [1].

Nanocarriers utilize various strategies to enhance drug delivery to brain tumors. The four primary strategies employed by nanocarriers for improved drug delivery to the brain tissue are discussed here. Firstly, by applying focused ultrasound waves, the tight junctions between endothelial cells in the blood–brain barrier (BBB) can be weakened. This enables better uptake of nanocarriers into the brain tissue. Then considering the enhanced permeability and retention (EPR) effect: While liposomes can pass through the intact BBB, the rate of penetration is generally low. However, in the presence of leaky tumor vasculature, such as in brain tumors, liposomes and exosomes can exploit the EPR effect, which enhances their penetration into the brain tissue.

Further, transporter substrate modification: Liposomes can be modified by attaching transporter substrates like glucose, transferrin, or glutathione. These modifications facilitate the crossing of liposomes through the BBB, improving drug delivery to the brain tissue. At last, Trojan Horse approach: Liposomes can be designed to target circulating cells that have the ability to penetrate the BBB. This approach involves using these cells as carriers to transport liposomes across the BBB and deliver drugs to the brain tissue. Additionally, it is important to note that once inside the brain tissue, drugs need to be released from the liposomes to exert their therapeutic effects. However, efflux pumps present in the brain parenchyma can remove many drugs, limiting their efficacy [9].

Various strategies have been employed for brain targeting using nanocarriers, including the incorporation of BBB receptor ligands, conjugation of antibodies, peptides, or aptamers with BBB receptor ligand delivery systems, and the utilization of transporter ligands coupled with micelle delivery systems [10]. BBB is composed of a specialized basal membrane with a number of pericytes embedded in this basal membrane, endothelial cells of the brain, and end feet astrocytes. Other than that, two types of tight paracellular and intercellular adherent junctions are also involved in BBB. Adherent junctions consist of actinin, catenin, vascular endothelium (VE), and cadherin, which plays an important role in maintaining functional integrity of BBB. Whereas the main role in controlling the permeability of the BBB is of paracellular tight junctions [11].

As soon as the nanoparticles enter intravenously into the bloodstream, there are higher chances of protein opsonization, which limits the bioavailability and reduces the retention time due to the nonspecific clearance of the nanoparticles by the immune system. Therefore, to avoid this development of safe and effective therapeutic nanocarriers is important for achieving the ultimate goal of nanomedicine, which is done by employing specific surface molecules such as carbohydrates, liposomes, aspartate-glycine-arginine peptide, acetyl groups, albumin, polyethyleneglycol (PEG) [12]. In a similar way to improve the bioavailability of nanoparticles, water-insoluble therapeutic agents can be used in combination with nanoparticles, which will provide protection from various physiological barriers leading to easy transmission of the nanoparticle to the targeted site. On the other hand, for easy imaging and pathway tracking to their delivery locations in in-vivo systems, specific contrasting agents in combination with therapeutic nanocarriers can be used [13].

In recent researches, nanomaterial-based therapeutics hold great value in the treatment of neurological disorders, however, there are also ethical constraints that need to be considered. These constraints include potential toxicity and technical challenges in fabricating them, and regulatory and ethical issues raised by the usage of nanomaterials. It is important to carefully evaluate the safety and efficacy of nanomaterial-based therapies and to ensure that they are accessible to all patients in an equitable manner. This comprehensive chapter gives a summary of diverse nano-carrier agents, with a specific focus on their therapeutic potential for various neurological diseases.

2 Smart Nanomaterials for Neuro-drug Delivery

2.1 Nanomaterial

A smart nanomaterial is a nanoscale material with the ability to respond and adapt to external stimuli, enabling functionalities such as sensing, actuation, or controlled release of substances. It combines the unique properties of nanomaterials with intelligent behavior for advanced applications in various fields [14]. Smart nanomaterials possess distinct characteristics that distinguish them from regular nanomaterials. These materials are designed to respond to external stimuli, such as changes in temperature, light, pH, or magnetic fields. They exhibit intelligent behavior by sensing, actuating, or releasing substances in a controlled manner. This responsiveness is achieved through the incorporation of stimuli-responsive elements, such as polymers or nanoparticles, into the nanomaterial structure. The ability of smart nanomaterials to adapt and self-regulate their properties enables advanced applications in areas such as drug delivery, sensing, and responsive coatings. [15]

Smart nanomaterials possess unique physical and chemical properties that enable their responsive behavior. Physically, they exhibit tunable sizes, shapes, and surface properties, allowing precise control over their interactions with the environment. Chemically, they can undergo reversible changes in their structure or properties in response to specific stimuli, such as pH, light, or temperature. These properties enable applications such as targeted drug delivery, stimuli-responsive sensors, and adaptive coatings for controlled release [16].

2.2 Types of Nanomaterials Used for Neuro-drug Delivery

Types of smart nanomaterials for neuro-drug delivery smart nanoparticles can be classified based on their interaction with the surrounding environment. The first class consists of environment-responsive nanoparticles, which have the ability to sense and react to changes in their environment. Various diseases are known to cause alterations in biochemical properties such as pH, redox potential, homeostatic pathways, and enzymatic activity. By utilizing these changes, nanoparticles can be designed to specifically target and immobilize pre-existing disease conditions [17]. The second class of nanoparticles, known as environment-primed nanoparticles, functions by manipulating the host environment. This can be achieved through the administration of different stimuli such as radiation (such as X-rays or infrared), heat, drugs, and additional nanoparticles. By employing these techniques, interactions between the host and nanoparticles and among nanoparticles can be facilitated and controlled [18]. Smart polymeric nanomaterials responsive to stimuli have been extensively studied for their potential in drug delivery. One particular area of investigation involves the development of redox-responsive polymeric micelles, taking advantage of the existing redox potential gradient between the intracellular and extracellular spaces. Polyphosphates, a class of biomaterials known for their biodegradability, biocompatibility, and structural similarity to nucleic and teichoic acids, have been successfully utilized for this purpose [19]. Different types of nanoparticles are illustrated in Fig. 1.

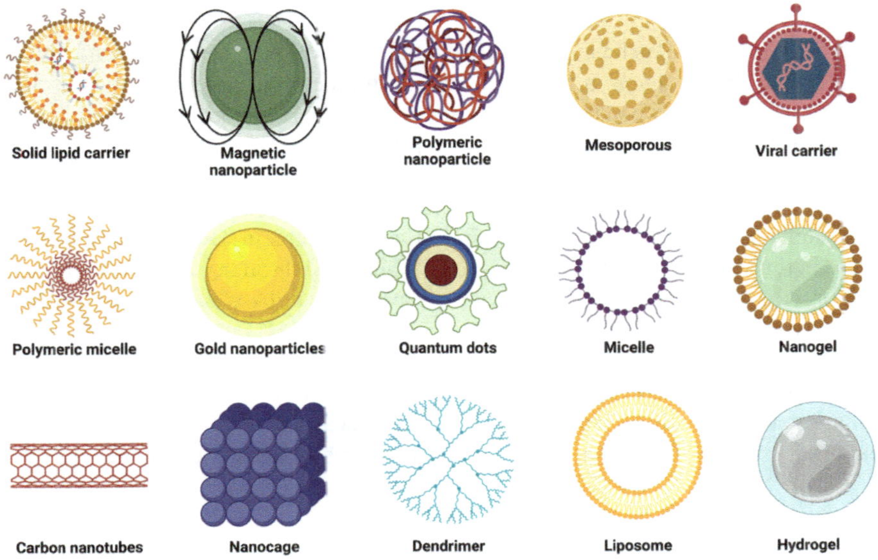

Fig. 1 Various types of nanoparticles used in nanodrug delivery

2.2.1 Micelle

A type of co-polyphosphate, which is amphiphilic (having both hydrophilic and hydrophobic parts), has been used to create tiny micellar structures for delivering drugs. These micelles have the unique property of being responsive to changes in the redox (oxidation–reduction) environment. They are also biocompatible and biodegradable and the micelles have many functional groups on their surface that can attach to drug molecules, targeting agents, or imaging agents. They respond to environmental cues and can release drugs, especially anticancer drugs, inside the nuclei of tumor cells. This inhibits the growth of cancer cells. By taking advantage of the sensitivity to redox conditions, these drug delivery systems can be designed effectively for the treatment of diseases [20]. In cellular and tissue environments, the decrease in pH has been utilized in different nanoparticle systems to induce various effects. These effects include altering the shape or solubility of nanoparticles, modifying the binding strength between receptor and ligand pairs, or initiating the breakdown of acid-sensitive bonds. In the field of pharmaceuticals, delivering antimicrobial peptides (AMPs) that have poor water solubility is a significant challenge. pH-sensitive nanomaterials can undergo changes in shape or solubility in response to acidic conditions, thereby facilitating the improved delivery of AMPs and enhancing their effectiveness in treating infections [21].

2.2.2 MicroRNAs

MicroRNAs (miRNAs) have gained considerable attention in cancer research due to their critical involvement in tumor formation and the noticeable variations in their expression levels between normal and cancerous cells. However, the limited quantities of miRNAs found in cancer cells create difficulties in utilizing them for triggering drug release [22]. To overcome this challenge, scientists have developed a unique DNA Y-motif that responds to specific stimuli. This Y-motif is designed to simultaneously deliver small interfering RNA (siRNA) and doxorubicin (Dox), a chemotherapy drug. In this design, the release of the cargo is achieved through a cascade amplification process that does not require enzymes. The process utilizes endogenous miRNAs found within the cells as triggers, along with ATP (or H^+) as a source of energy, through a mechanism called toehold-mediated strand displacement. By employing this strategy, therapeutic agents can be released in a controlled manner within tumor cells. To ensure specific release in tumor cells, nanocarriers are constructed with gold nanorods, stimuli-responsive Y-motifs, and temperature-sensitive polymers [23].

2.2.3 PEG (Polyethylene Glycol)

The nanocarriers used in this study have a surface that can be switched between two states: PEG (polyethylene glycol) and RGD. This switching is achieved through photothermal conversion. The PEG state acts as a protective coating on the nanocarrier surface, preventing the degradation of the Y-motifs coupled to it by nucleases. This protection allows the Y-motifs to accumulate at tumor sites. By combining stimuli-responsive Y-motifs, gold nanorods, and temperature-sensitive polymers, this approach enables the controlled release of drugs specifically within tumor cells. The use of endogenous miRNAs as triggers and NIR-induced heat allows for precise and targeted drug delivery. This strategy holds significant potential for enhancing the efficacy of cancer therapies by overcoming the limitations associated with low miRNA abundance and improving drug release specifically within tumor cells [24]. Neurological disorders present a significant challenge in drug delivery due to the complexities of the blood–brain barrier (BBB) and the need for precise targeting of specific brain regions. Smart nanomaterials have emerged as promising candidates for neuro-drug delivery due to their unique properties and ability to overcome these barriers.

2.2.4 Lipid-Based Nanoparticles

Lipid-based nanoparticles, such as liposomes and solid lipid nanoparticles (SLNs), have gained considerable attention for neuro-drug delivery [25]. These nanomaterials possess biocompatible and biodegradable properties, enabling efficient encapsulation and protection of neuroactive drugs. Furthermore, their surface can be modified to enhance BBB penetration, prolong circulation time, and target specific cell types or brain regions. Lipid-based nanoparticles offer controlled release and have demonstrated successful delivery of therapeutics to treat neurodegenerative diseases and brain tumors [26]. Polymer-based nanoparticles, including polymeric micelles and dendrimers, have shown promise for neuro-drug delivery. These nanomaterials possess high drug-loading capacity, stability, and the ability to encapsulate a wide range of drug molecules. Their surface can be functionalized to enhance BBB permeability and facilitate active targeting through ligand-receptor interactions.

2.2.5 Polymer-Based Nanoparticles

Polymer-based nanoparticles have demonstrated successful delivery of drugs for neuroprotection, pain management, and gene therapy in preclinical studies [27]. Scientists conducted a study on brain-targeting therapy for Alzheimer's disease using RIN administration. They developed Tween 80 coated methoxy poly (ethylene glycol) PLGA NPs to enhance RIN's activity and targeting abilities. The nanoparticles showed safety, improved permeation, and higher transport across the blood–brain barrier in vitro and in vivo, demonstrating their potential for neurodegenerative disease therapy [28].

2.2.6 Mesoporous Silica Nanoparticles

Mesoporous silica nanoparticles (MSNPs) offer unique features for neuro-drug delivery, including high surface area, tunable pore size, and excellent drug-loading capacity. MSNPs can encapsulate both hydrophilic and hydrophobic drugs within their porous structure, providing sustained release and protection against enzymatic degradation. Surface modifications with targeting ligands allow specific delivery to brain cells or regions. MSNPs have shown promise in delivering therapeutic agents for neurodegenerative disorders, neuroinflammation, and neurotrauma [29]. Thiol-functionalized mesoporous silica nanoparticles (HS-MSNPs) were employed in a method combining dispersive ionic liquid-micro-solid phase extraction (DIL-μ-SPE) with electrothermal atomic absorption spectrometry (ET-AAS). This technique enabled the detection and differentiation of Mo (II, VI) in human biological samples. HS-MSNPs, along with a hydrophobic ionic liquid and acetone, facilitated the separate extraction of Mo (II) and Mo (VI) ions from blood and serum samples, followed by their back-extraction and concentration determination using ET-AAS. [30].

2.2.7 Magnetic Nanoparticles

Magnetic nanoparticles, such as iron oxide nanoparticles, have attracted attention for their dual functionality in neuro-drug delivery. These nanoparticles can be guided and targeted using external magnetic fields, enabling precise localization within the brain. Additionally, they can serve as contrast agents for imaging, facilitating real-time monitoring of drug delivery. Magnetic nanoparticles have been explored for targeted drug delivery in neuro-oncology, neurodegeneration, and neuroimaging applications [31]. Different coatings have been used to develop iron nanoparticles (IONPs) as contrast agents for magnetic resonance imaging. When injected intravenously, these IONPs were observed to reach the brain by passing through the choroid plexus, as demonstrated in mice models with induced neuroinflammation [32].

2.2.8 Carbon-Based Nanoparticles

Carbon-based nanomaterials, including carbon nanotubes (CNTs) and graphene, offer unique properties for neuro-drug delivery. CNTs possess exceptional mechanical strength, high aspect ratios, and unique electrical conductivity, making them suitable for both drug delivery and neural tissue engineering. Functionalized CNTs can carry drugs and enhance their transport across the BBB. Graphene-based nanomaterials possess high drug-loading capacity, stability, and excellent biocompatibility, making them promising candidates for targeted neuro-drug delivery [33].

2.2.9 Quantum Dots

Quantum dots (QDs) are nanoparticles made of semiconducting materials that possess exceptional optical characteristics. They have a size-dependent bandgap that allows them to emit fluorescent light of various colors when excited by light or electricity. QDs can be engineered to encapsulate and deliver neuroactive drugs, acting as carriers for targeted drug delivery to specific brain regions. Their fluorescence properties enable real-time tracking and monitoring of drug release and distribution within the brain. Additionally, QDs can be functionalized with ligands for BBB penetration and targeted delivery to brain cells [34]. Researchers developed an innovative electrochemical sensor by modifying a carbon paste electrode (CPE) with an ionic liquid (IL) and carbon quantum dots (CQDs). This modified electrode exhibited excellent electrocatalytic activity for detecting dopamine (DA) even in the presence of uric acid and ascorbic acid. The sensor allowed for the accurate measurement of DA in a linear range of 0.1–50 μM, with a low limit of detection of 0.046 μM. The sensor's successful application in real samples highlights its potential for diagnosing neurological disorders through molecular analysis of DA [35].

2.2.10 Gold Nanoparticles

Gold nanoparticles (AuNPs) possess excellent biocompatibility, surface plasmon resonance, and the ability to carry therapeutic agents. They can be functionalized with various molecules to enhance their stability, target specific cell types, and facilitate BBB penetration. AuNPs can be used for controlled drug release triggered by external stimuli, such as heat or light, providing localized drug delivery to specific brain regions. Moreover, their unique optical properties enable them to act as imaging agents, allowing real-time visualization of drug delivery and distribution in the brain [36]. The nanoparticles were characterized using various analysis techniques, confirming their formation. In vitro studies using murine microglial BV2 cells demonstrated the cytotoxicity property and neuroprotective effect of the synthesized nanoparticles against inflammation. In vivo, experiments conducted on Parkinson-induced mice further validated the nanoparticles' ability to alleviate neuroinflammation and improve motor coordination. These findings highlight the potential of gold nanoparticles synthesized from Paeonia Mountain as an effective nanodrug for neurological disorders [37].

2.2.11 Stimuli-Responsive Nanoparticles

Stimuli-responsive nanoparticles are designed to release drugs in response to specific triggers in the target environment. For neuro-drug delivery, stimuli such as temperature, pH, enzyme activity, or magnetic fields can be employed to trigger drug release at the desired location. These nanoparticles can be engineered using materials that undergo structural changes or respond to external stimuli, leading to the release of encapsulated drugs. By incorporating stimuli-responsive elements into the nanomaterials, controlled drug release and targeted therapy can be achieved, improving the efficacy and reducing side effects of neuroactive drugs (X. [38]. Thermo-responsive hydrogels are extensively investigated stimuli-responsive hydrogels that typically incorporate various hydrophobic groups (such as ethyl, methyl, and propyl groups). These hydrophobic groups enable the hydrogels to undergo changes in their physical and conformational properties in response to temperature variations [39]. Photo-responsive hydrogels exhibit responsiveness to visible, near infrared (NIR), and ultraviolet (UV) light. These hydrogels consist of polymer networks that incorporate photosensitive components capable of reversible crosslinking and photothermal effects. When exposed to light, the photosensitive moieties within the hydrogel capture the light signal and undergo chemical reactions such as isomerization, cleavage, or dimerization, leading to structural or property changes such as swelling, shrinking, or cross-linking [40]. Magnetic-responsive hydrogels are created by incorporating magnetic nanoparticles into crosslinked polymers, allowing the nanoparticles to undergo structural, functional, and property changes when exposed to magnetic fields. Apart from Fe_3O_4, other commonly used magnetic nanoparticles include $Zn_{0.47}Mn_{0.53}Fe_2O_4$, $Fe_3O_4@SiO_2$, Co_3O_4, and γ-Fe_2O_3. The synthesis of magnetic-responsive hydrogels typically involves three methods: co-precipitation or embedding, grafting, and blending [41].

Electro-responsive hydrogels are created by incorporating electroactive materials into a hydrogel matrix. These electroactive materials can be categorized into two groups: natural materials, including metals, and inorganic or organic conductive materials such as graphene, polypyrrole (PPy), carbon nanotubes, ethylenedioxythiophene (PEDOT), polyaniline (PANI). When subjected to an electric field, electro-responsive hydrogels can undergo changes in their structures and properties, allowing them to perform specific functions [42]. Bio-responsive hydrogels have the ability to modify their structures or properties, such as swelling and contraction, when exposed to specific biological factors or changes in activity and concentration. These hydrogels can be broadly categorized into two types: hydrogels coated with antigens or antibodies that react to specific antigens or antibodies and hydrogels coated with enzyme reaction substrates that respond to enzymatic activity [43]. Scientists discovered a hydrogel composed of sodium alginate, collagen, stromal cell-derived factor-1 (SDF-1), loaded with bone marrow-derived mesenchymal stem cells (BMSCs/SA/Col/SDF-1), facilitated the recovery of neurological function following traumatic brain injury (TBI). This was achieved by promoting neurogenesis in the hippocampus, as indicated by an increase in the number of $EdU^+/NeuN^+$ cells and the expression of neurotrophic factors [44]. Zheng et al. developed an injectable hydrogel composed of polydopamine/stromal cell-derived factor-1α (PDA/SDF-1α) nanoparticles using imidazole-modified gelatin methacrylate (GelMA-imid). The study demonstrated that the GelMA-imid/SDF-1α hydrogel, when loaded with human amniotic mesenchymal stromal cells (hAMSCs), promoted the regeneration of endogenous neural cells. These regenerated cells exhibited high expression of neuronal nuclei (NeuN), brain-derived neurotrophic factor (BDNF), and neuron-specific enolase (NSE), suggesting significant potential for TBI recovery [45].

Smart nanomaterials hold immense potential for overcoming the challenges associated with neuro-drug delivery. Mesoporous silica nanoparticles, polymer-based nanoparticles, lipid-based nanoparticles, magnetic nanoparticles, and carbon-based nanomaterials offer unique properties that enable targeted and efficient drug delivery to the brain. Continued research and development in this field will further enhance the therapeutic efficacy of neuroactive drugs and pave the way for more effective treatments of neurological disorders. Incorporating these smart nanomaterials, such as gold nanoparticles, quantum dots, and stimuli-responsive nanoparticles, expands the arsenal of tools available for precise and targeted drug delivery to the brain. Further research and development in this field will continue to advance the field of neuro-drug delivery, enabling more effective treatments for neurological disorders [46].

2.3 Advantages of Nanomaterials

Smart nanomaterials offer numerous advantages and hold great potential for various applications due to their unique properties and responsive behavior. These have revolutionized drug delivery systems by offering precise and controlled release of therapeutic agents. These nanomaterials can be engineered to respond to specific triggers, such as changes in temperature, pH, or enzymatic activity, to release drugs at the desired site within the body [47]. This targeted drug delivery approach enhances therapeutic efficacy, minimizes side effects, and reduces the required dosage, thereby improving patient outcomes. It also offers numerous advantages in the field of neurological diseases, revolutionizing diagnosis, treatment, and monitoring. Their unique properties and functionalities make them highly promising tools for addressing the challenges associated with neurological disorders [48].

One of the primary benefits of smart nanomaterials is their ability to facilitate targeted drug delivery to the central nervous system (CNS). These nanomaterials can be engineered to carry therapeutic agents, such as drugs or gene therapies, specifically to the affected regions of the brain or spinal cord. By encapsulating these agents within nanocarriers, smart nanomaterials provide enhanced stability, protection, and controlled release. This targeted drug delivery approach minimizes off-target effects, reduces systemic toxicity, and maximizes the therapeutic efficacy of treatments for neurological diseases [49]. Functionalized nanomaterials can serve as biosensors, detecting specific biomarkers or abnormalities associated with these diseases. Their large surface area-to-volume ratio enhances the sensitivity and accuracy of these diagnostic tests, allowing for early and precise detection. This early detection facilitates timely interventions and improves patient outcomes [50]. Moreover, smart nanomaterials can be designed to cross the blood–brain barrier (BBB), a major challenge in treating neurological diseases. The BBB restricts the entry of therapeutic agents into the brain, posing challenges in the effective delivery of drugs. However, nanomaterials can be engineered to overcome this barrier by utilizing surface modifications and transport mechanisms. This breakthrough enables the delivery of drugs directly to the brain, improving their distribution and therapeutic impact [51].

Furthermore, smart nanomaterials offer opportunities for real-time monitoring and personalized treatment of neurological disorders. Nanosensors integrated into these materials can continuously monitor disease progression, biomarker levels, or treatment responses. This data can be wirelessly transmitted to healthcare providers, enabling timely adjustments to the treatment plan. Such personalized and adaptive approaches hold great potential for optimizing therapy and improving patient outcomes in neurological diseases [52]. The multifunctionality of smart nanomaterials also allows for combinational therapies. Multiple therapeutic agents can be co-loaded into nanocarriers, targeting different aspects of the disease simultaneously. This approach can enhance treatment efficacy by addressing complex disease mechanisms or overcoming drug resistance [53]. Furthermore, the biocompatibility and biodegradability of smart nanomaterials are crucial advantages in neurological applications. These materials can be designed to minimize immunogenic responses and promote safe interactions with the biological environment. Biodegradable nanomaterials eliminate the need for additional surgical procedures for removal, minimizing patient discomfort and complications [54]. Overall, smart nanomaterials hold great promise in advancing the diagnosis, treatment, and monitoring of neurological diseases. Their targeted drug delivery capabilities, non-invasive diagnostics, ability to cross the BBB, real-time monitoring, and combinational therapy options provide unprecedented opportunities for improved patient care and outcomes. While further research and development are needed, the potential impact of smart nanomaterials in the field of neurological diseases is immense, bringing hope for more effective and personalized approaches to combat these complex conditions [55].

2.4 Challenges and Limitations

While smart nanomaterials offer immense potential in the field of neurological diseases, there are also various obstacles and constraints that require attention for their successful translation into clinical applications. One of the primary challenges is ensuring the safety and biocompatibility of smart nanomaterials. As these materials are designed to interact with the intricate and sensitive structures of the central nervous system (CNS), it is crucial to thoroughly assess their toxicity, long-term effects, and potential immunological reactions. Understanding the biodistribution, clearance mechanisms, and potential accumulation of nanomaterials within the body is essential to mitigate any adverse effects on neuronal function or overall health [56]. Another challenge lies in the complex regulatory landscape surrounding the clinical translation of smart nanomaterials. The development and approval processes for these novel technologies require extensive preclinical and clinical studies to establish their safety, efficacy, and optimal dosing strategies. Regulatory agencies need to develop appropriate guidelines to evaluate and approve smart nanomaterial-based therapies, taking into account their unique characteristics and modes of action. The scalability and cost-effectiveness of smart nanomaterial production are additional challenges [57]. Many advanced nanomaterial fabrication techniques are still in the research and development stage and may not be easily scalable for large-scale manufacturing. The cost of production, including the synthesis of nanomaterials and functionalization processes, can be prohibitively high. Overcoming these challenges is crucial to ensure the affordability and accessibility of smart nanomaterial-based therapies for patients suffering from neuro diseases [58].

Furthermore, the heterogeneity and complexity of neurological diseases present a challenge for the design and application of smart nanomaterials. Neurological disorders often involve multiple pathological mechanisms, diverse cellular targets, and complex disease progression patterns. Developing nanomaterial-based therapies that can effectively address these complexities and deliver optimal outcomes for diverse patient populations remains a significant challenge [59]. The customization and personalization of smart nanomaterial-based treatments to suit the specific needs of individual patients add another layer of complexity to their development and implementation. Smart nanomaterials hold great promise in the field of neurological diseases, but several challenges and limitations need to be addressed. Ensuring the safety and biocompatibility of these materials, navigating the regulatory landscape, achieving scalability and cost-effectiveness in production, and addressing the complexities of neuro diseases pose significant hurdles. Nonetheless, with continued research, collaboration, and technological advancements, these challenges can be overcome, unlocking the full potential of smart nanomaterials for the diagnosis, treatment, and monitoring of neurological disorders [1].

3 Nanodrug Delivery Strategies for Neuro Diseases

Over the past few decades, there has been growing interest in utilizing nanomaterials for drug and gene delivery purposes. Various types of nanomaterials, such as micelles, polymeric nanoparticles, liposomes, nanofibers, and inorganic nanoparticles, have been engineered to serve as theranostics, offering unique advantages. These nanomaterial-based theranostics exhibit remarkable features, including high drug loading capacity, biocompatibility, efficient passive and active targeting abilities, excellent stability, controlled drug release, biodegradability, and low toxicity [60, 61]. The establishment of a drug delivery strategy can naturally vary based on the size, hydrophobicity, and hydrophilicity of the compounds being used. Extensive research has been dedicated to investigating local drug delivery systems for the central nervous system (CNS), leading to the development of numerous therapeutic strategies to enhance the targeted delivery of various nanodrugs to their specific sites within the CNS [62].

Drug-loaded nanoparticles can efficiently cross the blood–brain barrier (BBB) and deliver therapeutic agents to the brain. They can encapsulate various drugs, including small molecules, peptides, and nucleic acids, enhancing their stability, solubility, and targeted delivery to specific brain regions affected by neurodegenerative diseases [63]. Furthermore, strategies that prevent recognition by the reticuloendothelial system (RES) allow drug-containing nanomaterials to remain in the bloodstream for longer periods of time. This extended circulation greatly enhances the chances of nanomaterials crossing the blood–brain barrier (BBB), leading to a substantial accumulation of drugs in the brain tissue. These beneficial characteristics make nanomaterials highly valuable in facilitating the delivery of drugs across the BBB [62]. Various approaches utilizing nanotechnologies have been extensively employed to transport theranostic agents across the blood–brain barrier (BBB). Active targeted drug delivery to the brain for the treatment of various brain and central nervous system (CNS) diseases can be achieved using a wide range of biomolecule ligands, including sugars, proteins, peptides, or antibodies. Commonly employed strategies include receptor-mediated transcytosis, mechanical or ultrasound-induced disruption of the BBB, BBB-crossing facilitated by shutter peptides, and intranasal administration of nanomaterials [64]. Based on the nanomaterial-based strategies for transiting the blood–brain barrier (BBB) mentioned above, these mechanisms can be categorized into two main types: invasive mechanism and non-invasive mechanism. In the invasive mechanism, physical methods are employed to temporarily open the BBB, allowing nanomaterials to cross through the paracellular pathway. The strategies such as temporary BBB disruption and local delivery, fall under this category, which is also known as the paracellular mechanism.

On the other hand, the non-invasive mechanism involves delivering nanomaterials across the intact BBB via the transcellular pathway, without physically disrupting the barrier. The strategies mentioned, including intranasal delivery, cell-penetrating peptide (CPP) mediated BBB crossing, receptor-mediated BBB crossing, shuttle peptide mediated BBB crossing, and cell-mediated BBB crossing, all belong to the non-invasive mechanism (Fig. 2). This mechanism can also be referred to as the transcellular mechanism [62].

3.1 Receptor-Mediated Transcytosis

As the name suggests this drug delivery strategy is a non-invasive method based on the interaction between receptors present on the brain endothelial cells and their corresponding ligands. The process of receptor-mediated transcytosis facilitates the formation of corpuscles through the endocytosis pathway. Subsequently, these corpuscles release ligands, allowing them to cross the BBB and enter the central nervous system (CNS) through exocytosis. This mechanism enables the ligands to exert their bio functions within the CNS. In this manner, endogenous molecules get delivered into the brain through the receptor-mediated transcytosis pathway [1]. As a result, nanomaterials can be modified by attaching specific receptor ligands to enhance the transport of therapeutic agents loaded within them across the blood–brain barrier (BBB) through

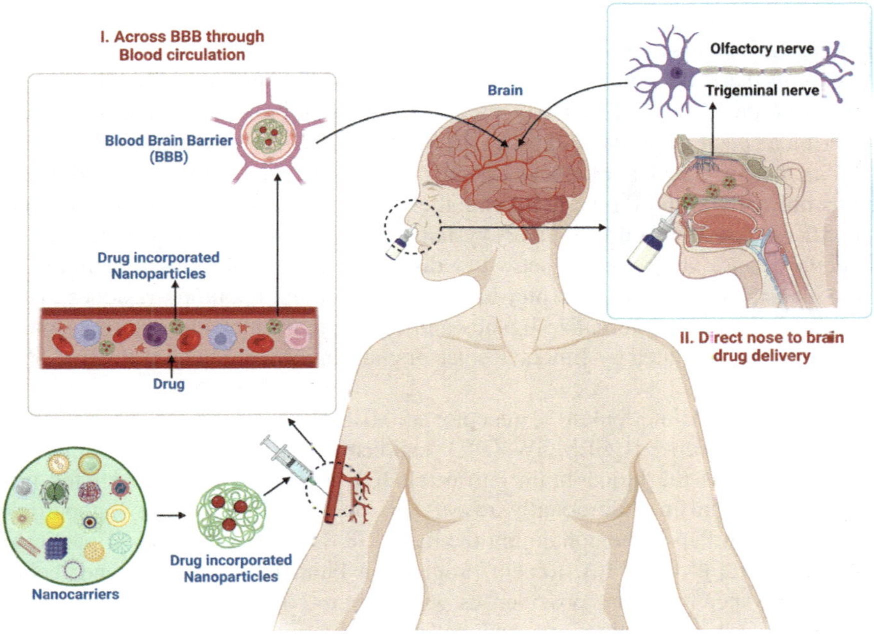

Fig. 2 Nanodrug delivery strategies for neuro diseases

receptor-mediated pathways. This approach holds great promise as a BBB-crossing strategy in the field of neuromedicine.

A recent study has shown that human serum albumin nanoparticles can be linked with insulin receptor monoclonal antibodies, such as 29B4. By conjugating these nanoparticles with therapeutic molecules, they can be effectively transported across the blood–brain barrier (BBB) [10]. Enhancing the density of ligands offers advantages in terms of polyvalency and avidity, leading to an increased likelihood of internalization by endothelial cells [65]. Nevertheless, an excessively high ligand density can introduce steric hindrance, reduce the diffusion coefficient, and increase the size of nanoparticles. Moreover, the density of ligands influences intracellular trafficking mechanisms, such as clathrin-mediated endocytosis and pinocytosis [66]. For example, a study demonstrated by Anraku et al. showed that a nanoparticle (NP) decorated with glucose molecules, which specifically recognize the glucose transporter-1 receptor on endothelial cells of the brain, demonstrated the highest permeability across the blood–brain barrier (BBB) when the surface density of glucose was at 25%. In comparison, surface densities of 10% or 50% did not exhibit the same optimal BBB permeability [67]. Another concept of the molecular Trojan horse delivery system involves associating drug compounds with high-affinity ligands for cellular transport. This approach can be utilized by incorporating drug molecules into liposomes, enabling their delivery through this mechanism [68]. Receptor-mediated transcytosis (RMT) serves as a mechanism for the transportation of essential nutrients like iron, leptin, lipoproteins, and insulin, maintaining equilibrium. In the context of nanoparticles (NPs), they can be conjugated with both natural and artificial ligands to exploit the RMT pathway. These ligands act as "Trojan horses," facilitating NP entry into the brain. RMT enables precise targeting of brain tissue and tumor cells, offering a specific approach for drug delivery [69].

Another special class of receptors known as scavenger receptors are the glycoproteins normally found on the brain endothelial cells surface of the BBB. They have significant potential as drug delivery systems because they do not require binding to a specific ligand. They can interact with a diverse range of molecules, including LDL (low-density lipoprotein) receptor-based molecules and apoptotic residues. These receptors primarily internalize ligands and carrier molecules through transcytosis, which can be mediated by either caveolae or clathrin, depending on the nature of the ligand [10].

In a study on interleukin-13 receptor a2 (IL-13Ra2), it was discovered that a peptide called Pep-1 (CGEMGWVRC) demonstrated the ability to facilitate drug transport across the blood–brain barrier (BBB) via the IL-13Ra2-mediated transcytosis mechanism. Additionally, researchers developed copolymer nanoparticles modified with Pep-1 and containing the ligand IL-13 for the delivery of paclitaxel, a chemotherapy drug [70]. Recent progress in biomedical sciences and technological advancements has provided us with a more comprehensive understanding of the underlying mechanisms and pathophysiology of central nervous system (CNS) diseases. This enhanced knowledge has shed light on the upregulation of various receptors that can be harnessed for the effective delivery of drugs across the blood–brain barrier (BBB).

3.2 *Transient Disruption of BBB*

The transient disruption of the blood–brain barrier (BBB) has been extensively investigated as a prominent strategy for delivering drugs from the circulatory system into the central nervous system (CNS) [71]. This paracellular pathway disruption can be caused by any of the methods such as ultrasound disruption, osmotic disruption, or magnetic disruption.

In recent studies it has been shown, focused ultrasound (FUS) in combination with nanodrug delivery systems utilizes targeted acoustic energy to reversibly open the blood–brain barrier (BBB), facilitating the delivery of therapeutics to specific regions of the brain [72]. Utilizing the focused ultrasound technique has shown the possibility of enhancing the delivery efficiency of liposomal doxorubicin. This approach resulted in significant advancement in median survival rates, with a 100% increase compared to the untreated control group and a 72% increase compared to the group treated with doxorubicin alone [62]. Furthermore, to improve the uptake of 10B enriched L-4-boronophenylalanine-fructose (BPA-f) used for the treatment of malignant glioma, a combination of focused ultrasound and microbubble injection was employed [73]. In a gliosarcoma-infected rat model, a 558 kHz transducer capable of producing pulsed ultrasound was used to disrupt the blood–brain barrier (BBB) along with microbubbles. The results demonstrated a 1.63-fold increase in 10B accumulation within the gliosarcoma tissue in the group treated with ultrasound and microbubbles compared to the control group [62].

Another method of temporary disruption of BBB is using magnetic fields, which has greatly enhanced the transportation rate of the nanoparticles. The application of magnetic fields induces thermal effects, which play a significant role in opening the blood–brain barrier (BBB). When exposed to radiofrequency electromagnetic fields, the brain temperature can increase by more than 1 °C. This temperature elevation leads to a reversible increase in BBB permeability specifically for macromolecules [74]. This method can also be used in combination with focused ultrasound for enhanced results. This mutual cooperative delivery technology has the potential to be employed in both healthy and infected brains, resulting in a significant enhancement in the collection of drug-loaded magnetic nanoparticles within the brain [75]. The technique of magnetic nanoparticle-based drug delivery involves several steps: firstly, the attachment of drugs to magnetic nanoparticles, then application of an external magnetic field to direct the nanoparticles to a specific location of the brain (such as a tumor), and the controlled release of drugs triggered by an external alternating magnetic field upon reaching the desired target [74]. In a study on blood–brain barrier (BBB) permeation, researchers investigated the use of ultra-small superparamagnetic iron oxide (USPIO) nanoparticles loaded into microbubbles (MB) based on poly(butyl cyanoacrylate). Initially, the USPIO-MB was directed magnetically to the desired tissue using an external magnetic field. Subsequently, the targeted BBB was locally disrupted through transcranial ultrasound pulse exposure [76]. Alternatively, IONPs can be transported across BBB by combining a magnetic field with osmotic disruption.

3.3 Shuttle Peptide Mediated

Shuttle peptides play a crucial role in facilitating the transport of various molecules across the blood–brain barrier (BBB), including small molecules, genetic material, proteins, and nanoparticles. Numerous BBB shuttle peptides have been developed specifically for delivering nanoparticles, aiming to enhance their distribution within the central nervous system (CNS) [62]. The majority of blood–brain barrier (BBB) shuttle peptides have been derived through methods such as phage display biopanning or identification of neurotropic biomolecules. In this process, specific receptors that are overexpressed in cells or in vivo are targeted. Phage that exhibits binding affinity to these receptors or accumulates in the brain is isolated, amplified through bacterial infection, and subsequently characterized through titration and sequencing [77]. Several BBB shuttle peptides have been also developed to facilitate the transport across the blood–brain barrier (BBB). Examples of these include B6, which specifically targets the transferrin receptor (TfR), and peptide-22, which exhibits a high affinity for the low-density lipoprotein receptor (LDLR). These shuttle peptides are designed to enhance the delivery of cargoes across the BBB for potential therapeutic applications [78].

In addition to it, through in vivo phage display biopanning, several BBB shuttle peptides with non-corresponding targeting receptors have been identified. One such example is the TGN shuttle peptide, a 12-amino acid peptide displayed by bacteriophage Clone 12–2. When conjugated to poly(ethylene glycol)-poly(lactic-co-glycolic acid) (PEG-PLGA) nanoparticles, the TGN shuttle peptide exhibited significantly higher uptake by bEnd.3 cells compared to unconjugated nanoparticles. Furthermore, in mouse models, administration of Pep TGN-conjugated nanoparticles resulted in enhanced accumulation within the brain, in contrast to unconjugated nanoparticles [62].

A glioma cascade delivery system, known as AsTNP, was developed by conjugating phage-displayed TGN peptide and AS1411 aptamer to nanoparticles. These ligands serve as specific targeting agents for both the blood–brain barrier (BBB) and cancer cells. In vitro cellular uptake studies demonstrated that AsTNP exhibited targeted uptake by brain endothelial cells (BECs) as well as tumor cells. Furthermore, 3-D tumor spheroid experiments confirmed that AsTNP was capable of penetrating both endothelial cell monolayers and tumor cells, reaching the core of the tumor spheroids. This capability is of significant importance for effective glioma therapy [79].

4 Applications of Nanomaterials in Neuro Diseases

Smart nanomaterials have emerged as promising tools in the field of neuro diseases, offering a wide range of applications for diagnosis, treatment, and monitoring. These nanomaterials possess unique properties and functionalities that enable precise targeting, enhanced therapeutic delivery, and real-time monitoring, addressing the challenges associated with neurodegenerative disorders, neuroinflammation, and neurological injuries (Fig. 3) [80].

4.1 Targeted Drug Delivery

One of the key applications of smart nanomaterials in neuro diseases is their role in targeted drug delivery. Neurological disorders often require specific treatment at the site of the affected regions in the brain or spinal cord. Smart nanocarriers can be designed to encapsulate therapeutic agents, such as drugs, genes, or proteins, and deliver them directly to the desired location. By functionalizing the nanomaterial surface with targeting ligands or peptides, these carriers can recognize and bind to specific receptors or biomarkers on diseased cells, improving the therapeutic efficacy

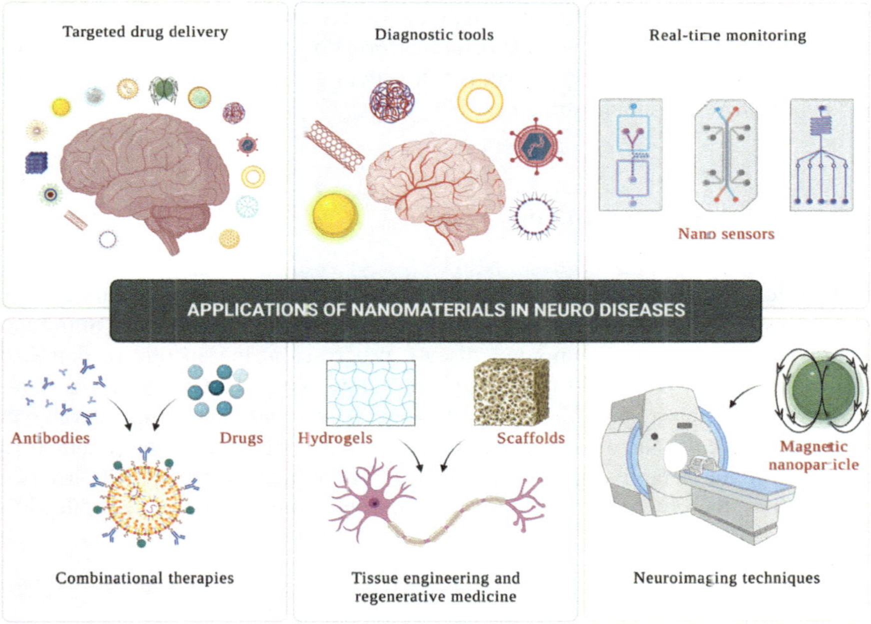

Fig. 3 Applications of nanomaterials in neuro diseases

and reducing off-target effects. This targeted approach enables higher drug concentrations at the site of action, leading to improved treatment outcomes [57]. Moreover, smart nanomaterials facilitate the delivery of neuroprotective agents across the blood–brain barrier (BBB), a major challenge in treating neuro diseases. The BBB limits the entry of therapeutic agents into the brain, restricting their efficacy. However, nanomaterials can be engineered with appropriate surface modifications and transport mechanisms to overcome this barrier. By leveraging their unique properties, such as small size, surface charge, or functionalization, nanomaterials can traverse the BBB and deliver therapeutic payloads directly to the brain, enhancing treatment efficacy for neurodegenerative disorders like Alzheimer's, Parkinson's, and Huntington's diseases.

4.2 Diagnostic Tools for Neuro Diseases

In addition to targeted drug delivery, smart nanomaterials play a significant role in the development of innovative diagnostic tools for neuro diseases. These nanomaterials can be functionalized with specific ligands or antibodies to detect disease-specific biomarkers or pathological aggregates associated with neurodegeneration [81]. By integrating nanosensors into diagnostic platforms, such as biosensors or imaging probes, smart nanomaterials enable highly sensitive and non-invasive detection of neuro disease markers. These diagnostic platforms offer the potential for early and accurate detection of neurodegenerative disorders, facilitating timely intervention and personalized treatment strategies.

4.3 Real-Time Monitoring

Furthermore, smart nanomaterials provide opportunities for real-time monitoring and personalized treatment of neuro diseases. Nanosensors integrated into nanomaterials can continuously monitor disease progression, therapeutic response, or biomarker levels. This real-time monitoring allows healthcare providers to make informed decisions regarding treatment adjustments, and optimizing therapy for individual patients. Nanomaterial-based monitoring systems offer the potential for personalized and adaptive approaches, tailoring treatments to the specific needs of each patient, thereby improving outcomes and reducing the risk of complications [82].

4.4 Combinational Therapies

The multifunctionality of smart nanomaterials also enables combinational therapies for neuro diseases. Multiple therapeutic agents, such as drugs, genes, or antibodies, can be co-loaded into nanocarriers, targeting different aspects of the disease simultaneously. Combinational therapies hold great potential for addressing the complex and multifactorial nature of neuro diseases. By simultaneously targeting neuroinflammation, oxidative stress, protein misfolding, or neuronal degeneration, these therapies can offer synergistic effects, improving treatment outcomes and potentially slowing disease progression [83].

4.5 Tissue Engineering and Regenerative Medicine

Additionally, smart nanomaterials contribute to tissue engineering and regenerative medicine approaches in neuro diseases. Nanomaterial-based scaffolds and matrices can mimic the extracellular matrix, providing structural support and guiding the growth and differentiation of neural cells. These scaffolds can be functionalized with growth factors, neurotrophic molecules, or stem cells to promote tissue repair and regeneration in conditions such as spinal cord injury or stroke. Smart nanomaterials offer precise control over the release of these bioactive agents, facilitating the restoration of neural circuits and enhancing functional recovery. Smart nanomaterials hold significant potential in the application of neuro diseases [84]. Their capabilities in targeted drug delivery, crossing the BBB, non-invasive diagnostics, real-time monitoring, and combinational therapies provide novel and effective approaches to tackle the complex challenges associated with neurodegenerative disorders, neuroinflammation, and neurological injuries. In the field of neurosurgery, smart nanomaterials offer significant advancements. These materials can be engineered to have unique properties, such as shape memory or self-healing capabilities, which can be beneficial for tissue repair and surgical interventions [27]. Nanomaterial-based implants and scaffolds provide mechanical support, promote neuronal regeneration, and facilitate the integration of new tissue into damaged areas. Additionally, smart nanomaterials can be designed to release antimicrobial agents or growth factors, reducing the risk of infection and enhancing the healing process after neurosurgical procedures.

4.6 Neuroimaging Techniques

Neuroimaging techniques greatly benefit from the application of smart nanomaterials. By incorporating contrast agents into nanomaterials, imaging modalities like magnetic resonance imaging (MRI) and positron emission tomography (PET) can be enhanced for improved resolution and sensitivity. Smart nanomaterials can specifically target areas of interest, enabling the visualization and tracking of disease progression or treatment response. Moreover, nanomaterial-based imaging probes can provide insights into the molecular and cellular processes associated with neuro diseases, aiding in diagnosis, treatment planning, and monitoring [85]. The development of neural interfaces and neuroprosthetic devices is another area where smart nanomaterials show promise. By combining nanomaterials with electrodes or sensors, it becomes possible to interface with the nervous system at the cellular or subcellular level. This opens avenues for precise stimulation and recording of neural activity, enabling the restoration of lost sensory or motor functions in neurodegenerative disorders or neurological injuries. The integration of smart nanomaterials with neural interfaces enhances their biocompatibility, electrical conductivity, and stability, improving the performance and longevity of these devices.

Overall, the application of smart nanomaterials in neuro diseases encompasses a wide range of areas, including targeted drug delivery, diagnostics, neurosurgery, neuroimaging, and neural interfaces. The unique properties and functionalities of these materials provide opportunities for personalized and precise interventions, leading to improved therapeutic outcomes, early diagnosis, and effective monitoring. As research and development in this field continue, smart nanomaterials hold great promise for addressing the complex challenges associated with neuro diseases, ultimately improving the quality of life for patients affected by these conditions [36].

5 Safety and Regulatory Considerations

The journey toward clinical translation of nanomedicines for brain drug delivery is filled with numerous obstacles. The process of scaling up a nanocarrier technology from a research/publication stage to a commercially viable product in clinical trials is highly challenging. Under ideal circumstances, it may take approximately 5 years to reach the clinical trial phase and a significant portion of a decade to achieve full clinical utilization [9]. Many publications rely on inadequate and non-predictive in vitro models, such as brain endothelial cell monolayers, or animal models like xenografts that may not accurately represent human physiology [87]. A study has revealed the permeability of drugs to the brain differs greatly when compared between different animal models which are the guinea pig, rat, monkey, minipig, and humans. It was found the drug concentrations differed by nine times between drugs and species [9].

In preclinical studies, there are substantial limitations in accurately measuring the distribution and uptake of nanocarriers in the brain. In the case of human trials, the concentration of cerebrospinal fluid (CSF) gives an idea for the measurement of drug delivery into the CNS but does not give the conformation of the target delivery site. Therefore, it is limited to clinical trials rather than long treatment courses [88]. For improving the penetration efficiency through brain tissues, PEG (polyethylene glycol) is generally used as a safe surface medium. However, in some cases, it was found it induces the formation of IgM and IgG which are anti-PEG antibodies and also activates the complement system resulting in reduced drug efficacy [89].

One of the most significant obstacles is regulatory uncertainty, which includes the lack of clear criteria for determining batch consistency and bioequivalence. The absence of a formal regulatory framework results in the lack of specific definitions for characterizing and reporting critical physicochemical properties of nanomedicines, such as size, charge, ligand density, and polydispersity, among others [90]. Consequently, establishing batch-to-batch consistency or determining bioequivalence becomes challenging since these properties significantly influence the behavior of nanomedicines within the body. Defining the "active ingredient" of nanomedicine is often imprecise as the drug molecule, carrier, and surface targeting molecules all play crucial roles in the functionality of the final product [91]. In light of these complexities, adopting a pragmatic and flexible "case-by-case" approach becomes necessary, enabling the assessment of potential benefits and risks associated with each individual nanomedicine product. A project "REFINE" has been developed in order to set up criteria for the advancement of the regulatory science of nanomaterials in clinical use [92]. The UK Medicines and Healthcare Products Regulatory Agency (MHRA) and the US Food and Drug Administration (FDA) adopt a case-by-case approach when evaluating new nanomedicine applications. This means that each nanomedicine product is assessed individually, taking into consideration its specific characteristics, intended use, and potential risks and benefits. Rather than implementing a standardized regulatory framework for nanomedicines, these regulatory agencies analyze and evaluate each case independently, considering the unique properties and requirements of the particular nanomedicine under review [93].

There is a need to evaluate nanomaterials separately for parameters such as toxicity and potential adverse effects on health. While certain agencies and regulatory organizations in various countries and globally have developed regulatory frameworks, there is still a lack of appropriate guidelines for ensuring the safe use of nanotechnology products [94]. To address these challenges, ongoing research and development efforts are focused on understanding the safety profiles of nanomaterials, improving manufacturing processes, optimizing drug formulations, and developing appropriate regulatory frameworks. Rigorous preclinical and clinical studies, as well as collaboration between researchers, clinicians, regulatory bodies, and industry stakeholders, are essential to ensure the safe and effective translation of nanomaterial-based drugs into clinical practice. While nanomaterials have unique properties that make them effective in the treatment of neurological disorders, they can also have unintended consequences. For example, carbon nanotubes have been shown to cause inflammation and oxidative stress in the brain, which can lead to neurodegeneration [95]. For nanosystems to have meaningful clinical applications, they should be designed to achieve regulated biodistribution, less frequent administration, decreased toxicity, and easy delivery methods that enhance patient benefits and compliance. Additionally, the development of standardized toxicological studies plays a crucial role in advancing applications based on nanoparticle (NP) technology. Considering that patients with neurodegenerative disorders (NDs) exhibit variations in their genetic backgrounds and clinical phenotypes, there is a growing need for personalized therapeutic doses and administration strategies [96]. Undoubtedly, ensuring the safety of a drug delivery system, particularly nanoparticulate systems, is of utmost importance during the design process. It is crucial to consider how nanoparticles (NPs) interact with living cells, tissues, and organs, making biocompatibility an essential requirement for both the NP and its components. The degradation time of the NP after administration and the behavior of its metabolites within living cells and tissues serve as indicators of the effectiveness of the drug delivery system [97]. Therefore, it is important to carefully evaluate the safety and efficacy of nanomaterial-based therapies and make sure that they are accessible to all patients in an equitable manner.

6 Conclusion and Future Prospective

Smart nanomaterials have emerged as a promising approach for drug delivery and managing neurological diseases. Neurodegenerative disorders pose significant challenges in terms of treatment due to the limited ability of drugs to cross the blood–brain barrier (BBB) and effectively reach the affected regions in the central nervous system (CNS). However, advancements in nanotechnology offer exciting opportunities to overcome these limitations by utilizing smart nanomaterials for targeted drug delivery. The unique properties of smart nanomaterials, such as their responsiveness to external stimuli, enable precise and controlled release of therapeutic agents at the desired site within the body. By engineering nanomaterials to respond to specific triggers, such as changes in temperature, pH, or enzymatic activity, drugs can be released in a controlled manner, enhancing therapeutic efficacy while minimizing side effects.

Moreover, functionalized nanomaterials can cross the BBB and deliver drugs to specific brain regions, improving the targeted treatment of neurological diseases. In addition to drug delivery, smart nanomaterials have significant applications in diagnosing and monitoring neuro diseases. These nanomaterials can be functionalized with specific ligands or antibodies to detect disease-specific biomarkers or pathological aggregates associated with neurodegeneration. Their high sensitivity and accuracy enable early detection, facilitating timely interventions and improving patient outcomes.

However, translating smart nanomaterials into clinical applications faces several challenges and limitations. Ensuring the safety and biocompatibility of nanomaterials is crucial, as they interact with sensitive structures within the CNS. A thorough evaluation of their toxicity, long-term effects, and potential immunological reactions is essential. Additionally, the complex regulatory landscape surrounding the clinical translation of nanomaterials needs to be navigated. The field of smart nanomaterials for drug delivery and neurological disease management holds immense potential for further advancements and applications. Future research should address the challenges and limitations associated with nanomaterials to facilitate their safe and effective clinical translation. Efforts should be made to enhance the understanding of nanomaterials' toxicity and long-term effects on the CNS. Comprehensive studies on the biodistribution, clearance mechanisms, and potential accumulation of nanomaterials within the body are necessary to ensure their safety and minimize any adverse effects on neuronal function and overall health.

Furthermore, research should aim to develop more accurate and predictive in vitro and animal models that closely resemble human physiology. These models will enable better evaluation of the efficacy and safety of smart nanomaterials, improving the success rate of clinical trials and accelerating their translation into clinical practice. Ethical considerations should also be a priority in developing and utilizing nanomaterial-based therapies. Ensuring equitable access to these therapies for all patients and addressing potential regulatory and ethical issues will be crucial in their widespread adoption.

References

1. Asil SM, Ahlawat J, Barroso GG, Narayan M (2020) Nanomaterial based drug delivery systems for the treatment of neurodegenerative diseases. Biomater Sci 8(15):4109–4128
2. Asil SM et al (2020) Nanomaterial based drug delivery systems for the treatment of neurodegenerative diseases. Biomater Sci 8(15):4109–4128. https://doi.org/10.1039/d0bm00809e

3. Andreone BJ, Larhammar M, Lewcock JW (2020) Cell death and neurodegeneration. Cold Spring Harb Perspect Biol 12(2):a036434
4. Guo ZH, Khattak S, Rauf MA, Ansari MA, Alomary MN, Razak S, Yang CY, Wu DD, Ji XY (2023) Role of nanomedicine-based therapeutics in the treatment of CNS disorders. Molecules 28(3):1283
5. Naqvi S, Panghal A, Flora SJ (2020) Nanotechnology: a promising approach for delivery of neuroprotective drugs. Front Neurosci 14:498007
6. Mitchell MJ, Billingsley MM, Haley RM, Wechsler ME, Peppas NA, Langer R (2021) Engineering precision nanoparticles for drug delivery. Nat Rev Drug Discovery 20(2):101–124
7. Farjadian F, Ghasemi A, Gohari O, Roointan A, Karimi M, Hamblin MR (2019) Nanopharmaceuticals and nanomedicines currently on the market: challenges and opportunities. Nanomedicine 14(1):93–126
8. Jhaveri J, Raichura Z, Khan T, Momin M, Omri A (2021) Chitosan nanoparticles-insight into properties, functionalization and applications in drug delivery and theranostics. Molecules 26(2):272
9. Lundy DJ, Nguy˜ên H, Hsieh PC (2021) Emerging nano-carrier strategies for brain tumor drug delivery and considerations for clinical translation. Pharmaceutics 13(8):1193
10. Anthony DP, Hegde M, Shetty SS, Rafic T, Mutalik S, Rao BS (2021) Targeting receptor-ligand chemistry for drug delivery across blood-brain barrier in brain diseases. Life Sci 274:119326
11. Babazadeh A, Mohammadi Vahed F, Jafari SM (2020) Nanocarrier-mediated brain delivery of bioactivesfor treatment/prevention of neurodegenerative diseases. J Control Release 321:211–221
12. Shreffler JW, Pullan JE, Dailey KM, Mallik S, Brooks AE (2019) Overcoming hurdles in nanoparticleclinical translation The influence of experimental design and surface modification. Int J Mol Sci 20(23):6056
13. Yetisgin AA, Cetinel S, Zuvin M, Kosar A, Kutlu O (2020) Therapeutic nanoparticles and their targeted delivery applications. Molecules 25(9):2193
14. Edoziuno FO et al (2023) Nanomaterials. In: Elsevier eBooks, pp 19–30. https://doi.org/10.1016/b978-0-323-95158-6.00023-0
15. Aflori M (2021) Smart nanomaterials for biomedical applications—a review. Nanomaterials 11(2):396. https://doi.org/10.3390/nano11020396
16. Lombardo D, Kiselev MA, Caccamo MT (2019) Smart nanoparticles for drug delivery application: development of versatile nanocarrier platforms in biotechnology and nanomedicine. J Nanomater:1–26. https://doi.org/10.1155/2019/3702518
17. Sharma D, Hussain CM (2020) Smart nanomaterials in pharmaceutical analysis. Arab J Chem 13(1):3319–3343. https://doi.org/10.1016/j.arabjc.2018.11.007.
18. Mao L et al (2021) A high-sensitivity flexible direct X-ray detector based on Bi2O3/PDMS nanocomposite thin film. Nanomaterials 11(7):1832. https://doi.org/10.3390/nano11071832
19. Mann GS, Singh L, Kumar P (2021) Potential applications of polymeric-nanomaterial as drug delivery carriers in the biomedical field. In: Elsevier eBooks, pp 109–134. https://doi.org/10.1016/b978-0-12-823152-4.00004-1
20. Sánchez-López E, Paús A, Pérez-Pomeda I, Calpena A., Haro I, Gómara MJ (2020) Lipid vesicles loaded with an HIV-1 fusion inhibitor peptide as a potential microbicide. Pharmaceutics 12(6):502
21. Fu Q et al (2022) Biomarker-responsive nanosystems for chronic disease theranostics. Adv Funct Mater 33(2):2206300. https://doi.org/10.1002/adfm.202206300
22. Rehman S et al (2020) Nanoparticle based gene therapy approach: a pioneering rebellion in the management of psychiatric disorders. Curr Gene Ther 20(3):164–173. https://doi.org/10.2174/1566523220666200607185903
23. Boca S et al (2019) Nanoscale delivery systems for microRNAs in cancer therapy. Cell Mol Life Sci 77(6):1059–1086. https://doi.org/10.1007/s00018-019-03317-9
24. Hosseinpour S, Walsh LJ (2020) Laser-assisted nucleic acid delivery: a systematic review. J Biophotonics 14(1).https://doi.org/10.1002/jbio.202000295

25. Burnouf T et al (2021) Solid lipid nanoparticles (SLNs): an advanced drug delivery system targeting brain through BBB. Pharmaceutics 13(8):1183. https://doi.org/10.3390/pharmaceutics13081183
26. Correia AMH et al (2022) Lipid nanoparticles strategies to modify pharmacokinetics of central nervous system targeting drugs: Crossing or circumventing the blood–brain barrier (BBB) to manage neurological disorders. Adv Drug Deliv Rev 189:114485. https://doi.org/10.1016/j.addr.2022.114485
27. Kumar AS, Fuh JYH, Dheen ST (2020) Functions and applications of metallic and metallic oxide nanoparticles in orthopedic implants and scaffolds. J Biomed Mater Res Part B Appl Biomater 109(2):160–179. https://doi.org/10.1002/jbm.b.34688
28. Xu R et al (2020) Rhynchophylline Loaded-mPEG-PLGA nanoparticles coated with Tween-80 for preliminary study in Alzheimer's disease. Int J Nanomedicine 15:1149–1160. https://doi.org/10.2147/ijn.s236922
29. Mehrasa M et al (2022) Silica nano particles embedded in random and aligned PLGA/gelatin electrospun nano fibers improve growth and differentiation of human adipose-derived stem cells into anterior neuroectodermal cells. Mater Today Commun 31:103461. https://doi.org/10.1016/j.mtcomm.2022.103461.
30. Ashori R, Mirzahosseini SAH (2020) In vitro speciation of molybdenum in human biological samples based on thiol functionalized mesoporous silica nanoparticles and hexylmethylimidazolium tris-pentafluoroethyl-trifluorophosphate. Anal Methods Environ Chem J 3(3):54–64. https://doi.org/10.24200/amecj.v3.i03.115
31. Sharma B, Pervushin K (2020) Magnetic nanoparticles as in vivo tracers for Alzheimer's disease. Magnetochemistry 6(1):13. https://doi.org/10.3390/magnetochemistry6010013
32. Hubert V et al (2019) MRI coupled with clinically-applicable iron oxide nanoparticles reveals choroid plexus involvement in a murine model of neuroinflammation. Sci Rep 9(1). https://doi.org/10.1038/s41598-019-46566-1
33. Xiang C et al (2020) Biomimetic carbon nanotubes for neurological disease therapeutics as inherent medication. Acta Pharm Sin B 10(2):239–248. https://doi.org/10.1016/j.apsb.2019.11.003
34. Perini G et al (2020) Unravelling the Potential of Graphene Quantum Dots in Biomedicine and Neuroscience. Int J Mol Sci 21(10):3712. https://doi.org/10.3390/ijms21103712
35. Nazari Z et al (2023) An electrochemical sensor based on carbon quantum dots and ionic liquids for selective detection of dopamine. Chem Sel 8(3).https://doi.org/10.1002/slct.202203630
36. Ko W-C et al (2022) pharmacological role of functionalized gold nanoparticles in disease applications. Molecules 27(5):1551. https://doi.org/10.3390/molecules27051551
37. Xue J et al (2019) Neuroprotective effect of biosynthesised gold nanoparticles synthesised from root extract of Paeonia moutan against Parkinson disease – In vitro & In vivo model. J Photochem Photobiol B-Biol 200:111635. https://doi.org/10.1016/j.jphotobiol.2019.111635
38. Li X et al (2022) Applications and mechanisms of stimuli-responsive hydrogels in traumatic brain injury. Gels 8(8):482. https://doi.org/10.3390/gels8080482
39. Avila-Salas F, Durán-Lara EF (2019) An overview of injectable thermo-responsive hydrogels and advances in their biomedical applications. Curr Med Chem 27(34):5773–5789. https://doi.org/10.2174/0929867325666190603110045
40. Mahlumba P et al (2021) Fabrication and characterisation of a photo-responsive, injectable nanosystem for sustained delivery of macromolecules. Int J Mol Sci 22(7):3359. https://doi.org/10.3390/ijms22073359
41. Shi W et al (2020) Imparting functionality to the hydrogel by magnetic-field-induced nano-assembly and macro-response. ACS Appl Mater & Interfaces 12(5):5177–5194. https://doi.org/10.1021/acsami.9b16770
42. Yan H et al (2019) An electrically and magnetically responsive nanocomposite of $GdPO_4 \cdot H_2O$/P_3HT/PLGA with electrical stimulation for synergistically enhancing the proliferation and differentiation of pre-osteoblasts. New J Chem 43(44):17315–17326. https://doi.org/10.1039/c9nj04167b

43. Shen K et al (2021) Anti-inflammatory nanotherapeutics by targeting matrix metalloproteinases for immunotherapy of spinal cord injury. Small 17(41):2102102. https://doi.org/10.1002/smll.202102102
44. Ma S et al (2021) Sodium alginate/collagen/stromal cell-derived factor-1 neural scaffold loaded with BMSCs promotes neurological function recovery after traumatic brain injury. Acta Biomaterialia 131:185–197. https://doi.org/10.1016/j.actbio.2021.06.038
45. Zheng Y-T et al (2021) Neuro-regenerative imidazole-functionalized GelMA hydrogel loaded with hAMSC and SDF-1α promote stem cell differentiation and repair focal brain injury. Bioact Mater 6(3):627–637. https://doi.org/10.1016/j.bioactmat.2020.08.026
46. Lee G et al (2022) Upconversion nanomaterials and delivery systems for smart photonic medicines and healthcare devices. Adv Drug Deliv Rev 188:114419. https://doi.org/10.1016/j.addr.2022.114419
47. G Wang et al (2020) Advances in nanotechnology-based strategies for the treatments of amyotrophic lateral sclerosis. Materials Today Bio 6:100055. https://doi.org/10.1016/j.mtbio.2020.100055
48. Bilal M et al (2020) Nanomaterials for the treatment and diagnosis of Alzheimer's disease: an overview. NanoImpact 20:100251. https://doi.org/10.1016/j.impact.2020.100251
49. Hanif S et al (2021) Nanotechnology-based strategies for early diagnosis of central nervous system disorders. Adv Nanobiomed Res 1(10):2100008. https://doi.org/10.1002/anbr.202100008.
50. Kerry RG et al (2021) A comprehensive review on the applications of nano-biosensor-based approaches for non-communicable and communicable disease detection. Biomater Sci 9(10):3576–3602. https://doi.org/10.1039/d0bm02164d
51. Yu S et al (2019) Chitosan and chitosan coating nanoparticles for the treatment of brain disease. Int J Pharm 560:282–293. https://doi.org/10.1016/j.ijpharm.2019.02.012
52. Moorthy H, Govindaraju T (2021) Dendrimer architectonics to treat cancer and neurodegenerative diseases with implications in theranostics and personalized medicine. ACS Appl Bio Mater 4(2):1115–1139. https://doi.org/10.1021/acsabm.0c01319
53. Wang Z et al (2023) Nanotechnology-empowered therapeutics targeting neurodegenerative diseases. Wiley Interdisciplinary Reviews-nanomedicine and Nanobiotechnology. https://doi.org/10.1002/wnan.1907
54. Kumar AS, Dheen ST, Fuh JYH (2021) A review of multi-functional ceramic nanoparticles in 3D printed bone tissue engineering. Bioprinting 23:e00146. https://doi.org/10.1016/j.bprint.2021.e00146
55. Ciceks H (2023) Treatment of brain tumors and age-dependent neurodegenerative diseases using nano medicine: advantages and limits. http://www.ijtos.com/index.php/journal/article/view/6
56. Akhtar A et al (2021) Neurodegenerative diseases and effective drug delivery: A review of challenges and novel therapeutics. J Control Release, 330:1152–1167. https://doi.org/10.1016/j.jconrel.2020.11.021
57. Naziris N, Demetzos C (2021) Advanced Health Technologies and Nanotechnologies in Neurodegenerative Diseases. In: Springer eBooks, p 317. https://doi.org/10.1007/978-3-030-78787-5_37
58. Singha S et al (2019) An endeavor in the reaction-based approach to fluorescent probes for biorelevant analytes: challenges and achievements. Acc Chem Res 52(9):2571–2581. https://doi.org/10.1021/acs.accounts.9b00314
59. Thangudu S (2020) Next generation nanomaterials: smart nanomaterials, significance, and biomedical applications. In: Springer eBooks, pp 287–312. https://doi.org/10.1007/978-981-15-4802-4_15
60. Ivask A, Pilkington EH, Blin T, Käkinen A, Vija H, Visnapuu M, Quinn JF, Whittaker MR, Qiao R, Davis TP, Ke PC (2018) Uptake and transcytosis of functionalized superparamagnetic iron oxide nanoparticles in an in vitro blood-brain barrier model. Biomater Sci 6(2):314–323
61. Tsai YC, Vijayaraghavan P, Chiang WH, Chen HH, Liu TI, Shen MY, Omoto A, Kamimura M, Soga K, Chiu HC (2018) Targeted delivery of functionalized upconversion nanoparticles for

externally triggered photothermal/photodynamic therapies of brain glioblastoma. Theranostics 8(5):1435
62. Xie J, Shen Z, Anraku Y, Kataoka K, Chen X (2019) Nanomaterial-based blood-brain-barrier (BBB) crossing strategies. Biomaterials 224:119491
63. Saeedi M, Eslamifar M, Khezri K, Dizaj SM (2019) Applications of nanotechnology in drug delivery to the central nervous system. Biomed Pharmacother 111:666–675
64. Hersh AM, Alomari S, Tyler BM (2022) Crossing the blood-brain barrier: advances in nanoparticle technology for drug delivery in neuro-oncology. Int J Mol Sci 23(8)
65. Johnsen KB, Bak M, Melander F, Thomsen MS, Burkhart A, Kempen PJ, Andresen TL, Moos T (2019) Modulating the antibody density changes the uptake and transport at the blood-brain barrier of both transferrin receptor-targeted gold nanoparticles and liposomal cargo. J Control Release 295:237–249
66. Alkilany AM, Zhu L, Weller H, Mews A, Parak WJ, Barz M, Feliu N (2019) Ligand density on nanoparticles: a parameter with critical impact on nanomedicine. Adv Drug Deliv Rev 143:22–36
67. Anraku Y, Kuwahara H, Fukusato Y, Mizoguchi A, Ishii T, Nitta K, Matsumoto Y, Toh K, Miyata K, Uchida S, Nishina K (2017) Glycaemic control boosts glucosylated nanocarrier crossing the BBB into the brain. Nat Commun 8(1):1001
68. Pardridge WM (2023) Brain gene therapy with Trojan horse lipid nanoparticles. Trends Mol Med 29(5):343–353
69. Markowicz-Piasecka M, Markiewicz A, Darłak P, Sikora J, Adla SK, Bagina S, Huttunen KM (2022) Current chemical, biological, and physiological views in the development of successful brain-targeted pharmaceutics. Neurotherapeutics 19(3):942–976
70. Wang B, Tang M, Yuan Z, Li Z, Hu B, Bai X, Chu J, Xu X, Zhang Q (2022) Targeted delivery of a STING agonist to brain tumors using bioengineered protein nanoparticles for enhanced immunotherapy. Bioactive Materials 16:232–248
71. Toccaceli G, Barbagallo G, Peschillo S (2019) Low-intensity focused ultrasound for the treatment of brain diseases: safety and feasibility. Theranostics 9(2):537–539
72. Duan L, Li X, Ji R, Hao Z, Kong M, Wen X, Guan F, Ma S (2023) Nanoparticle-based drug delivery systems: an inspiring therapeutic strategy for neurodegenerative diseases. Polymers 15(9):2196
73. Persano F, Batasheva S, Fakhrullina G, Gigli G, Leporatti S, Fakhrullin R (2021) Recent advances in the design of inorganic and nano-clay particles for the treatment of brain disorders. J Mater Chem B 9(12):2756–2784
74. Sun Y, Du L, Yang M, Li Q, Jia X, Li Q, Zhu L, Zhang Y, Liu Y, Liu S (2021) Brain-targeted drug delivery assisted by physical techniques and its potential applications in traditional Chinese medicine. J Tradit Chin Med Sci 8(3):186–197
75. Jones RM, Deng L, Leung K, McMahon D, O'Reilly MA, Hynynen K (2018) Three-dimensional transcranial microbubble imaging for guiding volumetric ultrasound-mediated blood-brain barrier opening. Theranostics 8(11):2909
76. Israel LL, Galstyan A, Holler E, Ljubimova JY (2020) Magnetic iron oxide nanoparticles for imaging, targeting and treatment of primary and metastatic tumors of the brain. Journal of Controlled Release 320:45–62
77. Majerova P, Hanes J, Olesova D, Sinsky J, Pilipcinec E, Kovac A (2020) Novel blood-brain barrier shuttle peptides discovered through the phage display method. Molecules (Basel, Switzerland) 25(4):874
78. McCully M, Sanchez-Navarro M, Teixido M, Giralt E (2018) Peptide mediated brain delivery of nano-and submicroparticles: a synergistic approach. Curr Pharm Des 24(13):1366–1376
79. Jafari B, Pourseif MM, Barar J, Rafi MA, Omidi Y (2019) Peptide-mediated drug delivery across the blood-brain barrier for targeting brain tumors. Expert Opin Drug Deliv 16(6):583–605
80. Ukhurebor KE et al (2022) A methodical review on the applications and potentialities of using nanobiosensors for disease diagnosis. BioMed Res Int 2022:1–20. https://doi.org/10.1155/2022/1682502

81. Kumar R et al (2020) Advances in nanotechnology and nanomaterials based strategies for neural tissue engineering. J Drug Deliv Sci Technol 57:101617. https://doi.org/10.1016/j.jddst.2020.101617
82. Behboudi H et al (2019) Carbon quantum dots in nanobiotechnology. In: Advanced structured materials. Springer International Publishing, pp 145–179. https://doi.org/10.1007/978-3-030-10834-2_6.
83. Angolkar M et al (2022) Nanotechnological advancements in the brain tumor therapy: a novel approach. Ther Deliv 13(11):531–557. https://doi.org/10.4155/tde-2022-0035
84. Jeong Y-C et al (2020) Progress in brain-compatible interfaces with soft nanomaterials. Adv Mater 32(35):1907522. https://doi.org/10.1002/adma.201907522
85. Sharma AK (2023) Current trends in nanotheranostics: a concise review on bioimaging and smart wearable technology. Nanotheranostics 7(3):258–269. https://doi.org/10.7150/ntno.82886
86. Sadeghi A et al (2023) Brainy biomaterials: latest advances in smart biomaterials to develop the next generation of neural interfaces. Curr Opin Biomed Eng 25:100420
87. Talele S, Mohammad AS, Schulz JA, Bauer B, Hartz AM, Sarkaria JN, Elmquist WF (2022) Drug delivery to primary and metastatic brain tumors: challenges and opportunities. In: Drug delivery to the brain: physiological concepts, methodologies and approaches, pp 723–762
88. Mainprize T, Lipsman N, Huang Y, Meng Y, Bethune A, Ironside S, Heyn C, Alkins R, Trudeau M, Sahgal A, Perry J (2019) Blood-brain barrier opening in primary brain tumors with non-invasive MR-guided focused ultrasound: a clinical safety and feasibility study. Sci Rep 9(1):321
89. Chen E, Chen BM, Su YC, Chang YC, Cheng TL, Barenholz Y, Roffler SR (2020) Premature drug release from polyethylene glycol (PEG)-coated liposomal doxorubicin via formation of the membrane attack complex. ACS Nano 14(7):7808–7822
90. Peltonen L (2018) Practical guidelines for the characterization and quality control of pure drug nanoparticles and nano-cocrystals in the pharmaceutical industry. Adv Drug Deliv Rev 131:101–115
91. Foulkes R, Man E, Thind J, Yeung S, Joy A, Hoskins C (2020) The regulation of nanomaterials and nanomedicines for clinical application: current and future perspectives. Biomater Sci 8(17):4653–4664
92. Zabeo A, Rosada F, Pizzol L, Caputo F, Borgos SE, Parot J, Geertsma RE, Pouw JJ, Vandebriel RJ, Moreno OI, Hristozov D (2022) A decision support system for preclinical assessment of nanomaterials in medical products: the REFINE DSS. Drug Deliv Transl Res 12(9):2101–2113
93. Đorđević S, Gonzalez MM, Conejos-Sánchez I, Carreira B, Pozzi S, Acúrcio RC, Satchi-Fainaro R, Florindo HF, Vicent MJ (2021) Current hurdles to the translation of nanomedicines from bench to the clinic. Drug Deliv Transl Res:1–26
94. Sahariah M, Sahariah JJ, Paul S, Sharma HK (2019) Nanomedicinal devices and nanomedicines: its challenges and regulations. Curr Trends Pharm Res 6(2)
95. Mohanta D, Patnaik S, Sood S, Das N (2019) Carbon nanotubes: evaluation of toxicity at biointerfaces. J Pharm Anal 9(5):293–300
96. Mistretta M, Farini A, Torrente Y, Villa C (2023) Multifaceted nanoparticles: emerging mechanisms and therapies in neurodegenerative diseases. Brain 146(6):2227–2240
97. Ayub A, Wettig S (2022) An overview of nanotechnologies for drug delivery to the brain. Pharmaceutics 14(2):224

Nanotechnology Approach for Nose-to-Brain Drug Delivery

Md. Meraj Ansari, Zamurrad Nayab, Faiyaz Ahmad Ansari, Manzar Alam, Rehan Khan, Syed Shadab Raza, Mohammad Waseem, Nazrul Islam, and Nemat Ali

Abstract Neurologists define neurological disorders (ND) medically as conditions that affect the brain, the nerves that run throughout the body, and the spinal cord. Treatment of neurological disease is still challenging. Whether given orally or intravenously, therapeutic medications need to penetrate the blood–brain barrier (BBB) in order to reach the brain. A rising number of therapeutic medications have the

Md. M. Ansari (✉)
Centre for Pharmaceutical Nanotechnology, Department of Pharmaceutics, National Institute of Pharmaceutical Education and Research, S.A.S Nagar, Sector 67, Mohali, Punjab 160062, India
e-mail: rajmeraj385@gmail.com

Z. Nayab
Department of Biotechnology, Science College Patna, Patna University, Patna, Bihar 800005, India

F. A. Ansari
Department of Medicine, Government Medical College and Hospital, Purnea, Bihar 854301, India

M. Alam
Centre for Interdisciplinary Research in Basic Sciences, Jamia Millia Islamia, New Delhi 110025, India

R. Khan
Department of Nano-Therapeutics, Institute of Nano Science and Technology, Knowledge City, Sector 81, SAS Nagar, Mohali, Punjab 140306, India

S. S. Raza
Laboratory for Stem Cell and Restorative Neurology, Department of Biotechnology, Era's Lucknow Medical College and Hospital, Sarfarazganj, Lucknow, Uttar Pradesh 226003, India

M. Waseem
Department of Pharmaceutical Sciences, University of Maryland Eastern Shore School of Pharmacy, Princess Anne, MD 21853, USA

N. Islam
Department of Chemistry, Jawahar Lal Nehru College, Chakradharpur, West Singhbhum, Jharkhand 833102, India

N. Ali
Department of Pharmacology and Toxicology, College of Pharmacy, King Saud University, Riyadh 11451, Saudi Arabia

S. K. Rath et al. (eds.), *Nanomaterials for Drug Delivery and Neurological Diseases Management*, Smart Nanomaterials Technology,
https://doi.org/10.1007/978-981-97-0308-1_9

potential to be used to treat neurological conditions. However, it has been realised that the potential of these drugs is being hampered by extraordinary difficulties in the delivery of therapeutically meaningful doses. As is well known, there is hope for the treatment of neurological illnesses in the developing field of nanotechnology in the biological sciences. Application of nanomedicine offer the bypassing of protective barriers during therapeutic medication via nose-to-brain (NTB). Additionally, the NTB route is currently being studied as a potential drug delivery technique for the treatment of neurological disorders because it avoids the BBB and delivers drugs straight to the target with the necessary concentration. Hence, regulated drug release can improve the delivery of nanoformulated medicines by NTB route in target concentration across BBB to the brain. The current chapter addresses the most recent developments in this field with a focus on nanotechnology-based methods and describes the mechanism of NTB route of drug delivery.

Keywords Neurological disorder · BBB · Nose-to-brain · Nanotechnology · Drug delivery

Abbreviations

PDI	Polydispersity index
NLC	Nanostructured lipid carrier
PF	Pluronic F
PLGA	Poly lactic-co-glycolic acid
PVA	Polyvinyl alcohol
SLN	Solid lipid nanoparticle

1 Introduction

Neurological illnesses have connections to both the central and peripheral nervous systems [1]. Among the common neurological disorders (ND) are brain tumours, epilepsy, Parkinson's disease, multiple sclerosis, Alzheimer's disease, and multiple sclerosis. Certain ND, such as Parkinson's disease, Alzheimer's disease, multiple sclerosis, and ischemic stroke, are more common than others in contemporary society. ND is the primary cause of human impairment and the second leading cause of death around the globe. In 2017, Neurologic Disorders Collaborator Group represented the mortality at a rate of 16.8% in worldwide regions. The overall concerns of neurodegenerative disease are gradually increasing and it has been expected that the unipolar and depressive disorders would become the second major reason for morbidity by 2030 [2]. Gradually, treatment of neurological disease is becoming very expensive. According to the report, expense on neurological disease treatment in Europe was about €798 billion in 2010, this scenario conferred both medical and nonmedical expenses and loss of production. Also, the ratio for both the display as a percentage of 60 and 40, respectively [3]. Furthermore, some neurological disorders have great socioeconomic impact on Europe Annual Health Budget such as anxiety, dementia, and addiction. Thus, it gives the opportunity to researcher and demand for clinician a new drug for better treatment of neurological disease. Furthermore, new drug synthesis/development for possible intervention of neurological disorders is expensive, challenging, and time-consuming. The BBB prevents medications from reaching the brain in the desired therapeutic quantities and is a key obstacle in the creation of innovative drug formulations for therapeutic intervention of neurological problems [4]. The BBB, an incredibly precise endothelial cell barrier, prevents unfettered passage of chemicals or treatments from the blood to the brain [5]. Alternative medication administration techniques are the current focus of research to improve drug delivery for central nervous system (CNS) targeting. The NTB route of drug delivery has emerged as a possible alternative route of drug administration since it can convey medications directly to the brain by circumventing the BBB in this circumstance. Using the NTB method of drug administration for the treatment of neurological diseases, medicines are deposited in the olfactory region of the aperture of the nasal cavity. The medications then go to the brain via perivascular and nerve fibre channels, but more study of these pathways is still required. The NTB route of drug delivery has been confirmed their potentiality in several preclinical studies, with both particulate formulations and solutions. This considerable route for drug administration required special device for drug deposition in nasal opening. Pharmaceutical industries are more eagerly interested in device production for NTB drug delivery that would be depicted for the possible convenience of this passage for drug delivery to captivating this way to get approval for the drugs and/or products.

The efficiency of drug delivery through the NTB route depends on a number of factors, such as drug delivery to the olfactory area of the nasal opening as opposed to the respiratory region, longer mucosal surface retention time, improved drug penetration via nasal epithelial cells, and reduced drug metabolism by enzyme present in the nasal cavity. The most recent advancements in the NTB route of drug delivery for the treatment of neurological illnesses are covered in this chapter. This particular method of drug delivery largely relies on the nasal cavity. The most recent advancements in the treatment of neurological illnesses using the NTB route of drug administration are covered in this chapter. The nasal cavity plays a significant role in this particular route of drug administration.

2 Nose and Nasal Cavity

The nose has been considered as a very complex architecture that has an importance in facial aesthetic and promising role in the physiological consequences in respiratory system [6]. It consists of the nasal skeleton, which houses the nasal cavity. Readers must comprehend the cellular makeup and physical layout of the nasal cavity in order

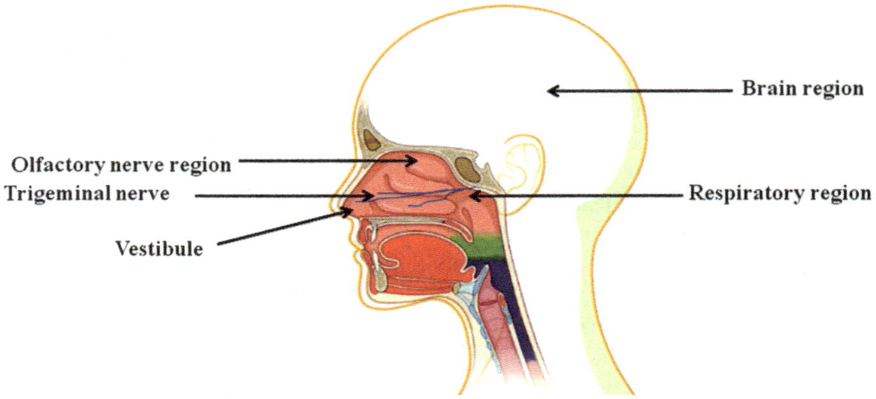

Fig. 1 Representative image of nasal cavity with its anatomical regions. Figure was created with BioRender.com

to better appreciate drug transport that starts in the nose and proceeds all the way to the brain. The nasal cavity measures 12–14 cm in length and 5 cm in height. Its surface area is 150–200 cm^2 and a total volume of 15–20 mL. To describe the anatomy of the nasal cavity, three divisions are used: nasal vestibule, olfactory, and respiratory portions (Fig. 1). The nasal vestibule, which has sebaceous and sweat glands as well as hair, is located in the anterior part of the nasal cavity. The respiratory system carries air to the lungs for breathing. The surface size of the olfactory region is roughly 10 cm^2. The olfactory area contains olfactory receptors, which are what give us our sense of smell. The absorption of intranasal drugs is significantly influenced by the respiratory and olfactory mucosa.

3 The NTB Route of Drug Delivery

Regardless of an emerging interest in NTB route of drugs delivery, the underlying mechanisms are limited or not yet elucidated. In another situation, researchers thought that medications given through the nose could get to the brain either directly or indirectly [7, 8]. Olfactory or trigeminal routes, as well as the possibility of the medications moving towards the brain following absorption in the blood and a subsequent cross-action in BBB, are also suggested by one pathway [9]. Figure 2 represents schematic possible pathway of drug transport from NTB route.

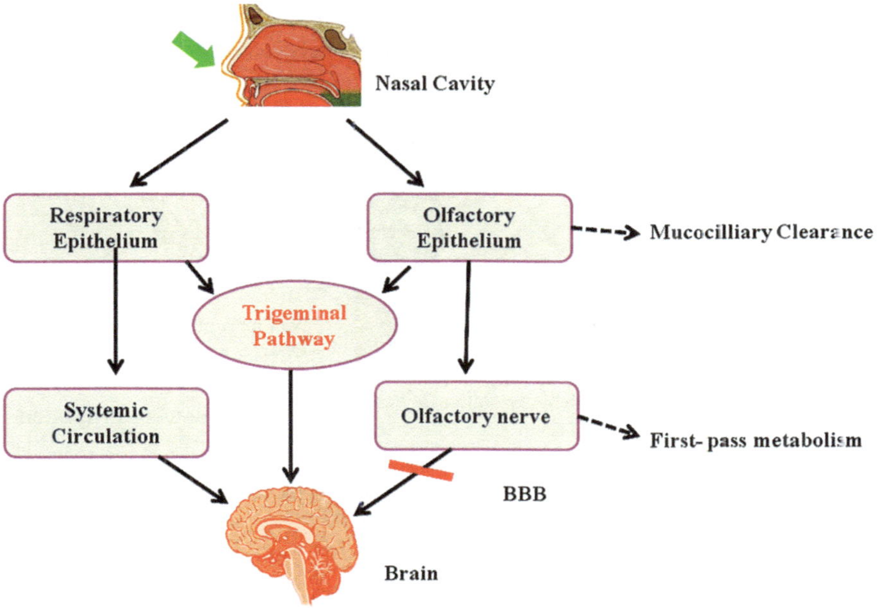

Fig. 2 Representative pathways of NTB route of drug delivery. Parts of the figure were created with BioRender.com

4 Nasal Drug Delivery Device

For NTB route of drug delivery, mucosal penetration and olfactory nerve uptakes of nanoparticles play a vital role. A particular medication delivery device is needed to deposit the desired amount of drug along this pathway in the olfactory area [10]. Among the very well-known brands of such devices being used for NTB technique of drug delivery are Impel Neuropharma's Precision Olfactory Device, Kurve Technologies' Vianase, and Alchemy Pharmatech's Naltos Device or Optinose device [11–13]. The promisible task for delivery of drugs from the nose to the brain is now possible because of nanomerics technology. The drug is inserted into the nostril's olfactory area, where the olfactory neurons may swiftly absorb it and convey it without passing through the BBB to the brain. Nanomerics nano-in-micro powder technology combined with Alchemy Pharmatech Naltos device enables reliable and targeted delivery of large microparticles to the nasal mucosal/olfactory area; these microparticles after disintegration to smaller nanoparticles can easily penetrate the nasal mucosal layer and facilitate mucosal and olfactory uptakes for medicine transport to the brain (Fig. 3). Even though the NTB route of medicine transport has been thoroughly demonstrated in a clinical trial, these devices are still not linked to approved medicines.

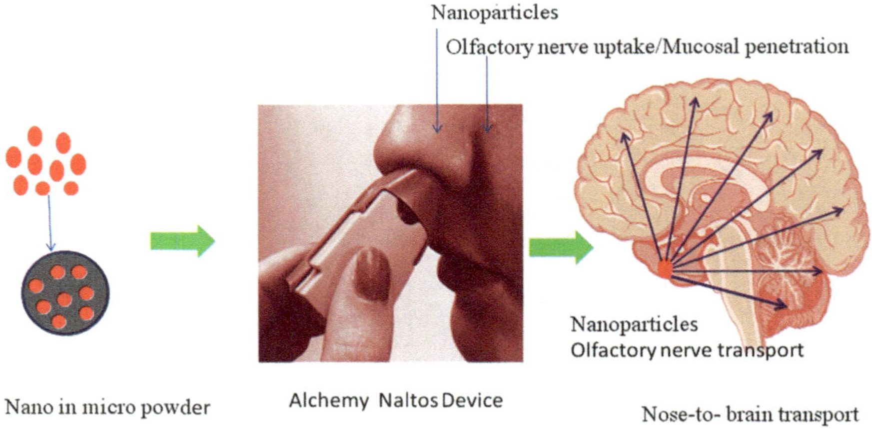

Fig. 3 Nano-in-micro powder technology combined with Alchemy Pharmatech Naltos device enables reliable and targeted delivery of large microparticles to the nasal mucosal/olfactory nerve transport. Parts of the figure were created with BioRender.com

5 Drug Formulations

Drug formulation strategies play a significant role in drug delivery. In the therapy of inflammatory illnesses, many types of nanoformulations have been employed. Despite the fact that medications and treatments have been utilised in numerous clinical studies [14], preclinical investigations in particle dispersion and solution have explored a variety of nanoformulations [15, 16]. Nasal drug delivery devices have been employed for the majority of formulation medication delivery in animal research and clinical studies.

6 Application of Pharmaceutical Nanotechnology for NTB Drug Transport

Nowadays, nanotechnology is the emerging field of nanomedicine and gained remarkable attention in diagnosis and therapy of disease [17]. NTB route has been extensively used to transport therapeutic drugs to desired targets. Pharmaceutical nanotechnology has a significant role in NTB drug transport. The most recent technology for the treatment of neurological diseases is the NTB medication delivery system. Pharmaceutical nanotechnology has great potential for use in NTB medication delivery [18]. The size range of nanoparticles (NPs) utilised to treat neurological illnesses is typically 1–1000 nm, and they typically take the form of colloidal dispersion [19]. Pharmaceutical nanotechnology's primary objectives are to extend the duration that a medicine remains in the body, make it more soluble, provide regulated

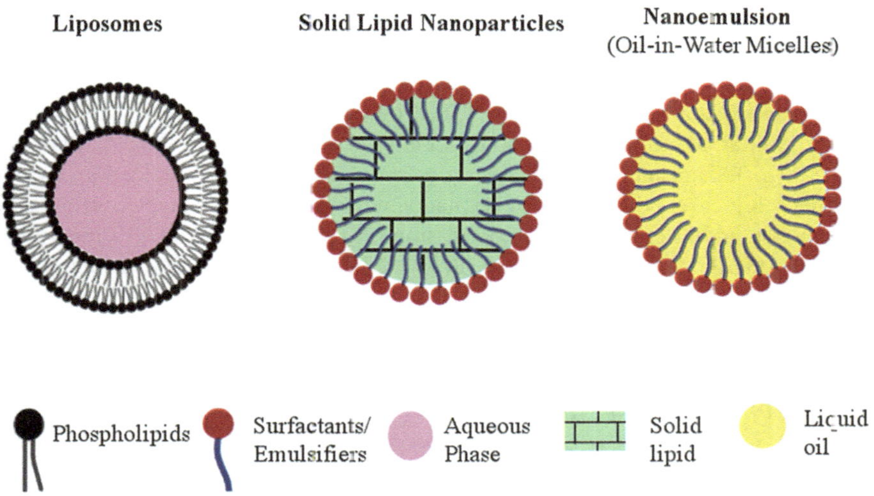

Fig. 4 Illustration of commonly used lipid-based NPs for NTB drug delivery. Using BioRender.com, the figures were produced

drug release, and minimise negative effects. As a result, all of the aforementioned traits make NPs a possible candidate for NTB drug transport [20]. NPs, such as lipid-based NPs and polymer-based NPs, are used for NTB medication delivery to treat neuroinflammatory diseases (Fig. 4). We have gone over each of these nanoparticles in detail in this section.

6.1 Lipid-Based NPs

Lipid-based NPs for NTB medication for the treatment of neurological conditions have been the subject of extensive research. Lipid-based NPs are appropriate for both hydrophilic and hydrophobic drug delivery since they are naturally amphiphilic in nature. Lipid-based nanoparticles have the properties of being cytocompatible and biodegradable. These properties of lipid-based NPs make it suitable to penetrate the cell efficiently without significant cellular toxicity. The most frequently used lipid-based NPs nowadays are solid lipid nanoparticles, liposomes, and nanoemulsions created with micelles (Fig. 3) [21]. PEG or poloxamers are polymers and are used for the modification of lipid-based nanoparticles. PEG is hydrophilic and biocompatible as well as acts as a nanoparticle stabiliser [22]. Poloxamers are generally used in the synthesis of lipid-based NPs as surfactant. It is water soluble and non-ionic in nature. Lipid-based NPs are cytocompatible, negligible toxicity, and excellent drug release properties make it potential candidature for NTB drug delivery. Furthermore, lipid-based NPs have the ability to carry the medicine over the respiratory epithelium and into the brain. This ability makes it a suitable candidature for NTB drug delivery.

Liposomes are the most frequently used lipid-based NPs for drug delivery purposes. In numerous studies, liposomes have been considered as potential NTB medication carriers for the treatment of neurological conditions [23]. Yet, SLNs are lipid-based nanocarriers that are appropriate for NTB drug delivery since they are emulsions in which liquid lipid has been replaced by solid lipid. They typically range in diameter from 100 to 300 nm and were effective delivery systems for NTB medications used to treat neurological conditions. However, nanoemulsions are of three types, water in oil, oil in water, and bi-continuous nanoemulsion [24]. The lipid-based NPs mentioned above are therefore appropriate nanocarriers for the delivery of NTB medicines for the treatment of neurological diseases.

6.2 Polymer-Based NPs

In the treatment of neurological illnesses, natural or synthetic polymer-based nanoparticles have been employed as promising nanocarriers for NTB drug delivery. These nanocarriers have some specific features such as cytocompatibility, increased stability, and controlled drug release patterns. Chitosan is a naturally occurring polymer made of D-glucosamine and N-acetyl-D-glucosamine, which are created when chitin is deacetylated [25]. The structural component of insects and crustaceans is chitin. The chitosan's acidic strength or pKa value has been noted as 6.5, and due to its pKa range, it has the capacity to get protonated in low and/or acidic pH environment. The potential of hydrogen ions in mucus has been recognised with a range of about 5.5–6.5 that is decisive to charged chitosan as positive leading to increase its stability [26]. Subsequently, both respiratory and olfactory epithelium have been known as chargeable with negative ions. This has been a speculation as chitosan encapsulated NPs has the capacity to survive for longer time in mucosa of both respiratory and olfactory regions. Increased bioavailability of the medicine and/or compounds included in NPs would be beneficial when contemplating nose-to-brain administration. In context of biochemistry investigations, several kinds of enzymes including cellulases, chitosanase, pepsin, and lipase have been known to deteriorate the chitosan-encapsulated NPs [27]. Synthetic polymers have also been extensively utilised in the creation of several drug delivery systems. The transmission of neuroprotective medications from the nose to the brain may be improved by the use of many synthetic polymers, which are regarded to be more cellularly friendly and may serve as superior nanocarriers. The nanocarriers of polymers like poly(L-lactide-co-glycolide), poly(lactic acid), and poly(glycolic acid) are particularly important for the transport of drugs from the nose to the brain for the therapeutic manifestation of neurological disorders, which piques the curiosity of nanobiologists. They are suitable for preventing drug degradation in the nasal cavity and increasing hydrophobic drug loading because of their hydrophobicity [21]. These synthetic polymer-mediated NPs may enhance the chance to encapsulate as drugs via single or double emulsion techniques [28]. Similar to PEG or poloxamers, various lipid-based NPs and synthesised polymeric NPs may exhibit a surface-based alteration. This may lead to improved stability, medication loading efficiency, and nasal mucosal penetration [29].

7 NTB Drug Delivery in Neurological Disorders

Neurological disorders have become global challenges for researchers. Epilepsy, Alzheimer's, Parkinson's, and strokes are just a few of the neurological disorders that plague people today. The specific cause is still unknown. The BBB is an extremely selective checkpoint for drug transport to the brain during the treatment of neurological disorders. Through the use of NTB drug delivery devices, researchers are attempting to overcome this obstacle. Several neurological illnesses will be briefly explained in this part, along with nanocarriers for effective drug administration via the NTB route.

7.1 Epilepsy

In recent years, epilepsy has been recognised as chronic neurological impairment known to cause seizures in patients. It has been manifested among all the ages and the maximum incidence of new cases is recorded mostly at childhood stage. This neurological disorder affects approximately 0.065 billion people at all over the globe [30]. Persistent seizures are critically linked with 20–40% risk of skeletal injuries. Such kinds of injuries are as fractures, burns, concussions and are observed in 1-year follow-up of a healthcare program. The primary target for epileptic therapy has been put as wipe off the seizures and its associated symptoms and also shut down the adverse effects of anti-seizure drugs or molecules. There is a limited advances have been noted in those countries with low sociodemographic indices. These incidences were recorded with higher numbers of epileptic mortality rate in the last 26 years [31]. There is no single specific aetiology of epilepsy as other factors may also be involved. The major common reasons for the occurrence of epilepsy are different as accordance with both population and area. The symptomatic factors of epilepsy could be different as at what type of threshold of seizures and affected region of brain? There has been a common movement disorders observed in epileptic patients. These symptoms include: shaking or twitching, numbness or tingling, and unconsciousness. Based on the symptoms, drug therapies of epilepsy include as benzodiazepines and antiseizure prescriptions to the affected patients. It has been known as antiepileptic drugs could show drug-drug interactions, and these are able to alter the activity of hepatic enzymes including CYP3A4 and CYP1A2. These alterations are more markedly concerns in the geriatric population as more drug consumers have been found to regulate their chronic disease [32]. In this era, nanotechnology-mediated drug formulations are more highlighted for the possible interventions of neurological impairments. For the best knowledge of the drug formulations, nose-to-brain exposures of antiepileptic drugs are safest and easy. And also, it has more beneficial actions including minimal drug-drug interactions, defence for the inactivation of hepatic enzymes and other possible factors as systemic side effects. Several types of nanoformulations are being discussed for better epilepsy treatment via nose-to-brain. In this regard, we have outlined a few typical drug nanoformulations that are applied to the nose-to-brain method of treating epilepsy (Table 1).

7.2 *Alzheimer's Disease*

Alzheimer's disease (AD) has been known as progressive neurodegenerative disorder [46]. Of course, it has brain disorder symptoms that gradually hinder the cognition and memory in affected population. As per the statistical incidence of United States, approximately 0.0058 billion people were considered for diagnosing of AD in 2020 [47]. There is one recent report indicating as the most prevalence of such kind of dementia disorder would be duplicated in Europe and triplicated at globally by 2050. Based on a biological definition of AD as opposed to the clinical definition, it is anticipated to be 3 times greater [48]. At early stage of AD, the accumulated or aggregated form of amyloid β has led the distribution of tau observed in pathological consequences. There is a high risk of AD and 60–80% are dependent on hereditary factors. There are many diagnosis or prognosis events for the confirmation of AD. Also, it was found that new biomarkers for AD included PET scans and blood tests for the harmful amyloid and the phosphorylated tau it associates with. This has generated strong attention for use in research and therapeutic settings. Genetic and environmental factors have been connected to AD, even if the exact causation is still up for debate. Presenilin1, 2, and Amyloid Precursor Proteins (APP) were studied as three genes. These three genes have been found to be the main contributors of early-onset familial AD through mutations or sudden changes. Contrarily, Apolipoprotein E is also a more promiscuous molecule that is linked to AD's late onset [49]. Such proteins are able to hyperphosphorylate the tau proteins and aggregation of beta-amyloid plaque. These are the most significant factors of AD onset [50]. Memory loss and aphasia are cognitive signs of Alzheimer's disease (AD), while depression, physical, or verbal violence are behavioural symptoms [51]. The two drugs that are most frequently used to treat AD are cholinesterase inhibitors and N-Methyl-D-aspartate (NMDA) receptor antagonists, however, it is recognised that these merely help patients with their symptoms and cannot stop neurodegeneration [52]. Most importantly, nanotechnology has been an emerging area of biological science and has great applications in pharmaceutical science for drug transport purposes. Nanotechnology-based nose-to-brain drug delivery offers many potential uses for the treatment of neurological diseases. In this regard, we've provided a summary of some popular drug nanoformulations used to treat AD via the NTB pathway (Table 1).

Table 1 A list of some typical nanoparticles used in nose-to-brain therapy for neurological diseases

Disease	Drug	Nanomaterials/ nanocarrier	Surfactant used	Size (nm)	Zeta potential (mV)	PDI	References
Epilepsy	Oxcarbazepine	PLGA NPs	Tween 80	256.16 ± 2.94	−15.12 ± 0.36	0.144 ± 0.024	Musumeci et al. [33]
Epilepsy	Carbamazepine	Nanoemulgel	Labrasol	45–146	–	–	Samia et al. [34]
Epilepsy	Diazepam	PLGA NPs	Poloxamer 407	183.2	–	–	Sharma et al. [35]
Epilepsy	Letrozole	Nanoemulsion	Tween 80	95.59 ± 2.34	–	0.162 ± 0.012	Iqbal et al. [36]
Epilepsy	Lamotrigine	Liposome	Tween 80	88.90 ± 1.56		0.247 ± 0.04	Praveen et al. [37]
Epilepsy	Lorazepam	PLGA NPs	Poloxamer 407	168.2	−18.4	0.08	Sharma et al. [38]
Alzheimer's disease	Pioglitazone	NLC	PF 68/Tween 80	211.4 ± 3.54	+14.9 ± 1.09	0.257 ± 0.108	Jojo et al. [39]
Alzheimer's disease	R-flurbiprofen	Albumin NPs	–	284.4 ± 14.9	–	0.404 ± 0.065	Wong and Ho [40]
Alzheimer's disease	Huperzine A	PLGA NPs	PVA	153.2 ± 13.7	+35.6 ± 5.2	0.229 ± 0.078	Meng et al. [41]
Alzheimer's disease	Memantine	Nanoemulsion	Tween 20/ Propylene glycol	~11	−19.6	0.080	Kaur et al. [42]
Alzheimer's disease	Galantamine	Liposome	–	112 ± 8	−49.2 ± 0.7	–	Li et al. [43]
Alzheimer's disease	Tarenflurbil	PLGA NPs	PF-68	133.13 ± 7.82	−30.25 ± 2.11	0.21 ± 0.02	Muntimadugu et al. [44]
Alzheimer's disease	Donepezil	Chitosan Nanosuspension	–	150–200	–	0.341	Bhavna et al. [45]

7.3 Parkinson's Disease

A neurological illness called Parkinson's disease (PD) affects both the brain and the part of the body that affects nerve controls. Movement is impacted, and tremors are frequently present. The most prevalent neurological ailment is Alzheimer's disease, followed by Parkinson's disease [53]. Ageing, genetic variation, and environmental variables are all risk factors for PD. The loss of dopaminergic neurons from the substantia nigra pars compacta is one of the clinical symptoms of PD, even if the true aetiology is currently unknown. PD symptoms may result from a 30% loss of dopamine neurons in the substantia nigra pars compacta, according to research [54]. Important pathological markers of PD include Lewy bodies, abnormal protein clusters linked to neuronal degeneration. PD is a disorder of bodily movement that is characterised by the presence of bradykinesia, stiffness, and tremor. Clinically, there are different ways to management of PD. In general, anticholinergic drugs are used to treat tremor while monoamine oxidase B (MAO-B) inhibitors are used to stop the breakdown of dopamine. Meantime, dopamine precursor and dopamine agonists are being used for satiation of dopamine. Unfortunately, these approaches of PD treatment give symptomatic relief to the patient not cure [55]. The distribution of NTB medicines used to treat neurological issues frequently makes use of nanotechnology. In this regard, we have included a number of popular medication nanoformulations that are used to treat PD via the NTB route (Table 2).

7.4 Stroke

In general, a stroke occurs when the blood flow to a specific region of the brain is halted or reduced, which lowers the amount of oxygen reaching that area of the brain. It is regarded as the second biggest global killer and a significant contributor to disability [56]. Strokes often come in two different forms: ischemic (87%) and haemorrhagic (13%) [57]. Local thrombus is the main factor blocking brain arteries in ischemic stroke. Blockage of artery hampers cerebral blood flow, which causes limited oxygen supply to the brain. In this condition, patients clinically required intervention within 2–3 h. Tissue plasminogen activator (tPA) is a serine protease, and it is being used to break down the blood clot and restore normal blood flow to the brain [58]. In contrast, haemorrhagic stroke occurs due to bleeding in the brain through rupture of cerebral blood vessels. Even though, currently several medications are being used in the management of haemorrhagic stroke such as osmotic agents, anticoagulants, and antihypertensive drugs. Unfortunately, no one drug has been approved for the treatment of hemorrhagic stroke [59]. There are currently relatively few options for stroke treatment. Nanotechnology-based NTB drug transport is a novel approach to stroke treatment, and certain drug nanoformulations that are employed in stroke management are compiled in Table 2.

Table 2 A list of some typical nanodrugs used in nose-to-brain delivery for treatment of epilepsy and alzheimer's disease

Diseases	Drug	Nanomaterials/ nanocarrier	Surfactant used	Size (nm)	Zeta potential (mV)	PDI	References
Parkinson's disease	Naringenin	Nanoemulsion	Tween 80/ Transcutol-HP	38.70 ± 3.11	−27.4 ± 0.14	0.14 ± 0.0024	Gaba et al. [60]
Parkinson's disease	Pramipexole	Chitosan NPs	–	292.5 ± 8.80	+14.0 ± 2.89	0.292	Raj et al. [61]
Parkinson's disease	Urocortin	PLGA NPs	Sodium cholate	114.8 ± 5.6	−24.7 ± 1.5	0.193	Wen et al. [62]
Parkinson's disease	Rasagiline	Chitosan glutamate NPs	–	151.1 ± 10.31	–	0.380 ± 0.01	Mittal et al. [63]
Parkinson's disease	Geraniol/ ursodeoxycholic acid conjugate	SLN	Span 85	121 ± 8.4	−22.5 ± 7.7	0.164 ± 0.03	de Oliveira Junior et al. [64]
Parkinson's disease	Bromocriptine	Chitosan NPs	–	161.3 ± 4.7	+40.32 ± 2.78	0.44 ± 0.03	Md et al. [65]
Parkinson's disease	Dopamine	PLGA NPs	PVA	175.3 ± 9.6	−15.7 ± 0.86	0.129 ± 0.011	Tang et al. [66]
Stroke	Thymoquinone	PLGA NPs	–	183.5 ± 8.2	+33.63 ± 2.25	0.257 ± 0.02	Xiao et al. [67]
Stroke	NR2B9c	PLGA NPs	Sodium cholate	~139	−23.3	<0.2	Li et al. [68]

8 Limitations

NTB drug delivery has some limitations. These limitations must be acknowledged while developing a new therapeutic drug for the delivery through NTB route. The recommended doses for various medication types vary, making the route only suitable for strong drugs. There are restrictions on dosage amounts, which range from 100 to 250 ml for liquid and 20–50 mg for powder [69–71]. Moreover, some drugs may be broken down by enzymes in the nose cavity, in this case, the drugs must be prevented from being broken down by nasal enzymes, and drug formulations should not irritate the nasal cavity. For NTB drug delivery, a nasal drug delivery system is also necessary.

9 Conclusion

Delivery of drugs hampers by BBB during the treatment of ND. NTB delivery of therapeutics drugs may be a future potential alternative because it increases the concentration of drugs into the brain by bypassing BBB through trigeminal and olfactory pathways. By the exploitation of nanotechnology techniques, we can deliver the drug through the NTB route by bypassing the BBB for the effective treatment of ND. Pharmaceutical nanotechnology's primary objectives are to extend the duration that a medicine remains in the body, make it more soluble, provide regulated drug release, and minimise negative effects. Several nanoformulations have been demonstrated in preclinical studies as well as clinical trial results for NTB drug transport for the treatment of ND. Solution forms are very effective clinically while solutions and NP formulations have been used in preclinical studies. The solution penetration enhancers and NPs use may be improving drug transport to the brain through NTB route due to its offer advantage over limitations in dose volume that can make it a future ray of hope for the treatment of neurological problems. NBT route of drug transport required nasal delivery device for the deposition of drugs in nasal opening. The Naltos Device from Alchemy Pharmatech and Optinose are two new device-makers that have recently joined the market. Notwithstanding these issues, NTB drug delivery has a lot of potential for the treatment of neurological disorders.

Conflict of Interest The author declares no competing interest.

References

1. Rinaldi S, Davies A, Fehmi J, Beadnall HN, Wang J, Hardy TA, Barnett MH, Broadley SA, Waters P, Reddel SW, Irani SR, Brilot F, Dale RC, Ramanathan S, Australian and New Zealand

MOG Study Group (2020) Overlapping central and peripheral nervous system syndromes in MOG antibody-associated disorders. Neurol (R) neuroimmunol neuroinflamm 8(1):e924
2. Mathers CD, Loncar D (2006) Projections of global mortality and burden of disease from 2002 to 2030. PLoS Med 3(11):e442
3. Gustavsson A, Svensson M, Jacobi F, Allgulander C, Alonso J, Beghi E, Dodel R, Ekman M, Faravelli C, Fratiglioni L, Gannon B, Jones DH, Jennum P, Jordanova A, Jönsson L, Karampampa K, Knapp M, Kobelt G, Kurth T, Lieb R, … CDBE2010Study Group (2011) Cost of disorders of the brain in Europe 2010. Eur Neuropsychopharmacol: J Eur Coll Neuropsychopharmacol 21(10):718–779
4. Pardridge WM (2005) The blood-brain barrier: bottleneck in brain drug development. NeuroRx: J Am Soc Exp NeuroThers 2(1):3–14
5. Daneman R, Prat A (2015) The blood-brain barrier. Cold Spring Harb Perspect Biol 7(1):a020412
6. Patel RG (2017) Nasal anatomy and function. Facial Plast Surg: FPS 33(1):3–8
7. Erdő F, Bors LA, Farkas D, Bajza Á, Gizurarson S (2018) Evaluation of intranasal delivery route of drug administration for brain targeting. Brain Res Bull 143:155–170
8. Crowe TP, Greenlee M, Kanthasamy AG, Hsu WH (2018) Mechanism of intranasal drug delivery directly to the brain. Life Sci 195:44–52
9. Illum L (2000) Transport of drugs from the nasal cavity to the central nervous system. Eur J Pharm Sci: Off J Eur Fed Pharm Sci 11(1):1–18
10. Lochhead JJ, Thorne RG (2012) Intranasal delivery of biologics to the central nervous system. Adv Drug Deliv Rev 64(7):614–628
11. Shrewsbury S, Swardstrom M, Satterly K, Campbell J, Tugiono N, Gillies J, and Hoekman J (2019) Placebo/active controlled, safety, pharmaco-kinetic/dynamic study of INP105 (POD® olanzapine) in healthy adults: western journal of emergency medicine: integrating emergency care with population health. West J Emerg Med 20(2):ix–x. https://escholarship.org/uc/item/86f519rb.1936-900X
12. Craft S, Claxton A, Baker LD, Hanson AJ, Cholerton B, Trittschuh EH, Dahl D, Caulder E, Neth B, Montine TJ, Jung Y, Maldjian J, Whitlow C, Friedman S (2017) Effects of regular and long-acting insulin on cognition and Alzheimer's disease biomarkers: a pilot clinical trial. J Alzheimer's Dis: JAD 57(4):1325–1334
13. Quintana DS, Westlye LT, Hope S, Nærland T, Elvsåshagen T, Dørum E, Rustan Ø, Valstad M, Rezvaya L, Lishaugen H, Stensønes E, Yaqub S, Smerud KT, Mahmoud RA, Djupesland PG, Andreassen OA (2017) Dose-dependent social-cognitive effects of intranasal oxytocin delivered with novel Breath Powered device in adults with autism spectrum disorder: a randomized placebo-controlled double-blind crossover trial. Transl Psychiatry 7(5):e1135
14. Craft S, Baker LD, Montine TJ, Minoshima S, Watson GS, Claxton A, Arbuckle M, Callaghan M, Tsai E, Plymate SR, Green PS, Leverenz J, Cross D, Gerton B (2012) Intranasal insulin therapy for Alzheimer disease and amnestic mild cognitive impairment: a pilot clinical trial. Arch Neurol 69(1):29–38
15. Godfrey L, Iannitelli A, Garrett NL, Moger J, Imbert I, King T, Porreca F, Soundararajan R, Lalatsa A, Schätzlein AG, Uchegbu IF (2018) Nanoparticulate peptide delivery exclusively to the brain produces tolerance free analgesia. J Control Release: Off J Control Release Soc 270:135–144
16. Thorne RG, Hanson LR, Ross TM, Tung D, Frey WH 2nd (2008) Delivery of interferon-beta to the monkey nervous system following intranasal administration. Neuroscience 152(3):785–797
17. Puri A, Loomis K, Smith B, Lee JH, Yavlovich A, Heldman E, Blumenthal R (2009) Lipid-based nanoparticles as pharmaceutical drug carriers: from concepts to clinic. Crit Rev Ther Drug Carrier Syst 26(6):523–580
18. Agrawal M, Dethe MR, Ahmed H, Yadav A, Gupta U, Alexander A (2022) Nose-to-brain drug delivery for the treatment of Alzheimer's disease: current advancements and challenges. Expert Opin Drug Deliv 19(1):87–102
19. Shen AM, Minko T (2020) Pharmacokinetics of inhaled nanotherapeutics for pulmonary delivery. J Control Release: Off J Control Release Soc 326:222–244

20. Sonvico F, Clementino A, Buttini F, Colombo G, Pescina S, Stanisçuaski Guterres S, Raffin Pohlmann A, Nicoli S (2018) Surface-modified nanocarriers for nose-to-brain delivery: from bioadhesion to targeting. Pharmaceutics 10(1):34
21. Wang Z, Xiong G, Tsang WC, Schätzlein AG, Uchegbu IF (2019) Nose-to-brain delivery. J Pharmacol Exp Ther 370(3):593–601
22. Chen W, Liu C, Ji X, Joseph J, Tang Z, Ouyang J, Xiao Y, Kong N, Joshi N, Farokhzad OC, Tao W, Xie T (2021) Stanene-based nanosheets for β-elemene delivery and ultrasound-mediated combination cancer therapy. Angewandte Chemie (International ed. in English) 60(13):7155–7164
23. Pashirova TN, Zueva IV, Petrov KA, Lukashenko SS, Nizameev IR, Kulik NV, Voloshina AD, Almasy L, Kadirov MK, Masson P, Souto EB, Zakharova LY, Sinyashin OG (2018) Mixed cationic liposomes for brain delivery of drugs by the intranasal route: the acetylcholinesterase reactivator 2-PAM as encapsulated drug model. Colloids Surf B, Biointerfaces 171:358–367
24. Hayes DG, Ye R, Dunlap RN, Anunciado DB, Pingali SV, O'Neill HM, Urban VS (2018) Bicontinuous microemulsions as a biomembrane mimetic system for melittin. Biochim Biophys Acta 1860(2):624–632
25. Ansari MM, Ahmad A, Mishra RK, Raza SS, Khan R (2019) Zinc gluconate-loaded chitosan nanoparticles reduce severity of collagen-induced arthritis in Wistar rats. ACS Biomater Sci Eng 5(7):3380–3397
26. Nurunnabi M, Revuri V, Huh KM, Lee Y-K (2017) Chapter 14—polysaccharide based nano/microformulation: an effective and versatile oral drug delivery system. In: Andronescu E, Grumezescu AM (eds) Nanostructures for oral medicine. Elsevier, Amsterdam, The Netherlands, pp 409–433
27. Gonçalves C, Ferreira N, Lourenço L (2021) Production of low molecular weight chitosan and chitooligosaccharides (COS): a review. Polymers 13(15):2466
28. McCall RL, Sirianni RW (2013) PLGA nanoparticles formed by single- or double-emulsion with vitamin E-TPGS. J Vis Exp: JoVE 82:51015
29. Suk JS, Xu Q, Kim N, Hanes J, Ensign LM (2016) PEGylation as a strategy for improving nanoparticle-based drug and gene delivery. Adv Drug Deliv Rev 99(Pt A):28–51
30. Kanner AM, Bicchi MM (2022) Antiseizure Medications for Adults With Epilepsy: A Review. JAMA 327(13):1269–1281
31. Singh G, Sander JW (2020) The global burden of epilepsy report: implications for low- and middle-income countries. Epilepsy Behav: E&B 105:106949
32. Johannessen SI, Landmark CJ (2010) Antiepileptic drug interactions—principles and clinical implications. Curr Neuropharmacol 8(3):254–267
33. Musumeci T, Serapide MF, Pellitteri R, Dalpiaz A, Ferraro L, Dal Magro R, Bonaccorso A, Carbone C, Veiga F, Sancini G, Puglisi G (2018) Oxcarbazepine free or loaded PLGA nanoparticles as effective intranasal approach to control epileptic seizures in rodents. Eur J Pharm Biopharm: Off J Arbeitsgemeinschaft fur Pharmazeutische Verfahrenstechnik e.V 133:309–320
34. Samia O, Hanan R, Kamal E (2012) Carbamazepine mucoadhesive nanoemulgel (MNEG) as brain targeting delivery system via the olfactory mucosa. Drug Deliv 19(1):58–67
35. Sharma D, Sharma RK, Sharma N, Gabrani R, Sharma SK, Ali J, Dang S (2015) Nose-to-brain delivery of PLGA-diazepam nanoparticles. AAPS PharmSciTech 16(5):1108–1121
36. Iqbal R, Ahmed S, Jain GK, Vohora D (2019) Design and development of letrozole nanoemulsion: a comparative evaluation of brain targeted nanoemulsion with free letrozole against status epilepticus and neurodegeneration in mice. Int J Pharm 565:20–32
37. Praveen A, Aqil M, Imam SS, Ahad A, Moolakkadath T, Ahmad FJ (2019) Lamotrigine encapsulated intra-nasal nanoliposome formulation for epilepsy treatment: formulation design, characterization and nasal toxicity study. Colloids Surf B, Biointerfaces 174:553–562
38. Sharma D, Maheshwari D, Philip G, Rana R, Bhatia S, Singh M, Gabrani R, Sharma SK, Ali J, Sharma RK, Dang S (2014) Formulation and optimization of polymeric nanoparticles for intranasal delivery of lorazepam using Box-Behnken design: in vitro and in vivo evaluation. BioMed Res Int 2014:156010

39. Jojo GM, Kuppusamy G, De A, Karri V (2019) Formulation and optimization of intranasal nanolipid carriers of pioglitazone for the repurposing in Alzheimer's disease using Box-Behnken design. Drug Dev Ind Pharm 45(7):1061–1072
40. Wong LR, Ho PC (2018) Role of serum albumin as a nanoparticulate carrier for nose-to-brain delivery of R-flurbiprofen: implications for the treatment of Alzheimer's disease. J Pharm Pharmacol 70(1):59–69
41. Meng Q, Wang A, Hua H, Jiang Y, Wang Y, Mu H, Wu Z, Sun K (2018) Intranasal delivery of Huperzine A to the brain using lactoferrin-conjugated N-trimethylated chitosan surface-modified PLGA nanoparticles for treatment of Alzheimer's disease. Int J Nanomed 13:705–718
42. Kaur A, Nigam K, Srivastava S, Tyagi A, Dang S (2020) Memantine nanoemulsion: a new approach to treat Alzheimer's disease. J Microencapsul 37(5):355–365
43. Li W, Zhou Y, Zhao N, Hao B, Wang X, Kong P (2012) Pharmacokinetic behavior and efficiency of acetylcholinesterase inhibition in rat brain after intranasal administration of galanthamine hydrobromide loaded flexible liposomes. Environ Toxicol Pharmacol 34(2) 272–279
44. Muntimadugu E, Dhommati R, Jain A, Challa VG, Shaheen M, Khan W (2016) Intranasal delivery of nanoparticle encapsulated tarenflurbil: a potential brain targeting strategy for Alzheimer's disease. Eur J Pharm Sci: Off J Eur Fed Pharm Sci 92:224–234
45. Bhavna MS, Ali M, Ali R, Bhatnagar A, Baboota S, Ali J (2014) Donepezil nanosuspension intended for nose to brain targeting: in vitro and in vivo safety evaluation. Int J Biol Macromol 67:418–425
46. Yu TW, Lane HY, Lin CH (2021) Novel therapeutic approaches for Alzheimer's disease: an updated review. Int J Mol Sci 22(15):8208
47. Mebane-Sims I (2020) 2020 Alzheimer's disease facts and figures. Alzheimers Dement 16:391–460
48. Scheltens P, De Strooper B, Kivipelto M, Holstege H, Chételat G, Teunissen CE, Cummings J, van der Flier WM (2021) Alzheimer's disease. Lancet (London, England) 397(10284):1577–1590
49. Williamson J, Goldman J, Marder KS (2009) Genetic aspects of Alzheimer disease. Neurologist 15(2):80–86
50. Bloom GS (2014) Amyloid-β and tau: the trigger and bullet in Alzheimer disease pathogenesis. JAMA Neurol 71(4):505–508
51. Peron EP, Zimmerman KM, Crouse EL, Slattum PW, Hobgood SE (2020) Alzheimer disease. In: DiPiro JT, Yee GC, Posey L, Haines ST, Nolin TD, Ellingrod V (eds) Pharmacotherapy: a pathophysiologic approach, 11e; McGraw Hill, New York, NY, USA
52. Sadowsky CH, Galvin JE (2012) Guidelines for the management of cognitive and behavioral problems in dementia. J Am Board Fam Med: JABFM 25(3):350–366
53. Orozco JL, Valderrama-Chaparro JA, Pinilla-Monsalve GD, Molina-Echeverry MI, Pérez Castaño AM, Ariza-Araújo Y, Prada SI, Takeuchi Y (2020) Parkinson's disease prevalence, age distribution and staging in Colombia. Neurol Int 12(1):8401
54. Fearnley JM, Lees AJ (1991) Ageing and Parkinson's disease: substantia nigra regional selectivity. Brain: J Neurol 114(Pt 5):2283–2301
55. Jankovic J, Aguilar LG (2008) Current approaches to the treatment of Parkinson's disease. Neuropsychiatr Dis Treat 4(4):743–757
56. Johnson W, Onuma O, Owolabi M, Sachdev S (2016) Stroke: a global response is needed. Bull World Health Organ 94(9):634-634A
57. Virani SS, Alonso A, Aparicio HJ, Benjamin EJ, Bittencourt MS, Callaway CW, Carson AP, Chamberlain AM, Cheng S, Delling FN, Elkind M, Evenson KR, Ferguson JF, Gupta DK, Khan SS, Kissela BM, Knutson KL, Lee CD, Lewis TT, Liu J, … American Heart Association Council on Epidemiology and Prevention Statistics Committee and Stroke Statistics Subcommittee (2021) Heart disease and stroke statistics-2021 update: a report from the American heart association. Circulation 143(8):e254–e743
58. Powers WJ, Rabinstein AA, Ackerson T, Adeoye OM, Bambakidis NC, Becker K, Biller J, Brown M, Demaerschalk BM, Hoh B, Jauch EC, Kidwell CS, Leslie-Mazwi TM, Ovbiagele B, Scott PA, Sheth KN, Southerland AM, Summers DV, Tirschwell DL (2019) Guidelines for the

early management of patients with acute ischemic stroke: 2019 update to the 2018 guidelines for the early management of acute ischemic stroke: a guideline for healthcare professionals from the American heart association/American stroke association. Stroke 50(12):e344–e418
59. Hemphill JC 3rd, Greenberg SM, Anderson CS, Becker K, Bendok BR, Cushman M, Fung GL, Goldstein JN, Macdonald RL, Mitchell PH, Scott PA, Selim MH, Woo D, American Heart Association Stroke Council, Council on Cardiovascular and Stroke Nursing & Council on Clinical Cardiology (2015) Guidelines for the management of spontaneous intracerebral hemorrhage: a guideline for healthcare professionals from the American heart association/ American stroke association. Stroke 46(7):2032–2060
60. Gaba B, Khan T, Haider MF, Alam T, Baboota S, Parvez S, Ali J (2019) Vitamin E loaded naringenin nanoemulsion via intranasal delivery for the management of oxidative stress in a 6-OHDA Parkinson's disease model. BioMed Res Int 2019:2382563
61. Raj R, Wairkar S, Sridhar V, Gaud R (2018) Pramipexole dihydrochloride loaded chitosan nanoparticles for nose to brain delivery: Development, characterization and in vivo anti-Parkinson activity. Int J Biol Macromol 109:27–35
62. Wen Z, Yan Z, Hu K, Pang Z, Cheng X, Guo L, Zhang Q, Jiang X, Fang L, Lai R (2011) Odorranalectin-conjugated nanoparticles: preparation, brain delivery and pharmacodynamic study on Parkinson's disease following intranasal administration. J Control Release: Off J Control Release Soc 151(2):131–138
63. Mittal D, Md S, Hasan Q, Fazil M, Ali A, Baboota S, Ali J (2016) Brain targeted nanoparticulate drug delivery system of rasagiline via intranasal route. Drug Deliv 23(1):130–139
64. de Oliveira Junior ER, Truzzi E, Ferraro L, Fogagnolo M, Pavan B, Beggiato S, Rustichelli C, Maretti E, Lima EM, Leo E, Dalpiaz A (2020) Nasal administration of nanoencapsulated geraniol/ursodeoxycholic acid conjugate: towards a new approach for the management of Parkinson's disease. J Control Release: Off J Control Release Soc 321:540–552
65. Md S, Khan RA, Mustafa G, Chuttani K, Baboota S, Sahni JK, Ali J (2013) Bromocriptine loaded chitosan nanoparticles intended for direct nose to brain delivery: pharmacodynamic, pharmacokinetic and scintigraphy study in mice model. Eur J Pharm Sci: Off J Eur Fed Pharm Sci 48(3):393–405
66. Tang S, Wang A, Yan X, Chu L, Yang X, Song Y, Sun K, Yu X, Liu R, Wu Z, Xue P (2019) Brain-targeted intranasal delivery of dopamine with borneol and lactoferrin co-modified nanoparticles for treating Parkinson's disease. Drug Deliv 26(1):700–707
67. Xiao XY, Zhu YX, Bu JY, Li GW, Zhou JH, Zhou SP (2016) Evaluation of neuroprotective effect of thymoquinone nanoformulation in the rodent cerebral ischemia-reperfusion model. BioMed Res Int 2016:2571060
68. Li R, Huang Y, Chen L, Zhou H, Zhang M, Chang L, Shen H, Zhou M, Su P, Zhu D (2019) Targeted delivery of intranasally administered nanoparticles-mediated neuroprotective peptide NR2B9c to brain and neuron for treatment of ischemic stroke. Nanomedicine: Nanotechnol Biol Med 18:380–390
69. Djupesland PG, Messina JC, Mahmoud RA (2014) The nasal approach to delivering treatment for brain diseases: an anatomic, physiologic, and delivery technology overview. Ther Deliv 5(6):709–733
70. Santos-Morales O, Díaz-Machado A, Jiménez-Rodríguez D, Pomares-Iturralde Y, Festary-Casanovas T, González-Delgado CA, Pérez-Rodríguez S, Alfonso-Muñoz E, Viada-González C, Piedra-Sierra P, García-García I, Amaro-González D, NeuroEPO Study Group, García-Rodríguez JC, Sosa-Testé I, Lagarto-Parra A, Barrero-Viera L, David-Baldo M, Tamayo-Rodríguez M, Rivero-Vázquez I et al (2017) Nasal administration of the neuroprotective candidate NeuroEPO to healthy volunteers: a randomized, parallel, open-label safety study. BMC Neurol 17(1):129
71. Tepper SJ, Johnstone MR (2018) Breath-powered sumatriptan dry nasal powder: an intranasal medication delivery system for acute treatment of migraine. Med Devices (Auckland, N.Z.) 11:147–156. https://doi.org/10.2147/MDER.S130900

Nanocarriers and Nano Drug Delivery Therapy in Neuro Diseases

Palak Rana, Gursharan Kaur, Aleena James Chirayimmel, Anupama Rajput, Santosh Kumar Rath, and Vagish Dwibedi

Abstract Neurological diseases pose significant challenges in drug delivery due to the complex and delicate nature of the central nervous system (CNS). Nanotechnology has opened up new avenues for targeted drug delivery and therapy in neuro diseases. This book chapter provides a comprehensive overview of nanocarriers and nano-drug delivery therapy in neuro diseases, focusing on their applications, challenges, and prospects. The book chapter's first section explores various nanocarriers, including liposomes, polymeric nanoparticles, dendrimers, and carbon-based nanomaterials, highlighting their characteristics and advantages. We discuss how these nanocarriers can overcome the blood–brain barrier and deliver therapeutic agents to specific brain regions affected by neuro diseases. Additionally, the challenges and limitations in nanocarriers development are addressed. The book chapter's next section focuses on nanocarriers' specific applications in neuro diseases. We examine the role of nanocarriers in delivering therapeutic agents for Alzheimer's disease, Parkinson's disease, and multiple sclerosis. Targeted drug delivery approaches and strategies to enhance drug delivery efficacy are discussed in each case. Furthermore, we explore the applications of nanocarriers in neuroimaging, including the use of contrast agents and targeted imaging of specific brain regions. We also highlight the potential of multifunctional nanocarriers for theranostic applications. The safety and regulatory considerations associated with nanocarrier-based therapies are addressed, including the biocompatibility and toxicity of nanocarriers, approaches for evaluating safety and efficacy, and regulatory challenges in their development. This book chapter provides valuable insights into the potential impact of nanocarrier-based therapies in

---

P. Rana · G. Kaur · A. J. Chirayimmel · A. Rajput · V. Dwibedi (✉)
University Institute of Biotechnology, Chandigarh University, Mohali 140413, India
e-mail: vagishdwibedi@gmail.com; vagish.lcc@gmail.com

S. K. Rath
School of Pharmaceuticals and Population Health Informatics, Faculty of Pharmacy, DIT University, Dehradun, Uttarakhand 248009, India

V. Dwibedi
Institute of Soil, Water and Environmental Sciences, Volcani Research Center, Agricultural Research Organization, 7528809 Rishon Lezion, Israel

S. K. Rath et al. (eds.), *Nanomaterials for Drug Delivery and Neurological Diseases Management*, Smart Nanomaterials Technology,
https://doi.org/10.1007/978-981-97-0308-1_10

neuro diseases and sets the stage for further research and development in this exciting field.

Keywords Nanocarriers · Nano-drug delivery · Alzheimer's disease · Parkinson's disease · Biocompatibility

1 Introduction

The human nervous system is incredibly intricate, consisting of billions of neurons (nerve cells) that transmit electrical and chemical signals. These neurons form intricate networks and pathways, allowing for the transmission of information and coordination of various bodily functions. Neurological diseases, also known as neurological disorders or nervous system disorders, can be defined as a wide range of conditions that affect the central nervous system (CNS) which includes the brain and spinal cord, peripheral nervous system (nerves outside the brain and spinal cord), or both. These disorders can result in abnormalities in the structure, function, or chemistry of the nervous system, leading to various neurological symptoms and impairments. Neurological diseases pose significant challenges to human health and well-being, requiring effective management strategies to relieve symptoms, enhance the quality of life, and slow disease progression. It also has significant implications in today's life due to its prevalence, impact on individuals, families, and society, and the associated healthcare and economic burden. The management of human neurological diseases provides critical approaches and emerging trends with nano-based materials which have emerged as promising tools in human neurological disorders, offering new avenues for diagnosis, treatment, and management. Neurological diseases can have diverse causes, including genetic factors, infections, autoimmune reactions, traumatic injuries, tumors, vascular disorders, degenerative processes, and metabolic abnormalities. Neurological diseases are complex and have multiple etiologies and pathogenesis that are not yet fully understood [1]. The dysfunction, degeneration, or injury of nerve cells can result in neurological disorders, which currently have no cure [2]. Neurological diseases account for a large and increasing health burden worldwide and are among the most vexing afflictions known to mankind [3].

Neurodegenerative diseases, which comprise a prominent class of neurological diseases, include the continuous loss of neurons and synapses in the brain and the spinal cord [4]. Neuroinflammation plays an important role in the pathogenesis of many neurodegenerative diseases [5]. Astrocytes, a type of glial cell in the brain, play a central role in neurological diseases. They have multiple roles in the healthy central nervous system (CNS) and exhibit diverse responses to neurological disorders. Astrocytes could be a promising therapeutic target for treating diseases like Alexander disease, neurotrauma, stroke, epilepsy, Alzheimer's disease, and various other neurodegenerative conditions [6]. While currently there is no effective cure for neurological diseases, bioactive compounds such as triptolide and celastrol are found in Tripterygium wilfordii Hook. F. (TWHF) a traditional Chinese medicine, has been identified as a potential therapeutic agent for treating neurological diseases. These compounds have been found to show anti-inflammatory, anti-tumor, and immunosuppressive activities [1]. Similarly, the amount of dopamine in the body is related to neurological diseases. Neurological disorders such as Schizophrenia and Parkinson's arise from a decrease in dopamine secretion due to damage to brain cells, as dopamine is a molecule produced by these cells [7]. In some cases, neurodegenerative diseases have a genetic component. Mutations or variations in specific genes can increase an individual's susceptibility to these disorders. For example, mutations in the genes associated with Parkinson's disease, Huntington's disease, and Alzheimer's disease, can play a role in their development. Genetic predisposition can increase susceptibility to certain disorders, but environmental factors, such as exposure to toxins or infections, can also play a role [8]. Furthermore, the interaction between genetic and environmental factors is intricate and not fully understood, making it challenging to unravel the precise mechanisms of disease development.

Neurological disorders encompass a broad range of conditions with diverse symptoms, underlying causes, and disease progression patterns. Each disorder may affect different parts of the nervous system, leading to a wide array of symptoms and manifestations. Additionally, individuals with the same diagnosis may exhibit variations in symptoms and disease progression, making it challenging to develop standardized approaches for diagnosis and treatment. The disease progression can vary widely between individuals, making it difficult to predict the course of the disease and the effectiveness of treatments. Monitoring disease progression, adjusting treatment strategies, and providing ongoing care for individuals with progressive neurological disorders pose significant challenges [9].

Many neurological disorders lack specific biomarkers or definitive diagnostic tests, making diagnosis complex. Healthcare professionals often rely on a combination of clinical evaluations, medical history, neurological examinations, imaging techniques (such as MRI or CT scans), and specialized tests to arrive at a diagnosis [10]. The overlapping symptoms and similarities between different neurological disorders further complicate the diagnostic process. The treatment of neurological disorders is often complex due to the intricate nature of the nervous system and the diverse manifestations of these disorders. Treatment approaches may involve a combination of medications, physical therapy, occupational therapy, speech therapy, assistive devices, and surgical interventions, depending on the specific condition and symptoms. Developing effective treatments that can halt or reverse disease progression remains a major challenge in many neurological disorders. Each person's response to neurological disorders and treatments can vary greatly [11]. Factors such as age, overall health, genetic makeup, and environmental influences can influence disease progression and treatment outcomes. Personalized approaches to diagnosis and treatment are increasingly recognized as essential to address the individual variations observed in neurological disorders [12]. Addressing the complexity of neurological disorders requires ongoing research, collaboration among multidisciplinary healthcare teams, advancements in diagnostic tools, and a comprehensive understanding of the underlying mechanisms. Continued efforts are needed to improve diagnostic accuracy, develop targeted therapies, enhance supportive care, and promote early intervention strategies for better management of these complex conditions. Treatment options for neurodegenerative diseases aim to alleviate symptoms, slow down disease progression, and improve the quality of life for affected individuals. It's important to note that specific treatments vary depending on the neurodegenerative disease. It's worth noting that ongoing research and clinical trials continuously explore new treatment approaches, including disease-modifying therapies and innovative interventions such as gene therapies, immunotherapies, and stem cell-based treatments [13, 14].

These advancements promise the future management and potential cure of neurodegenerative diseases. The available treatments only help to alleviate some of the physical or mental symptoms associated with them. However, recent advancements in the field of nanotechnology have led to the emergence of innovative methods for transporting drug molecules at their specific site of action through nanoformulations also known as smart nanocarriers which are designed effectively for the transportation of drug molecules. These nanocarriers have opened up numerous opportunities for various applications in the field of biotechnology. Although significant progress has been made in recent methodologies, the effectiveness of nanocarriers in nanomedicine is often hindered by undesirable side effects. This underscores the crucial challenges in designing and engineering nanocarrier systems for biotechnology applications, which stem from the intricate environment and diverse interactions occurring within specific biological media [15]. Indeed, the delivery of drugs to the brain continues to pose a challenge in the treatment of neurodegenerative disorders. To address this issue, various strategies have been proposed out of which is the use of chemically stable nanoparticles. Despite the relatively abundant blood flow in the central nervous system (CNS), drug delivery to this region remains a significant challenge. This is primarily due to a series of protective barriers that have evolved within the CNS, including the blood-cerebrospinal fluid (CSF) barrier, blood-retinal barrier, blood–brain barrier (BBB), and blood-spinal cord barrier. These physiological barriers separate the brain from its blood supply and include the BBB and the blood-cerebrospinal fluid barrier (BCSFB) [16].

This chapter is based on the latest studies of nano-fabricated smart drug delivery systems which hold promising results for facilitating neurological brain repair.

2 Nanocarriers for Neuro Drug Delivery

A. **Types of Nanocarriers Used in Neuro Drug Delivery**:

Neurological disorders are mainly caused by the loss in function of nerve cells and ultimately neuronal death. Alzheimer's disease, Huntington's disease, Parkinson's disease, etc., are some of the neuro diseases affecting a large number of the population globally. Drug delivery is the process of transferring of drug with the help of a carrier under optimal pharmacokinetics inside the body so that it creates the desired therapeutic effect. In the case of neurological diseases, the significant challenges associated with drug delivery are the P-glycoproteins, blood–brain barrier [BBB], and the blood-cerebrospinal fluid barrier [BCFB]. But currently through recent research on several approaches associated with drug delivery, these limitations have been overcome by employing receptor-mediated transcellular transport, by physiochemical methods to disrupt the BBB, using protein transduction domains (PTDs) and magnetic field-induced disruption [17]. However, with the advancement in nanotechnology, nanocarriers are being widely employed as novel, effective, and specific tools for delivering pharmaceutical products, for treating various contagious neuro diseases. This type of drug delivery method has been found effective not only in animals but also in humans [18]. In order to reduce the side effects associated with treatment, the use of nanocarriers allows efficient and targeted interactions with biomolecules. Nanocarriers can be defined as inactive colloidal nanoparticles of size usually between 1 and 100 nm (nm) (so that they can pass through thin microcapillaries of the human body) which are used for the transportation of therapeutic agents to the target site. Although different types of nanocarriers have been made, only a few have the extraordinary capability of reaching the infected site. The properties that make a nanocarrier different from other drug delivery agents are- High stability, low toxicity, prolonged and on-target drug delivery, improved biodistribution, and pharmacokinetics [19].

1. **Liposomes**:

Liposomes are microscopic vesicles composed of lipid bilayers, which are similar to the structure of cell membranes. These vesicles can be artificially prepared and are commonly used in various scientific and medical applications. Liposomes have a hydrophilic (water-loving) outer surface and a hydrophobic (water-repelling) inner core, allowing them to encapsulate and deliver hydrophilic or hydrophobic substances, such as drugs, genes, or cosmetic ingredients. The lipid bilayers of liposomes can self-assemble into closed spherical structures, creating an inner compartment that can hold the desired substances [20]. This characteristic makes liposomes useful as drug delivery systems, as they can protect the encapsulated substances from degradation or premature release, and deliver them to specific target tissues or cells. Liposomes offer several advantages in drug delivery and research applications. They can improve the solubility, stability, and bioavailability of drugs, enhance their therapeutic efficacy, and reduce their toxicity [21]. Liposomes are versatile and biocompatible structures composed of phospholipids, resembling natural cell membranes. They can efficiently encapsulate drugs, genes, proteins, and other bioactive compounds, protecting them during delivery (Fig. 1). Liposomes can be tailored to different sizes, allowing precise control over their properties and stability. Through surface modification, liposomes can be equipped with targeting ligands to deliver cargo specifically to desired cells or tissues. By altering the lipid composition and encapsulated cargo, liposomes exhibit controlled release profiles, offering sustained or triggered release of therapeutics. Additionally, liposomes are biodegradable, minimizing long-term accumulation and toxicity risks. With broad applications in drug delivery, gene

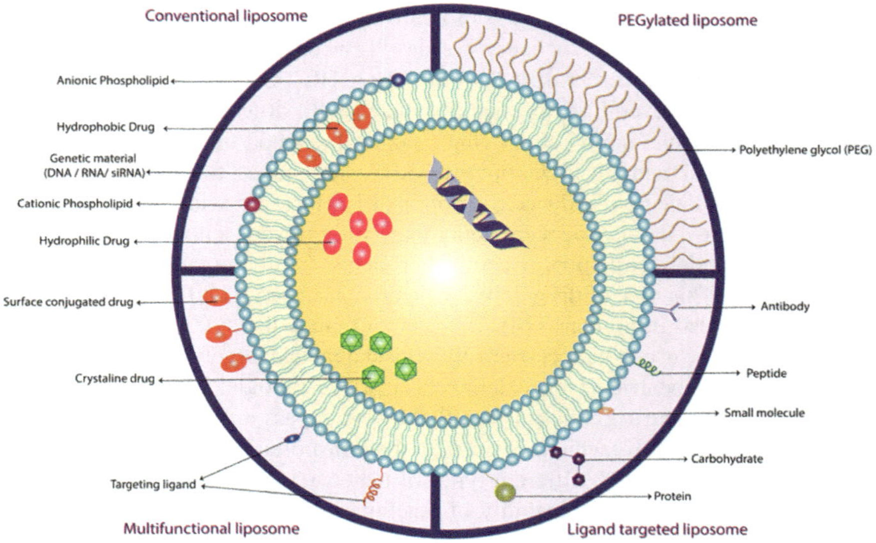

Fig. 1 Structure of liposome

therapy, cosmetics, and research, liposomes offer a versatile platform that can be administered via various routes to meet specific requirements [22].

According to the study of [23], an example is given that αvβ3 is a specific vector that is conjugating integrin attached to liposomes carrying paclitaxel, overexpress on glioma cells to target integrin receptors and improves survival in mice. Conjugation of tamoxifen to liposomes carrying topotecan to brain tumors whereas Rhenium-186 is a radionucliosides that is encapsulated by liposomes to target gliomas with radiation therapy. The experimental research of [24] found that docetaxel present in liposomes known as anti-cancer drugs, RGD-TGPs functionalized a radioactive drug and quantum dots were developed for brain cancer imaging. [25] studied that doxorubicin (Caelyx®/Doxil® and Myocet®) and daunorubicin (Daunosome®) are anticancer drugs for liposomal conceptualization include clinical approval. In a study by [26] a targeted long-circulating thermosensitive smart-release liposome (LCTL) system was developed to improve therapeutic effectiveness and reduce toxicity. The findings demonstrated that LCTL exhibited an extended circulation time and enhanced accumulation at tumor sites, enabling selective drug release. The results suggest that LCTL holds great potential as a carrier for delivering oxaliplatin to effectively treat solid tumors. In a study by [27], a brain-targeted liposomal system was used in a Parkinson's disease mouse model. The administration of liposomes loaded with dopamine (DA) resulted in a significant increase in striatal DA levels with a lower dose compared to commonly used levodopa. The liposomal delivery system shows promise for treating PD and other brain diseases by enabling efficient penetration through the blood–brain barrier (BBB).

2. **Polymeric Nanoparticles:**

Polymeric nanoparticles are microscopic particles made up of polymers, which are large molecules composed of repeating subunits. These nanoparticles are engineered structures that can be designed to have specific functions and properties. They are widely used in various scientific and medical applications, including drug delivery, imaging, diagnostics, and tissue engineering. These nanoparticles are typically fabricated using techniques such as emulsion/solvent evaporation, nanoprecipitation, or self-assembly [28]. The choice of polymer and fabrication method allows for precise control over the size, shape, surface properties, and drug-loading capacity of the nanoparticles. The polymeric matrix of these nanoparticles can be composed of natural or synthetic polymers. Natural polymers, such as chitosan, alginate, or gelatin, offer biocompatibility and biodegradability. Synthetic polymers, such as polyethylene glycol (PEG), poly (lactic-co-glycolic acid) (PLGA) or poly(caprolactone) (PCL), provide tunability of physicochemical properties and degradation rates [29]. Polymeric nanoparticles can encapsulate a wide range of therapeutic agents, including small molecule drugs, proteins, genes, or imaging agents. The encapsulation provides protection to the cargo, enhances its stability, and controls its release kinetics. This enables targeted delivery, sustained release, and improved therapeutic efficacy while minimizing side effects. The surface of these nanoparticles can be modified by targeting ligands, antibodies, or other functional molecules to achieve site-specific delivery to cells or tissues of interest. These modifications facilitate interactions with target receptors, enhance cellular uptake, and improve the accumulation of nanoparticles at the desired site [30]. The research of Rabiee et al. [31] gives the statement that polymeric Nanoparticles (TFB-NPs) are synthesized by the integration solvent technique with qualified surfactants. For example, Muntimadugu group reported that in both vitro and in vivo SD rat models, TFB commonly known as the name of tarenflurbil, a γ-secretase modulator is carried by polymeric carriers which transfuse in their body via the intranasal route. Ojha et al. [32] studied SH-SY5Y cells that is the neuroprotective capacity of polymeric nanoparticles and the formulation has proved its neuroprotective potential was further assigned to approach its pharmacodynamic potential using the cuprizone model of Wistar rats. Zhang et al. [33] stated that significant higher brain activity can be exhibited by conjugating polymeric nanoparticle systems consisting of a block copolymer of 10% hyperbranched polyglycerol (PLA-HPG), polylactic acid and adenosine modified PLA-HPG nanoparticles were compared to similar sized PLGA-DSPE-PEG nanoparticles through the BBB. In the study, Zhao et al. [34] developed nanoparticles (NPs) capable of efficiently encapsulating a significant amount of GB (ginkgolide B) using an antisolvent precipitation method. These GB-NPs demonstrated enhanced uptake in MDCK cells and were found to traverse various barriers, including the chorion, GI barrier, BRB, and BBB, in zebrafish. The results indicate the potential of GB-NPs as an oral delivery system for GB, improving its bioavailability and brain delivery for the treatment of PD.

3. **Dendrimers**:

Dendrimers are highly branched synthetic polymers with a well-defined and symmetric structure. They consist of a central core from which multiple branches radiate, forming successive layers or generations. Their unique architecture offers precise control over size, shape, and surface functionality, making them valuable in applications such as drug delivery, diagnostics, and nanotechnology. They possess unique characteristics that make them highly attractive in scientific and technological fields. Their highly branched and symmetric structure allows for precise control over size, shape, and surface functionality. Dendrimers exhibit mono-dispersity, meaning that individual molecules within a generation are nearly identical, ensuring consistent behavior [35]. With their multivalency, dendrimers offer multiple reactive sites for encapsulating or conjugating diverse molecules, such as drugs or imaging agents. Their tunable solubility in both aqueous and organic solvents expands their applicability in various environments. Additionally, dendrimers can be surface-functionalized by targeting ligands or biomolecules, allowing for specific interactions and tailored properties. These characteristics, including their precise architecture, monodispersity, multivalency, solubility, and surface functionalization, make dendrimers promising candidates for drug delivery, diagnostics, and nanotechnology applications (Fig. 2) [36].

Scientists developed a nanocarrier system based on a fourth-generation PAMAM dendrimer, designed to penetrate the blood–brain barrier (BBB) and target gliomas. The system was modified by incorporating an angiopep-2 peptide and an additional peptide to enhance the targeting effect through epidermal growth factor receptor (EGFR) penetration [37]. In another study doxorubicin (DOX), an anticancer medication, was loaded into the internal compartments of dendrimers through non-covalent interactions. The dendrimer's channels exhibited controlled release of the encapsulated drugs in response to the acidic environment of tumors, resulting in reduced toxic effects on normal tissues both in vivo and in vitro. Furthermore, the incorporation of peptides into the dendrimer carriers showed significant improvement in their ability to penetrate the blood–brain barrier (BBB) and enhanced their effectiveness in combating tumors after crossing the BBB [38]. Scientists highlighted an alternative method for drug delivery to the brain through the nasal route, utilizing dendrimers in combination with in-situ gel formation. This approach involved the administration of an in-situ stable gel, which enhanced the nasal transport efficiency of PAMAM nanocomposites. The PAMAM dendrimer nanocomposite combined with DGG (dextran-grafted gelatin) represents a promising system for nasal delivery of drugs to the brain, offering potential as a nasal brain transport system [39].

4. **Nanoparticles**:

Quantum dots are nanoscale semiconductor particles with unique optical and electronic properties, making them valuable for imaging, sensing, and targeted drug delivery applications. Dendrimers, highly branched synthetic polymers, serve as

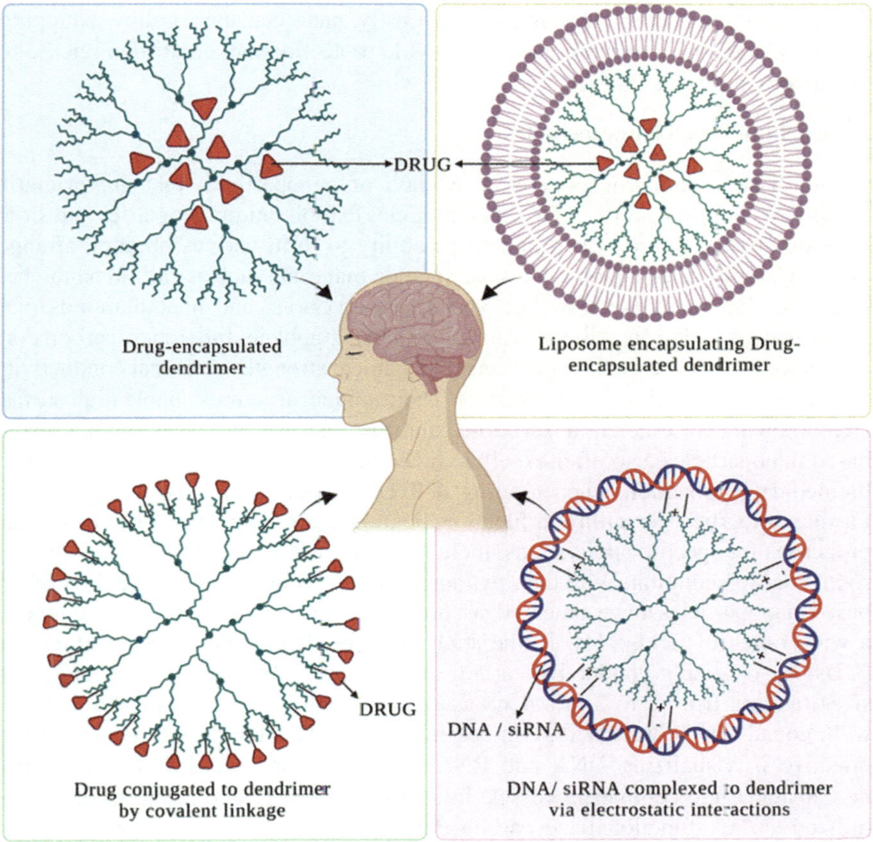

Fig. 2 Structure of different types of dendrimers

effective carriers to encapsulate and deliver drugs or biomolecules precisely to desired targets. Magnetic nanoparticles (NPs) possess magnetic properties, enabling targeted drug delivery through the application of external magnetic fields [40]. Modified viruses are utilized as carriers to deliver therapeutic genes or drugs specifically to selected cells or tissues. Gold nanoparticles find applications in drug delivery, imaging, and photothermal therapy, while core–shell nanoparticles, commonly composed of gold or silver, are employed in imaging and photothermal therapy. Liposomes, lipid-based nanoparticles, improve drug stability and efficacy by encapsulating and delivering drugs to specific sites. Self-assembled nanoparticles formed by amphiphilic molecules are used for drug delivery and solubilization of hydrophobic drugs [41]. Crystalline nanoparticles exhibit size-dependent properties and are utilized in imaging, diagnostics, and drug delivery. Cylindrical nanoparticles with a tubular structure find applications in drug delivery, biosensing, and tissue engineering. Polyethylene glycol (PEG) polymer-based nanoparticles are used for drug delivery and enhancing biocompatibility. Lastly, nano capsules, hollow nanoparticles enclosing drugs or biomolecules, provide protection and controlled release for therapeutic purposes [42].

5. **Carbon-Based Nanoparticles**:

Carbon-based nanoparticles refer to a class of nanoparticles that are primarily composed of carbon atoms. These nanoparticles exhibit unique properties and structures due to the nature of carbon and its ability to form various bonding arrangements. Carbon-based nanoparticles can include materials such as carbon nanotubes, graphene, fullerenes (such as buckyballs), carbon dots, and nanodiamonds [43]. These nanoparticles, including carbon nanotubes, graphene, fullerenes, carbon dots, and nanodiamonds, exhibit exceptional mechanical strength, electrical conductivity, thermal stability, and optical properties. Their unique structures enable high surface area, allowing for efficient adsorption, catalysis, and sensing capabilities. Carbon-based nanoparticles also offer excellent biocompatibility, making them suitable for biomedical applications such as drug delivery, imaging, and tissue engineering. Furthermore, their versatility in functionalization and modification enables tailored properties for specific applications, including energy storage, electronics, and environmental remediation. With their extraordinary combination of properties, carbon-based nanoparticles have emerged as promising materials with vast potential in a wide range of fields [44]. In the study, Han et al. [45] developed carbon dots (CDs) by oxidizing conductive carbon nanoparticles. The synthesized CDs, with sizes ranging from 2 to 3 nm, demonstrated the ability to penetrate the intestinal wall, gonad vesicle wall, and germ-cell membrane. This unique CD system proved effective in visualizing DNA and RNA structures during cell division, offering new insights into cellular processes. In a separate investigation, Shoval et al. [46] utilized surface-functionalized carbon dots (CDs) with a size of 8 nm to effectively penetrate various ocular structures, including the epithelial layer, cornea, eye cavity, and lens. Their study demonstrated the potential of these functionalized CDs in targeted delivery and imaging applications within the eye. Chung et al. [47] employed polymerized CDs derived from OPD (ortho-phenylenediamine) to interact with copper ions, resulting in the reduction of amyloid-beta (Aβ) aggregation in Alzheimer's disease. This study highlights the potential of these polymerized CDs as a means to counteract Aβ aggregation, offering potential therapeutic implications for Alzheimer's disease. Hettiarachchi et al. [48] developed a triple-conjugated drug delivery system (DDS) based on cyclodextrins (CDs) for the targeted treatment of glioblastoma. The results demonstrated that the triple-conjugated system (C-dots-transferrin-epirubicin-temozolomide, C-DT) required a significantly lower concentration to reduce tumor cell viability compared to non-transferrin systems (NT) and C-TT, dual-conjugated systems (CDs-transferrin-temozolomide, and CDs-transferrin-epirubicin, C-ET). This highlights the potential of CDs for the simultaneous loading of multiple therapeutic agents, which can synergistically enhance the effectiveness of anti-tumor treatments.

B. **Characteristics and Advantages of Nanocarriers:**

Nanocarriers are also known as colloidal nano-scale devices, designed in modular form from a variety of materials in numerous different shapes. The size of nanocarriers (10–400 nm) could also be useful in the resolution of conventional drug limitations, involving weak aqueous solubility, undesirable drug pharmacokinetic characteristics, and poor bioavailability. The size of nanocarriers is capable of a medication carrier that contains small weights of macromolecules as genetic enzymes. They have the benefits of carrying big amounts of drugs, transiting anticancer agents, and particular cells focusing on stronger pharmacokinetics and pharmacodynamic models [49]. The physio-chemical characteristics of the different nanocarriers can be designed by modifying their composition, shape, and dimensions as well as by varying their surface. Nanocarriers can provide benefits that are reduced toxicity, improved pharmacokinetics, protection from degradation, and site-specific delivery of drug molecules [50]. Inorganic nanocarriers lack biodegradability, abundantly from Protein coronas, or have a short range of drugs that could be linked via covalent bonds to the more limited number of functional groups whereas organic nanocarriers including liposomes and albumin provide many advantages also used in clinical practice. The most studied natural nanocarriers are the special types of protein nanocages, virus-like particles, or even whole viral capsids [51]. Nanocarriers with conjugated drugs can improve the biological distribution of medications as well as enhance their circulation in the bloodstream. Nanocarriers deliver drugs to the ailment site either actively or passively. They enhance the solubility of hydrophobic drugs. Preparation of such nanocarriers is crucial because most of the new and upcoming drug products have low bioavailability or less soluble in water. The latest advancements in modifications of nanocarriers for application as targeted dialysis disequilibrium syndrome (DDS). High surface-to-volume proportions and controllable shapes make NPs as incredible candidates for drug delivery applications [52]. Nanocarriers are preferred to gel formulations or conventional solutions, stabilizers, and enzyme inhibitors. They protect drugs from chemical and metabolic degradation, improve their solubility, or enable transport through biological barrier membranes to achieve improved targeting and reduced systemic side effects [53]. Lipids such as butter oil, fish oil, and various surfactants used in nanocarrier formulation have the ability to fluidize cell membranes, change permeability, and open the tight junction of the epithelial layers. The associated advantages include the encapsulation and delivery of hydrophobic drugs, increased therapeutic efficacy, decreased therapeutic dose, and reduced systemic side effects. Nanocarriers can efficiently overcome the BBB and control the release of the therapeutic drug at the destined location while minimizing the toxic effects of the encapsulated or adsorbed therapeutic agents [54]. Nanocarriers besides the usual forms of anxiolytics could help to prevent aggravation into depression or a severe generalized form and to improve the treatment of anxiety disorders. Systematic studies are required to determine the long-term toxicity of nanocarriers as a whole system to neuronal transport pathway (the trigeminal nerve and the trigeminal nerve) and the brain, which could provide guidance for their clinical application [55].

C. **Challenges and Limitations in Nanocarrier Development**:

Nanocarriers, including liposomes, can be susceptible to instability during storage and transportation. Factors such as aggregation, fusion, leakage, or degradation of the carrier system can affect their performance and compromise their efficacy. The production of nanocarriers on a large scale can be challenging [54]. Maintaining consistent quality, reproducibility, and batch-to-batch uniformity is important for their successful translation into clinical or commercial use. Efficient encapsulation of drugs within nanocarriers is crucial for their effective delivery. However, certain drugs may exhibit low encapsulation efficiency or have difficulties in being released from the carriers in a controlled manner, limiting their therapeutic benefits [56]. While liposomes are generally considered biocompatible, some formulations or modifications may lead to toxicity concerns. Ensuring the safety and minimizing potential adverse effects is essential for clinical applications. Achieving efficient targeting of specific cells or tissues can be challenging. The modification of nanocarriers with targeting ligands or antibodies requires careful selection, optimization, and validation to ensure effective binding and internalization at the desired site. Nanocarriers, once administered, can be cleared from the body by various mechanisms, such as renal filtration or phagocytosis by macrophages. Understanding their biodistribution and clearance pathways is important for optimizing their therapeutic efficacy and minimizing off-target effects [57]. The development and commercialization of nanocarriers face regulatory challenges. Ensuring compliance with safety, efficacy, and quality standards set by regulatory authorities requires extensive preclinical and clinical studies, which can be time-consuming and costly. The production and formulation of nanocarriers can be expensive, limiting their accessibility in resource-limited settings or for certain patient populations. Cost-effective manufacturing processes and strategies are essential for their widespread adoption. Addressing these challenges and limitations requires interdisciplinary research, optimization of formulation parameters, robust characterization techniques, and close collaboration between academia, industry, and regulatory bodies. Overcoming these hurdles will further advance the field of nanocarrier development and enhance their potential for effective drug delivery and therapeutic applications [58].

3 Nano Drug Delivery Strategies for Specific Neuro Diseases

Nano drug delivery strategies can be classified into two categories namely Blood Brain Barrier drug delivery and Nano pharmaceutical routes (Fig. 3).

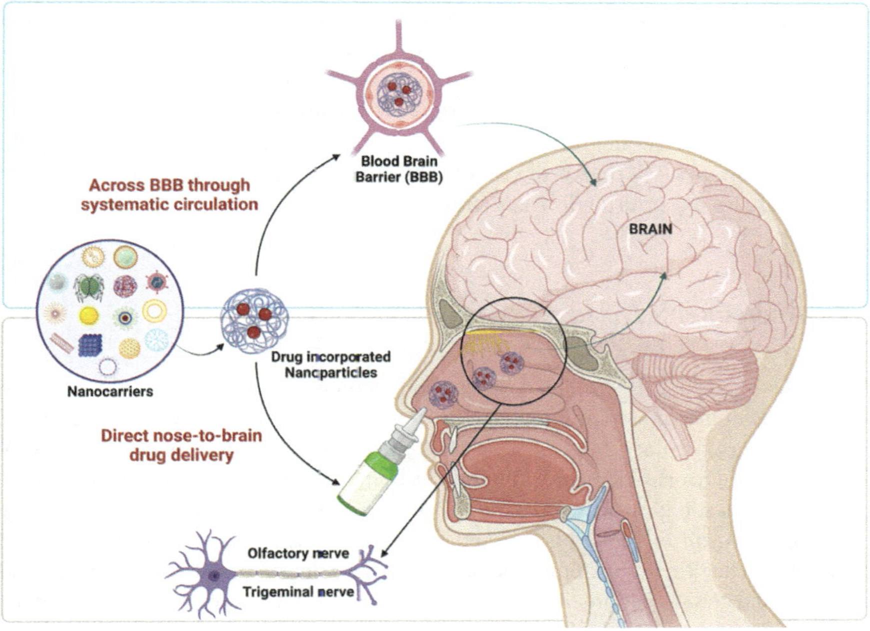

Fig. 3 Nano drug delivery strategies for neuro diseases

Blood Brain Barrier Targeted Drug Delivery:

The blood–brain barrier is a highly selective and protective barrier formed by specialized cells in the blood vessels of the brain. It restricts the passage of substances from the bloodstream into the brain, maintaining a stable and controlled environment for proper brain function. Targeted drug delivery is an approach that focuses on delivering medications or therapeutic substances to specific sites in the body. This technique involves developing delivery systems that can precisely target the intended location, leading to improved treatment effectiveness, reduced side effects, and optimal therapeutic results [59].

Nano Pharmaceutical Routes:

Intravenous administration involves directly introducing a substance into a vein, allowing it to be distributed throughout the body systemically. In contrast, intranasal delivery refers to the administration of a substance through the nasal route, bypassing the blood–brain barrier and gaining direct access to the brain. For localized treatment, intracerebral administration entails injecting a substance into specific regions or target areas of the brain. Intrathecal administration involves introducing a substance into the cerebrospinal fluid (CSF), enabling it to reach the brain and spinal cord [60]. Intraventricular delivery entails introducing a substance into the ventricular system of the brain, facilitating wide distribution within the brain. By injecting a substance into the peritoneal cavity, intraperitoneal administration ensures systemic distribution throughout the body. Transcranial delivery involves non-invasive stimulation or administration of a substance to the brain through the skull, commonly used in imaging or therapy. Oral administration refers to the ingestion of a substance through the mouth, typically in the form of pills or liquids, for systemic distribution. Ocular administration involves delivering a substance to the eye, targeting ocular tissues for localized treatment or drug delivery [61].

3.1 Alzheimer's Disease

Alzheimer's disease is the most prominent dementia causing neurodegenerative disorder. Primary histopathological features of Alzheimer's disease are Senile Plaques, neurofibrillary tangles, and Synoptic loss. Currently, approximately 50 million people worldwide are affected by dementia. However, due to rising life expectancy rates, it is projected that by 2050, the number of individuals with dementia will reach 139 million globally. This anticipated increase will have significant socioeconomic and healthcare system implications [62]. Memory loss, disorientation, mood changes, and the development of depression are the early symptoms of AD while progressive memory loss, difficulty recognizing loved ones, loss of impulse control, and impairment in communication, lead to severe functional and cognitive decline, eventually resulting in death due to complications like swallowing and urination difficulties are the more severe symptoms of AD [63]. Some histopathological features of AD are Senile plaques, Neurofibrillary tangles, and Synoptic loss. Senile plaques are deposits of beta-amyloid protein (Aβ) that accumulate outside of nerve cells and they can take on various morphological forms, including compact, dense-cored, neuritic, diffuse, and classic-type plaques. The accumulation of more compact and dense plaques in the brain can result in the activation of astrocytes and microglia, leading to damage to axons, dendrites, and the loss of synapses and these pathological changes contribute to cognitive impairments [64]. Neurofibrillary tangles (NFTs) are abnormal filamentous structures composed of hyperphosphorylated tau protein these filaments can intertwine and form paired helical filaments (PHFs) and they accumulate in the cytoplasm of dendrites, axons, and neural cell bodies, leading to the loss of cytoskeletal microtubules and proteins associated with tubulin. In the early stages of Alzheimer's disease, memory impairment is often associated with synaptic damage in the limbic system and neocortex, and this damage involves various mechanisms such as defects in axonal transport, oxidative stress, mitochondrial damage, and other processes. These mechanisms can contribute to the accumulation of beta-amyloid (Aβ) and tau proteins at synaptic sites, leading to synaptic loss [65].

Therapeutic Approaches:

One therapeutic approach to enhance cognitive and neural cell function is to increase cholinergic levels by inhibiting the enzyme acetylcholinesterase (AChE). Acetylcholinesterase inhibitors (AChEIs) are utilized to block the degradation of acetylcholine in synapses, leading to the continuous buildup of acetylcholine and subsequent activation of cholinergic receptors [62]. Tacrine, donepezil, rivastigmine, and galantamine are used for the symptomatic treatment of AD. Donepezil binds reversibly to the enzyme acetylcholinesterase, inhibiting its activity and preventing the breakdown of acetylcholine and Rivastigmine prevents ACh metabolism [66]. Galantamine functions as a competitive inhibitor of acetylcholinesterase (AChE), blocking its activity and preventing the degradation of acetylcholine. And also, it has the ability to bind to the α-subunit of nicotinic acetylcholine receptors in an allosteric manner. Stimulation of NMDAR (N-methyl-D-aspartate receptor) causes an influx of calcium ions (Ca^{2+}), initiating signal transduction pathways that ultimately trigger gene transcription. This process is crucial for the establishment of long-term potentiation (LTP), which plays a significant role in synaptic neurotransmission, plasticity, and the formation of memories [67]. Memantine is utilized as a therapeutic option for moderate to severe Alzheimer's disease, either as a standalone treatment or in combination with acetylcholinesterase inhibitors (AChEIs) [68]. Disease-modifying treatments or therapies (DMTs) aim to modify the progression of Alzheimer's disease by targeting various underlying pathophysiological mechanisms. Protein misfolding and aggregation are common causes of neurodegenerative diseases, ultimately resulting in cell death. Molecular chaperones, including intracellular ones like heat shock proteins (Hsp40, Hsp60, Hsp70, Hsp90, Hsp100, and Hsp110) and extracellular ones like clustering and alpha-macroglobulin, play a critical role in facilitating proper protein folding and safeguarding cells against stress-related damage. Hsp60 plays a crucial role in facilitating the folding of proteins within mitochondria. In the pursuit of future therapies, disease-modifying treatments show potential for altering the progression of Alzheimer's disease by targeting the Aβ pathway [69]. Several drugs, including AN-1792, solanezumab, semagacestat, avagacestat, bapineuzumab, and tarenflurbil, have undergone clinical trials but failed to demonstrate efficacy in the final stages. Other DMTs, such as aducanumab, crenezumab, tideglusib, gantenerumab, lithium, and others, continue to be investigated for their ability to target Aβ and tau pathologies. Additionally, chaperones like heat shock proteins and vacuolar sorting protein 35 (VPS35) hold promise as they assist other proteins in functioning properly and reaching their intended destinations within cells, making them potential treatments for neurodegenerative diseases [70].

Examples of Target Drug Delivery in Alzheimer's:

The researchers successfully formulated curcumin-loaded PLGA nanoparticles using an emulsification solvent evaporation method, and administered them intravenously to Sprague–Dawley rats, resulting in sustained curcumin concentration in the brain. In another experiment, the researchers utilized di-block PEG-PLA nanoparticles loaded with curcumin, prepared through nanoprecipitation, and administered them orally to Tg2576 Alzheimer's model mice [64]. The nanocurcumin formulations showed a significant improvement in cue and working memory compared to the placebo control group. The study involved administering quercetin-loaded zein nanoparticles orally to SAMP8 mice, resulting in enhanced memory impairments and cognition characteristics in these mice. Researchers also conducted experiments in liposomes, liposomes loaded with quercetin were administered intranasally to Wistar rats, leading to an improvement in the cognitive functions of the rats. In another study, quercetin-loaded PLGA nanoparticles were prepared using a double emulsion solvent evaporation method and administered intravenously to APP/PS1 transgenic mice. The PLGA nanoparticles successfully alleviated cognition and memory deficits in the APP/PS1 mice [60]. In another research, ginsenoside Rg3-loaded PLGA nanoparticles formulated as a nanoemulsion with Angiopep-2 attached to them demonstrated enhanced penetration across an in vitro blood–brain barrier (BBB) model. The researchers utilized emulsion solvent evaporation to prepare huperzine A-loaded PLGA nanoparticles, which were administered intranasally to KM mice. These nanoparticles exhibited higher fluorescence intensity and prolonged residence time in the brain. In the study, epigallocatechin-3-gallate (EGCG) was formulated as nano lipidic particles through co-solubilization, and orally administered to Sprague–Dawley rats. These nano lipidic particles demonstrated a significant improvement in the α-secretase enhancing ability of EGCG in vitro. In the experiment, bacoside-A-loaded PLGA nanoparticles were prepared using an oil-in-water emulsion solvent evaporation method and administered intravenously to Wistar rats [68]. The use of Ps-80 coated PLGA nanoparticles resulted in a significant increase in the concentration of bacoside-A in the brain. In the study, polymeric micelles loaded with resveratrol were prepared through nanoprecipitation. These resveratrol-loaded nanoparticles demonstrated a protective effect on PC12 cells against amyloid-β induced toxicity. In the research, chitosan nanoparticles loaded with piperine were prepared using the ionic gelation method and administered intranasally to Wistar rats. The administration of these nanoparticles via the intranasal route significantly enhanced the cognitive functions of the rats [71].

3.2 Parkinson's Disease

Parkinson's disease is a degenerative neurological condition that progresses over time. It is characterized by the gradual loss of specific brain cells called dopaminergic neurons in an area known as the substantia nigra and individuals with Parkinson's disease exhibit the presence of abnormal protein clumps called Lewy bodies. Parkinson's disease is a condition that impacts a significant number of people globally. Recent estimates indicate that around 2–3% of individuals who are 65 years or older are affected by Parkinson's disease [72]. Parkinson's disease presents a range of symptoms that can differ among individuals. Some common symptoms include tremors, muscle stiffness, Bradykinesia, Changes in Speech and Writing, Loss of Smell, etc. Tremor is another distinct motor symptom associated with Parkinson's disease, primarily affecting areas of the brain such as the cerebellum, brainstem, and basal ganglia. These regions play a crucial role in motor control and are significantly impacted by the disease [73]. A significant histopathological characteristic of Parkinson's disease is the occurrence of abnormal protein clusters known as Lewy bodies. These clusters consist mainly of a protein called alpha-synuclein and are found within the brain cells of individuals diagnosed with Parkinson's and the protein aggregates are believed to contribute to the degeneration of neurons in the disease. Neuroinflammation, characterized by inflammation in the brain, is a significant feature observed in Parkinson's disease. The activation of immune cells and the release of inflammatory molecules contribute to the degeneration of dopaminergic neurons and the advancement of the disease. In PD, the loss of dopaminergic neurons is a prominent characteristic [74]. However, the disease can also lead to the loss of other neurotransmitters, such as norepinephrine, serotonin, and acetylcholine. This disruption in the balance of neurochemicals contributes to the diverse range of motor and non-motor symptoms observed in individuals with Parkinson's disease [75].

Various Treatments and Their Drawback:

Parkinson's disease often requires medications like levodopa, dopamine agonists, and MAO-B inhibitors. Although these medications are effective in relieving motor symptoms, their long-term efficacy may diminish, and individuals may experience fluctuations in their response, resulting in periods of symptom re-emergence ("on–off" periods). Prolonged use of levodopa can also lead to dyskinesias, which are involuntary movements [76]. Deep Brain Stimulation (DBS) is a surgical intervention that involves the implantation of electrodes in precise brain regions to administer electrical impulses and it can be beneficial in managing motor symptoms for certain individuals. But the DBS comes with inherent surgical risks, including the possibility of infection, bleeding, and potential side effects like speech or cognitive alterations and it may not be an appropriate treatment option for everyone [77]. Physical and Occupational Therapy focuses on enhancing mobility, muscle strength, balance, and daily functioning in individuals with Parkinson's disease. While these therapies offer benefits, it's important to recognize that they require consistent dedication and may not entirely eliminate symptoms [78]. Parkinson's disease can impact speech and swallowing abilities. Speech therapy aims to enhance speech clarity and improve swallowing techniques. However, the effectiveness of therapy may vary, and individuals may continue to encounter difficulties in communication and eating [79]. The medications utilized in the treatment of Parkinson's disease can produce side effects including nausea, dizziness, sleep disturbances, hallucinations, and mood changes. Striking a balance between the medication's benefits and its potential side effects is vital, necessitating attentive monitoring [80].

Therapeutic Approaches Using Various Drugs

Parkinson's disease treatment involves medication such as levodopa, MAO-B inhibitors, and dopamine agonists, aiming to address the deficiency of dopamine. Levodopa, the primary choice in early treatment, crosses the blood–brain barrier (BBB) and is converted to dopamine in the basal ganglia and it is effective for motor symptoms, long-term levodopa therapy can lead to levodopa-induced dyskinesia [81]. Dopamine agonists are a group of medications that simulate dopamine by stimulating the receptors in the brain, compensating for the deficiency of dopamine. These drugs bind to dopamine receptors in cases where dopamine levels are insufficient. Dopamine receptor agonists can be categorized into two main classes: ergot derivatives and non-ergot derivatives [82]. Ergot derivatives encompass medications such as bromocriptine, lisuride, cabergoline, and pergolide. On the other hand, non-ergot derivatives include pramipexole, apomorphine, ropinirole, and rotigotine. Ropinirole, classified as a non-ergot derivative among dopamine agonists, demonstrates a notable preference for D2 receptors, exhibiting high selectivity toward them. The exact mechanism of action of Pramipexole is not fully understood, but it is believed to involve the stimulation of dopamine receptors within the striatum. This hypothesis is supported by physiological studies conducted on animals, which demonstrate the activation of dopamine receptors in the substantia nigra and striatum regions [83].

Apomorphine, a non-ergoline dopamine agonist, exhibits dopamine-like effects by directly stimulating both pre and postsynaptic dopamine receptors, specifically the D1 and D2 receptors. This direct activation contributes to its anti-Parkinsonian effect. Nausea and vomiting are the most commonly observed side effects of apomorphine therapy. To minimize these effects, Parkinson's disease patients should receive anti-emetic treatment three days before initiating apomorphine therapy [84]. Rotigotine, which belongs to the non-ergoline class of dopamine agonists, is utilized for the treatment of Parkinson's disease and is also employed off-label for Willis-Ekbom Disease. It has the capability to stimulate dopamine receptors, specifically the D2 receptors, in the caudate-putamen region [85].

Anti-cholinergics work by inhibiting the activity of the neurotransmitter acetylcholine, which plays a role in controlling movement, rather than directly affecting dopaminergic pathways. However, a significant disadvantage of using these parasympatholytic medications is the occurrence of adverse effects such as hallucinations, confusion, drowsiness, as well as blurred vision, constipation, and tachycardia [86]. MAO inhibitors have a longstanding history as one of the earliest medications used in the treatment of Parkinson's disease. Combining MAO inhibitors with levodopa enhances the effects of levodopa therapy. Selegiline, an MAO enzyme inhibitor, is an amphetamine derivative that undergoes metabolism to form L-amphetamine and L-methamphetamine during first-pass metabolism [87]. Rasagiline, often considered a follow-up to selegiline, is an MAO-B inhibitor. This second-generation MAO-B inhibitor, characterized by an N-propargyl-R-amidoindan ring arrangement in its molecular structure, exhibits a neuroprotective effect that is independent of the inhibitory effects of MAO inhibition. Rasagiline can be used as both a monotherapy and as an adjunct to levodopa therapy by interfering with the breakdown of dopamine [88].

Examples of Target Drug Delivery in Parkinson's Disease

Zhao and colleagues synthesized a novel nanoparticle (BMM NP) using a polymer composition of PEI-PEG and catalyze and this composition allowed for the development of nanoparticles with a Poly Ethylene Glycol corona and an enzyme attached via a polyion complex. The experimental results demonstrated that the presence of macrophages facilitated the transportation of nanozymes, and the BMM nanoparticles loaded with nanozymes acted as carriers for the enzyme, enabling a prolonged release rate and circulation. Yang and colleagues developed a sustained-release formulation using polymeric nanoparticles (PLGA) loaded with benserazide or levodopa methyl ester (LDME). The formulation was tested on rats that were induced with dyskinesia through continuous administration of LD. The researchers observed that LD treatment led to dyskinesia in rats, accompanied by increased levels of p-ERK1/2, p-DARPP-32, and ΔfosB. However, the administration of nanoparticles loaded with LDME/benserazide effectively prevented the onset of LD-induced dyskinesia. Trapani and colleagues conducted a study in which dopamine (DA) was incorporated into chitosan-based nanoparticles (CSNP) with the aim of developing a targeted carrier system for Parkinson's disease. The results demonstrated a rapid interaction between DA and CSNPs, confirming the successful formulation of an effective nanocarrier for DA. Ray and colleagues employed a conventional emulsification crosslinking method to develop chitosan-based nanoparticles loaded with ropinirole hydrochloride. The purpose of this formulation was to enhance the uptake of ropinirole hydrochloride by the brain. Tzeyung and colleagues utilized the ionic gelation method to develop and assess chitosan-based nanoparticles loaded with rotigotine. Their research focused on optimizing and characterizing the formulation for intranasal administration and investigating the potential of rotigotine as a therapeutic option for Parkinson's disease. Esposito and colleagues conducted a study where they developed solid lipid nanoparticles (SLN) containing bromocriptine. The SLN was formulated using a mixture of tristearin and tricaprin to achieve stable plasma levels and an extended drug half-life. The results showed that the release of bromocriptine from the encapsulated formulation was slower compared to free bromocriptine, and the SLN containing the tristearin/tricaprin mixture exhibited the slowest release in in-vivo studies. Álvarez and colleagues investigated the impact of gold nanoparticles (NPs) capped with citrate on the aggregation activity of α-Synuclein. Gao et al. evaluated gold NP clusters for their activity against Parkinson's induced in mice using MPTP. The research showed that these NP formulations effectively inhibited fibrosis and accumulation of α-Synuclein, as demonstrated in in-vitro analysis. Furthermore, promising neuroprotective properties were observed in in-vivo studies. Kaushik and co-researchers used computational biology to study the activity of α-Synuclein in the presence of cerium oxide nanoparticles (CeO_2NP) as an inhibitor. CeO_2NP exhibited superior metal interaction and affinity toward the α-Synuclein residue compared to other nanoparticles [89].

Future Scope of Nanoparticles in PD

Nanoparticles (NPs) offer several beneficial features in the treatment of Parkinson's disease (PD), including targeted drug release, reduced drug dosage leading to decreased toxicity, controlled drug release, enhanced bioavailability, and improved biodistribution [90]. Numerous research studies have demonstrated their significant impact on incorporating drugs into nanocarriers, facilitating drug transport across the blood–brain barrier (BBB), achieving optimal drug distribution in the brain, and controlling the release of drugs from NP formulations [91]. Additionally, NPs have provided the opportunity to administer drugs through alternative routes, bypassing the need to penetrate the BBB. Exciting advancements in the field of Parkinson's disease (PD) treatment include the use of drug carrier nanoparticles that target specific intracellular pathways, interventions that promote structural changes in tangled proteins, and the introduction of reprogramming genes. These innovative approaches hold great potential and are expected to lead to more customized and effective treatments for PD in the future [92].

3.3 Multiple Sclerosis

Multiple sclerosis (MS) is a chronic neurological condition that affects the central nervous system (CNS), which comprises both brain and spinal cord. It is characterized by the immune system mistakenly attacking the protective covering of myelin, a nerve fiber. This damage disrupts the normal flow of electrical impulses along the nerves, leading to a wide range of symptoms. Globally, multiple sclerosis (MS) affects around 2.3 million individuals, with an incidence rate ranging from approximately 50–300 per 100,000 people. The majority of MS cases (about 80–85%) follow a relapse-remitting course (RR-MS), while a smaller percentage experience primary progressive MS (PP-MS), which is characterized by a continuous progression of symptoms without distinct relapses and remissions. It is more prevalent in certain regions such as North America, Western Europe, and Australasia, with over 100 cases per 100,000 population [93]. Multiple sclerosis (MS) is characterized by two distinct pathological features. Firstly, there is inflammation accompanied by demyelination, which refers to the loss of the protective covering around nerve fibers. Secondly, there is astroglia proliferation, also known as gliosis, and neurodegeneration, which involves the proliferation of certain types of brain cells and the progressive loss of nerve cells. The tissue damage caused by MS is limited to the central nervous system (CNS), which includes the brain and spinal cord [94]. The peripheral nervous system, which consists of nerves outside the CNS, remains unaffected. In a clinical context, multiple sclerosis (MS) can manifest in two ways: progressive or relapsing. The relapsing form, known as relapsing MS (RMS), is the most common type, characterized by episodes of neurological dysfunction that can be followed by complete, partial, or no remission. As time passes, the frequency of relapses tends to decrease, but a gradual deterioration often occurs, leading to uninterrupted progression, which is termed secondary progressive MS [95]. Common symptoms of multiple sclerosis (MS) include sensory loss or tingling sensations, unilateral painful visual loss (optic neuritis), limb weakness accompanied by hyperreflexia and the Babinski sign, facial weakness resembling Bell's palsy, ataxia, visual blurring leading to double vision (diplopia), vertigo, Lhermitte's symptom (electric shock-like sensations triggered by neck flexion), paroxysmal symptoms, trigeminal neuralgia, hemifacial spasm, and glossopharyngeal neuralgia. Additional symptoms may include bladder dysfunction, facial myokymia (rapid flickering contractions of the facial muscles), bladder dysfunction, heat sensitivity, sexual dysfunction, mild cognitive dysfunction referred to as “brain fog” with difficulties in multitasking, and fatigue [96].

Highly Effective Drugs:

Ocrelizumab is a first-line treatment for both primary progressive multiple sclerosis (PPMS) and relapsing multiple sclerosis (RMS). It is administered via intravenous (IV) infusion every 6 months. Common side effects include upper respiratory tract infections, headache, infusion-related reactions, nasopharyngitis, urinary tract infections for RMS, and infusion-related reactions, upper respiratory tract infections, and oral herpes infections for PPMS [97]. Ofatumumab, another first-line treatment for RMS, is administered through subcutaneous (SC) injection every 4 weeks. Common side effects include injection-related reactions, nasopharyngitis, headache, upper respiratory tract infections, and urinary tract infections [98]. Natalizumab, a second-line treatment for RMS, is administered via IV infusion every 4 weeks. Common side effects include fatigue and allergic reactions [99]. Alemtuzumab, a first-line treatment for RMS, is administered through IV infusion once daily Common side effects include headache, rash, nausea, and pyrexia [100]. Mitoxantrone, used as a second or third-line treatment for RMS and secondary progressive multiple sclerosis (SPMS), is administered every month or 3 months via IV infusion. However, it is associated with dose-related cardiomyopathy and an increased risk of developing promyelocytic leukemia [101]. Some moderately effective drugs include Fingolimod is taken once orally daily, as a second-line treatment for relapsing multiple sclerosis (RMS). However, it is associated with side effects such as atrioventricular conduction block, bradycardia, elevated liver-enzyme levels, macular edema, and mild hypertension [102]. Siponimod, a first-line treatment for the clinically isolated syndrome (CIS), RMS, and active secondary progressive multiple sclerosis (SPMS), is taken orally once daily. Common side effects include headache, nasopharyngitis, urinary tract infections, and falls [103]. Ozanimod, another sphingosine 1-phosphate receptor modulator, is used as a treatment for CIS, RMS, and active SPMS. Side effects may include headache and elevated liver aminotransferase levels [104]. Dimethyl fumarate and diroximel fumarate, which are inhibitors of the nuclear factor (erythroid-derived 2)-like 2 pathways, are first-line treatments for RMS. Side effects may include upper abdominal pain, flushing, decreased lymphocyte counts, diarrhea, nausea, and elevated liver aminotransferase levels [105]. Cladribine, although its exact mode of action is not fully known, is a second or third-line treatment for RMS. It is taken orally over 4–5 days in 2-week treatment courses. Common side effects include headache, nausea, lymphocytopenia, nasopharyngitia, and upper respiratory tract infections [106].

Nano-Targeted Drug Delivery and Their Examples

The treatment of MS encounters challenges in terms of low efficacy due to the presence of the blood–brain barrier (BBB) and the occurrence of side effects caused by the limited dispersion of drugs into the CNS. Additionally, it is essential to administer therapeutic agents specifically to MS lesions located in different areas of the CNS, while minimizing any potential damage to normal CNS tissues [107].

The utilization of nanoscale materials is expected to offer unique opportunities to address these challenges by improving drug solubility and bioavailability, enabling targeted delivery and controlled release, increasing effective routes of administration, and reducing toxicity. Nanoparticles (NPs) have the ability to utilize various materials, such as metals, synthetic polymers, and natural polymers. The engineering of nanoscale materials holds great potential in enhancing the stability, solubility, and bioavailability of encapsulated molecules [108]. This enables targeted delivery and controlled release, facilitates transportation across physiological barriers, extends the half-life of drugs, improves the routes of administration, and enhances the safety and effectiveness of treatments. Hunter et al. have developed biodegradable nanoparticles using poly (lactic-co-glycolic acid) (PLGA) that carry myelin antigens (Ags). These nanoparticles have demonstrated the ability to effectively induce strong tolerance and provide long-term protection against the development of comprehensive disease in the mouse model of relapse-remitting experimental autoimmune encephalomyelitis (RR-EAE). Montes-Cobos and colleagues developed hybrid inorganic–organic nanoparticles (NPs) that displayed potent activity against human macrophages. Their findings indicated that these NPs successfully delivered glucocorticoids specifically to macrophages in the multiple sclerosis (MS) model, while preserving their therapeutic effectiveness. Additionally, gold nanoparticles loaded with MOG35-55 and ITE demonstrated greater efficiency in inducing functional regulatory T-cells in the animal model of MS compared to particles loaded only with MOG. The clinical condition, including locomotor activity, coordination, and balance, as well as remyelination, was enhanced by orally administering nanolipidic carriers loaded with DMF and coated with vitamins such as tocopherol acetate, cholecalciferol, and retinol acetate in a cuprizone-induced demyelination model. To enhance the effectiveness of nanocarriers for the treatment of multiple sclerosis (MS), the surface of PEGylated solid lipid nanoparticles (SLNs) was modified by incorporating anti-Contactin-2 or anti-Neurofascin, which are antigens found at the Ranvier node. The results of brain uptake studies in a mouse model of MS showed that the modified SLNs achieved greater uptake in the brain compared to the unmodified SLNs. In the mouse model of demyelination induced by ethidium bromide treatment, the administration of chitosan nanoparticles (NPs) loaded with siRNA LINGO-1, a protein that inhibits myelination and axonal regeneration, resulted in the downregulation of LINGO-1 expression. This downregulation was associated with increased expression of myelin basic protein (MBP) and reduced activity of caspase-3. These effects demonstrated neuroprotection and promoted remyelination. In the future, collaborative efforts across disciplines such as materials science, bioengineering, biology, medicine, and drug discovery will undoubtedly facilitate the practical application of nanotechnology in multiple sclerosis (MS) treatments. This interdisciplinary synergy will lead to significant advancements in utilizing nanotechnology for the effective management of MS [109].

4 Applications of Nanocarriers in Neuroimaging

Neuroimaging plays a crucial role in early detection and monitoring of neurological diseases. Conventional techniques for neuroimaging include computed tomography (CT), magnetic resonance imaging (MRI), positron emission tomography (PET), optical imaging, functional ultrasound (fUS), etc., and each technique depending upon the requirements provides a detailed evaluation of the brain. But with different advantages, these techniques also offer many limitations like low sensitivity, limited soft tissue contrast, low resolution, suboptimal signal-to-noise ratio, high cost of radioisotopes, and prolonged scanning duration [24].

With the advancement in the field of neuroimaging, nowadays the use of nanotechnology-based nanocarriers combined with conventional techniques gives promising results in the precise imaging of tumors for evaluation and surgical excision. The small size (typically 1–100 nm in largest diameter) of nanoparticles along with their wide range of chemical configurations make them appealing as carriers that enable target delivery by crossing the blood–brain barrier [110].

Contrast agents can be defined as substances employed to modify the passage of electromagnetic radiation through the body, aiming to intensify the radiodensity of a specific tissue [111]. Nanotechnology-based neuroimaging mainly focuses on the incorporation of contrast agents into nanocarriers such as liposomes, nanobodies, quantum dots, etc., or their use as imaging agents [24]. The nanostructured contrast agents have the ability to capture images at different time points using multiple imaging techniques. This multimodal imaging enables the utilization of the strengths of each neuroimaging technique while overcoming their drawbacks [112].

A study by Li et al. [113] has shown that heptamethine cyanine dye IR780 in combination with various specifically modulated nanocarriers has amazing specific tumor targeting and near-IR fluorescence imaging potential. They experimented in vivo on nude mice infected with glioblastoma and utilized liposomes as the nanocarrier which showed enhanced Near-IR fluorescence (NIRF) imaging.

In recent years, metal-based nanoparticles have been found as a capable theranostic agent for the treatment of neurodegenerative diseases. Gold nanoparticles (GNPs) have gained great popularity in the field of neuroimaging. It provides multimodal and wider imaging not only in the presurgical stage but also in the intra and postsurgical stages because of its extended time of motion in the body [114]. This statement has been confirmed by showing precision targeted fluorescence signal-based neuroimaging for identifying glioma stem cell CD133 biomarker through peptide-coated GNPs [115]. In addition to it, the stem cells that have been reimplanted in the brain can be easily observed and diagnosed with the help of GNPs labeled with gadolinium as a contrast agent for T1 MR imaging [116]. The principle behind the bright contrast of T1 images using gadolinium complexes is based on its paramagnetic nature which causes the shortening of the longitudinal relaxation time of hydrogens present in the neighboring H_2O molecules [117].

Polymer-based nanoparticles have recently gained popularity as a potential theranostic system for drug delivery. Research by Cahalane et al. [118] showed the delivery of rolipram an anti-inflammatory drug encapsulated in polymer-based nanoparticles with the MRI contrasting agent gadolinium-diethylenetriaminepentaacetic acid (Gd[DTPA]) in the specific microglial cells of the central nervous system (CNS). The uptake of nanoparticles by the microglial cells showed no indication of toxicity as well as it did not result in the release of proinflammatory cytokines. These results clearly indicate that polymer-based nanoparticles can be used as a versatile platform for delivering contrast agents and therapeutic drugs to the target site of neuroinflammation.

Similarly, potential strategies have been developed for the early imaging and diagnosis of Alzheimer's disease first is using carbon nanotubes combined with gadolinium complex and Pittsburgh compound B that binds to Aβ plaques and can be observed in the CT images [119]. Another strategy is using nanobodies linked to anti-Aβ and anti-pTau imaging probes that show the fluorescence with amyloid plaques which are the aggregations developed in the interstitial spaces between nerve cells and neurofibrillary tangles which are intricate bundles within brain cells using the two-photon fluorescence imaging (2PFI) technique [120].

Another useful theranostic technique associated with liposomes, having docetaxel (an anti-cancer drug) and quantum dots, was developed for brain tumor neuroimaging and diagnosis. These liposomes were adapted with RGD-TPGS, which enabled active targeting of tumors and gets internalized through receptor-mediated endocytosis. In in vivo studies conducted on Charles Foster rats, these RGD-TPGS-functionalized theranostic liposomes demonstrated higher delivery efficiency in comparison to commercially available docetaxel formulations [121].

For the treatment and diagnosis of glioblastoma, a useful theranostic strategy is used based on nanoparticles composed of polysiloxane. This technique involves the combination of nanoparticles with a contrast agent that is gadolinium (AGulX), 5-(4-carboxyphenyl)-10,15,20-triphenylporphyrin that acts as a photosensitizer and peptide motif as a ligand. This system is used in targeting the neuropilin-1 receptor a transmembrane receptor that gets overexpressed in the tumor vascular network [122].

All the above-discussed strategies for neuroimaging offer a promising alternative to chemotherapy with minimum side effects in future healthcare applications.

5 Safety and Regulatory Considerations

The evaluation of the nano-particulate system for estimating its toxicity plays a vital role in determining its suitability for biomedical applications. Considering the nano size of nanoparticles, they possess the ability to penetrate physiological barriers and potentially accumulate within the body. The accumulation of the components integrated into the formulation development may or may not generate toxic effects, thereby posing significant health risks [123]. As a result, it becomes imperative to assess the toxic characteristics of these nanocarrier-based delivery systems specifically in the case of treating neurological diseases [124].

A. **Biocompatibility and Toxicity of Nanocarriers**:

The inherent potential to control the characteristics and biocompatibility on the nanoscale ultimately influences the interaction with the surrounding environment. According to the European Society of Biomaterials, biocompatibility can be defined as the ability of a material or molecule to elicit a response within a specific host during a particular application [125]. The biocompatibility of nanocarriers can be analyzed by considering some specific properties such as toxicity, cell viability, inflammatory response, uncontrolled proliferation, cell structure distortion, apoptosis, oxidative pressure, and hematotoxicity [126]. Solid lipid-based nanoparticles are based on oil-in-water emulsification and are colloidal carriers on which the drugs are loaded over the lipid matrix. They are being widely used as nanocarriers and are proven to be safe for use in therapeutics but it has been reported in a study that L1210 cells DNA shows inhibition of 3-H thymidine uptake in vitro which serves as an indicator of liposome toxicity. Interestingly it was discovered that no inhibitory effect on 3-H-thymidine was observed in the case of phosphatidylcholine and cholesterol [125]. Stearylamine which is used as a positive charge inducer in lipid nanocarriers was investigated and observed to be cytotoxic when administered for neurological disorders [127].

During the interaction between a nanocarrier and the cellular membrane, a number of promotive and resistive forces are acting. Promotive forces include free energy, ligand-receptor binding interactions, optimal size, particle surface characteristics, and shape. All these factors facilitate cell binding at the membrane surface and aid in the traversal of biological barriers for particulate delivery. On the other hand, resistive forces, such as cell membrane stretching, elasticity, thermal fluctuations, and bond elasticity in receptor-ligand stretching, hinder internalization. Therefore, achieving a delicate balance between these two forces is crucial to facilitate particle internalization [128].

Additionally, interactions with protein domains or negatively charged phospholipids on cell surface are significantly influenced by the surface charge of nanocarriers [123]. Positively charged surfaces have a more pronounced effect compared to anionic groups. For instance, studies suggest that positively charged nanocarriers like PAMAM and poly(ethylene imine) (PEI) can physically disrupt the plasma membrane, leading to transient holes. However, such disruptions are considered as necrotic toxicity associated with these nanocarriers [129].

B. **Approaches for Evaluating Safety and Efficacy**:

Surface modifications of nanocarriers are one of the widely used procedures for enhancing or adding new useful properties for using them in biomedical applications [126]. The surface modification of nanoparticles can be accomplished through two distinct methods: non-covalent conjugation and covalent conjugation. The non-covalent approach relies on a multitude of weak interactions, such as van der Waals, absorption, hydrophobic interactions, electrostatic, ionic, and hydrogen bonds. This strategy is particularly employed with metallic nanoparticles [130]. For covalent conjugation, many different alternative processes are used depending on the configuration of nanoparticles. Furthermore, this approach enables modifications at various stages through sequential (Świetek et al., 2019). By utilizing this methodology, it becomes possible to create multifunctional structures capable of combining diagnostic and therapeutic capabilities and thus can be easily applied for medical use [131].

Various techniques have been employed to assess the internalization of nanoparticles within specific cellular contexts, which can be categorized as label-free and label-based methods. Label-free techniques, such as scanning electron microscopy (SEM), transmission electron microscopy (TEM), and Raman microscopy, are commonly utilized. These approaches offer the advantage of not requiring the use of fluorophores that may potentially alter the size (physical property) or chemical properties of nanoparticles. Moreover, label-free methods facilitate the differentiation between internalized nanoparticles and those attached to the cell membrane. In contrast, label-based techniques can complicate this discrimination. However, it is important to note that TEM and SEM imaging, while providing high-resolution images down to the cellular organelle level, are relatively time-consuming, expensive and destructive in nature, unlike Raman microscopy [132, 126].

6 Conclusion

Nanocarriers and nano-drug delivery therapy have shown great promise in neurodiseases. Nanocarriers' unique properties and capabilities have enabled targeted drug delivery to the central nervous system, overcoming the challenges posed by the blood–brain barrier. The prospects of nanocarriers and nano drug delivery therapy in neurodiseases are promising. Ongoing clinical trials and emerging trends indicate a growing interest in this field. Advancements in nanotechnology, including developing novel nanocarriers and improved drug delivery systems, will further enhance the efficacy and specificity of neurodisease treatments. Additionally, integrating nanocarriers with other therapeutic modalities, such as gene therapy and immunotherapy, holds the potential for synergistic effects and improved outcomes. However, several challenges lie ahead. The scale-up of nanocarrier production, cost-effectiveness, and long-term stability must be addressed for widespread clinical adoption. Furthermore, collaboration between researchers, clinicians, regulatory agencies, and industry partners is crucial to accelerate the translation of nanocarrier-based therapies from bench to bedside. Nanocarriers and nano-drug delivery therapy have emerged as promising approaches for effectively treating neurodiseases. Integrating nanotechnology with neuroscience can revolutionize the field, offering targeted and personalized therapies with enhanced efficacy and reduced side effects. Continued research and development efforts and close collaborations among various stakeholders will drive future advancements in this exciting field and pave the way for improved neurodisease management and patient outcomes.

References

1. Cui Y, Jiang X, Feng J (2022) The therapeutic potential of triptolide and celastrol in neurological diseases. Front Pharmacol 13:1024955
2. Toricelli M, Pereira AAR, Abrao GS, Malerba HN, Maia J, Buck HS, Viel TA (2021) Mechanisms of neuroplasticity and brain degeneration: strategies for protection during the aging process. Neural Regen Res 16(1):58
3. Chikkara G, Mittal P, Chikara SK (2022) Neurological diseases: a perspective genetic approach & dietary intervention. Int J Appl Res
4. Hashempour-Baltork F, Farshi P, Alizadeh AM, Eskandarzadeh S, Abedinzadeh S, Azadmard-Damirchi S, Torbati M (2022) Effect of refined edible oils on neurodegenerative disorders. Adv Pharm Bull
5. Francelle L, Mazzulli JR (2022) Neuroinflammation in aucher disease, neuronal ceroid lipofuscinosis, and commonalities with Parkinson's disease. Brain Res 147798
6. Chen Y, Qin C, Huang J, Tang X, Liu C, Huang K, Xu J, Guo G, Tong A, Zhou L (2020) The role of astrocytes in oxidative stress of central nervous system: a mixed blessing. Cell Prolif 53(3):e12781
7. Yanik S, Kurt SB, Ari B, Demirci S, Yilmaz S (2020) Development of electrochemical sensors for quantitative analysis of methyldopa at modified-Gce and Pge electrodes by voltammetry. J Sci Perspect. https://doi.org/10.26900/jsp.4.019
8. Mohd Murshid N, Aminullah Lubis F, Makpol S (2020) Epigenetic changes and its intervention in age-related neurodegenerative diseases. Cell Mol Neurobiol 1–19
9. Burtchell J, Fetty K, Miller K, Minden K, Kantor D (2019) Two sides to every story: perspectives from four patients and a healthcare professional on multiple sclerosis disease progression. Neurol Ther 8:185–205
10. Hussain S, Mubeen I, Ullah N, Ud Din Shah SS, Khan BA, Zahoor M, Ullah R, Khan FA, Sultan MA (2022) Modern diagnostic imaging technique applications and risk factors in the medical field: a review. BioMed Research International
11. Anestis E, Eccles FJ, Fletcher I, Triliva S, Simpson J (2022) Healthcare professionals' involvement in breaking bad news to newly diagnosed patients with motor neurodegenerative conditions: a qualitative study. Disabil Rehabil 44(25):7877–7890
12. Kölker S, Gleich F, Mütze U, Opladen T (2022) Rare disease registries are key to evidence-based personalized medicine: highlighting the European experience. Front Endocrinol 13
13. Rosser AE, Busse ME, Gray WP, Badin RA, Perrier AL, Wheelock V, Cozzi E, Martin UP, Salado-Manzano C, Mills LJ, Drew C (2022) Translating cell therapies for neurodegenerative diseases: Huntington's disease as a model disorder. Brain 145(5):1584–1597
14. Weninger S, Sperling B, Alexander R, Ivarsson M, Menzies FM, Powchik P, Weber CJ, Altar CA, Crystal RG, Haggarty SJ, Loring J (2020) Active immunotherapy and alternative therapeutic modalities for Alzheimer's disease. Alzheimer's & Dement Transl Res Clin Interv 6(1):e12090
15. Lombardo D, Kiselev MA, Caccamo MT (2019) Smart nanoparticles for drug delivery application: development of versatile nanocarrier platforms in biotechnology and nanomedicine. J Nanomater
16. Akhtar A, Andleeb A, Waris TS, Bazzar M, Moradi A, Awan NR, Yar M (2021) Neurodegenerative diseases and effective drug delivery: a review of challenges and novel therapeutics. J Control Release 330:1152–1167
17. Asil SM et al (2020) Nanomaterial based drug delivery systems for the treatment of neurodegenerative diseases. Biomater Sci 8(15):4109–4128. https://doi.org/10.1039/d0bm00809e
18. Hussein HA, Abdullah MZ (2021) Novel drug delivery systems based on silver nanoparticles, hyaluronic acid, lipid nanoparticles and liposomes for cancer treatment. Appl Nanosci 12(11):3071–3096. https://doi.org/10.1007/s13204-021-02018-9
19. Chamundeeswari M, Jeslin J, Verma ML (2019) Nanocarriers for drug delivery applications. Environ Chem Lett 17(2):849–865. https://doi.org/10.1007/s10311-018-00841-1

20. Almeida B et al (2020) Recent progress in bioconjugation strategies for liposome-mediated drug delivery. Molecules 25(23):5672. https://doi.org/10.3390/molecules25235672
21. Large DE et al (2021) Liposome composition in drug delivery design, synthesis, characterization, and clinical application. Adv Drug Deliv Rev 176:113851. https://doi.org/10.1016/j.addr.2021.113851
22. Guimarães DIP, Cavaco-Paulo A, Nogueira E (2021) Design of liposomes as drug delivery system for therapeutic applications. Int J Pharm 601:120571. https://doi.org/10.1016/j.ijpharm.2021.120571
23. Hersh A, Alomari S, Tyler B (2022) Crossing the blood-brain barrier: advances in nanoparticle technology for drug delivery in neuro-oncology. Int J Mol Sci 23(8):4153. https://doi.org/10.3390/ijms23084153
24. Teleanu DM, Chircov C, Grumezescu AM, Volceanov A, Teleanu RI (2019) Contrast agents delivery: an up-to-date review of nanodiagnostics in neuroimaging. Nanomaterials 9(4):542. https://doi.org/10.3390/nano9040542
25. Khan AA, Khan M, Cho MH, Khan MM (2020) Selected nanotechnologies and nanostructures for drug delivery, nanomedicine and cure. Bioprocess Biosyst Eng 43(8):1339–1357. https://doi.org/10.1007/s00449-020-02330-8
26. Li Y et al (2020) Long-circulating thermosensitive liposomes for the targeted drug delivery of oxaliplatin. Int J Nanomed 15:6721–6734. https://doi.org/10.2147/ijn.s250773
27. Kahana M et al (2020) Liposome-based targeting of dopamine to the brain: a novel approach for the treatment of Parkinson's disease. Mol Psychiatry 26(6):2626–2632. https://doi.org/10.1038/s41380-020-0742-4
28. Begines B et al (2020) Polymeric nanoparticles for drug delivery: recent developments and future prospects. Nanomaterials 10(7):1403. https://doi.org/10.3390/nano10071403
29. Gagliardi A et al (2021) Biodegradable polymeric nanoparticles for drug delivery to solid tumors. Front Pharmacol 12. https://doi.org/10.3389/fphar.2021.601626
30. Calzoni E et al (2019) Biocompatible polymer nanoparticles for drug delivery applications in cancer and neurodegenerative disorder therapies. J Funct Biomater 10(1):4. https://doi.org/10.3390/jfb10010004
31. Rabiee N, Ahmadi S, Afshari R, Khalaji S, Rabiee M, Bagherzadeh M, Fatahi Y, Dinarvand R, Tahriri M, Tayebi L, Hamblin MR, Webster TJ (2021) Polymeric nanoparticles for nasal drug delivery to the brain: relevance to Alzheimer's disease. Adv Therapeutics 4(3):2000076. https://doi.org/10.1002/adtp.202000076
32. Ojha S, Kumar B, Chadha H (2019) Neuroprotective potential of dimethyl fumarate-loaded polymeric nanoparticles against multiple sclerosis. Indian J Pharm Sci 81(3). https://doi.org/10.36468/pharmaceutical-sciences.535
33. Zhang WS, Mehta A, Tong Z, Esser L, Voelcker NH (2021) Development of polymeric nanoparticles for blood-brain barrier transfer—strategies and challenges. Adv Sci 8(10):2003937. https://doi.org/10.1002/advs.202003937
34. Zhao Y et al (2020) Polymeric nanoparticles-based brain delivery with improved therapeutic efficacy of Ginkgolide B in Parkinson's disease. Int J Nanomed 15:10453–10467. https://doi.org/10.2147/ijn.s272831
35. Zhu Y, Liu C-Y, Pang Z (2019) Dendrimer-based drug delivery systems for brain targeting. Biomolecules 9(12):790. https://doi.org/10.3390/biom9120790
36. Gauro R et al (2021) Advances in dendrimer-mediated targeted drug delivery to the brain. J Nanopart Res 23(3). https://doi.org/10.1007/s11051-021-05175-8
37. Liu C et al (2019) Enhanced blood-brain-barrier penetrability and tumor-targeting efficiency by peptide-functionalized poly(amidoamine) dendrimer for the therapy of gliomas. Nanotheranostics 3(4):311–330. https://doi.org/10.7150/ntno.38954
38. Singh AK et al (2020) Machine-learning-based approach to decode the influence of nanomaterial properties on their interaction with cells. ACS Appl Mater Interfaces 13(1):1943–1955. https://doi.org/10.1021/acsami.0c18470
39. Xie H et al (2019) An available strategy for nasal brain transport of nanocomposite based on PAMAM dendrimers via in situ gel. Nanomaterials 9(2):147. https://doi.org/10.3390/nano9020147

40. Alotaibi BS et al (2021) Potential of nanocarrier-based drug delivery systems for brain targeting: a current review of literature. Int J Nanomed 16:7517–7533. https://doi.org/10.2147/ijn.s333657
41. Panda MK et al (2020) Role of nanoparticles and nanomaterials in drug delivery: an overview. Springer eBooks, pp 247–265. https://doi.org/10.1007/978-981-15-2195-9_19
42. Han L, Jiang C (2020) Evolution of blood–brain barrier in brain diseases and related systemic nanoscale brain-targeting drug delivery strategies. Acta Pharm Sin B. https://doi.org/10.1016/j.apsb.2020.11.023
43. Da Ros T, Martín N, Nierengarten J-F (2021) Carbon nanostructures for biomedical applications. Royal Society of Chemistry
44. Maiti D et al (2019) Carbon-based nanomaterials for biomedical applications: a recent study. Front Pharmacol 9. https://doi.org/10.3389/fphar.2018.01401
45. Han G et al (2019) Membrane-penetrating carbon quantum dots for imaging nucleic acid structures in live organisms. Angew Chem 58(21):7087–7091. https://doi.org/10.1002/anie.201903005
46. Shoval A et al (2019) Anti-VEGF-aptamer modified C-Dots—a hybrid nanocomposite for topical treatment of ocular vascular disorders. Small 15(40):1902776. https://doi.org/10.1002/smll.201902776
47. Chung YC, Lee BS, Park CB (2019) Multifunctional carbon dots as a therapeutic nanoagent for modulating Cu(ii)-mediated β-amyloid aggregation. Nanoscale 11(13):6297–6306. https://doi.org/10.1039/c9nr00473d
48. Hettiarachchi SD et al (2019) Triple conjugated carbon dots as a nano-drug delivery model for glioblastoma brain tumors. Nanoscale 11(13):6192–6205. https://doi.org/10.1039/c8nr08970a
49. Huda S, Alam A, Sharma P (2020) Smart nanocarriers-based drug delivery for cancer therapy: an innovative and developing strategy. J Drug Deliv Sci Technol 60:102018. https://doi.org/10.1016/j.jddst.2020.102018
50. Mura P (2020) Advantages of the combined use of cyclodextrins and nanocarriers in drug delivery: a review. Int J Pharm 579:119181. https://doi.org/10.1016/j.ijpharm.2020.119181
51. Tesarova B, Musilek K, Dostalova S, Heger Z (2020) Taking advantage of cellular uptake of ferritin nanocages for targeted drug delivery. J Control Release 325:176–190. https://doi.org/10.1016/j.jconrel.2020.06.026
52. Shah A, Aftab S, Nisar J, Ashiq MN, Iftikhar FJ (2021) Nanocarriers for targeted drug delivery. J Drug Deliv Sci Technol 62:102426. https://doi.org/10.1016/j.jddst.2021.102426
53. Emad NA, Ahmed BMA, Alhalmi A, Alzobaidi N, Al-Kubati S (2021) Recent progress in nanocarriers for direct nose to brain drug delivery. J Drug Deliv Sci Technol 64:102642. https://doi.org/10.1016/j.jddst.2021.102642
54. Ahlawat J et al (2020) Nanocarriers as potential drug delivery candidates for overcoming the blood–brain barrier: challenges and possibilities. ACS Omega 5(22):12583–12595. https://doi.org/10.1021/acsomega.0c01592
55. Zorkina Y, Abramova O, Ushakova VM, Morozova AL, Zubkov EA, Valikhov MP, Mel'nikov PA, Majouga AG, Chekhonin VP (2020) Nano carrier drug delivery systems for the treatment of neuropsychiatric disorders: advantages and limitations. Molecules 25(22):5294.https://doi.org/10.3390/molecules25225294
56. Dahiya S, Dahiya R, Hernandez E (2021) Nanocarriers for anticancer drug targeting: recent trends and challenges. Crit Rev Therapeutic Drug Carrier Syst 38(6):49–103. https://doi.org/10.1615/critrevtherdrugcarriersyst.2021035650
57. Agrahari V et al (2019) Nanoformulation properties, characterization, and behavior in complex biological matrices: challenges and opportunities for brain-targeted drug delivery applications and enhanced translational potential. Adv Drug Deliv Rev 148:146–180. https://doi.org/10.1016/j.addr.2019.02.008
58. Alshawwa SZ et al (2022) Nanocarrier drug delivery systems: characterization, limitations, future perspectives and implementation of artificial intelligence. Pharmaceutics 14(4):883. https://doi.org/10.3390/pharmaceutics14040883

59. Sweeney MD, Zhao Z, Montagne A, Nelson AR, Zlokovic BV (2019) Blood-brain barrier: from physiology to disease and back. Physiol Rev 99(1):21–78. https://doi.org/10.1152/physrev.00050.2017
60. Cunha SC et al (2021) Improving drug delivery for Alzheimer's disease through nose-to-brain delivery using nanoemulsions, nanostructured lipid carriers (NLC) and in situ hydrogels. Int J Nanomed 16:4373–4390. https://doi.org/10.2147/ijn.s305851
61. Ramalho MJ et al (2020) Nanotechnology to improve the Alzheimer's disease therapy with natural compounds. Drug Deliv Transl Res 10(2):380–402. https://doi.org/10.1007/s13346-019-00694-3
62. Andrade-Guerrero J et al (2023) Alzheimer's disease: an updated overview of its genetics. Int J Mol Sci 24(4):3754. https://doi.org/10.3390/ijms24043754
63. Cheng Y, Tian D-Y, Wang Y-J (2020) Peripheral clearance of brain-derived Aβ in Alzheimer's disease: pathophysiology and therapeutic perspectives. Transl Neurodegener 9(1). https://doi.org/10.1186/s40035-020-00195-1
64. Doifode T et al (2021) The impact of the microbiota-gut-brain axis on Alzheimer's disease pathophysiology. Pharmacol Res 164:105314. https://doi.org/10.1016/j.phrs.2020.105314
65. Breijyeh Z, Karaman R (2020) Comprehensive review on Alzheimer's disease: causes and treatment. Molecules 25(24):5789
66. Pooladgar P et al (2022) Donepezil Beyond Alzheimer's disease? A narrative review of therapeutic potentials of Donepezil in different diseases. Iranian J Pharm Res 21(1). https://doi.org/10.5812/ijpr-128408
67. Metz CN, Pavlov VA (2021) Treating disorders across the lifespan by modulating cholinergic signaling with galantamine. J Neurochem 158(6):1359–1380. https://doi.org/10.1111/jnc.15243
68. Shafiei-Irannejad V et al (2021) Memantine and its benefits for cancer, cardiovascular and neurological disorders. Eur J Pharmacol 910:174455. https://doi.org/10.1016/j.ejphar.2021.174455
69. Abelein A, Johansson J (2023) Amyloid inhibition by molecular chaperones in vitro can be translated to Alzheimer's pathology in vivo. RSC Med Chem 14(5):848–857. https://doi.org/10.1039/d3md00040k
70. Hettiarachchi SD, Zhou Y, Seven E, Lakshmana MK, Kaushik AK, Chand HS, Leblanc RM (2019) Nanoparticle-mediated approaches for Alzheimer's disease pathogenesis, diagnosis, and therapeutics. J Control Release 314:125–140. https://doi.org/10.1016/j.jconrel.2019.10.034
71. Wilson B, Geetha KM (2020) Neurotherapeutic applications of nanomedicine for treating Alzheimer's disease. J Control Release 325:25–37. https://doi.org/10.1016/j.jconrel.2020.05.044
72. Tansey MG, Wallings RL, Houser MC, Herrick MK, Keating CE, Joers V (2022) Inflammation and immune dysfunction in Parkinson disease. Nat Rev Immunol 1–17. https://doi.org/10.1038/s41577-022-00684-6
73. Rektorová I (2019) Current treatment of behavioral and cognitive symptoms of Parkinson's disease. Parkinsonism Relat Disord 59:65–73. https://doi.org/10.1016/j.parkreldis.2019.02.042
74. Castillo-Rangel C et al (2023) Neuroinflammation in Parkinson's disease: from gene to clinic: a systematic review. Int J Mol Sci 24(6):5792. https://doi.org/10.3390/ijms24065792
75. Aarsland D et al (2021) Parkinson disease-associated cognitive impairment. Nat Rev Dis Primers 7(1). https://doi.org/10.1038/s41572-021-00280-3
76. Finberg JPM (2019) Inhibitors of MAO-B and COMT: their effects on brain dopamine levels and uses in Parkinson's disease. J Neural Transm 126(4):433–448. https://doi.org/10.1007/s00702-018-1952-7
77. Limousin P, Foltynie T (2019) Long-term outcomes of deep brain stimulation in Parkinson disease. Nat Rev Neurol 15(4):234–242. https://doi.org/10.1038/s41582-019-0145-9
78. Tofani M et al (2020) Efficacy of occupational therapy interventions on quality of life in patients with Parkinson's disease: a systematic review and meta-analysis. Mov Disord Clin Pract 7(8):891–901. https://doi.org/10.1002/mdc3.13089

79. Hidecker MJC et al (2022) Coordinated speech therapy, physiotherapy, and pharmaceutical care telehealth for people with Parkinson disease in rural communities: an exploratory, 8-week cohort study for feasibility, safety, and signal of efficacy. Rural and Remote Health [Preprint]. https://doi.org/10.22605/rrh6679
80. Armstrong MJ, Okun MS (2020) Diagnosis and treatment of parkinson disease. JAMA 323(6):548. https://doi.org/10.1001/jama.2019.22360
81. Draoui A, El Hiba O, Aimrane A, El Khiat A, Gamrani H (2020) Parkinson's disease: from bench to bedside. Rev Neurol Fr. https://doi.org/10.1016/j.neurol.2019.11.002
82. Latt MD et al (2019) Factors to consider in the selection of dopamine agonists for older persons with Parkinson's disease. Drugs Aging 36(3):189–202. https://doi.org/10.1007/s40266-018-0629-0
83. Cerri S, Blandini F (2020) An update on the use of non-ergot dopamine agonists for the treatment of Parkinson's disease. Expert Opin Pharmacother 21(18):2279–2291. https://doi.org/10.1080/14656566.2020.1805432
84. Montecucco F et al (2019) Apomorphine for Parkinson's disease: efficacy and safety of current and new formulations. CNS Drugs 33(9):905–918. https://doi.org/10.1007/s40263-019-00661-z
85. Raeder V et al (2021) Rotigotine transdermal patch for motor and non-motor Parkinson's disease: a review of 12 years' clinical experience. CNS Drugs 35(2):215–231. https://doi.org/10.1007/s40263-020-00788-4
86. Rajan R et al (2020) Anticholinergics may carry significant cognitive and gait burden in Parkinson's disease. Mov Disord Clin Pract 7(7):803–809. https://doi.org/10.1002/mdc3.13032
87. Müller T, Möhr J-D (2019) Pharmacokinetics of monoamine oxidase B inhibitors in Parkinson's disease: current status. Expert Opin Drug Metab Toxicol 15(5):429–435. https://doi.org/10.1080/17425255.2019.1607292
88. Paul A, Yadav KS (2020) Parkinson's disease: current drug therapy and unraveling the prospects of nanoparticles. J Drug Deliv Sci Technol 58:101790. https://doi.org/10.1016/j.jddst.2020.101790
89. Ghazy E et al (2021) Nanomaterials for Parkinson disease: recent progress. J Mol Struct 1231:129698. https://doi.org/10.1016/j.molstruc.2020.129698
90. Phuna ZX et al (2021) Recent development in nanocrystal based drug delivery for neurodegenerative diseases: scope, challenges, current and future prospects. J Drug Deliv Sci Technol 68:102921. https://doi.org/10.1016/j.jddst.2021.102921
91. Sharma S, Rabbani SA, Agarwal T, Baboota S, Pottoo FH, Kadian R (2021) Nanotechnology driven approaches for the management of Parkinson's disease: current status and future perspectives. Curr Drug Metab 22(4):287–298
92. Baskin J, Jeon JY, Lewis SJG (2020) Nanoparticles for drug delivery in Parkinson's disease. J Neurol 268(5):1981–1994. https://doi.org/10.1007/s00415-020-10291-x
93. Hughes SE, Macaron G (2021) Fast facts: multiple sclerosis, 5th ed. A new era of disease modification and treatment. Karger Medical and Scientific Publishers
94. Faissner S et al (2019) Progressive multiple sclerosis: from pathophysiology to therapeutic strategies. Nat Rev Drug Discov 18(12):905–922. https://doi.org/10.1038/s41573-019-0035-2
95. Buscarinu MC et al (2019) The contribution of gut barrier changes to multiple sclerosis pathophysiology. Front Immunol 10.https://doi.org/10.3389/fimmu.2019.01916
96. Rayatpour A, Javan M (2021) Targeting the brain lesions using peptides: a review focused on the possibility of targeted drug delivery to multiple sclerosis lesions. Pharmacol Res 167:105441. https://doi.org/10.1016/j.phrs.2021.105441
97. Amirov CB et al (2023) Ocrelizumab in pediatric multiple sclerosis. Eur J Paediatr Neurol 43:1–5. https://doi.org/10.1016/j.ejpn.2023.01.011
98. Kang C, Blair HA (2021) Ofatumumab: a review in relapsing forms of multiple sclerosis. Drugs 82(1):55–62. https://doi.org/10.1007/s40265-021-01650-7
99. Khoy K et al (2020) Natalizumab in multiple sclerosis treatment: from biological effects to immune monitoring. Front Immunol 11. https://doi.org/10.3389/fimmu.2020.549842

100. Scappaticcio L et al (2020) Alemtuzumab-induced thyroid events in multiple sclerosis: a systematic review and meta-analysis. J Endocrinol Investig 43(2):219–229. https://doi.org/10.1007/s40618-019-01105-7
101. Foo EC et al (2020) Mitoxantrone in relapsing-remitting and rapidly progressive multiple sclerosis: ten-year clinical outcomes post-treatment with mitoxantrone. Mult Scleros Related Disord 44:102330. https://doi.org/10.1016/j.msard.2020.102330
102. Chun J et al (2019) Fingolimod: lessons learned and new opportunities for treating multiple sclerosis and other disorders. Ann Rev Pharmacol Toxicol 59(1):149–170. https://doi.org/10.1146/annurev-pharmtox-010818-021358
103. Scott LJ (2020) Siponimod: a review in secondary progressive multiple sclerosis. CNS Drugs 34(11):1191–1200. https://doi.org/10.1007/s40263-020-00771-z
104. Fronza M et al (2021) An overview of the efficacy and safety of Ozanimod for the treatment of relapsing multiple sclerosis. Drug Des Dev Ther 15:1993–2004. https://doi.org/10.2147/dddt.s240861
105. Naismith RT et al (2020) Diroximel fumarate demonstrates an improved gastrointestinal tolerability profile compared with dimethyl fumarate in patients with relapsing–remitting multiple sclerosis: results from the randomized, double-blind, phase III EVOLVE-MS-2 study. CNS Drugs 34(2):185–196. https://doi.org/10.1007/s40263-020-00700-0
106. Hauser SL, Cree BAC (2020) Treatment of multiple sclerosis: a review. Am J Med 133(12):1380–1390.e2. https://doi.org/10.1016/j.amjmed.2020.05.049
107. Saeedi M et al (2019) Applications of nanotechnology in drug delivery to the central nervous system. Biomed Pharmacother 111:666–675. https://doi.org/10.1016/j.biopha.2018.12.133.
108. Liu R et al (2022) Advances of nanoparticles as drug delivery systems for disease diagnosis and treatment. Chin Chem Lett 34(2):107518. https://doi.org/10.1016/j.cclet.2022.05.032
109. Nuzzo D, Picone PM (2021) Multiple sclerosis: focus on extracellular and artificial vesicles, nanoparticles as potential therapeutic approaches. Int J Mol Sci 22(16):8866. https://doi.org/10.3390/ijms22168866
110. Faiz K, Lam F, Chen J, Kasper E, Salehi F (2022) The emerging applications of nanotechnology in neuroimaging: a comprehensive review. Front Bioeng Biotechnol 1111
111. Kaller MO, An J (2023) Contrast agent toxicity. StatPearls Publishing, In StatPearls
112. Zhao W, Yu X, Peng S, Luo Y, Li J, Lu L (2021) Construction of nanomaterials as contrast agents or probes for glioma imaging. J Nanobiotechnol 19(1):1–31
113. Li S, Johnson J, Peck A, Xie Q (2017) Near-infrared fluorescent imaging of brain tumor with IR780 dye incorporated phospholipid nanoparticles. J Transl Med 15(1):1–12
114. Meola A, Rao J, Chaudhary N, Sharma M, Chang SD (2018) Gold nanoparticles for brain tumor imaging: a systematic review. Front Neurol 9:328
115. Zare I, Yaraki MT, Speranza G, Najafabadi AH, Shourangiz-Haghighi A, Nik AB, Manshian BB, Saraiva C, Soenen SJ, Kogan MJ, Lee JW (2022) Gold nanostructures: synthesis, properties, and neurological applications. Chem Soc Rev 51(7):2601–2680
116. Imran M, Kumar A, Vyawahare A, Saha P, Ahmad A, Ansari MM, Mishra RK, Ali A, Khan AQ, Khan R (2022) Nanotechnology: a daydream for advanced imaging, diagnosis, and therapeutic approach for cerebral ischemia. In: Regenerative therapies in ischemic stroke recovery. Springer Nature Singapore, Singapore, pp 53–83
117. Haribabu V, Girigoswami K, Sharmiladevi P, Girigoswami A (2020) Water–nanomaterial interaction to escalate twin-mode magnetic resonance imaging. ACS Biomater Sci Eng 6(8):4377–4389
118. Cahalane C, Bonezzi J, Shelestak J, Clements R, Boika A, Yun YH, Shriver LP (2020) Targeted delivery of anti-inflammatory and imaging agents to microglial cells with polymeric nanoparticles. Mol Pharm 17(6):1816–1826
119. Costa PM, Wang JTW, Morfin JF, Khanum T, To W, Sosabowski J, Tóth E, Al-Jamal KT (2018) Functionalised carbon nanotubes enhance brain delivery of amyloid-targeting Pittsburgh compound B (PiB)-derived ligands. Nanotheranostics 2(2):168
120. Vander Zanden CM, Chi EY (2020) Passive immunotherapies targeting amyloid beta and tau oligomers in Alzheimer's disease. J Pharm Sci 109(1):68–73

121. d'Angelo M, Castelli V, Benedetti E, Antonosante A, Catanesi M, Dominguez-Benot R, Pitari G, Ippoliti R, Cimini A (2019) Theranostic nanomedicine for malignant gliomas. Front Bioeng Biotechnol 7:325
122. Choi J, Kim G, Cho SB, Im HJ (2020) Radiosensitizing high-Z metal nanoparticles for enhanced radiotherapy of glioblastoma multiforme. J Nanobiotechnol 18(1):1–23
123. Patnaik S, Gorain B, Padhi S, Choudhury H, Gabr GA, Md S, Mishra DK, Kesharwani P (2021) Recent update of toxicity aspects of nanoparticulate systems for drug delivery. Eur J Pharm Biopharm 161:100–119
124. Sarwal A, Singh G, Prasad P, Sharma S, Ali W (2020) Recent advances in nanocarrier-based brain-targeted drug delivery for effective treatment of central nervous system disorders. Nanoformul Human Health Chall Approach 187–203
125. Oladipo AO, Lebelo SL, Msagati TA (2023) Nanocarrier design–function relationship: the prodigious role of properties in regulating biocompatibility for drug delivery applications. Chem Biol Interact 377:110466
126. Sanità G, Carrese B, Lamberti A (2020) Nanoparticle surface functionalization: how to improve biocompatibility and cellular internalization. Front Mol Biosci 7
127. Shah S, Chougule MB, Kotha AK, Kashikar R, Godugu C, Raghuvanshi RS, Singh SB, Srivastava S (2021) Nanomedicine based approaches for combating viral infections. J Control Release 338:80–104
128. de Almeida MS, Susnik E, Drasler B, Taladriz-Blanco P, Petri-Fink A, Rothen-Rutishauser B (2021) Understanding nanoparticle endocytosis to improve targeting strategies in nanomedicine. Chem Soc Rev 50(9):5397–5434
129. Dabbaghi M, Kazemi Oskuee R, Hashemi K, Afkhami Goli A (2018) Evaluating polyethyleneimine/DNA nanoparticles-mediated damage to cellular organelles using endoplasmic reticulum stress profile. Artif Cells Nanomed Biotechnol 46(1):192–199
130. Yue L, Sun C, Cheng Q, Ding Y, Wei J, Wang R (2019) Gold nanorods with a noncovalently tailorable surface for multi-modality image-guided chemo-photothermal cancer therapy. Chem Commun 55(90):13506–13509
131. Zhao S, Yu X, Qian Y, Chen W, Shen J (2020) Multifunctional magnetic iron oxide nanoparticles: an advanced platform for cancer theranostics. Theranostics 10(14):6278
132. Malatesta M (2021) Transmission electron microscopy as a powerful tool to investigate the interaction of nanoparticles with subcellular structures. Int J Mol Sci 22(23)

Novel Nano Delivery Strategies in Targeted Neurological Diseases Management

Nanocarriers for Tracking and Treating Epilepsy, and Seizures Management

Arya Swati, Shraddha Singh Raghav, Kangkan Sarma, and Neha Pathak

Abstract Epilepsy, the neurological disorder causes abnormal electrical discharge of the brain that leads to seizures, is a severe healthcare problem. The treatment options available are antiepileptic drugs, surgery, antiepileptic devices, and ketogenic diets. The common adverse effects of antiepileptic drugs are cognitive disorders, dizziness, abdominal pain, hypersomnia, etc. To overcome the adverse effects, the antiepileptic drugs are loaded with suitably modified nanocarriers. It enhances the drug's efficacy to the targeted site at a minimum concentration. Even a few nanocarriers are suitable for diagnosis purpose. A few reported nanocarrier systems used for treatments and diagnostic purposes are micelles, polymeric ligands, liposomes, solid lipid nanoparticles, dendrimers, quantum dots, silver, gold nanoparticles, nanoconjugates, nanosponges, etc. Nanocarrier's physicochemical properties influence its invading nature to the targeted site, circulation lifetime, and retention time of active drugs within. Strategically different attempts are made to modify the nanocarriers to overcome barriers like mononuclear phagocytes of the immune system. Biofunctionalization or functionalization or functional modification of the nanocarriers not only helps to overcome the barriers but also enhances the permeability and retention time of nanocarriers to the targeted site. Mostly, epilepsy causes unconsciousness, so treatment automation is another aspect of epilepsy treatment. So, attempts like implantable devices like bio-physiochemical responsive nanotheranostic system, magnetic field responsive nanoparticles system, thermo responsive, electro responsive discrete release of doses via self-triggered drug injection during seizure systems are useful to treat epilepsy.

A. Swati (✉)
SGT College of Pharmacy, SGT University, Gurugram, Haryana 122505, India
e-mail: aryaswati2020@gmail.com

S. S. Raghav · K. Sarma
School of Pharmaceutical and Population Health Informatics (SoPPHI), DIT University, Mussoorie Diversion Road, Makkawala, Dehradun, Uttarakhand 248009, India

N. Pathak
Department of Pharmacy, School of Medical Allied Sciences, GD Goenka University, Sohna, Gurugram 122103, India

S. K. Rath et al. (eds.), *Nanomaterials for Drug Delivery and Neurological Diseases Management*, Smart Nanomaterials Technology,
https://doi.org/10.1007/978-981-97-0308-1_11

Keywords Nanocarrier · Epilepsy · Seizures

1 Introduction

1.1 Epileptic Seizures

As per the world health organization (WHO), a seizure event occurs when a unit of brain cells experiences a massive electrical discharge. These outbursts can occur anywhere in the brain. There may be one seizure per year to several per day due to these discharges [1]. Epilepsy refers to neuronal activity within the brain that is abnormally excessive or synchronized, resulting in rapid onset of symptoms. Séizure is a Greek word that means "to take hold" [2]. Paroxysmal symptoms and indicators of increased brain electrical activity are the typical clinical manifestation of dysfunctional neural circuits. Seizures can be caused by various neurological conditions and are associated with a wide range of expressions since they originate from any part of the cerebral cortex [3]. Most unexpected physical or psychological episodes, some of which are not even pathogenic, resemble epileptic seizures. Epileptic seizures are regular, unpredictable disturbances of normal brain function [2]. Over 50 million people, or 1% of the world's population, deal with epilepsy. Antiepileptic medications are used to treat seizures in two-thirds of those who are affected.

Over 50 million people, or 1% of the world's population, deal with epilepsy. Antiepileptic medications are used to treat seizures in two-thirds of those who are affected. As a result, none of the known therapies can control seizures in roughly 25% of people. The seemingly random unpredictability of seizures is one of the most traumatic aspects of epilepsy. Episodes of gazing, aimless walking, or lack of awareness that could be unimportant if they happen at home might be catastrophic when the patient is operating a motor vehicle, crossing a busy street, or swimming alone [4].

1.2 Categorization of Epileptic Seizures

In 2001, the International League against Epilepsy (ILAE) proposed a new diagnosis system to address the limitations of the seizure categorization published in 1981 [5, 6]. Seizures can still be classified by semiological characteristics or by preexisting distinctions between focalized and generalized seizures. Clinically, focal and generalized seizure classifications are often based on EEG and imaging data rather than semiological criteria. Another method of seizure classification relies solely on semiological criteria [7]. The classification of epileptogenic zones/epilepsy symptoms differentiates between focal and generalized seizures instead of focusing on the extent of the epileptic seizure. An expert visual assessment is traditionally used to analyze seizures and focuses primarily on apparent ictal features. Based on their ictal manifestations, epileptic seizures fall into four categories. A. Sensorial sphere, B. Autonomic sphere, C. Motor sphere, D. Consciousness.

The category "special seizures" refers to seizures that cannot be categorized into any of the four above mentioned categories. The majority of the seizures listed in this category are classified as "negative" ictal phenomena (atonic seizures, adverse myoclonic seizures, etc.). The semiological seizure categorization allows for the most accurate classification of seizures in the context of the available information (Table 1) [8].

2 Pathology of Epileptic Seizures

In the brain, the intense and irregular electrical activity is the principal cause of epileptic seizures [2]. Different parts of the brain, including temporal, frontal, parietal, and occipital lobes, reflect this pathological condition [9, 10]. Epilepsy can have multiple causes, even though its exact etiology is not yet established. In addition to factors like birth abnormalities, brain infections, brain tumors, strokes, and brain damage [2], genetic mutations seem to have a significant influence on the development of the condition [1]. Antiepileptic medicines are typically used as prophylactic therapy before seizures arise but are not used as on-demand treatments since seizures frequently start suddenly and unexpectedly [11].

3 Smart Nano-materials for the Treatment and Management of Epilepsy and Seizures

The main obstacle to this illness's treatment is the lack of an accurate diagnosis, which can be caused by several issues, including a lack of clinical experts' knowledge and training, their inability to recognize symptoms, or their common symptoms being misinterpreted by other conditions like migraine, movement disorders, psychosis, hysteria, and brain injuries that are erratically labelled as epilepsy [12–14].

The term "nanotheranostics," which offers improved structural qualities, non-invasive ways for better distribution, and faster therapeutic action, has been developed for the frequent and extensive use of nanotechnology in theranostics. Nanotheranostics, which provides a platform to distribute, actives while concurrently monitoring their therapeutic impact at diseased locations, helps establish a relationship between the human biological system and associated disorders. Numerous nanocarriers, like micelles, solid lipid nanoparticles, polymeric ligands, liposomes, dendrimers, quantum dots, nanosponges, nanoconjugates, silver and gold nanoparticles, and others [14–18], can be used for targeted distribution with diagnostic features.

Table.1 The semiological classification of epilepsy

Sl. no.	Seizure types	Characteristic
1	Auras	Auras, often known as "warning symptoms," typically appear at the start of a seizure and can endure for several minutes or a few seconds
1.1	Somatosensory aura	Somatosensory auras comprise somatosensory signals localized to a specific body area, like tingling on one side of the face or arm
1.2	Autonomic aura	Tachycardia, sweating, and altered breathing are associated with autonomic auras. Autonomic symptoms can be brought on by epileptic activation of the anterior cingulated gyrus and the basal frontal area
1.3	Visual aura	Visual auras, caused by visual cortex epileptic activity, typically appear as "bright spots" or occasionally as "black spots"
1.4	Olfactory aura	Olfactory auras are generally uncommon and a sign of amygdale or, less frequently, orbitofrontal region of gyrus rectus activation during epilepsy
1.5	Auditory aura	As a result of the epileptic activation of Heschl's gyrus, auditory auras include auditory hallucinations like sounds. This symptom is associated with the temporal association cortex
1.6	Gustatory aura	Auras that cause the feeling of taste are known as gustatory auras and are uncommon
1.7	Abdominal aura	A confused, uncomfortable feeling in the stomach, as if something were rising, is among the most common characteristic of abdominal auras. It is most likely that epileptic activation of the insula is the cause of this aura's frequent association with temporal lobe epilepsy
1.8	Psychic aura	Psychic auras are characterized by a "weird feeling" that appears whenever the internal or external world is interpreted incorrectly. Psychic auras are caused by temporal association and cortex stimulation during epilepsy
2	Autonomic seizures	These unusual seizures are captured on polygraphic recordings and show distinct EEG seizure patterns. However, they only negatively affect the autonomic nervous system without the patient knowing it, such as tachycardia or ictal pallor
3	Dialeptic seizures	Dialeptic seizures are connected to a state of altered awareness during which patients cannot respond to outside stimuli or only partially and cannot be recalled later. Dialeptic seizures accompany numerous focal and generalized epilepsies
4 4.1	Motor seizures Simple motor seizures	Electrical stimulation of the primary and supplementary sensorimotor areas can mimic the abnormal, generally basic movements that define these seizures. Based on the muscles involved, duration of the muscle contraction, and rhythm of recurrence of the action, simple motor seizures can be classified into the following subtypes: Epileptic spasm, versive, tonic, clonic, hypermotor, automotor, gelastic, myoclonic and tonic–clonic seizure

(continued)

Table.1 (continued)

Sl. no.	Seizure types	Characteristic
4.2	Complex motor seizures	These are characterized by relatively complex motions that mimic regular movements (sometimes known as "automatisms") and frequently involve multiple body parts moving in various planes. Depending on the nature of the automatisms, three categories of complex motor seizures are subdivided: Hypermotor, Gelastic, and Automotor seizures
5	Special seizures	Most of these seizures certainly influence motor (atonic, akinetic) or cognitive (aphasic) activity in a negative aspect
5.1	Atonic seizure	A transient collapse of postural tone that causes a loss of posture (head drop, falls, etc.) is a marker of atonic seizures. The axial muscles are predominantly affected
5.2	Astatic seizure	Atonic, myoclonic, or tonic seizures can cause atonic seizures, characterized by epileptic falls
5.3	Akinetic seizure	The difficulty in making voluntary movements is a characteristic of akinetic seizures. The whole body or just some parts of it may be affected by the inability to start and maintain voluntary movements
5.4	Hypomotor seizure	In these seizures, the level of motor activity is diminished or completely absent
5.5	Negative myoclonic seizure	A negative myoclonic seizure, also known as epileptic negative myoclonus, consists of brief episodes of muscular atonia lasting between 30 and 400 ms. The seizure does not happen when the patient is at rest; instead, it manifests clinically during muscle contractions
5.6	Aphasic seizure	This seizure causes inability to speak or understand language. Most likely, aphasic seizures are caused by epileptic activation of language-processing regions in the hemisphere that control speech

Recently, huge developments in the field of delivery systems, which provide therapeutically active agents or naturally occurring compounds that are effective for specific targeted drug delivery. This is for the treatment of various neurodisorders like epilepsy, seizures, etc. [19, 20]. At present, there are different types of drug delivery systems that are very efficient, but they still face many challenges that must be addressed and advanced technologies must be developed to improve drug delivery. Biomedical nanocarriers are typically sized between 1 and 1000 nm and can carry therapeutics and diagnostics, individually or in combination, to specific biological targets [21]. Bio-distribution and bioavailability of these compounds are often determined by their size, morphology, charge, and surface chemistry [22]. Physiochemical properties, formation methods, and cargo loading characteristics determine the classification of nanocarriers [23]. It is popular for nanomedicine strategies to deliver both hydrophilic and hydrophobic payloads simultaneously [24].

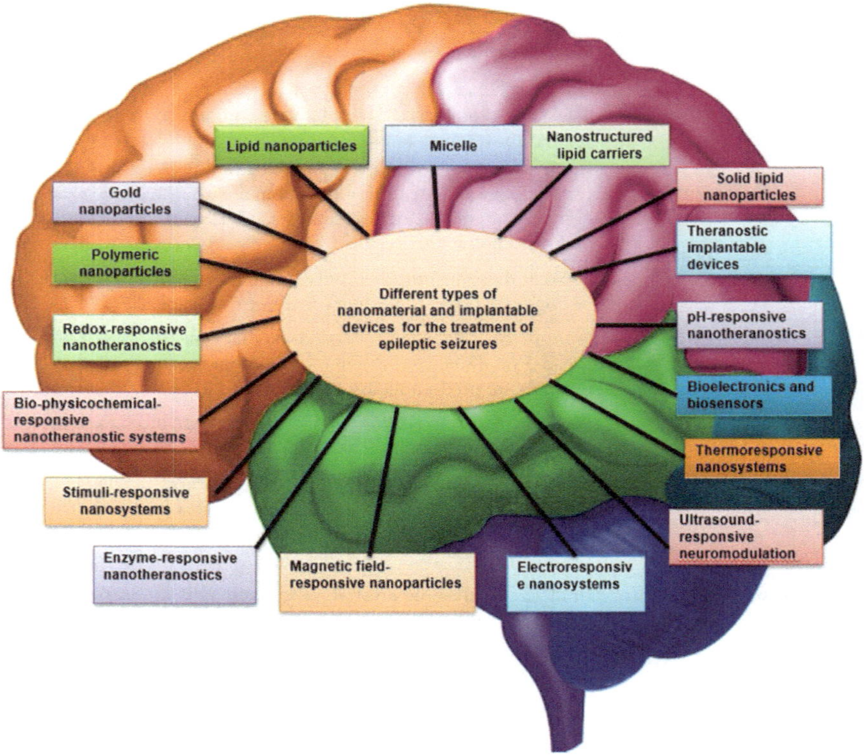

Fig. 1 Different types of nanomaterial and implantable devices for the treatment of epileptic seizure

There are currently insufficient, temporary, and noneffective methods and medications available for preventing and treating epilepsy. Thus, smart nanomaterial-based drug delivery systems are currently studied that will surely facilitate advanced drug delivery systems [25]. Here, we present some updated smart nanomaterial and implantable devices for delivering therapeutic moieties in the treatment and management of epileptic seizures in Fig. 1.

3.1 Polymeric Nanoparticle

Polymeric nanoparticles (PNPs) are currently one of the Control Drug Delivery System used most frequently [26]. These nanocarriers, whose sizes range from 10 to 1000 nm, are made of polymeric structures, as their name implies. PNPs can have both positive and negative surface charges depending on their natural or synthetic polymer composition. This characteristic significantly influences biological behaviour, mucoadhesion, and cell penetration. PNPs can also be formed as nanospheres or nanocapsules. In vesicular nanocapsules, the drug is dissolved in a liquid core enclosed in a polymer shell. In contrast, nanospheres consist of a polymer matrix in which drugs are dispersed in the gaps of the matrix. They are also adsorbed on their spherical surfaces. The latter PNP encapsulates large amounts of drugs [27, 28]. PNP can cross physiological barriers such as BBB, improving drug bioavailability and biodistribution [29]. They simultaneously enable drug release kinetics control, thereby, consequently, extending therapeutic action [30, 31].

Furthermore, PNP protects drugs from enzymatic degradation and immune system action. PNP characteristics are determined by the polymeric matrix. This matrix can be formed from a wide range of polymers or polymer combinations. The polymers that are most frequently employed for the production of PNP include polylactide (PLA), poly(lactide-co-glycolide) (PLGA), chitosan, polyethyleneimine (PEI), polycaprolactone (PCL), and chitosan, all of which have received FDA approval for use in biomedical applications [21, 32, 33]. Polymeric matrix surface functionalization enables selective PNP targeting to therapeutic targets. Many efforts have been made in recent years to enable these drugs' administration. PNP enhances the pharmacological treatment of epilepsy and decreases the number of patients with ASM resistance. A study by Musumeci et al. They developed PNP for the intranasal (IN) administration of oxcarbazepine as an illustration of this (OXC). A PLGA polymeric matrix was used to encapsulate the OXCs in these nanoparticles. They showed that PLGA-NP could reduce drug administration poses up to a single dose every 24 h. Consequently, multiple administrations were reduced, and seizures were controlled more effectively. They also showed that these PNP accumulated in the brain after Intranasal (IN) administration and had a neuroprotective effect [34].

In a different study, Zybina et al. In 2018, PNP was successfully encapsulated with carbamazepine (CBZ). These NPs showed that encapsulated CBZ was 30 times more effective against seizures than free CBZ. They also demonstrated that encapsulating CBZ into PNP overcomes drug resistance mediated by Pgp. PGP is one of the main transporters that restricts drug entry into the brain. While Pgp is responsible for some patients' resistance to ASM treatment, it is extremely promising that PLGA NP has overcome this complication [35]. Kaur et al. [36] developed chitosan-coated PLGA PNP with high mucoadhesive properties to contain these TRH analogs for IN administration. In vivo studies showed that thyrotropin-releasing hormone (TRH) NP significantly reduced seizures and neuronal death in the pentylenetetrazole (PTZ)—induced seizures model, demonstrating not only that TRH PNP could reach the brain after IN administration [36].

According to Zhu et al. [37], a further study found that piperine-loaded PNP that was functionalized with copper oxide quantum dots and coated with hyaluronic acid significantly reduced convulsions after IN administration [37]. Moreover, piperine has also been encapsulated into chitosan PNP for IP administration, showing increased neuroprotectant properties against free piperine [38]. Furthermore, Cano et al. [39] formulate PNP capable of encapsulating epigallocatechin-3-gallate (EGCG), one of the most common catechins in tea. Although EGCG reduces seizure episodes, the mechanism is unclear [32, 40]. Additional research, like that done by Bohrey et al. [41], has developed PNP with therapeutic potential for epilepsy treatment. The authors observed diazepam, which is used to treat seizures while an epileptic episode occurs. Though their size is much larger than 200 nm, which may make it difficult for them to penetrate the BBB, in vitro and in vivo, testing is required in this study to confirm that diazepam-loaded PNP is effective and can cross the BBB [41]. In addition, Lopalco et al. [42] developed a formulation of PNP that contained OXC and used PLGA as a polymer as a therapeutic tool to treat epilepsy in pregnant women. In this scenario, increased efforts are needed to optimize the formulation to produce a targeted drug delivery carrier beneficial for pregnant women [42].

3.2 Lipid Nanoparticles

Lipid nanoparticles (LNP) are one of the most adaptable nanoparticulate drug delivery systems because they have low toxicity and a high loading capacity. These nanocarriers can pass through the BBB through transcellular pathways due to structural similarities between NP (often derived from natural sources) and the endothelial cells of the BBB. Additionally, because of their biocompatibility and low immunogenicity, they are a suitable candidate for treating CNS diseases.

LNPs are classified into two types, solid lipid nanoparticles (SLNs), the first generation of lipid nanoparticles, and nanostructured lipid carriers (NLCs), the second generation. NLC offers improved stability, enhanced loading capacity, and the prevention of drug expulsion during storage [43]. Several studies have demonstrated that SLN and NLC have anticonvulsant properties. Additionally, they can deliver medications deep into the brain because of their physicochemical properties. Therefore, SLN and NLC are the most widely used lipid-based nanocarriers for neurological disorders.

3.2.1 Solid Lipid Nanoparticles

SLNs are biocompatible and biodegradable lipid-based colloidal carriers stabilized by a suitable surfactant. At body temperature, SLN has a solid structure with an average size between 50 and 1000 nm [32, 33, 44, 45]. Some advantages of SLN as pharmaceutical drug delivery carriers include the use of safe, recognized excipients (which is not the case with the organic solvents used in the fabrication of PNP); protection of the chemical compounds incorporated; high physical stability in comparison to liposomes; a propensity to incorporate both lipophilic and hydrophilic molecules; sustained release of the drugs; simplicity in fabrication; and targeting mechanisms. Research shows that SLN is mostly used to treat epilepsy. Curcumin-containing synthetic SLN, used to treat epilepsy, was developed by Huang et al. Curcumin is a naturally occurring antioxidant and neuroprotectant that was found in 2020. Curcumin SLN's potential as an acid sphingomyelinase (ASM) was demonstrated in fascinating in vitro studies developed by researchers. In vivo, tests are required to confirm the efficacy of this strategy, even though the results were very positive

[46]. Alprazolam-loaded SLN (APZ) was discovered to be distributed throughout the body, according to Singh et al. [47]. Glyceryl monostearate develops the SLN. By combining radioactive tracers with APZ and SLN loaded with APZ, their biodistribution was investigated in rats. Intranasal (IN) and intravenous (IV) routes were used to administer these formulations. According to the author's observations, the brain concentration was shown to be substantially higher following IN administration than after IV administration. Second, they observed that, as compared to SLN administered via the same route, the concentration of APZ solution by the IN route remained much lower. Because of the enhanced bioavailability, we were able to confirm that loading APZ into SLN could reduce the APZ dose. The SLN formulation also shows improved targeting efficiency. The blood–brain barrier's low-density lipid receptors, according to the authors, maybe the cause of this fact [47]. Nair et al. [48] also did a study that demonstrated that SLN is coated with chitosan and includes CBZ created by phospholipid R80H. They investigated whether CBZ-loaded SLN displayed anticonvulsant activity in rats following administration of CBZ solution, CBZ-loaded SLN without chitosan, and CBZ-loaded SLN with chitosan (dose of 1 mL/100 mg body weight). According to the authors' evaluations, CBZ SLN with and without chitosan had varying therapeutic activity levels. The maximal electro-shock (MES) method, which applies an electrical stimulus through ear electrodes, showed better activity in SLN with chitosan. However, when applied to the isoniazid-induced convulsions (INH) method, SLN without chitosan showed superior anticonvulsant activity. Chitosan-loaded SLN has a better chance of success due to its higher CBZ encapsulation and improved physical stability. The investigation will, however, be illuminated by additional analyses [48].

3.2.2 Nanostructured Lipid Carriers

The purpose of creating nanostructured lipid carriers was to overcome the drawbacks of SLN. The nanostructure contains liquid and solid lipids in a matrix. NLC over SLN has several advantages, including a better crystallinity index and a slower polymorphic transition. These advantages lead to higher loading capacity (due to liquid oil droplets embedded in the matrix), greater drug immobilization, and fewer molecules expelled during storage. In contrast to PNP, SLN, and NLC cannot entrap hydrophilic drugs like PNP due to their partitioning effects during production. As Scioli Montoto et al. [49] demonstrated, biodegradable lipids can be loaded into NLCs, including Crodamol®, cetyl esters wax, and lipid myristyl myristate. During their preliminary study, IP was administered along with CBZ controls (30 mg/kg of CBZ solution), two negative controls (empty NLC and physiological solution), and an IP NLC containing CBZ. It was shown that the CBZ control and CBZ NLC exhibited anticonvulsant activity for 4 h. Despite this, only the CBZ NLC showed effective therapeutic activity after four hours, likely due to the prolonged release of CBZ from the core of the NLC. Scioli Montoto et al. [50] have synthesized OXCBZ NLC for in vitro experiments. It was found that free OXCBZ had less permeability to MDCK-MDR1 cells than free OXCBZ. They concluded that the developed NLC did not interact with the investigated immunoglobulin or bovine serum albumin. However, in vivo studies are required for this research [50]. Eskandari et al. [51] found that sodium valproate (VPA) loaded into NLC administered by the IN route exhibited comparable neuroprotective activity to VPA control. This study showed that IN administration of VPA into NLC might be an effective epilepsy treatment [51].

3.3 Liposome

Liposomes are spherical vesicles with an aqueous core surrounded by phospholipids, artificial amphiphiles, and sterols. They are found in one or more bilayers with particle sizes ranging from 25 to 2500 nm. They form reversible structures due to noncovalent interactions between molecules. This lipid-based drug delivery carrier is suitable for hydrophilic and lipophilic drugs as it has aqueous and lipidic layers. Liposomes are nontoxic, stable, have high vascular density, and have adjustable surface nanocarriers with a high retention time at the targeted site. It can deliver macromolecules like DNA, proteins, imaging agents, and active chemotherapeutic agents. Liposome preparation generally begins with drying lipids in organic solvents, dispersing them in aqueous media, followed by purification and analysis. Phospholipids like phosphatidylethanolamine and phosphatidylcholine are commonly used in liposome preparation. Limitations and benefits of liposome drug carriers depend on liposome interaction with cells and their fate in vivo after administration. Liposomes interact with cell surfaces through adsorption and endocytosis. A functional modification of the liposomal drug delivery system is necessary to overcome the bio-physiochemical difficulties active medicaments face in reaching their targeted sites and the need to remain in the circulation cycle [52–56].

A variety of modifications are made to liposomes to improve their ability to cross the blood–brain barrier and enhance circulation. Generally, unmodified liposomes can recognize reticuloendothelial cells for phagocytosis [56].

A hollow gold nanoparticle-tethered liposome formulation loaded with Muscimol causes rapid hyperpolarization in neurons and suppresses seizures. It acts like a physiological inhibitory post-synaptic potential [43]. A seizure occurs when epileptic neurons undergo prolonged depolarization with continuous action potential bursts. The GABA-A agonist (Muscimol) controls hyperpolarization in seizures and Parkinson's. Another drug commonly used for convulsions is valproic acid. Jufri et al. [57] have found that intranasal valproic acid-loaded liposomes have better brain uptake than plasma [57]. In another study, tocopherol (Toc) and omega-3 fatty acid-enriched liposomes loaded with tacrine, an anti-Alzheimer drug, showed better drug permeability and cellular uptake when given through the intranasal route [58].

3.4 Micelles

The micelle is a colloidal dispersion formed by supramolecular assemblies of surfactant phospholipids in water. It is about 10–100 nm in size spherical-shaped compound that contains hydrophilic regions (polar head groups) and hydrophobic regions (the long hydrophobic chain). Micelle may be of two types-polymeric and nonpolymeric. Polymeric or nonpolymeric micelles containing amphiphilic surfactants are more effective at delivering drugs to the central nervous system. But nonpolymeric micelle is better biodistribution and stability. As a result of the external hydrophilic shell, micelles are stable in an aqueous environment and can circulate longer in the bloodstream. It further facilitates their accumulation in areas with leaky vessels by protecting them from reticuloendothelial (RES) attacks. A micelle can carry low molecular mass hydrophobic drugs, proteins, and genes. Micelles are stable at high polymer concentrations but become unstable when diluted below a critical micelle concentration and release the loaded drug prematurely. Even micelle releases the drugs when it comes to contact with systemic circulation [59–62].

A variety of modifications are made to micelles to improve their ability to cross the blood–brain barrier. In one attempt, a polyclonal antibody attaches to a micelle against 2-GP or insulin to attack the luminal side of BBB. In this attempt, the researchers have found that drug delivery to the brain increases[63]. In another study, transferrin-modified cyclopeptide conjugated micelles were found to increase Paclitaxel uptake by brain microvascular endothelial cells [64]. Recently, Wu et al. [65] found that thermo-sensitive micelle loaded with caspase-1 inhibitor CZL80 reduces caspase-1 enzyme activity. This modified treatment profile was implanted on febrile seizures attenuated mice. A febrile seizure is an unpredictable convulsive seizure associated with hyperthermia. The incorporation of thermo-sensitive micelles that release drugs upon local heat stimulation extends the therapeutic window [65]. In a reported case study by Sun et al. [66] have found that Cremophor EL-free polymeric micelle loaded with paclitaxel can be useful for nonconvulsive seizure patients [66].

In preclinical studies for the treatment of epilepsy and seizure, some effective antiepileptic drugs are used as nanocarriers:

Table.1 Some implantable devices are also used in epileptic seizures

Drug	Nanocarriers	Outcome	References
Oxcarbazepine	Polymeric nanoparticles	Oxcarbazepine with PLGA showed a potent neuroprotective effect when administered intranasal	[34]
Piperine	Polymeric nanoparticles	Have potent anticonvulsant activity in PTZ	[37]
Epigallocatechin	Polymeric nanoparticle	Polylactic glycolic acid conjugated with polyethylene glycol polymeric nanoparticles given intranasally showed potent neuroprotective activity	[39]

(continued)

(continued)

Drug	Nanocarriers	Outcome	References
Diazepam	Polymeric nanoparticles	Diazepam conjugated with PLGA nanoparticles showed a potent neuroprotective response	[41]
Curcumin	Solid Lipid nanoparticle	Have neuroprotective activity and also have potential efficiency against oxidative damage	[46]
Alprazolam	Solid Lipid Nanoparticles	At lower doses, the SLN increased bioavailability Administration of SLN through intranasal route, higher concentration of drug reaches into the brain	[47]
Carbamazepine	Solid Lipid nanoparticle (SLN)	It shows better anticonvulsant activity when solid lipid nanoparticles conjugated with chitosan and showed good activity against convulsion	[48]
Valproic acid	Nanostructured Lipid carriers (NLC)	When taken in intranasal route, higher concentration of drug reaches into the brain and in same protective effect as systemic administration was observed with lower doses	[51]
Clonazepam Lipid nanoparticle	Solid Lipid Nanoparticle and Nanostructured Lipid Carrier	Formulation was incorporated into a thermosensitive mucoadhesive gel NLC significantly protects the animals against chemically induced convulsions	[67]
Catechin hydrate	Polymeric nanoparticle	Improved brain biodistribution in brain	[68]
Lamotrigine	Nanostructured Lipid nanoparticles (NLC)	Compared to intrasnasal or oral administration, intranasal administration maintained the effects of Lamotrigine, crossing the brain in a higher concentration, and increasing residence time in the brain	[69]
TRH analogues (NP355 and NP 647)	Polymeric nanoparticles	TRH analogues conjugate with PLGA and chitosan taken intranasally showed anticonvulsant efficacy and also decreased neuronal damage	[70]
Lacosamide conjugated glucose coated gold nanoparticles	Gold nanoparticles	Decrease seizure severity and frequency Glucose-coated gold nanoparticles can efficiently transfer antiepileptic drugs into the brain in drug-resistant epilepsy	[71]

4 Nanotheranostics Strategies in Epilepsy

Currently, antiepileptic medications are ineffective, short-lived, and incapable of relieving epileptic patients. An exciting new field is theranostics, which addresses the problems of real-time physiological change detection in early disease development, biomarker location, and subsequent applications using novel approaches, such as bioelectronics, biosensors, implantable devices, stimuli-responsive devices, and so on, to stop epilepsy from progressing further.

4.1 Theranostic Implantable Devices

Various body components have been implanted with theranostics over the past 20 years, including pacemakers, bone implants, dental implants, brain stimulation models, and signal monitoring methods. Researchers are currently studying implantable devices like nanobots and biodegradable polymer implants equipped with nanocarriers to help improve bioavailability and concentrate the action of epilepsy medications. In neuromodulation, bioelectronics is used to integrate electroencephalogram (EEG) data, process and amplify the signals, then deliver AEDs concurrently in response to seizures that are detected through transducers. Researchers have developed an energy-saving device with seizure detection and a neuronal signal amplifier for temporal lobe epilepsy treatment (TLE). As a result of this asynchronous design, the device was adapted for use in neurophysiology diagnosis and was stable in a transient state until epilepsy changed the physiological conditions. Through self-triggered drug injections, the drug was released in discrete doses after detection by a micro pump-based unit [70]. According to the experiments, seizures were detected 8 s before the time when the seizure progression time (22 s) ended, and they were suppressed within five seconds of detection, indicating fast activity. Although this study did not use nanotechnology-based medicine, the advantages still include a 49% reduction in power consumption and a low dose of parenteral medication (35–50 μL). Thus, extending the use of nanocarriers is crucial in the development of new theranostic devices. A flexible implantable chip with silicon dioxide nanoparticles dispersed in a core of iron oxide has been composed of an indium tin oxide-coated PET substrate. This device generated gradual changes in drug elution profiles in the presence of an external magnetic field, indicating a burst release of ethosuximide. The in-vitro investigations showed that 100% of the medication was released in an hour when a high magnetic field (2.5 kA m^{-1}) was applied, but only 10% when there was no magnetic induction. The anti-epileptic activity was determined by lowering the number of spike-wave discharges (by roughly 30 to 50%) and their length in in-vivo tests using an external magnetic field [72]. The amount of drug released was not quantified. A study focused on adenosine molecules that had been entrapped and were delivered to the brain at specific doses for sustained delivery. This was done using a biodegradable matrix made up of silk fibroin. This device was developed as a 3D nanofilm-coated, water-porous silk scaffold. This device released target doses of adenosine (40, 200, and 1000 ng adenosine day^{-1}) in the hippocampus. In focal or partial seizures, an adenosine deficiency is treated with focal Adenosine Augmentation Therapy (AAT). The rats received doses of 1000 ng of adenosine, which showed a delayed onset of epilepsy by preventing seizures during the first 23 stimulations. Additionally, the amount of kindling stimulation required to cause partial seizures to progress to stages 1 or 2 increased at this dose, exhibiting anti-epileptic effects. Although seizure suppression was not the primary goal of this study, it was noticed that the after-discharge period was shorter (less than 100 s for a 1000 ng dose) [73].

4.2 Bioelectronics and Biosensors

Various bioelectronics or bio-electrochemical techniques can detect neurotransmitters, physiological biomarkers, or epilepsy-specific proteins and amino acids. As an alternative to conventional diagnostic tools, bio-electrode microarrays contain silicon-modified platinum metal nanoparticles and enzymes that have been specially formulated. These arrays demonstrated impressive diagnostic results and potentially complicated focal seizure mechanisms. [74] Such "on-demand" and desirable drug release mechanisms have the potential to be modified in the future to develop theranostic systems at the nanoscale level for epilepsy treatment. By changing surface properties, increasing polymer biocompatibility, and improving drug loading capabilities, biosensors [75–78] have an advantage over other implants. In response to a seizure attack, multipurpose in vivo treatments like self-powered triboelectric nanogenerators release the medication at the targeted site when employing nanobiosensors.

5 Bio-physicochemical-Responsive Nanotheranostics Systems

Epilepsy nanodiagnostic systems emphasize two distinct aspects: (1) the presence of biomarkers as important tools for detection and treatment that play a crucial role in the pathogenesis, progression, and dangerous effects of seizures; and (2) pathways involved in the stimulation and prolonged duration of epileptic seizures. When choosing nanosystems for epilepsy treatment, oxidation, energy metabolism, amino acid transport, and other physiological processes must be taken into account. The presence of excessive amounts of neurotransmitters, the breakdown of the blood–brain barrier, the dysfunction of ion channels, the existence of excessive numbers of tight junctions, or the overexpression of receptors are just a few examples of how brain chemistry affects physiological processes like oxidation, energy metabolism, amino acid transport, and other processes [79, 80]. Nanosystems work on the brain to treat epilepsy. Bio-physicochemical-responsive nanotheranostics devices enhance conditions in afflicted areas by altering biomolecules such as peptides, amino acids, antibodies, mRNAs, and others for "on-demand use."

5.1 Stimuli-Responsive Nanosystems Used in Epilepsy

Epilepsy treatment methods like ultrasound, laser ablation, radiosurgery, heat-reduction therapy, and others are now being transformed into noninvasive in-situ theranostics using nanotechnology. Currently, there are two types of stimuli-responsive systems: (1) external stimuli like magnetic, electrical, ultrasonic, heat, NIR radiations, and UV; and (2) internal (physiological) stimuli where the body itself acts as a reservoir for activating sources like oxidative state, pH, enzymes, ionic potential, etc. [81–83].

5.2 Magnetic Field-Responsive Nanoparticles

Iron oxide, a superparamagnetic nanoparticle (SPION), is impacted by an external magnetic field for therapeutic and diagnostic applications. It is made up of two unpaired electrons. Depending on their structural make-up, superparamagnetic iron oxide nanoparticles (SPIONs) are either coated with medications to serve as MRI contrast agents or serve as a vehicle for a variety of therapeutic substances, including medications, antibodies, and nucleic acids (primarily miRNA) for effective delivery. SPION size, drug delivery place, targeted receptors, contrast intensity, and epilepsy type are all considered important variables. This can be between 10 and 100 nm. Better absorption by individual cells, increased drug availability at the targeted region, and biocompatibility are the best ways to illustrate their superior qualities for nanocarrier manufacturing [60, 61]. Additionally, carriers made of biodegradable polymeric SPIONs or SPIONs with surface alterations demonstrated increased performance. For generating heat from a magnetic field to release medicines, they were regarded as stimuli-responsive systems [17, 84, 85]. Iron oxide nanoparticles can be modified with fluorescent dyes to enable fluorescent imaging, which enables the creation of optically active nanoparticles that detect antigens in epilepsy [17]. The effects of SPION on epilepsy were demonstrated using electrophysiological and EEG recordings, and their route was studied using an MRI scan [86].

5.3 Thermoresponsive Nanosystems

One of the most distinctive areas of epileptic seizure initiation. This uses an MRI and an ultrasound-guided probe to eliminate seizure-focal areas. However, this procedure is incredibly invasive and comes with risks like bleeding, infection, brain damage, and more. Innovative and noninvasive techniques are required to suppress epilepsy progression in order to prevent such complications. Temperature-responsive or thermoresponsive systems alter their physical properties in response to temperature [87]. Thermoresponse is a special characteristic that releases medication in a controlled way and can help febrile seizures. Photothermal therapy relies on external sources such as radiation and heat to release drugs [83]. Thermoresponsive nanocarriers are polymers that respond to temperatures above their lower critical solution temperature (LCST), including poly(N-isopropylacrylamide-co-acrylic acid), poly(vinylcaprolactam), poly(N,N-diethylacrylamide), and pluronics. In order to release the drug in a controlled and temperature-dependent manner, the hydrophilicity of the polymeric nanocarriers is reduced at temperatures above this range, and structural swelling or shrinkage results from hydrophobic interactions [81–83]. The concept of increased heat or temperature produced by excessive neuronal firing or inflammation in epilepsy is used with absorptive nanomaterials and polymers. This is used to develop internally triggered drug release systems for acute epilepsy. Similar to this, nanocarriers are subjected to external heat stimulations like magnetic fields, ultrasound, and UV radiation to potentiate their antiepileptic effects. When exposed to temperatures of 37°C or higher, self-assembling ethosuximide-loaded nanocapsules made of glycerolphosphate-modified chitosan formed a gel. The glycerolphosphate was attached to reduce the repulsive forces between the chitosan nanocapsules, which made the sol–gel transition visible. By the third day of administration, this special injectable thermo-gelling nanogel with 10 mg/mL of the drug suppressed abnormal neuronal firings and decreased spike wave discharges to 50% as visually observed using MRI in a partial seizure animal model [88].

5.4 Electro-responsive Nanosystems

Electric potentials are used as a source to show the sustained or pulsatile release kinetics of a medication. This is done to alter the mechanical structure of nanotheranostic systems. Electrical impulses serve as excellent stimuli in epilepsy, leading to significant attention to neuronal signaling pathways in neuroscience. This kind of stimuli-responsive mechanism often releases drugs via an external electrical field [82]. However, in neurological diseases like epilepsy, excessive electrical signals are generated in-vivo without the usage of external electrical sources. the application of outside electrical sources to treat neurological disorders like epilepsy. In excess neuronal signals in electroresponsive theranostic systems, materials with ionizable groups in their structures, such as electroactive polymers or polyelectrolytes, such as polyaniline, polyphenylacetylene, polypyrrole, polythiophene, polyaniline, ethylene vinyl acetate, and polyethylene, as well as ionic polymer gels, change in volume, size, and shape[82, 83]. These polymers are included into different nanostructures, such as self-assembling micelles, nanohydrogels, and others, to increase stability and solubility. These substances act as a biotransducer or biosensor to detect the presence of neurotransmitters, ionic potential, and membrane flow in the brain. They appear to be perfect for identifying specific physiological and serological indicators, including high levels of electrolytes or brain vibrational excitation. Currently available electroresponsive systems function through a variety of neurostimulating mechanisms. One of these involves the prompt release of an anti-epileptic medicine after the automatic gathering of electrical data from an epileptic brain to identify and record from EEG, as stated in the case of closed-loop implantable devices. One epileptic study created protein-bound phenytoin sodium-loaded nanoparticles (doses 10–20 mg kg^{-1}) with the help of an electroresponsive sodium 4-vinylbenzene sulfonate (NaSS) hydrogel to ensure better brain-plasma concentration ratios and higher drug release for "on-demand" treatment of tonic–clonic seizures[89].

5.5 *PH-Responsive Nanotheranostics*

pH-responsive carriers are crucial for site-specific drug release with few side effects. In pathological conditions, the pH value of the diseased site changes from neutral (7–7.2) to acidic or alkaline. Similar to this, pH values between 6.8 and 7.8 fluctuate in epilepsy for a variety of reasons, including hypoxia, inflammation, ionic gradients, carbonic acid presence, GABA-receptor dysfunction, and more [90, 91]. pH-responsive nanomedicines recognize the microenvironment in pathological conditions and ensure drug release at the targeted site without affecting healthy tissues. For instance, astrocytes are represented by a basic environment while neurons are represented by an acidic environment in epilepsy [92]. In addition to pH-sensitive quantum dots, other types of nanomedicine include polymer-modified hydrogels, liposomes, micelles, and nanoparticles loaded with pH-sensing actives used for epilepsy and seizures. A pH-responsive nanomedicine or polymer exhibits a therapeutic effect in acidic or basic conditions based on their functional groups. When carboxyl or amino groups are protonated in nanocarrier structures at a particular pH, solubility, volume, swelling, and conformation change [82] and the bonds between the drug and polymer weaken, allowing the drug to be released at the targeted site [93]. In order to provide pregabalin with a controlled release for five hours, a pH-sensitive nanohydrogel was found to serve as a delivery vehicle in epilepsy. Through photopolymerization using UV and visible light, a nontoxic, biocompatible, pH-responsive macromer called poly (methacrylic acid-g-ethylene glycol) was developed. According to this study, a polymer breaks down in an acidic environment. This results in only a ~15–16% drug release in the gastric environment, compared to ~70–80% in the intestinal environment with high pH. The researchers demonstrated that pH-sensitive nanocarriers could be used to treat partial seizures by showing that pregabalin (AED for partial seizures) showed swelling behavior under basic (intestinal) pH conditions while Fickian diffusion was observed under acidic (gastric) pH conditions [94]. Additionally, nanohydrogels or micelles made of these polymers, like polyethylene glycol diacrylate or amphiphilic block polymers, play a crucial role as an "on–off" switch by restoring structure after early drug release. By absorbing, recycling, and transporting glutamate, the primary neurotransmitter, endosomal systems demonstrate synaptic plasticity. As a result, endosomal pH can also be considered in epilepsy.

6 Some Other Potential Strategies for Epilepsy

6.1 Ultrasound-Responsive Neuromodulation

Focused ultrasound (FUS) therapy, a noninvasive method to control epilepsy progression without the use of ionizing radiation to minimize side effects and improve therapeutic outcomes, uses ultrasound, an imaging tool and medical device, in medicine. This method demonstrated benefits for a variety of cancers as well as neurodegenerative conditions like schizophrenia, depression, Alzheimer's disease, Parkinson's, and epilepsy [95]. With micro bubbles, it was also used to open the BBB's tight junctions so that medications could enter to treat CNS disorders [96]. As the name implies, a pulsed ultrasonic beam is directed at the targeted region or portion of the brain in order to modify synaptic transmission and modify neuronal activity. FUS modulates acoustic wave propagation with a single, concave, or phased array of waves. This reduces the frequency and duration of seizures in epileptic discharges, which is a similar principle to that used in ultrasound machines [95]. Additionally, controlled drug delivery systems have applications in theranostic nanosystems where they combine MRI guided scanners with ultrasonic energy. Nanomedicines cause biochemical changes and greater permeation to tissues in a shorter amount of time when the dose is released at a higher rate using low- and high-frequency ultrasound [95–97]. However, due to their increased susceptibility to ultrasound, polymeric nanocarriers like liposomes, dendrimers, hydrogels, and micelles demonstrated higher intracellular uptake [96, 98]. Drug release from nanocarrier centres is triggered by ultrasound-responsive polymers like Pluronic micelles, ethylene vinyl acetate copolymer, chitosan, PEG-PLA copolymers, poly (methacrylic acid), and others [81–83, 87, 99]. Drugs that contain ultrasound contrast agents offer a way to capture drug release pathways on an optical device. However, the conventional method of using an EEG or other similar instrument to identify epilepsy onset is possible. By coupling ligands, such as antibodies or peptides, to specific receptors that bind magnetic nanoparticles, the diagnostic properties of the nanocarriers are improved [86, 100]. In monkey models, low-intensity ultrasound waves were applied for 16 h. This resulted in a two-fold decrease in seizure count and seizure frequency. It prevented epileptic activities by rearranging excitatory and inhibitory synaptic responses [101]. Therefore, even though the applications of such nanosystems in epilepsy treatment have not yet been fully investigated, ultrasound-responsive nanosystems offer a novel method for enhancing drug release kinetics and achieving deep penetration effects, providing a route to creating systems with theranostic effects in the future.

6.2 Redox-Responsive Nanotheranostics

Epilepsy mechanisms are complicated and often involve looping steps. High levels of polyunsaturated fatty acids and oxidative stress may result from the brain's high oxygen requirement combined with neuronal damage. This is in cases of brain injury, hypoxia, infections, and other conditions. Reactive oxygen species (ROS) are released by oxidative stress, including peroxide, superoxide, hydroxyl oxide, nitric oxide, and others [102–104]. ROS alters the cellular functions and structures of essential enzymes involved in aerobic metabolism, resulting in brain damage. Overproduction of metabolites, especially neurotransmitters, changes ionic gradients. This activates enzymes and generates ROS while enhancing synaptic transmission. Thus, oxidative stress and metabolic dysfunction work together in a loop to increase neuronal excitability and occasionally neuronal death in epilepsy [102, 103]. In one study, patients with tonic–clonic seizures had significantly higher levels of ROS, MDA, and nitric oxide than healthy patients [103]. Antioxidants like vitamin E and ascorbic acid significantly reduced oxidation in epileptic patients [105]. As a result, ROS and molecules with redox potential like glutathione, the NADP-NADPH system, and others are studied in focused theranostic systems and are regarded as excellent biomarkers for epilepsy development as well as for diagnostic aids. Glutathione (GSH) is an antioxidant amino acid present in the brain for removing peroxidases from brain tissues, and its concentration typically ranges from 0.2 to 10 mM [82, 106, 107]. To improve visual detection or imaging of the theranostic system, many radioactive, fluorescent, or magnetic molecules can be coupled to the surface of this system. These molecules include redox-responsive gold nanoparticles with organic fluorescent dyes attached as ligands.

6.3 Enzyme-Responsive Nanotheranostics

Epilepsy is characterized by complex networks that move chemicals in the form of neurotransmitters, proteins, amino acids, glucose, and other substances from one part of the brain to another part of the brain. The creation of the major neurotransmitter glutamate by the enzyme glutaminase and the amino acid glutamine by glutamine synthethase are two examples of how enzymes are important indicators in epilepsy [108]. The enzyme glutamate opens the sodium and calcium channels in the brain, whereas the enzyme gamma-amino butyric acid transaminase (GABA-T) is in charge of breaking down the inhibitory neurotransmitter gamma-amino butyric acid. The Krebs or glucose cycle in the mitochondria helps produce energy with the assistance of oxidases and hydrolases. The functions and concentration levels of enzymes alter in the epileptic state due to the absence or overexpression of certain enzymes such glutaminase, glutamine synthase, lactase, or oxidase [108–110]. Targeting high concentrations of enzymes at a specific area in the brain is an intriguing strategy for the production of sophisticated nanocarriers. The cleavage of polymeric materials and the activation of overexpressed enzymes are brought about by a substrate or component contained in the polymeric carriers that react to enzymes [82]. In order to guarantee delivery at the intended place and prevent medication pre-systemic metabolism brought on by harmful environmental interactions, this theranostic technique also incorporates safe transport in specific brain regions. Several other processes are carried out by enzymes, such as the opening of sodium and calcium channels in the brain, which is mediated by glutamate. The majority of theranostic systems for treating epilepsy are classified as dual or multimodal-responsive systems because they use various stimuli-response methods. Better therapeutic effects are produced by nanosystems that combine two or three physiological reactions to circumstances. Multi-stimuli nanomaterials are hence ideal theranostic carriers in epilepsy and simultaneously profile multiple elements of the illness.

7 Conclusion

An epileptic seizure, the intense and irregular electrical activity in the brain, is caused by nonspecific characteristics like birth abnormalities, brain infections, tumors, strokes, damage in parts, and genetic mutations, that have limited treatment profiles. Fewer drugs can bypass the BBB and reach a targeted site in the concentration required. In the era of nanotherapeutics, different nanocarriers have been developed to bypass biological barriers. Optimization of the physical properties of nanocarriers facilitates the delivery of drugs at a specific rate and time to the desired sites. In addition to protecting the active medicament from premature degradation, nanocarriers control and improve drug distribution with intracellular accumulation, penetration, and shelf-life. Nanobiocarriers are the bioactive or targeting vectors or ligands to deliver active pharmaceutical moiety to mimic and control unnecessary cellular extravasations, growth, and cellular events. Additionally, nanobiocarriers enable the delivery of drugs with optimal bio-compatibility, bio-interaction, safety, and efficacy. A few reported nanocarriers used for the treatment of epileptic seizure are polymeric nanoparticles, solid lipid nanoparticles, liposomes, nanostructured lipid nanoparticles, and micelle. Further, theranostic implant devices and bioelectrical biosensors also can help to treat epileptic seizures by reacting to bio-physiologic changes during the epileptic seizure. Depending upon the response of these biosensors- magnetic field-responsive, thermo-responsive, electro-responsive, and pH-responsive nanoparticles can be used by loading active pharmaceutical ingredients onto them. Moreover, ultrasound response neuro-modulators, redox-responsive neurotheranostic, and enzyme-responsive neuro theranostic can be used to treat epilepsy.

References

1. Yavuz B, Yildirim O, Yilmaz AG (2021) A new approach in epilepsy treatment: nanocarrier systems. Aurum J Health Sci 3:33–44
2. Fisher RS, Boas WVE, Blume W, Elger C, Genton P, Lee P, Engel J Jr (2005) Epileptic seizures and epilepsy: definitions proposed by the International League Against Epilepsy (ILAE) and the International Bureau for Epilepsy (IBE). Epilepsia 46:470–472
3. Reichard M, Cellerino A, Valenzano DR (2015) Turquoise killifish. Curr Biol 25:R741–R742
4. Litt B, Echauz J (2002) Prediction of epileptic seizures. Lancet Neurol 1:22–30
5. Angeles D (1981) Proposal for revised clinical and electroencephalographic classification of epileptic seizures. Epilepsia 22:489–501
6. Engel J Jr, International League Against Epilepsy (ILAE) (2001) A proposed diagnostic scheme for people with epileptic seizures and with epilepsy: report of the ILAE Task Force on Classification and Terminology. Epilepsia 42:796–803
7. Noachtar S, Rosenow F, Arnold S, Baumgartner C, Ebner A, Hamer H, Holthausen H, Meencke HJ, Müller A, SakamotoA C, Steinhoff BJ, Tuxhorn I, Werhahn KJ, Winkler PA, Lüders HO (1998) Semiologic classification of epileptic seizures. Nervenarzt 69:117–126
8. Noachtar S, Peters AS (2009) Semiology of epileptic seizures: a critical review. Epilepsy Behav 15:2–9
9. Kwan P, Schachter SC, Brodie MJ (2011) Drug-resistant epilepsy. N Engl J Med 365:919–926
10. Aronica E, Mühlebner A (2018) Neuropathology of epilepsy. Handb Clin Neurol 145:193–216
11. Wang Y, Ying X, Chen L, Liu Y, Wang Y, Liang J, Xu C, Guo Y, Wang S, Hu W, Du Y, Chen Z (2016) Electroresponsive nanoparticles improve antiseizure effect of phenytoin in generalized tonic-clonic seizures. Neurotherapeutics 13:603–613
12. Goldenberg MM (2010) Pharm Ther 35:392
13. Billakota S, Devinsky O, Kim KW (2020) Neuropharmacology 170:107855
14. Kevadiya BD, Ottemann BM, Thomas MB, Mukadam I, Nigam S, Mcmillan J, Gorantla S, Bronich TK, Edagwa B, Gendelman HE (2019) Adv Drug Deliv Rev 148:252
15. Sudhakar CK, Upadhyay N, Verma A, Jain A, NarayanaCharyulu R, Jain S (2015) Nanotechnology applications for tissue engineering. William Andrew Publishing, Cambridge, USA, pp 1–19
16. Kalash RS, Lakshmanan VK, Cho C, Park I (2016) Biomaterials nanoarchitectonics. William Andrew Publishing, Cambridge, USA, pp 197–215
17. Bai RG, Muthoosamy K, Manickam S (2015) Nanotechnology applications for tissue engineering. William Andrew Publishing, Cambridge, USA, pp 195–213
18. Vogenberg FR, Isaacson C, Pursel BMPT (2010) 35:560
19. Obeid MA, Al-Qaraghuli MM, Alsaadi M, Alzahrani AR, Niwasabutra K, Ferro VA (2017) Delivering natural products and biotherapeutics to improve drug efficacy. Ther Deliv 8:947–956
20. Miele E, Spinelli GP, Miele E, Fabrizio ED, Ferretti E, Tomao S, Gulino A (2012) Nanoparticle-based delivery of small interfering RNA: challenges for cancer therapy. Int J Nanomed 7:36–37
21. Wagner V, Dullaart A, Bock AK, Zweck A (2006) Nat Biotechnol 24:1211
22. Scott EA, Karabin NB, Augsornworawat P (2017) Annu Rev Biomed Eng 19:57–84
23. Sangtan A, Nag OK, Field LD, Breger JC, Delehanty JB (2017) Wiley Interdiscip Rev: Nanomed Nanobiotechnol 9:e1466

24. Parhi P, Mohanty C, Sahoo SK (2012) Drug Discov Today 17:1044–1052
25. McNamara K, Tofail SA (2015) Nanosystems: the use of nanoalloys, metallic, bimetallic, and magnetic nanoparticles in biomedical applications. Phys Chem Chem Phys 17:27981–27995
26. Kumari A, Yadav SK, Yadav SC (2010) Biodegradable polymeric nanoparticles based drug delivery systems. Colloids Surf B Biointerfaces 75:1–18
27. Deng S, Gigliobianco MR, Censi R, Di MP (2020) Polymeric nanocapsules as nanotechnological alternative for drug delivery system: current status, challenges and opportunities. Nanomaterials 10:847
28. Adhikari C (2021) Polymer nanoparticles- preparations, applications and future insights: a concise review. Polym Technol Mater 60:1–29
29. Calzoni E, Cesaretti A, Polchi A, DiMichele A, Tancini B, Emiliani C (2019) Biocompatible polymer nanoparticles for drug de-livery applications in cancer and neurodegenerative disorder therapies. J Funct Biomater 10:1–15
30. Soppimath KSK, Aminabhavi TMTM, Kulkarni ARAR, Rudzinski WE (2001) Biodegradable polymeric nanoparticles as drug delivery devices. J Control Release 70:1–20
31. Wischke C, Schwendeman SP (2008) Principles of encapsulating hy-drophobic drugs in PLA/ PLGA microparticles. Int J Pharm 364:298–327
32. Marin E, Briceño MI, Caballero-George C (2013) Critical evaluation of biodegradable polymers used in nanodrugs. Int J Nanomedicine 8:3071–3091
33. Zielińska A, Carreiró F, Oliveira AM, Neves A, Pires B, Venkatesh DN, Durazzo A, Lucarini M, Eder P, Silva Amélia M, Santini A, Souto Eliana B (2020) Polymeric nanoparticles: production, characterization, toxicology and ecotoxicology. Molecules 25:3731
34. Musumeci T, Francesca M, Pellitteri R, Dalpiaz A, Ferraro L, Dal R, Bonaccorso A, Carbone C, Veiga F, Sancini G, Giovanni Puglisi G (2018) Oxcarbazepine free or loaded PLGA nanoparticles as effective intranasal approach to control epileptic seizures in rodents. Eur J Pharm Biopharm 133:309–320
35. Zybina A, Anshakova A, Malinovskaya J, Melnikov P, Baklaushev V, Chekhonin V, Maksimenko O, Titov S, Balabanyan V, Kreuter J, Gelperina S, Abbasova K (2018) Nanoparticle-based delivery of carbamazepine: a promising approach for the treatment of refractory epilepsy. Int J Pharm 547:10–23
36. Kaur S, Manhas P, Swami A, Bhandari R, Sharma KK (2018) Bioengineered PLGA-chitosan nanoparticles for brain targeted intranasal delivery of antiepileptic TRH analogues. Chem Eng J 346:630–639
37. Zhu D, Zhang WG, Nie XD, Ding SW, Zhang DT, Yang L (2020) Rational design of ultra-small photoluminescent copper nano- dots loaded PLGA micro-vessels for targeted co-delivery of natural piperine molecules for the treatment for epilepsy. J Photochem Photobiol B Biol 205:1–8
38. Anissian D, Ghasemi-Kasman M, Khalili-Fomeshi M (2018) Piperine- loaded chitosan-STPP nanoparticles reduce neuronal loss and astrocytes activation in chemical kindling model of epilepsy. Int J Biol Macromol 107:973–983
39. Cano A, Ettcheto M, Espina M, Auladell C, Calpena AC, Folch J, Barenys M, Sánchez-López E, Camins A, García ML (2018) Epigallocatechin-3-gallate loaded PEGylated- PLGA nanoparticles: a new anti-seizure strategy for temporal lobe epilepsy. Nanomed Nanotechnol Biol Med 14:1073–1085
40. Kim J, Park H, Jeong M, Kang T (2020) Epigallocatechin-3-gallate and PEDF 335 peptide, 67LR activators, attenuate vasogenic edema, and astroglial degeneration following status epilepticus. Antioxidants 9:854
41. Bohrey S, Chourasiya V, Pandey A (2016) Polymeric nanoparticles containing diazepam: preparation, optimization, characteri-zation, in-vitro drug release and release kinetic study. Nano Converg 3:3–9
42. Lopalco A, Ali H, Denora N, Rytting E (2015) Oxcarbazepine- loaded polymeric nanoparticles: development and permeability studies across in vitro models of the blood– brain barrier and human placental trophoblast. Int J Nanomedicine 10:1985–1996

43. Nakano T, Rizwan SB, Myint DMA, Gray J, Mackay SM, Harris P, Perk CG, Hyland BI, Empson R, Tan EW, Dani KM, Reynolds JN, Wickens JR (2022) An on-demand drug delivery system for control of epileptiform seizures. Pharmaceutics 14:468
44. Sánchez-López E, Espina M, Doktorovova S, Souto EB, García ML (2017) Lipid nanoparticles (SLN, NLC): overcoming the anatomical and physiological barriers of the eye—Part I—barriers and determining factors in ocular delivery. Eur J Pharm Biopharm 110:70–75
45. Sánchez-López E, Espina M, Doktorovova S, Souto EB, García ML (2017) Lipid nanoparticles (SLN, NLC): overcoming the anatom-ical and physiological barriers of the eye—Part II—ocular drug- loaded lipid nanoparticles. Eur J Pharm Biopharm 110:58–69
46. Huang R, Zhu Y, Lin L, Song S, Cheng L, Zhu R (2020) Solid lipid nanoparticles enhanced the neuroprotective role of curcumin against epilepsy through activation of Bcl-2 Family and P38 MAPK pathways. ACS Chem Neurosci 11:1985–1995
47. Singh AP, Saraf SK, Saraf SA (2012) SLN approach for nose- to- brain de-livery of alprazolam. Drug Deliv Transl Res 2:498–507
48. Nair R, Kumar AC, Priya VK, Yadav CM, Raju PY (2012) Formulation and evaluation of chitosan solid lipid nanoparticles of carba-mazepine. Lipids Health Dis 11:72
49. Scioli Montoto S, Sbaraglini ML, Talevi A, Couyoupetrou M, Di Ianni M, Pesce GO, Alvarez VA, Bruno-Blanch LE, Castro GR, Ruiz ME, Islan GA (2018) Carbamazepine- loaded solid lipid nanoparticles and nanostructured lipid carriers: physicochemical characterization and in vitro/in vivo evalua-tion. Colloids Surf B Biointerfaces 167:73–81
50. Scioli Montoto S, Muraca G, Di Ianni M, Couyoupetrou M, Pesce G, Islan GA, Chain CY, Vela ME, Ruiz ME, Talevi A, Castro GR (2021) Preparation, physicochemical and biopharmaceutical characterization of oxcarbazepine- loaded nanostructured lipid carriers as potential antiepileptic devices. J Drug Deliv Sci Technol 63:102470
51. Eskandari S, Varshosaz J, Minaiyan M, Tabbakhian M (2011) Brain delivery of valproic acid via intranasal administration of nano-structured lipid carriers: in vivo pharmacodynamic studies using rat electroshock model. Int J Nanomedicine 6:363–371
52. Munusamy C, John J, Verma ML (2018) Nanocarriers for drug delivery applications. Environ Chem Lett
53. Sercombe L, Veerati T, Moheimani F, Wu SY, Sood AK, Hua S (2015) Advances and challenges of liposome assisted drug delivery. Front Pharmacol 6:286
54. Skupin-Mrugalska P (2019) Nanotechnology-based targeted drug delivery systems for lung cancer. Liposome-Based Drug Deliv Lung Cancer 2019:123–160
55. Akbarzadeh A, Rezaei-Sadabady R, Davaran S, Joo SW, Zarghami N, Hanifehpour Y, Samiei M, Kouhi M, Nejati-Koshki K (2013) Liposome: classification, preparation, and applications. Nanoscale Res Lett 8(1):102
56. Naqvi S, Panghal A, Flora SJS (2020) Nanotechnology: a promising approach for delivery of neuroprotective drugs. Front Neurosci 14:494
57. Jufri M, Yuwanda A, Surini S, Harahap Y (2022) Study of valproic acid liposomes for delivery into the brain through an intranasal route. Heliyon. 8:e09030
58. Corace G, Angeloni C, Malaguti M, Hrelia S, Stein PC, Brandl M, Gotti R, Luppi B (2014) Multifunctional liposomes for nasal delivery of the anti-Alzheimer drug tacrine hydrochloride. J Liposome Res 24:323–335
59. Ozkizilcik A, Davidson P, Turgut H, Sharma HS, Sharma A, Tian ZR (2017) Nanocarriers as CNS drug delivery systems for enhanced neuroprotection. In: Sharma H, Muresanu D, Sharma A (eds) Drug and gene delivery to the central nervous system for neuroprotection. Springer, Cham, p 2017
60. Lu Y, Zhang E, Yang J, Cao Z (2018) Strategies to improve micelle stability for drug delivery. Nano Res 11:4985–4998
61. Hanafy NAN, El-Kemary M, Leporatti S (2018) Micelles structure development as a strategy to improve smart cancer therapy. Cancers (Basel) 10:238
62. Park JH, Lee S, Kim JH, Park K, Kim K, Kwon IC (2008) Polymeric nanomedicine for cancer therapy. Prog Polym Sci (Oxford) 33:113–137

63. Kabanov AV, Chekhonin VP, Alakhov VY, Batrakova EV, Lebedev AS, Melik-Nubarov NS, Arzhakov SA, Levashov AV, Morozov GV, Severin ES, Kabanov VA (1989) The neuroleptic activity of haloperidol increases after its solubilization in surfactant micelles. Micelles as microcontainers for drug targeting. FEBS Lett 258:343–345
64. Zhang P, Hu L, Yin Q, Feng L, Li Y (2012) Transferrin-modified c[RGDfK]-paclitaxel loaded hybrid micelle for sequential blood-brain barrier penetration and glioma targeting therapy. Mol Pharm 9:1590–1598
65. Wu D, Tang Y, Li W, You Y, Shi J, Xu C, Du Y, Chen Z, Wang Y (2021) Thermo-sensitive micelles extend therapeutic potential for febrile seizures. Signal Transduct Target Ther 6:296
66. Sun SY, Jin MK, Young CS, Woo LN (2018) Non-convulsive seizure related to Cremophor EL™-free, polymeric micelle formulation of paclitaxel: a case report. Obstet Gynecol Sci 61:421. https://doi.org/10.5468/ogs.2018.61.3.421
67. Abbas H, Refai H, El-Sayed N (2018) Superparamagnetic iron oxideloaded lipid nanocarriers incorporated in thermosensitive in situ gel for magnetic brain targeting of clonazepam. J Pharm Sci 107:2119–2127
68. Ahmad N, Ahmad R, Alrasheed RA, Almatar HMA, AlRamadan AS, Amir M, Sarafroz M (2020) Quantification and evaluations of catechin hydrate polymeric nanoparticles used in brain targeting for the treatment of epilepsy. Pharmaceutics 12:203
69. Alam T, Pandit J, Vohora D, Aqil M, Ali A, Sultana Y (2015) Optimization of nanostructured lipid carriers of lamotrigine for brain delivery: in vitro characterization and in vivo efficacy in epilepsy. Expert Opin Drug Deliv 12:181–194
70. Salam MT, Mirzaei M, Ly MS, Nguyen DK, Sawan M (2012) IEEE Trans Neural Syst Rehabil Eng 20:432
71. Yilmaz CU, Emik S, Orhan N, Temizyurek A, Atis M, Akcan U, Khodadust R, Arican N, Kucuk M, Gurses C, Ahishali B, Kaya M (2020) Targeted delivery of lacosamide-conjugated gold nanoparticles into the brain in temporal lobe epilepsy in rats. Life Sci
72. Huang WC, Hu SH, Liu KH, Chen SY, Mo D, Liu J (2009) Control Release 139:221
73. Wilz A, Pritchard EM, Li T, Lan JQ, Kaplan DL, Boi-sona D (2008) Biomaterials 23:1
74. Li Z, Song Y, Xiao G, Gao F, Xu S, Wang M, Zhang Y, Guo F, Liu J, Xia CX (2018) Anal Biochem 550:123
75. Shende P, Prabhakar B, Patil A (2019) TrAC - Trends Analyt Chem 121:115687
76. Shende P, Sahu MP, Gaud R (2017) Ther Deliv 8:411
77. Takke A, Shende P (2019) Curr Pharm Des 25:4108
78. Shende P, Vaidya J, Kulkarni YA, Gaud RS (2017) J Control Release 268:282
79. Raedt R, Durand DM, Boon P, Vonck K, Krames ES (2018) Neuromodulation. Academic Press, London, UK, pp 987–997. Goldenberg MM (2010) Pharm Ther 35:392
80. Vliet AV, Araujo SDC, Redeker S, Schaik RV, Aronica E, Gorter JA (2007) Brain 130:521
81. Pamfil D, Vasile C (2019) Polymeric nanomaterials in nanotherapeutics. Elsevier, Cambridge, US, pp 67–121
82. Rasheed T, Bilal M, Abu-Thabit NY, Iqbal HM (2018) Responsive polymeric nanocarriers for drug delivery applications. Woodhead Publishing, Cambridge, US, pp 61–99
83. Wells CM, Harris M, Choi L, Murali VP, Guerra FD, A Jennings (2019) J J Funct Biomater 10:34
84. Kalash RS, Lakshmanan VK, Cho ICP (2016) Biomaterials Nanoarchitectonics, William Andrew Publishing, Cambridge, USA, pp 197–215
85. Enrico C (2018) Design of nanostructures for theranostics applications. William Andrew Publishing, Cambridge, US, pp 41–68
86. Fu T, Kong Q, Sheng H, Gao L (2016) Neural Plast, 1
87. Sahle FF, Gulfam M, Lowe TL (2018) Drug Discov Today 23:992
88. Hsiao MH, Larsson M, Larsson A, Evenbratt H, Chen YY, Liu DM (2012) Design and characterization of a novel amphiphilic chitosan nanocapsule-based thermo-gelling biogel with sustained in vivo release of the hydrophilic anti-epilepsy drug ethosuximide. J Control Release 161:942–948

89. Wang Y, Ying X, Chen L, Liu Y, Wang Y, Liang J, Xu C, Guo Y, Wang S, Hu W, Du Y, Chen Z (2016) Neurotherapeutics 13:603
90. Xiong ZQ, Saggau P, Stringer JLJ (2000) Neurosci 20:1290
91. Pasternack M, Voipio J, Kaila K (1993) Acta Physiol Scand 148:229
92. Raimondo JV, Tomes H, Irkle A, Kay L, Kellaway L, Markram H, Millar RP, Akerman CJ (2016) J Neurosci 36:7002
93. Reyes-Ortega F (2014) PH-responsive polymers: properties, synthesis and applications. Woodhead Publishing Limited, Cambridge,UK
94. Cevik O, Gidon D, Kizilel S (2015) Acta Biomater 11:151
95. Konofagou EE (2012) Theranostics 2:1223
96. Chen KT, Wei KC, Liu HL (2019) Front Pharmacol 10:86
97. Zhang N, Yan F, Liang X, Wu M, Shen Y, Chen M, Xu Y, Zou G, Jiang P, Tang C, Zheng H, Dai Z (2018) Theranostics 8:2264
98. Negishi Y, Yamane M, Kurihara N, Endo-Takahashi Y, Sashida S, Takagi N, Suzuki R, Maruyama K (2015) Pharmaceutics 7:344
99. Sabourian P, Tavakolian M, Yazdani H, Frounchi M, VanDeVen TGM, Maysinger D, Kakkar AJ (2020) Controll Release 317:216
100. Wang Y, Wang Y, Sun R, Wu X, Chu X, Zhou S, Hu X, Gao L, Kong Q (2018) J Transl Med 16:337
101. Lin Z, Meng L, Zou J, Zhou W, Huang X, Xue S, Bian T, Yuan T, Niu L, Guo Y, Zheng H (2020) Theranostics 10:5514
102. Pearson-Smith J, Patel M (2017) Int J Mol Sci 18:2365
103. Prasad DKV (2017) J Clin Diagn Res 11:BC05
104. Yu L, Chen Y, Chen H (1841) Chin Chem Lett 2017:28
105. Santos MS, Tomé ADR, Saldanha GB, Ferreira PMP, Militão GCG, Freitas RMD (2009) Oxid Med Cell Longev 2:214
106. Cárdenas-Rodríguez N, Coballase-Urrutia E, Pérez-Cruz C, Montesinos-Correa H, Rivera-Espinosa L, Sampieri A, Carmona-Aparicio L (2014) Oxid Med Cell Longev 2014:1
107. Rao NV, Ko H, Lee J, Park JH (2018) Front Bioeng Biotechnol 6:110
108. Eid T, Gruenbaum SE, Dhaher R, Lee TSW, Zhou Y, Danbolt NC (2016) The glutamate/GABA-glutamine cycle. Springer Inter-national Publishing, Cham. The Glutamate–GlutamineCycle in Epilepsy
109. Eid T, Hammer J, Rundén-Pran E, Roberg B, Thomas MJ, Osen K, Davanger S, Laake P, Torgner IA, Lee TSW, Kim JH, Spencer DD, Ottersen OP, De Lanerolle NC (2007) Acta Neuropathol 113:137
110. Sada N, Lee S, Katsu T, Otsuki T, Inoue T (2015) Science 347:1362

Targeted Nano-based Drug Delivery in Alzheimer's Disease and Dementia

Payel Mal, Santosh Kumar Rath, and Tripti Halder

Abstract Alzheimer's disease (AD), the utmost widespread neurodegenerative illness, contributes to an enormous and expanding healthcare burden and impairs cognitive function in more than 50 million people globally. It is an irreversible form of dementia that primarily affects older people. Its typical clinical signs include memory loss and deteriorating cognitive abilities. The highly varied nature of AD, with various underlying hypotheses and complex pathophysiology, is blamed for the failure to produce effective medications, although this is not the only explanation. In addition, the difficulties posed by blood–brain interfaces surrounding the CNS, reducing the bioavailability of therapies, limit targeted drug delivery to the central nervous system (CNS) for the diagnosis and management of neurological illnesses like AD. Few attempts at designing a sensible pharmacological therapy have been successful, despite tremendous work in the field of nano-based drug delivery. As a potent substitute for current medication delivery methods, nanotechnology offers fresh promise for the treatment of AD.

Keywords Alzheimer's diseases · Amyloid beta · Neuroinflammations · Polymeric nanoparticles · Lipid based nanoformulations

1 Introduction

1.1 Alzheimer's Disease

Alzheimer's disease (AD) describes a specific onset and progression of cognitive and functional deterioration driven on by aging that ultimately causes death. The term was given regarding Alois Alzheimer, who specified AD for the first time in 1906

Payel Mal · S. K. Rath · T. Halder (✉)
School of Pharmaceuticals and Population Health Informatics, Faculty of Pharmacy, DIT University, Dehradun, Uttarakhand 248009, India
e-mail: tripti.halder@dituniversity.edu.in

S. K. Rath et al. (eds.), *Nanomaterials for Drug Delivery and Neurological Diseases Management*, Smart Nanomaterials Technology,
https://doi.org/10.1007/978-981-97-0308-1_12

[1]. As a result of pathological and morphological alterations that consist of cortical degeneration, neuroinflammation, impairment of synapses, and premature death of cells, AD lowers the patient's standard of life because their memories and motor skills degrade and they develop a dependency on intensive care. Amyloid plaques, clusters of erratically folded proteins, and neurofibrillary tau tangles (NFTs), which are present throughout the brain, are its defining features. The triggering factors of AD are thought to be hereditary and societal [2, 3]. A significant percentage of AD cases are sporadic, with no specific genetic origin, while there are only a handful of instances caused by dominant genetic changes. The chance of developing dementia is enhanced by environmental and metabolic risk factors like diabetes, cerebrovascular condition, unhealthy diet, brain injuries, and anxiety [4, 5]. Despite being broadly supported, the amyloid hypothesis, the dominant theory for how AD develops, has many unanswered challenges. While beta-amyloid peptide detected in deposits and hyperphosphorylated tau protein located in neurofibrillary tangles (NFTs), the two pathologies that define Alzheimer's disease were subjectively described by Alzheimer in 1906, their chemical origins were not discovered till the second half of the 1980s [6].

Alzheimer's disease is a progressive illness that causes impairments in memory, speech, thinking, and ability to resolve issues as well as behavioral alterations and finally fatalities. Although memory loss and executive dysfunction are the main symptoms, speech, and visual abnormalities are frequently present before these symptoms. Furthermore, not every kind of cognition is impacted in the same way. However, persistent memory, such as operational memory, is often unaffected by AD [1]. Patients with Dementia have substantially degraded sporadic, linguistic, and functional memory. There seemed to be 7 phases of AD identified medically. Considering the consequences of incapacity, such as pneumonia or thrombosis, patients frequently pass away 3–10 years beyond the first signs of indications [7, 8].

1.2 Established Hypotheses

1. Neurofibrillary tangles
2. Amyloid plaques
3. Cholinergic insufficiency
4. Autophagy dysfunction
5. Mitochondrial dysfunction
6. Neuroinflammation

1. **Neurofibrillary tangles**:

The microtubule-associated protein tau (MAPT) gene, which is responsible for encoding NFTs, acquires hyperphosphorylated tau protein within neurons [9].

- **Tau**

Tau fibril-coupled helical segments with a diameter of 20 nm are the basis for NFTs. It is believed that tau primarily functions as a cytoskeletal protein that interacts with tubulin to facilitate the formation and stabilization of microtubules. Six variants of tau are produced through different splicing of exons 10, 3, and 2 in human beings [10]. Exon 10's insertion results in quadruple microtubule-binding repetitions (4R tau) as compared to triple (3R tau), which affects the protein's ability to associate with microtubules and its inclination to combine. Human adults in good physical condition show equivalent levels of 3R and 4R tau [11, 12].

- **Tau Phosphorylation**

According to investigations, a balance between the two can influence health issues, with elevated levels of 4R isoforms causing severe neurodegeneration. Tau phosphorylation not only has an essential role in controlling tau functionality but may also be the fundamental alteration causing tau aggregation and possible neurotoxicity [13]. Tau gets hyperphosphorylated just before NFT formation. Interestingly, tau becomes more easily phosphorylated as a result of numerous tauopathy alterations. It has been proposed that tau causes neurodegeneration by altered localization, augmentation of activity, and/or impairment of activity [14, 13].

- **Tau Dysfunction**

Once tau loses its ability to maintain microtube stability, which affects the cytoskeleton of neurons, this is known as tau dysfunction. Tau dysfunction may also result in errors in axonal communication. Higher amounts of tau have also been demonstrated to affect axonal movement, block vesicles and organelles, particularly those containing APP, and boost levels of oxidative stress in the brain [15]. In vivo studies have demonstrated that tau's incorrect positioning to dendritic fibres affects memory and synapses. Symptoms start close to the entorhinal cortex and then propagate across the brain resembling plaques as the disease worsens [16].

On the other side, the course of the disorder demonstrated by the pathology of Tau is frequently articulated using Braak staging [17]. Tangles first emerge in the trans-entorhinal area in stages I & II; they subsequently travel to the limbic tract and begin to manifest in the neural cortex in stages III and IV; and finally, they develop across the neural cortex in stages V and VI [18]. As a result, one of the most significant indicators of dementia in Alzheimer's disease is the degeneration of synapses. Researchers have been able to detect alterations in both Amyloid and tau before variations in brain function and the development of symptoms through familial instances and PET scans [19].

2. **Amyloid precursor proteins**:

The breakdown of the amyloid precursor protein (APP) via the b-site of APP cleaving enzyme 1 as well as secretase results in the formation of plaques of amyloid, or the insoluble α peptides, in the cerebral cortex [20]. A class I transmembrane protein associated with secretory and endocytic activities; APP is encoded on the 21st chromosome [21]. Heparin, laminin, collagen a protease inhibitor region, and a metal-binding region are all present within it. The ectodomain of APP might play a role in cell binding, mechanical support, proliferation, and division of stem cells from neurons, however, the exact purpose of APP is unknown. On the other hand, the domain located within the cell might alter mitochondrial activity [22, 23].

- **Metabolic Pathways**

The amyloidogenic pathway & the non-amyloidogenic pathway are 2 distinct metabolic routes for APP. α-secretase, a single-pass transmembrane family member that releases zinc-bearing endopeptidases, cleaves APP amid amino acid 671 in the amyloidogenic pathway, generating APP (sAPP) [24]. Subsequently, the four-subunit -secretase, which includes the catalytic regions of the Presenilin1 gene (PS1) & Presenilin2 gene, cleaves the CTF99 contained in the layer. α-secretase cleaves APP amid amino acid 687 in the nonamyloidogenic pathway, yielding soluble APP (sAPPα) [25, 26]. A dissoluble p3 remnant is produced when α-secretase cleaves the rest of the polypeptide. Gathered Aβ role in healthy homeostasis is still unclear, nevertheless it interferes with postsynaptic transportation at glutamate receptors including NMDA and AMPA. Their responses could be crucial for plasticity of synapses, acquiring knowledge, and remembrance. GABA, a neurotransmitter that inhibits impulses, was previously found to be modulated by Aβ through its connection with KCC2 [27].

- **BACE1**

The expression of BACE1 corresponds not just with the start of AD but additionally with insulin resistance, it serves as a major pharmacological potential for treatment. The amino acid sequence of Sez6 is also enriched in regions linked to phenotypic adaptability. This covers regions of the postnatal brain's hippocampus and cerebellum. Sez6 regulates dendritic arbor in cortical neurons, is considered essential for neuronal communication, and is likewise broken by BACE1 [28, 29]. Therefore, impaired BACE1 results in impaired balance, poor motor coordination, and dementia. Finally, Jagged-1 (Jag1), which controls astrogenesis and neurogenesis employing the Notch signaling cascade and is involved in building memories, is also impacted by BACE1 loss. Hence, this enzyme's inhibition is a two-edged sword, and further exploration is required to assist AD victims [30, 31].

According to data, amyloid plaques, and soluble Aβ are equally harmful [32]. They are considered to affect cellular processes in a way that causes collateral or downhill events such as oxidative stress, inflammation, excitotoxicity, and hyperphosphorylation of the tau protein, which results in the formation of NFTs. These occurrences result in apoptosis and impairments in neurotransmitters, particularly ACh, and its absence is a contributing factor of certain AD's indications. Some people speculate that these latter mechanisms could cease to be reliant on the original Ab-related trigger [33, 32].

- **Zinc and Amyloid**

Zinc functions in enzymatic and protein structure-stabilizing events in tissues and cells, and it is crucial for neurological wellness [34]. It is mostly found in grey matter, where between 20 and 30 percent of brain zinc is found in glutamatergic Zn^{2+} vesicles. This leads to an exceptionally high concentration within the synaptic gap throughout neurological transmission [35]. Long-term potentiation (LTP) in the hippocampus CA3 area is influenced by Zn at presynaptic and postsynaptic sites due to a large influx of it into synapses. As a result, synaptic zinc revenue is extremely active yet becomes less so during aging, raising the possibility that zinc disequilibrium contributes to memory loss in AD [36, 35, 37].

Molecules promoting Aß accumulation emerged as significant once it was discovered that Aß is routinely produced by neurons in the form of soluble peptides. Zn2 + was observed to adhere to Aß with selectivity in the large nM to small μM range and to promote its fast ag Zn2 + accumulation and deposition [38, 36]. These deposits are reversibly assembled by the use of histidine bridges, and Asp7 is necessary for the interaction, although can be broken down through phosphorylation. Because the Aß-zinc combination is proteolysis-resistant, Aß aggregate reliability is enhanced. Hence, it serves as a potential target for therapeutic agents [38, 39].

3. **Cholinergic insufficiency**:

Another of the earliest hypotheses regarding how AD manifests was the cholinergic theory. This resulted from abnormally high amounts of acetylcholine in AD neural tissue [40]. The basal forebrain's cholinergic neurons are among the first to be impacted by AD, and the rest of the neurons' choline acetyltransferase (ChAT) transcription and functioning is reduced. A link involving acetylcholinesterase (AChE) and Aβ buildup has also been demonstrated by research. Connecting cholinergic with other AD diseases has been challenging as AD scientific research has advanced. The biggest number of pyramidal neurons mostly glutamatergic neurons are destroyed in areas with plaques and tangles [41, 42].

4. **Autophagy dysfunction**:

Other suggested pathways for the development of AD include autophagy and lysosomal failure. Tau removal is aided by autophagy, which also contributes to the production and elimination of Aβ. The report suggested that by upregulating the expression of brain CYP27A1 and elevating the levels of 27-OHC and 24S-hydroxycholesterol (24S-OHC), dietary cholesterol causes learning and memory impairment in male C57BL/6 J mice. They observed the total-tau (t-tau), phosphorylated-tau (p-tau), glycogen synthase kinase-3 (GSK-3), and cyclin-dependent kinase 5 (CDK5) protein expressions are all noticeably increased in the same population. In mice given the CYP27A1-shRNA + 2% cholesterol diet, reduced expressions of the proteins t-tau and p-tau, as well as lower 27-OHC levels in serum and the brain, were seen [43]. Processing of APP that results in amyloid genesis includes transportation through the endo-lysosomal route. BIN1, SORL1, and PICALM are three markers linked to AD that contribute to endosomal recycling, and research suggests that every one of these genes may directly affect how the APP is processed in endosomes [44, 45].

5. **Mitochondrial dysfunction and oxidative stress**:

The mitochondrial pathway is just one of many that AD compromises. In AD, modifications in the membrane potential of mitochondrial cells, variations in mitochondrial construction, quantity, and movement, decreased cytochrome oxidase action, impairments in metabolic proteins, and an upsurge in oxidative stress have all been documented. Since mitochondria are so important to neurons, they build up at junctions, which helps to meet their high metabolic needs. Oxidative stress can result from the terminals' elevated rate of ROS generation, a lack of antioxidants, and other factors [46]. The nervous system also contains significant amounts of cholesterols, which make it extremely susceptible to damage caused by oxidation. As a result, the brain has high energy requirements and a high lipid level, which puts it in jeopardy of oxidative harm [47]. Abnormal glucose metabolism is connected to phosphorylated tau and amyloid beta accumulation in AD brain. The relationship between insulin signaling and AD has brought attention to the role of GLUTs and IRS/PI3K/Akt/AMPK signaling in the development of the illness [48]. The mitochondrial cascade hypothesis contends both environmental as well as genetic factors establish the progression of mitochondrial loss, which in response controls the rate of aging and ultimately AD, instead of aging leading to amyloid pathology as in the case of the amyloid hypothesis [49, 50].

6. **Neuroinflammation**:

A current area of focus in the realm of AD is inflammatory conditions. As was previously said, impaired cognition is more prevalent among individuals with inflammation, and individuals with dementia who have higher concentrations of inflammatory indicators tend to decline quicker. Inflammation has been linked to brain damage, neuronal injury, and synaptic degeneration both in vivo and in addition to vitro, according to studies in experimental animals [51–53]. Essentially inflammation and stimulation of microglia are known to have a protective impact on the brain in short-term situations, over time they may cause neurodegeneration and an increase in Aβ burden. The activation of microglia by Aβ is considered to draw them together in plaques and promote scavenging. Possibly, the microglial response to Aβ is safeguarding, but after prolonged stimulation, the microglia start to behave negatively, creating a destructive feedback loop [54, 55]. In a similar vein, it has been demonstrated that immune cells can impact the formation of ROS and that a rise in ROS can raise inflammatory indicators, highlighting the intricate relationship between inflammation, oxidative stress, and Aβ [56, 57].

Inflammation certainly seems to influence and have an impact on tau pathogenesis. Studies on microglia's capacity to eliminate tau clumps have produced inconsistent results, possibly because microglia initially contributed to elimination but then lost the capacity to do so over time. Ultimately, it has been observed that modifying

TREM2 transcription might have an impact on Aβ levels and plaque-associated macrophages [58, 59].

2 Pharmacological Aspects

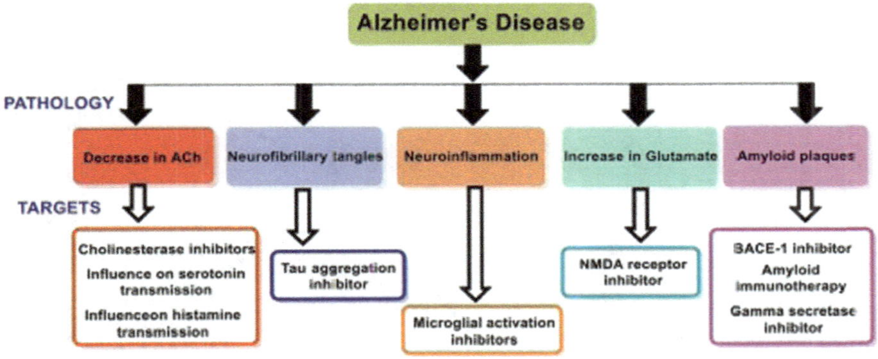

2.1 *Current Ongoing Treatments and Status of AD Management*

For the treatment of mild to severe AD, the US-FDA has approved few drugs including acetylcholine esterase inhibitors (Rivastigmine, galantamine, donepezil, tacrine), NMDA receptor agonists (Memantine), and, most recently, aducanumab (monoclonal antibody) [60, 61]. However, after enhancing the drug dose, the usual medication delivery method fails to deliver therapeutic doses to the target site in the AD brain due to its systemic adverse effects. Tacrine was the first acetylcholine esterase inhibitor which was approved for the treatment of Alzheimer's disease by the US Food and Drug Administration [60]. But it was banned due to the occurrence of severe hepatotoxicity. Next, the Donepezil tablets (5 mg/day) are used to treat the early stages of Alzheimer's disease. It was suggested, after one month, that the dose is increased to 10 mg/day. Further, it was observed that donepezil is frequently associated with agitation, nausea, fatigue, diarrhoea, gastrointestinal issues, and muscle cramps [62]. Next, the Galantamine capsules came at a dose of 8 mg/day for one month, followed by a month of 16 mg/day, and are used to treat mild to moderately severe AD and dementia [63]. Galantamine has cholinergic side effects, as do donepezil and rivastigmine. Memantine frequently causes dizziness, constipation, dizziness, weight gain, somnolence, hypertension, headache, and an increased risk of developing CNS disorders [64]. A novel molecule, Ladostigil, a dual reversible acetylcholine esterase and butyrylcholine esterase inhibitor, is being studied in phase II clinical trials for dementia and AD. It is a neuroprotective medication that increases the expression of brain derived neurotrophic factor (BDNF) and glial cell-line derived neurotropic factor (GDNF). Because of its permanent inhibition of the monoamine oxidase A and B enzymes, it also has anti-anxiety and anti-depressant characteristics [65, 60].

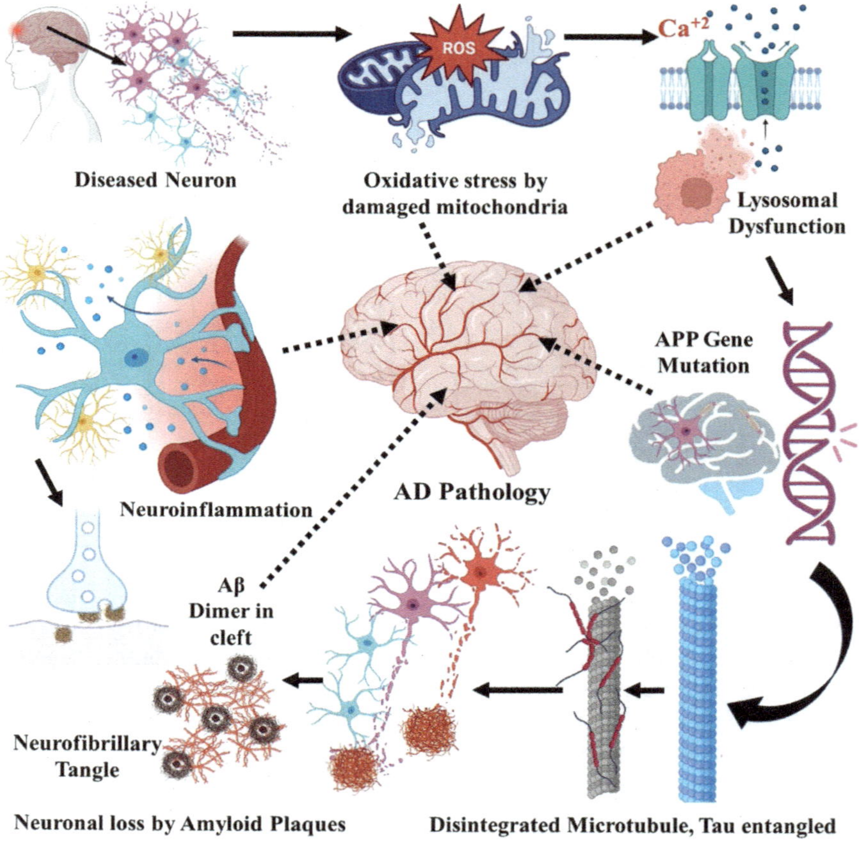

2.2 *Challenges for Drug Delivery at the Targeted Site for AD Treatment*

Unfortunately, no therapies are now available to cure neurodegeneration, present drugs can only able to relieve symptoms and are sometimes linked with unanticipated adverse effects, therefore a nonstop advancement of the degenerative process going on. Furthermore, the discovery of effective preventative or protective medicines has been hampered by our limited understanding of the causes and mechanisms by which neurons die in neurodegenerative illnesses, as well as the difficulty of delivering therapeutic agents across the BBB to the CNS [66]. The CNS system has a number of barriers that protect it from invading pathogens, neurotoxic molecules, and circulating blood cells, preventing therapeutic interventions. These barriers include the blood-cerebrospinal fluid barrier (CSFB), the blood–brain barrier (BBB), the blood-retinal barrier, and the blood-spinal cord [67, 68].

There are three methods for delivering a nanomaterial-based BBB across the brain: noninvasive, invasive, or identifying other pathways for drug delivery. Noninvasive approaches are commonly utilized, which are based on endogenous cellular mechanisms that promote drug transport over the BBB via a transcellular channel [67, 69]. The intranasal administration method efficiently carries NPs to the CNS via the olfactory epithelium or the trigeminal nerves, bypassing the previously described BBB. For a while, intranasal administration has been utilized to administer medications for both local and systemic effects since, after passing through the nasal mucosa, these medications can enter the bloodstream immediately. The direct connection between the olfactory and trigeminal areas through the sub-mucosa space of the nose into the CSF compartment of the brain has also been acknowledged as a means of improving targeting to the brain [70]. The principal location for systemic medication distribution is the respiratory system; here, drug absorption into the systemic circulation avoids hepatic first-pass metabolism. Drug absorption into the systemic circulation through the nasal mucosa has been theorized to occur by a number of processes; the most prevalent include paracellular passive absorption, transcellular pathways, and transcytosis pathways by vesicle carriers. The majority of low molecular weight, lipid-soluble medications are quickly and effectively absorbed from the nasal cavity and can pass across the BBB to reach the brain [71]. The primary place from which a medication can be absorbed directly into the brain via the olfactory and trigeminal neuronal pathways is the olfactory area, which is located in the upper section of the nasal cavity [72, 73]. Furthermore, medications transported by NPs can cross the BBB via receptor and adsorption-mediated endocytosis and the carrier-mediated pathway, which are used by a variety of endogenous compounds for delivery into the brain [74, 73]. The BBB can be broken or drugs can be administered directly into the brain tissue using invasive techniques, such as intracerebral implants, intraventricular/intrathecal/interstitial delivery, convection-enhanced delivery, osmotic BBB disruption (BBBD), biochemical strategy, or ultrasound (US)-mediated BBBD. Numerous endogenous compounds use carrier-mediated pathways, as well as, to deliver chemicals into the brain [71, 75, 76].

3 Inorganic Nanoparticle

3.1 Gold Nanoparticles

Because of their multifunctional properties in treatments, imaging, and surface modification, gold nanoparticles (AuNPs) have been widely exploited as nanomaterials for theranostic applications in AD therapy. AuNPs were discovered to suppress the production of amyloid fibrils. This protective effect could be caused by an increase in protein adsorption to the surface of the nanoparticles, preventing structural alterations [77]. By attaching to the monomer, the nanoparticle prevented them from coming together and elongating the core of amyloid fibrils. As a result, it can be employed as an effective therapeutic agent for preventing amyloid development and treating amyloid illness [78]. Huo et al. reported L and D glutathione stabilized gold nanoparticles were able to inhibit amyloid $beta_{1\text{-}42}$ and also penetrate through BBB. Enhanced binding affinity and brain distribution were also observed after intravenous administration [79]. Zang et al. explored a novel self-assembled nano-peptide from maize tetrapeptide anchored gold nanoparticle for the treatment of AD. The results revealed that the nanopeptide antioxidant was able to inhibit ROS accumulation and promote cell differentiation. Moreover, the levels of acetylcholinesterase were also reduced and in parallel superoxide dismutase and glutathione peroxidase were enhanced [80]. Ali et al. also highlighted, the anthrocyanin-loaded polyethylene glycol gold nanoparticle for increasing the neuroprotective effects in AD rats. This nanoparticle was able to regulate PI3K, p-Akt, and GSK3beta pathways and also inhibit neurodegeneration and apoptosis in AD-induced rats [81]. Feng et al. prepared transmembrane peptide and chondroitin sulphate conjugated gold nanoparticle, which exhibited excellent cellular uptake along with inhibition of amyloid beta accumulation. It also reduced oxidative stress and cholinergic injury by regulating the levels of glutathione, acetylcholine, malondialdehyde, etc [82]. Geng et al. reported that gold nanoparticles capped with mesoporous silica-based controlled system for targeted delivery of metal chelator ciloquinol were developed for AD treatment through reduction of cell membrane disruption, microtubular defects and ROS mediated apoptosis. This nanoparticle showed high BBB permeability and anti-amyloid beta aggregation properties [83].

3.2 Silver Nanoparticles

Silver nanoparticles (SNPs) travel through the blood to the brain after in-vivo implantation through vascular endothelial cell transcytosis and BBB disruption by weakening of the tight connections or by dissolving the membrane of the endothelial cells are the proposed methods of admission of SNPs into the brain through rupture of the BBB [60]. Popli et al. evaluated Cladosporium mediated silver nanoparticle for its neuroprotective potential in AD. Prepared nanoparticles showed antioxidant and significant inhibitory effect of both acetylcholine and butyrylcholine [84]. Huda et al. also prepared silver nanoparticles loaded with *Kickxia elatine* extract. Green extract and nanoparticle revealed significant anticholinesterase activity and the author also suggested it can be used as cheaper medicine for the treatment of AD [85]. Huda et al. also reported silver nanoparticles loaded with *Hypecoum pendulum* showed antioxidant as well as neuroprotective effects for AD management. Several characterization studies manifested, its crystalline properties and particle size nearly 80 nm. Its antioxidant and anti-acetyl cholinesterase activities suggested it a neuroprotective potential properties [85, 86]. Parveen et al. reported that silver and gold nanoparticles entrapped with *Accacia auriculiformis* leaves showed efficacy against AD. Prepared nanoparticles revealed smaller particle size and thermally stable. Thiflavin T assay showed better inhibitory properties and also revealed antioxidant activity with DPPH assay [87]. Azeem et al. highlighted, novel microalges *Galaxaura elongata, Turbinaria ornata,* and *Enteromorpha flexuosa* macroalgae loaded silver nanoparticles for AD treatment. All the bioalgae capped silver nanoparticles showed neuroprotective potential effects for safe biomedical application [88, 89].

3.3 Polymeric Nanoparticles

The polymeric NPs, a smart nanosystem offers a novel and secure approach for enhancing the pharmacokinetics and biodistribution effectively after administration. In the body frequently, simple monomers of natural and synthetic origin, such as albumin and polysaccharides, are combined to form polymeric NPs, which are mainly biocompatible, biodegradable, and readily excretable. There are also other natural and synthetic polymers including, chitosan, poly(butyl-cyanoacrylate), polylactic acid (PLA), polylactic glycolic acid (PLGA), polyethylene glycol (PEG), and polyethyleneimine (PEI) are some of the most often used polymers in the manufacture of these NPs [90]. To facilitate BBB entry, various ligands can be conjugated to the surface of NPs. These molecules can be divided into four categories: (i) ligands that can adsorb proteins from the bloodstream and interact with receptors or transporters directly expressed on the endothelial compartment of the BBB, such as T80; (ii) ligands that directly bind BBB receptors or transporters, such as targeting ligands or absorption specific for the transferrin, insulin receptor, or glucose transporter; (iii) amphiphilic peptides are an example of a ligand that can increase charge and hydrophobicity, while (iv) PEG is an example of a ligand that can speed up blood circulation [91]. Lopez et al. explored, memantine-loaded PEG-PLGA loaded polymeric nanoparticle was developed for AD treatment. The negatively charged particle size was nearly 200 nm. Developed nanoparticles were non-toxic and permeate through bEnd3 cell lines [92]. Yusuf et al. reported thymoquinone PLGA nanoparticle using polysorbate 80 surfactant was able to treat AD. This nanoparticle was able to reduce amyloid beta accumulation and hypo-phosphorylated tau protein through antioxidative properties [93]. Tripathi et al. showed that donepezil-loaded PLGA nanoparticle was also developed for AD treatment. Several characterization studies showed particle size was 40.8 nm with 74% entrapment efficiency. Pharmacokinetic studies showed the developed nanoparticle revealed the sustained release properties following the Hixon crowel model [94]. Zou et al. highlighted rifampicin loaded RVG-29 loaded PLGA nanoparticle for AD treatment. Formulation was non-toxic and easily enhanced cellular uptake. In pharmacodynamics studies, the nanoparticle-treated rats showed better spatial learning memory in MWM studies also with the reduction of amyloid beta deposition in hippocampal and cortex areas [95].

3.4 *Lipid Based Nanoparticles*

Nanoparticles have been designated as superior nose-to-brain transporters due to their ability to shield the encapsulated drug from biological and chemical degradation, as well as extracellular transport by P-gp efflux proteins. The safety and toxicity assessment of the matrix is one of the most important factors in their creation as nasal dosage forms. Among colloidal carriers, lipid-based nanoparticles (LNs) are seen to be the most promising for nasal medication administration, particularly in terms of biocompatibility. They range in size from 50 to 1000 nm. So far, LNs have been described as excellent carriers when compared to other colloidal systems [96].

3.5 *Liposomes*

Liposomes are spherical organic nanoparticle forms, made up of lipid bilayer encompassing an aqueous core and an impermeable lipophilic phospholipid layer on the outside. Liposome formulation is one method for classifying different types of liposome vesicles. Multilamellar vesicles (MLVs), small unilamellar vesicles (SUVs), and big unilamellar vesicles are the three types of liposomes. Liposomes are distinguished by their ability to transport amphipathic, hydrophilic, and hydrophobic drugs, as well as their low toxicity, excellent compatibility with their external environment, lack of immune system activation, and ability to target the site of action for effective drug delivery [97]. Kuo et al. reported glutathione and apolipoprotein E conjugated liposomes were developed to mitigate the cognitive deficits. This liposomes were entrapped with curcumin, quercetin and epigallocatechin. It was functioned against hypophosphorylated mitogen-activated protein kinase, tau protein, and up-regulate p cyclic adenosine monophosphate [98]. Wang et al. explored, icariin, and tanshinone IIA-loaded liposomes were used for AD treatment. Formulation was stable and nano ranged and uniform distribution was observed through several characterization studies. In pharmacodynamics studies, the nanoparticle was able to reduce neuroinflammation and oxidative stress [99]. Arora et al. developed a novel liposome surface functionalized with glucose transporter and cell penetrating peptide to enhance the cellular internalization in brain cells. Results manifested, higher protein expression of apolipoprotein E2 in bend3 cells and also showed higher transfection in p-apolipoproteinin C57BL/6 mice after single iv administration [100]. Kong et al. observed transferrin modified pegylated osthole-loaded liposomes were able to cross BBB and also cure the AD-related pathology. It was prepared by thin film hydration technique and it was able to enhance cellular uptake in hCMEC/D3 cells and APP-SH-SY5Y cells. Moreover, pharmacokinetic data revealed the liposomes prolonged the retention time into the mice brain [101]. Li et al. evaluated hydroxyl alpha sanshool loaded liposome for its potential in AD treatment. The particle sizes were in nano-ranged and stable for one week in 4 and 8 degree temperature. It showed neuroprotective potential by protecting hippocampal neuronal cells in d galactose induced learning memory deficits [102]. Andrade et al. reported vitamin B12 loaded transferrin conjugated liposomes were developed for AD therapy. The developed nanoparticles showed required entrapment efficiency and stable up to 2 months. Moreover, it showed sustained release properties for 9 days also which might be delayed the amyloid beta fibril formation [103].

3.6 Nanoemulsions

Nanoemulsions are ultra-fine colloidal dispersions of dispersed droplets that include an immiscible liquid phase and are stabilized by the addition of surfactants or surface-active chemicals, resulting in particles ranging in size from 20 to 500 nm. Biphasic systems (oil-in-water or water-in-oil) and multiphasic systems [water-in-oil-in-water (w/o/w) or oil-in-water-in-oil (o/w/o). Nanoemulsions are widely characterized depending on their external and internal phases. The relative volume of internal and exterior phases determines the kind of nanoemulsions. Furthermore, the relative volume determines the droplet number of the nanoemulsions as well as the system's stability. Because of the steric stability and electrostatic hindrance, nanoemulsions contain ionic or non-ionic surfactants to prevent flocculation. Ostwald ripening is the cause of nanoemulsions instability, in which big particles form agglomerates and detach from the phase [104]. These nanocarriers have been demonstrated to increase the bioavailability and permeability of anti-Alzheimer's medication. In various stages of clinical trials, new drug delivery systems for anti-AD medicines are being investigated. The intranasal drug delivery technique for the treatment of AD is highlighted in the current article [105]. Roy et al. developed citicoline-loaded D alpha tocopherol enriched nanoemulsion for crossing the BBB and targeted drug delivery. Bovin serum albumin and PLGA conjugated this novel formulation exhibited significant satisfactory results to achieve therapeutic benefits in AD patients [106]. Ahmad et al. reported curcumin-piperine loaded nanoemulsion for the management of AD and this formulation helped to overcome its poor bioavailability and permeability [107]. Vasdev et al. reported that rosemary oil loaded nanoemulsion (particle size 16 nm) revealed more penetration in ex-vivo permeation studies and it was stable for 3 months as per ICH guidelines [108]. Kotta et al. reported coconut oil based resveratrol nanoemulsion was prepared using pluronic 107 and cremophor EL and optimized with response surface methodology. Brain concentration of resveratrol was significantly higher than blood which confirms its brain targeting efficiency [109]. Ovais et al. highlighted, osthol loaded nanoemulsion enhanced the brain concentration after intranasal administration. It also showed neuroprotective effects by inhibiting apoptosis and oxidative stress and balanced cholinergic system [110]. Kaur et al. reported that donepezil nanoemulsion was evaluated in AD through nasal route and showed maximum uptake in brain. Results manifested, dose-dependent cytotoxicity and antioxidative properties [111]. Patil et al. showed quercetin entrapped nanoemulsion for treatment of aluminium chloride induced AD rats. Results showed the mitigating effects of AD induced animals and antioxidant and anti-inflammatory activities were also found. Neurotransmitter levels were also balanced and histochemical changes were also recovered after treatment with this formulation [112]. Kaur et al. also prepared memantine loaded nanoemulsion with ultrasonication method and it showed 80% drug release in simulated nasal fluid. Biodistribution results also revealed higher uptake and 3.6% of radioactivity at 1.5 h in the brain [113].

3.7 Solid Lipid Nanoparticles

SLNs are a type of colloidal particle composed of lipids that are solid at both room and body temperatures and have unique size-dependent properties in the 50–80 to 1000 nm range, combining the benefits of lipid-based nanocarriers and polymeric nanoparticles while avoiding their limitations. When compared to the free drug form, drug-loaded SLNs have preferred BBB penetration [114]. The increased BBB permeability of SLNs may be owing to their high lipid content, which promotes transcellular diffusion across the BBB. Surfactants included in SLNs can also act as absorption enhancers, decreasing nanoparticle clearance by the reticuloendothelial system and inhibiting the efflux system, particularly P-glycoprotein, boosting transport across the BBB. They are tiny biodegradable particles with simple surface functionalization for both hydrophobic and hydrophilic medicines, and they aid in increasing drug solubility, allowing for tailored drug release and stability in the solid lipid matrix [115]. Arora et al. reported rivastigmine tartrate loaded solid lipid nanoparticle was prepared with glyceryl monostearate as solid lipid and polysorbate 80 as surfactant and further optimized with central composite design. This SLN was stable in various conditions and bioavailability was also improved as compared to normal rivastigmine treatment [116]. Campisi et al. prepared curcumin-loaded solid lipid nanoparticle for AD treatment using wild and TgCRND8 mice model. Behavioral studies revealed different expression levels like Bcl-2, Cyclin-D1, and caspase-3 evaluated and it allows differently modulated TG2 isoforms [117]. Hinge et al. highlighted the rivastigmine docosahexaenoic acid loaded pair complex improved drug loading and was able to more inhibit amyloid after administration. It also improves drug retention at targeted site and significantly improves pharmacokinetic parameters as compared to other rivastigmine formulations. Saini et al. reported, chitosan coated ferulic acid loaded SLN for AD management. It was prepared with compritol as solid lipid and polysorbate 80 as a surfactant and followed by optimized using 3^2 central composite design. Several characterization studies like SEM studies revealed uniform spherical shaped nanoparticles. In vivo studies it has been observed, that the AD induced mice were taken minimum escape latency in behavioral studies [118].

3.8 Nano Structured Lipid Carrier

NLCs are a new class of solid lipid nanoparticles that were created primarily to solve their limitations. NLCs exist as solid lipid matrices at room and body temperature, but the fundamental difference between them and SLNs is that a portion of the solid lipids are replaced with oil, resulting in a less ordered lipid matrix. NLCs have been demonstrated to inhibit the Pgp efflux pump, resulting in increased drug concentrations in the brain and the potential for longer drug circulation [119–121]. They are made of FDA and/or EMA-approved surfactants and lipids, may be synthesized in the absence of an organic solvent, and the method is easily scalable into large batch quantities by high pressure homogenization. NLCs are regarded as prospective drug carriers due to their biocompatibility and greater formulation qualities than SLNs, as their components are more flexible and contain lipids in both liquid and solid phases [122]. Salvi et al. described that the NLCs are one of the lipid-based drug delivery systems and as an alternating approach to polymeric NPs, liposomes, emulsion, etc., is suitable for hydrophobic drugs for enhancing the targeting efficiencies. He also suggested that DDS is compatible, better stable, enhanced drug loading, and can be considered as a potent lipid nanocarrier for the treatment of various diseases [115]. Rajput et al. developed resveratrol loaded NLC with sonication method and observed nanosized particles, stable negative ranged ZPs with 9.26% of DL. Moreover, it showed significant improvement in memory function against free drug administration [123]. Raju et al. prepared berberine-loaded NLCs for the treatment of AD and the achieved particle sizes were in nano range and optimized with 32 factorial designs. It showed 82% of release within 24 h. Moreover, it is significantly effective in AD model [124]. Halder et al. reported myricetin loaded NLCs were developed and optimized for the treatment of AD. Brain targeting efficiency was 127.05% enhanced as compared to normal myricetin suspension administration [125]. Halder et al. highlighted that asiatic acid loaded with NLCs was developed using stearic acid and labrafac lipophile as solid lipid and liquid lipid respectively. The cytotoxicity was observed as dose dependent and the cellular internalization was time dependent. The Asiatic acid concentration was 2.99-fold enhanced after administration against normal drug suspension. Pharmacodynamics studies also revealed significant neuroprotective effect in amyloid beta induced AD brain [126]. Gabal et al. prepared and evaluated cationic as well as anionic NLCs for brain targeting drug delivery of Ropinirole HCl. Results showed absolute bioavailability of both NLCs in situ gels was enhanced compared to that of the intranasal solution of the drug. But anionic NLCs showed highest drug targeting efficiency nearly 1.2 times more than cationic NLCs in the brain.

4 Conclusion

In this chapter, it has been explored that nano-based several polymeric, metallic, and lipid-based approaches were successfully employed for the treatment of AD. However, the multi-targeted drug delivery systems are more fruitful than the single targeted approach. Nonetheless, because this study is concerned with the central nervous system as well as the treatment of AD, it has been proposed that we should focus more on pharmacokinetic and pharmacodynamic evaluation investigations. Several cellular pathways for the medication and the targeted areas for AD treatment should also be highlighted. However, based on this discussion, we can conclude that combinational and ligand-based methods of AD therapy are productive and efficacious.

References

1. Lopez JA, González HM, Léger GC (2019) Alzheimer's disease. Handb Clin Neurol 167:231–255
2. Nie J (2023) Exposure to aluminum in daily life and Alzheimer's disease. In: Neurotoxicity of aluminum. Springer, pp 107–121
3. Villemagne VL, Doré V, Burnham SC, Masters CL, Rowe CC (2018) Imaging tau and amyloid-β proteinopathies in Alzheimer disease and other conditions. Nat Rev Neurol 14(4):225–36
4. Loera-Valencia R, Goikolea J, Parrado-Fernandez C, Merino-Serrais P, Maioli S (2019) Alterations in cholesterol metabolism as a risk factor for developing Alzheimer's disease: potential novel targets for treatment. J Steroid Biochem Mol Biol 190:104–114
5. Podcasy JL, Epperson CN (2022) Considering sex and gender in Alzheimer disease and other dementias. Dialogues Clin Neurosci
6. Morató X, Pytel V, Jofresa S, Ruiz A, Boada M (2022) Symptomatic and disease-modifying therapy pipeline for Alzheimer's disease: towards a personalized polypharmacology patient-centered approach. Int J Mol Sci 23(16):9305
7. Alzheimer's Association (2015) Alzheimer's disease facts and figures. Alzheimer's & Dementia 11(3):332–384
8. Rogers SL, Friedman RB (2008) The underlying mechanisms of semantic memory loss in Alzheimer's disease and semantic dementia. Neuropsychologia 46(1):12–21
9. Idda ML, Munk R, Abdelmohsen K, Gorospe M (2018) Noncoding RNAs in Alzheimer's disease. Wiley Interdisciplinary Reviews: RNA 9(2):e1463
10. McMillan P, Korvatska E, Poorkaj P, Evstafjeva Z, Robinson L, Greenup L, Leverenz J, Schellenberg GD, D'Souza I (2008) Tau isoform regulation is region-and cell-specific in mouse brain. J Comp Neurol 511(6):788–803
11. LaFerla FM, Oddo S (2005) Alzheimer's disease: Aβ, tau and synaptic dysfunction. Trends Mol Med 11(4):170–176
12. Roberts M, Sevastou I, Imaizumi Y, Mistry K, Talma S, Dey M, Gartlon J, Ochiai H, Zhou Z, Akasofu S, Tokuhara N (2020) Pre-clinical characterisation of E2814, a high-affinity antibody targeting the microtubule-binding repeat domain of tau for passive immunotherapy in Alzheimer's disease. Acta Neuropathol Commun 8:1–24
13. Wang Y, Mandelkow E (2016) Tau in physiology and pathology. Nat Rev Neurosci 17(1):22–35
14. Abey A, Davies D, Goldsbury C, Buckland M, Valenzuela M, Duncan T (2021) Distribution of tau hyperphosphorylation in canine dementia resembles early Alzheimer's disease and other tauopathies. Brain Pathol 31(1):144–162

15. Kuznetsov IA, Kuznetsov AV (2015) A coupled model of fast axonal transport of organelles and slow axonal transport of tau protein. Comput Methods Biomech Biomed Eng 18(13):1485–1494
16. Van der Jeugd A, Hochgräfe K, Ahmed T, Decker JM, Sydow A, Hofmann A, Wu D, Messing L, Balschun D, D'Hooge R, Mandelkow EM (2012) Cognitive defects are reversible in inducible mice expressing pro-aggregant full-length human Tau. Acta Neuropathol 123:787–805
17. Leuzy A, Chiotis K, Lemoine L, Gillberg PG, Almkvist O, Rodriguez-Vieitez E, Nordberg AJM (2019) Tau PET imaging in neurodegenerative tauopathies—still a challenge. Mol Psychiatry 24(8):1112–1134
18. Jellinger KA (2016) A view on early diagnosis of dementias from neuropathology. In: The dementias. CRC Press, pp 329–446
19. Barthélemy NR, Li Y, Joseph-Mathurin N, Gordon BA, Hassenstab J, Benzinger TL, Buckles V, Fagan AM, Perrin RJ, Goate AM, Morris JC (2020) A soluble phosphorylated tau signature links tau, amyloid and the evolution of stages of dominantly inherited Alzheimer's disease. Nat Med 26(3):398–407
20. Behl T, Kaur D, Sehgal A, Singh S, Sharma N, Zengin G, Andronie-Cioara FL, Toma MM, Bungau S, Bumbu AG (2021) Role of monoamine oxidase activity in Alzheimer's disease: an insight into the therapeutic potential of inhibitors. Molecules 26(12):3724
21. Sisodia SS, St George-Hyslop PH (2002) γ-Secretase, Notch, Aβ and Alzheimer's disease: where do the presenilins fit in? Nat Rev Neurosci 3(4):281–290
22. Masi M, Biundo F, Fiou A, Racchi M, Pascale A, Buoso E (2023) The Labyrinthine landscape of APP processing: state of the art and possible novel soluble APP-related molecular players in traumatic brain injury and neurodegeneration. Int J Mol Sci 24(7):6639
23. Reinhard C, Hébert SS, De Strooper B (2008) The amyloid-β precursor protein: integrating structure with biological function. EMBO J 24(23):3996–4006
24. Seegar TC, Killingsworth LB, Saha N, Meyer PA, Patra D, Zimmerman B, Janes PW, Rubinstein E, Nikolov DB, Skiniotis G, Kruse AC (2017) Structural basis for regulated proteolysis by the α-secretase ADAM10. Cell 171(7):1638–1648, e1637
25. Da Costa Dias B, Jovanovic K, Gonsalves D, Weiss SF (2011) Structural and mechanistic commonalities of amyloid-β and the prion protein. Prion 5(3):126–137
26. Van De Craen M, de Jonghe C, van den Brande I, Declercq W, van Gassen G, Van Criekinge W, Vanderhoeven I, Fiers W, van Broeckhoven C, Hendriks L, Vandenabeele P (1999) Identification of caspases that cleave presenilin-1 and presenilin-2: five presenilin-1 (PS1) mutations do not alter the sensitivity of PS1 to caspases. FEBS Lett 445(1):149–154
27. Wu QL, Gao Y, Li JT, Ma WY, Chen NH (2022) The role of AMPARs composition and trafficking in synaptic plasticity and diseases. Cell Mol Neurobiol 42(8):2489–2504
28. Chapman NH, Nato AQ, Bernier R, Ankenman K, Sohi H, Munson J, Patowary A, Archer M, Blue EM, Webb SJ, Coon H (2015) Whole exome sequencing in extended families with autism spectrum disorder implicates four candidate genes. Hum Genet 134:1055–1068
29. Mir GH (2017) BACE1 is a novel regulator of Th17 function in EAE. University of Pittsburgh
30. Sarlak G, Vincent BJ (2016) The roles of the stem cell-controlling Sox2 transcription factor: from neuroectoderm development to Alzheimer's disease? Mol Neurobiol 53:1679–1698
31. Taylor HA, Przemylska L, Clavane EM, Meakin PJ (2022) BACE1: more than just a β-secretase. Obes Rev 23(7):e13430
32. Edrey YH, Medina DX, Gaczynska M, Osmulski PA, Oddo S, Caccamo A, Buffenstein R (2013) Amyloid beta and the longest-lived rodent: the naked mole-rat as a model for natural protection from Alzheimer's disease. Neurobiol Aging 34(10):2352–2360
33. Chen ZR, Huang JB, Yang SL, Hong FF (2022) Role of cholinergic signaling in Alzheimer's disease. Molecules 27(6):1816
34. Chasapis CT, Ntoupa PS, Spiliopoulou CA, Stefanidou ME (2020) Recent aspects of the effects of zinc on human health. Arch Toxicol 94:1443–1460
35. Que EL, Domaille DW, Chang CJ (2008) Metals in neurobiology: probing their chemistry and biology with molecular imaging. Chem Rev 108(5):1517–1549

36. Li Y, Hough CJ, Frederickson CJ, Sarvey JM (2001) Induction of mossy fiber→ Ca3 long-term potentiation requires translocation of synaptically released Zn2+. J Neurosci 21(20):8015–8025
37. Takeda A, Fuke S, Ando M, Oku N (2009) Positive modulation of long-term potentiation at hippocampal CA1 synapses by low micromolar concentrations of zinc. Neuroscience 158(2):585–591
38. Datki Z, Galik-Olah Z, Janosi-Mozes E, Szegedi V, Kalman J, Hunya ÁG, Fulop L, Tamano H, Takeda A, Adlard PA, Bush AI (2020) Alzheimer risk factors age and female sex induce cortical Aβ aggregation by raising extracellular zinc. Mol Psychiatry 25(11):2728–2741
39. Lu N, Li J, Gao Z (2015) Key roles of Tyr 10 in Cu bound Aβ complexes and its relevance to Alzheimer's disease. Arch Biochem Biophys 584:1–9
40. Anand A, Patience AA, Sharma N, Khurana N (2017) The present and future of pharmacotherapy of Alzheimer's disease: a comprehensive review. Eur J Pharm 815:364–375
41. Nordberg A (2006) Mechanisms behind the neuroprotective actions of cholinesterase inhibitors in Alzheimer disease. Alzheimer Dis Assoc Disord 20:S12–S18
42. Walton HS, Dodd PR (2007) Glutamate–glutamine cycling in Alzheimer's disease. Neurochem Int 50(7–8):1052–1066
43. Wang T, Zhang X, Wang Y, Liu W, Wang L, Hao L, Ju M, Xiao R (2022) High cholesterol and 27-hydroxycholesterol contribute to phosphorylation of tau protein by impairing autophagy causing learning and memory impairment in C57BL/6J mice. J Nutr Biochem 106:109016
44. Li Y, Laws SM, Miles LA, Wiley JS, Huang X, Masters CL, Gu BJ (2021) Genomics of Alzheimer's disease implicates the innate and adaptive immune systems. Cell Mol Life Sci:1–30
45. Wang Z, Lei H, Zheng M, Li Y, Cui Y, Hao F (2016) Meta-analysis of the association between Alzheimer disease and variants in GAB2, PICALM, and SORL1. Mol Neurobiol 53:6501–6510
46. Reddy PH, Tripathi R, Troung Q, Tirumala K, Reddy TP, Anekonda V, Shirendeb UP, Calkins MJ, Reddy AP, Mao P, Manczak M (2012) Abnormal mitochondrial dynamics and synaptic degeneration as early events in Alzheimer's disease: implications to mitochondria-targeted antioxidant therapeutics. Biochim Biophys Acta (BBA)-Mol Basis Dis 1822(5):639–649
47. Lane RK, Hilsabeck T, Rea SL (2015) The role of mitochondrial dysfunction in age-related diseases. Biochim et Biophys Acta (BBA)-Bioenerg 1847(11):1387–1400
48. Dewanjee S, Chakraborty P, Bhattacharya H, Chacko L, Singh B, Chaudhary A, Javvaji K, Pradhan SR, Vallamkondu J, Dey A, Kalra RS (2022) Altered glucose metabolism in Alzheimer's disease: role of mitochondrial dysfunction and oxidative stress. Free Radic Biol Med
49. Franceschi C, Garagnani P, Morsiani C, Conte M, Santoro A, Grignolio A, Monti D, Capri M, Salvioli S (2018) The continuum of aging and age-related diseases: common mechanisms but different rates. Front Med 5:61
50. John A, Reddy PH (2021) Synaptic basis of Alzheimer's disease: focus on synaptic amyloid beta, P-tau and mitochondria. Ageing Res Rev 65:101208
51. Daulatzai MA (2016) Fundamental role of pan-inflammation and oxidative-nitrosative pathways in neuropathogenesis of Alzheimer's disease in focal cerebral ischemic rats. Am J Neurodegener Dis 5(2):102
52. Ivanova N, Liu Q, Agca C, Agca Y, Noble EG, Whitehead SN, Cechetto DF (2020) White matter inflammation and cognitive function in a co-morbid metabolic syndrome and prodromal Alzheimer's disease rat model. J Neuroinflammation 17(1):1–18
53. Licastro F, Candore G, Lio D, Porcellini E, Colonna-Romano G, Franceschi C, Caruso C (2005) Innate immunity and inflammation in ageing: a key for understanding age-related diseases. Immun Ageing 2:1–14
54. Ennerfelt HE, Lukens JR (2020) The role of innate immunity in Alzheimer's disease. Immunol Rev 297(1):225–246
55. Leng F, Edison P (2021) Neuroinflammation and microglial activation in Alzheimer disease: where do we go from here? Nat Rev Neurol 17(3):157–172

56. Bhatt S, Nagappa AN, Patil CR (2020) Role of oxidative stress in depression. Drug Discov Today 25(7):1270–1276
57. Rojas-Gutierrez E, Muñoz-Arenas G, Treviño S, Espinosa B, Chavez R, Rojas K, Flores G, Díaz A, Guevara J (2017) Alzheimer's disease and metabolic syndrome: a link from oxidative stress and inflammation to neurodegeneration. Synapse 71(10):e21990
58. Jay TR, Hirsch AM, Broihier ML, Miller CM, Neilson LE, Ransohoff RM, Lamb BT, Landreth GE (2017) Disease progression-dependent effects of TREM2 deficiency in a mouse model of Alzheimer's disease. J Neurosci 37(3):637–647
59. Ulrich JD, Finn MB, Wang Y, Shen A, Mahan TE, Jiang H, Stewart FR, Piccio L, Colonna M, Holtzman DM (2014) Altered microglial response to Aβ plaques in APPPS1-21 mice heterozygous for TREM2. Mol Neurodegener 9(1):1–9
60. Taliyan R, Kakoty V, Sarathlal KC, Kharavtekar SS, Karennanavar CR, Choudhary YK, Singhvi G, Riadi Y, Dubey SK, Kesharwani P (2022) Nanocarrier mediated drug delivery as an impeccable therapeutic approach against Alzheimer's disease. J Control Release 343:528–550
61. Verma A, Waiker DK, Bhardwaj B, Saraf P, Shrivastava SK (2022) The molecular mechanism, targets, and novel molecules in the treatment of Alzheimer's disease. Bioorganic Chem 119:105562
62. Gauthier S, Feldman H, Hecker J, Vellas B, Emir B, Subbiah P, Donepezil MSAD Study Investigators' Group (2002) Functional, cognitive and behavioral effects of donepezil in patients with moderate Alzheimer's disease. Curr Med Res Opin 18(6):347–354
63. Hsieh YH, Yang YH, Yeh HH, Lin PC, Chen SH (2009) Simultaneous determination of galantamine, rivastigmine and NAP 226-90 in plasma by MEKC and its application in Alzheimer's disease. Electrophoresis 30(4):644–653
64. Benninghoff J, Perneczky R (2022) Anti-dementia medications and anti-alzheimer's disease drugs: side effects, contraindications, and interactions. In: NeuroPsychopharmacotherapy. Springer, pp 1–10
65. Ouyang Q, Meng Y, Zhou W, Tong J, Cheng Z, Zhu Q (2022) New advances in brain-targeting nano-drug delivery systems for Alzheimer's disease. J Drug Target 30(1):61–81
66. Valasaki M (2022) Young onset Parkinson's disease: Biographical disruption as a repetitive process. Sociol Health Illn 44(4–5):798–814
67. Nguyen TT, Nguyen TT, Vo TK, Nguyen MK, Van Vo T, Van Vo G (2021) Nanotechnology-based drug delivery for central nervous system disorders. Biomed Pharmacother 143:112117
68. Van Giau V, An SS, Hulme JP (2018) Mitochondrial therapeutic interventions in Alzheimer's disease. J Neurol Sci 395:62–70
69. Xie J, Shen Z, Anraku Y, Kataoka K, Chen X (2019) Nanomaterial-based blood-brain-barrier (BBB) crossing strategies. Biomaterials 224, 119491
70. Zha S, Wong KL, All AH (2022) Intranasal delivery of functionalized polymeric nanomaterials to the brain. Adv Healthc Mater 11(11):2102610
71. Ayub A, Wettig S (2022) An overview of nanotechnologies for drug delivery to the brain Pharmaceutics 14(2):224
72. Md S, Bhattmisra SK, Zeeshan F, Shahzad N, Mujtaba MA, Meka VS, Radhakrishnan A, Kesharwani P, Baboota S, Ali J (2018) Nano-carrier enabled drug delivery systems for nose to brain targeting for the treatment of neurodegenerative disorders. J Drug Deliv Sci Technol 43:295–310
73. Wong LR, Ho PC (2018) Role of serum albumin as a nanoparticulate carrier for nose-to-brain delivery of R-flurbiprofen: implications for the treatment of Alzheimer's disease. J Pharm Pharmacol 70(1):59–69
74. Shehata MK, Ismail AA, Kamel MA (2023) Nose to brain delivery of astaxanthin–loaded nanostructured lipid carriers in rat model of Alzheimer's Disease: preparation, in vitro and in vivo evaluation. Int J Nanomed:1631–1658
75. Bourganis V, Kammona O, Alexopoulos A, Kiparissides C (2018) Recent advances in carrier mediated nose-to-brain delivery of pharmaceutics. Eur J Pharm Biopharm 128:337–362
76. Mittal D, Ali A, Md S, Baboota S, Sahni JK, Ali J (2014) Insights into direct nose to brain delivery: current status and future perspective. Drug Deliv 21(2):75–86

77. Sibuyi NR, Moabelo KL, Fadaka AO, Meyer S, Onani MO, Madiehe AM, Meyer M (2021) Multifunctional gold nanoparticles for improved diagnostic and therapeutic applications: a review. Nanoscale Res Lett 16:1–27
78. Khongkow M, Yata T, Boonrungsiman S, Ruktanonchai UR, Graham D, Namdee K (2019) Surface modification of gold nanoparticles with neuron-targeted exosome for enhanced blood–brain barrier penetration. Sci Rep 9(1):8278
79. Hou K, Zhao J, Wang H, Li B, Li K, Shi X, Wan K, Ai J, Lv J, Wang D, Huang Q (2020) Chiral gold nanoparticles enantioselectively rescue memory deficits in a mouse model of Alzheimer's disease. Nat Commun 11(1):4790
80. Zhang J, Liu R, Zhang D, Zhang Z, Zhu J, Xu L, Guo Y (2021) Neuroprotective effects of maize tetrapeptide-anchored gold nanoparticles in Alzheimer's disease. Colloids Surf B Biointerfaces 200:111584
81. Ali T, Kim MJ, Rehman SU, Ahmad A, Kim MO (2017) Anthocyanin-loaded PEG-gold nanoparticles enhanced the neuroprotection of anthocyanins in an Aβ 1–42 mouse model of Alzheimer's disease. Mol Neurobiol 54:6490–6506
82. Feng Y, Li X, Ji D, Tian J, Peng Q, Shen Y, Xiao Y (2023) Functionalised penetrating peptide-chondroitin sulphategold nanoparticles: synthesis, characterization, and applications as an anti-Alzheimer's disease drug. Int J Biol Macromol 230:123125
83. Geng J, Li M, Wu L, Chen C, Qu X (2012) Mesoporous silica nanoparticle-based H2O2 responsive controlled-release system used for Alzheimer's disease treatment. Adv Healthc Mater 1(3):332–336
84. Popli D, Anil V, Subramanyam AB, MN N, VR R, Rao SN, Rai RV, Govindappa M (2018) Endophyte fungi, Cladosporium species-mediated synthesis of silver nanoparticles possessing in vitro antioxidant, anti-diabetic and anti-Alzheimer activity. Artif Cells NanomedBiotechnol 46(1):676–683
85. Huda NU, Ghneim HK, Fozia F, Ahmed M, Mushtaq N, Sher N, Khan RA, Ahmad I, Al-Sheikh YA, Giesy JP, Aboul-Soud MA (2023) Green synthesis of Kickxia elatine-induced silver nanoparticles and their role as anti-acetylcholinesterase in the treatment of Alzheimer's disease. Green Process Synth 12(1):20230060
86. Kang Y, Miyamoto Y, Muraoka Y, Yamaguchi O (1995) Fabrication and characterization of MoSi2/Al2O3/Ni/Al2O3/MoSi2 FGMs; MoSi2/Al2O3/Ni/Al2O3/MoSi2 keikeisha kino zairyo no sakusei to hyoka. Zairyo (J Soc Mater Sci, Japan) 44
87. Parveen M, Kumar A, Khan MS, Rehman R, Furkan M, Khan RH, Nami SA (2022) Comparative study of biogenically synthesized silver and gold nanoparticles of Acacia auriculiformis leaves and their efficacy against Alzheimer's and Parkinson's disease. Int J Biol Macromol 203:292–301
88. Abdel Azeem MN, Hassaballa S, Ahmed OM, Elsayed KNM, Shaban M (2021) Photocatalytic activity of revolutionary *Galaxaura elongata Turbinaria ornata, and Enteromorpha flexuosa's* bio-capped silver nanoparticles for industrial wastewater treatment. Nanomaterials 11(12):3241
89. Azeem MN, Ahmed OM, Shaban M, Elsayed KN (2022) In vitro antioxidant, anticancer, anti-inflammatory, anti-diabetic and anti-Alzheimer potentials of innovative macroalgae bio-capped silver nanoparticles. Environ Sci Pollut Res 29(39):59930–59947
90. La Barbera L, Mauri E, D'Amelio M, Gori M (2022) Functionalization strategies of polymeric nanoparticles for drug delivery in Alzheimer's disease: current trends and future perspectives. Front Neurosci 16:939855
91. Asil SM, Ahlawat J, Barroso GG, Narayan M (2020) Nanomaterial based drug delivery systems for the treatment of neurodegenerative diseases. Biomater Sci 8(15):4109–4128
92. Sánchez-López E, Ettcheto M, Egea MA, Espina M, Cano A, Calpena AC, Camins A, Carmona N, Silva AM, Souto EB, García ML (2018) Memantine loaded PLGA PEGylated nanoparticles for Alzheimer's disease: in vitro and in vivo characterization. J Nanobiotechnol 16:1–16
93. Yusuf M, Khan M, Alrobaian MM, Alghamdi SA, Warsi MH, Sultana S, Khan RA (2021) Brain targeted Polysorbate-80 coated PLGA thymoquinone nanoparticles for the treatment of Alzheimer's disease, with biomechanistic insights. J Drug Deliv Sci Technol 61:102214

94. Tripathi SK, Patel B, Shukla S, Pachouri C, Pathak S, Pandey A (2021) Donepezil loaded PLGA nanoparticles, from modified nano-precipitation, an advanced drug delivery system to treat Alzheimer disease. J Phys Conf Ser
95. Zhou R, Zhu L, Zeng Z, Luo R, Zhang J, Guo R et al (2022) Targeted brain delivery of RVG29-modified rifampicin-loaded nanoparticles for Alzheimer's disease treatment and diagnosis. Bioeng Transl Med 7(3):e10395
96. Akel H, Ismail R, Csoka I (2020) Progress and perspectives of brain-targeting lipid-based nanosystems via the nasal route in Alzheimer's disease. Eur J Pharm Biopharm 148:38–53
97. Hernandez C, Shukla S (2022) Liposome based drug delivery as a potential treatment option for Alzheimer's disease. Neural Regener Res 17(6):1190
98. Kuo YC, Ng IW, Rajesh R (2021) Glutathione-and apolipoprotein E-grafted liposomes to regulate mitogen-activated protein kinases and rescue neurons in Alzheimer's disease. Mater Sci Eng C 127:112233
99. Wang J, Kong L, Guo RB, He SY, Liu XZ, Zhang L, Liu Y, Yu Y, Li XT, Cheng L (2022) Multifunctional icariin and tanshinone IIA co-delivery liposomes with potential application for Alzheimer's disease. Drug Deliv 29(1):1648–1662
100. Arora S, Singh J (2021) In vitro and in vivo optimization of liposomal nanoparticles based brain targeted vgf gene therapy. Int J Pharm 608:121095
101. Kong L, Li XT, Ni YN, Xiao HH, Yao YJ, Wang YY, Ju RJ, Li HY, Liu JJ, Fu M, Wu YT (2020) Transferrin-modified osthole PEGylated liposomes travel the blood-brain barrier and mitigate Alzheimer's disease-related pathology in APP/PS-1 mice. Int J Nanomed:2841–2858
102. Li R, Lu F, Sun X, He L, Duan H, Peng W, Wu C (2022) Development and in vivo evaluation of hydroxy-α-sanshool intranasal liposomes as a potential remedial treatment for Alzheimer's disease. Int J Nanomed:185–201
103. Andrade S, Ramalho MJ, Loureiro JA, Pereira MC (2022) Transferrin-functionalized liposomes loaded with vitamin VB12 for Alzheimer's disease therapy. Int J Pharm 626:122167
104. Handa M, Tiwari S, Yadav AK, Almalki WH, Alghamdi S, Alharbi KS, Shukla R, Beg S (2021) Therapeutic potential of nanoemulsions as feasible wagons for targeting Alzheimer's disease. Drug Discov Today 26(12):2881–2888
105. Bahadur S, Sachan N, Harwansh RK, Deshmukh R (2020) Nanoparticlized system: promising approach for the management of Alzheimer's disease through intranasal delivery. Curr Pharm Des 26(12):1331–1344
106. Roy H, Srungarapati S, Gade NJ, Gummadi A, Karunasree BK, Dakkumalla M, Maddiboyina B (2023) Citicoline loaded nanoemulsion enriched with D-alpha-Tocopherol acetate and protein: formulation and in-silico study. J Drug Deliv Sci Technol 82:104340
107. Ahmad S, Hafeez A (2023) Formulation and development of curcumin–piperine-loaded S-SNEDDS for the treatment of Alzheimer's disease. Mol Neurobiol 60(2):1067–1082
108. Vasdev N, Handa M, Kesharwani P, Shukla R (2022) Rosemary oil low energy nanoemulsion: optimization, μrheology, in silico, in vitro, and ex vivo characterization. J Biomater Sci Polym Ed 33(15):1901–1923
109. Kotta S, Aldawsari HM, Badr-Eldin SM, Alhakamy NA, Md S (2021) Coconut oil-based resveratrol nanoemulsion: optimization using response surface methodology, stability assessment and pharmacokinetic evaluation. Food Chem 357:129721
110. Ovais M, Zia N, Ahmad I, Khalil AT, Raza A, Ayaz M, Sadiq A, Ullah F, Shinwari ZK (2018) Phyto-therapeutic and nanomedicinal approaches to cure Alzheimer's disease: present status and future opportunities. Front Aging Neurosci 10:284
111. Kaur A, Nigam K, Bhatnagar I, Sukhpal H, Awasthy S, Shankar S, Tyagi A, Dang S (2020) Treatment of Alzheimer's diseases using donepezil nanoemulsion: an intranasal approach. Drug Deliv Transl Res 10:1862–1875
112. Patil P, Killedar S (2021) Formulation and characterization of gallic acid and quercetin chitosan nanoparticles for sustained release in treating colorectal cancer. J Drug Deliv Sci Technol 63:102523
113. Kaur A, Nigam K, Srivastava S, Tyagi A, Dang S (2020) Memantine nanoemulsion: a new approach to treat Alzheimer's disease. J Microencapsul 37(5):355–365

114. Saini S, Sharma T, Jain A, Kaur H, Katare OP, Singh B (2021) Systematically designed chitosan-coated solid lipid nanoparticles of ferulic acid for effective management of Alzheimer's disease: a preclinical evidence. Colloids Surf B Biointerfaces 205:111838
115. Salvi VR, Pawar P (2019) Nanostructured lipid carriers (NLC) system: a novel drug targeting carrier. J Drug Deliv Sci Technol 51:255–267
116. Arora D, Bhatt S, Kumar M, Verma R, Taneja Y, Kaushal N, Tiwari A, Tiwari V, Alexiou A, Albogami S, Alotaibi SS (2022) QbD-based rivastigmine tartrate-loaded solid lipid nanoparticles for enhanced intranasal delivery to the brain for Alzheimer's therapeutics. Front Aging Neurosci 14:960246
117. Campisi A, Sposito G, Pellitteri R, Santonocito D, Bisicchia J, Raciti G, Russo C, Nardiello P, Pignatello R, Casamenti F, Puglia C (2022) Effect of unloaded and curcumin-loaded solid lipid nanoparticles on tissue transglutaminase isoforms expression levels in an experimental model of Alzheimer's disease. Antioxidants 11(10):1863.
118. Hinge NS, Kathuria H, Pandey MM (2023) Rivastigmine-DHA ion-pair complex improved loading in hybrid nanoparticles for better amyloid inhibition and nose-to-brain targeting in Alzheimer's. Eur J Pharm Biopharm
119. Chandu AN, Singh S, Rath SK (2022) Antimicrobial resistance: meaning and developing realization. In: Emerging modalities in mitigation of antimicrobial resistance. Springer, pp 315–331
120. Jnaidi R, Almeida AJ, Gonçalves LM (2020) Solid lipid nanoparticles and nanostructured lipid carriers as smart drug delivery systems in the treatment of glioblastoma multiforme. Pharmaceutics 12(9):860
121. Rath SK, Singh S, Kumar S, Wani NA, Rai R, Koul S, Khan IA, Sangwan PL (2019) Synthesis of amides from (E)-3-(1-chloro-3, 4-dihydronaphthalen-2-yl) acrylic acid and substituted amino acid esters as NorA efflux pump inhibitors of Staphylococcus aureus. Bioorganic Med Chem 27(2):343–53
122. Tomsen-Melero J, Merlo-Mas J, Carreño A, Sala S, Córdoba A, Veciana J, González-Mira E, Ventosa N (2022) Liposomal formulations for treating lysosomal storage disorders. Adv Drug Deliv Rev:114531
123. Rajput AP, Butani SB (2019) Resveratrol anchored nanostructured lipid carrier loaded in situ gel via nasal route: formulation, optimization and in vivo characterization. J Drug Deliv Sci Technol 51:214–23
124. Raju M, Kunde SS, Auti ST, Kulkarni YA, Wairkar S (2021) Berberine loaded nanostructured lipid carrier for Alzheimer's disease: design, statistical optimization and enhanced in vivo performance. Life Sci 285:119990
125. Halder T, Patel B, Acharya N (2022) Design and optimization of myricetin encapsulated nanostructured lipid carriers: in-vivo assessment against cognitive impairment in amyloid beta (1–42) intoxicated rats. Life Sci 297:120479
126. Halder T, Patel B, Acharya N (2023) Asiatic acid fabricated nanoconstructs to mitigate amyloid beta1–42 induced injury in SH-SY5Y cells in-vitro and ameliorates cognitive impairment by dual cholinesterase inhibition and attenuation of oxidative stress in-vivo. Pharm Res 40(1):197–213

Nanomaterials as Drug Delivery Vehicles for Therapy of Parkinson's Disease

Aleena James Chirayimmel, Gursharan Kaur, Palak Rana, Santosh Kumar Rath, Sudip Kumar Mandal, and Vagish Dwibedi

Abstract Parkinson's disease is a prevalent neurodegenerative disorder characterized by motor impairments and coordination difficulties. With a significant number of individuals affected worldwide, the need for innovative therapies is paramount. Nanomaterials have emerged as promising drug delivery vehicles to address the challenges in Parkinson's disease therapy. This article provides an overview of the potential of nanomaterials in improving therapeutic outcomes while reducing side effects. Current treatment options for Parkinson's disease primarily involve dopaminergic medications, such as dopamine agonists and levodopa. However, these treatments have limitations, including fluctuating efficacy and adverse effects. To overcome these challenges, nanomaterial-based drug delivery systems offer several advantages. Nanomaterials, including lipid-based nanoparticles, polymer-based nanoparticles, inorganic nanomaterials, and carbon-based nanomaterials, provide opportunities for targeted delivery, controlled release, and improved bioavailability. Lipid-based nanocarriers, such as liposomes, solid lipid nanoparticles (SLNs), and nanostructured lipid carriers (NLCs), can enhance drug stability, encapsulation, and controlled release. Polymer-based nanoparticles and inorganic nanomaterials, such as mesoporous silica nanoparticles (MSN) and magnetic nanoparticles, offer

---

Aleena James Chirayimmel and Gursharan Kaur are the authors contributed equally.

A. J. Chirayimmel
School of Biosciences and Technology, Vellore Institute of Technology, Vellore 632014, India

G. Kaur · P. Rana · V. Dwibedi (✉)
University Institute of Biotechnology, Chandigarh University, Mohali 140413, India
e-mail: vagish.lcc@gmail.com; vagishdwibedi@gmail.com

S. K. Rath
School of Pharmaceuticals and Population Health Informatics, Faculty of Pharmacy, DIT University, Dehradun 248009, Uttarakhand, India

S. K. Mandal · V. Dwibedi
Dr. B. C. Roy College of Pharmacy and AHS, Durgapur 713206, West Bengal, India

V. Dwibedi
Institute of Soil, Water and Environmental Sciences, Volcani Research Center, Agricultural Research Organization, 7528809 Rishon Lezion, Israel

S. K. Rath et al. (eds.), *Nanomaterials for Drug Delivery and Neurological Diseases Management*, Smart Nanomaterials Technology,
https://doi.org/10.1007/978-981-97-0308-1_13

targeted drug delivery and imaging capabilities. Carbon-based nanomaterials, such as carbon nanotubes and graphene, demonstrate unique properties for drug delivery applications.

Keywords Parkinson's disease · Drug delivery vehicles · Solid lipid nanoparticles · Nanostructured lipid carriers · Mesoporous silica nanoparticles

1 Introduction

Parkinson's disease is one of the most prominent neurodegenerative diseases that induce convulsions such as stiffness, tremor, and imparted coordination. Recent cases revealed that about 10 million people worldwide are living with Parkinson's disease and about one million people in the United States are living with PD, estimated to be 1.2 million by 2030. Approximately 4% of individuals with Parkinson's disease (PD) receive a diagnosis prior to reaching the age of 50, and it is observed that men have a higher susceptibility to PD compared to women. Parkinson's disease (PD) is primarily characterized by the buildup of misfolded α-synuclein and the degeneration of dopaminergic neurons in the substantia nigra (SN) pars compacta (SNpc), which are observed in the formation of Lewy bodies (LBs) [1]. As Parkinson's disease advances from stage 1 to stage 2, individuals may experience sleep disorders or depression as a result of changes in the lower brainstem. Additionally, a decrease in the sense of smell can be observed due to the impact on the olfactory bulb. During the transition from stage 3 to stage 4 of Parkinson's disease, the midbrain substantia nigra is affected. In stages 5 to 6 of Parkinson's disease, the pathology extends to the cerebral cortex, resulting in symptoms such as hallucinations and dementia (Fig. 1) [2]. Parkinson's disease is also characterized by four primary symptoms. These include tremors occurring in the hands, arms, legs, jaw, or head. The disease also leads to muscle stiffness, causing prolonged muscle contractions. The slowness of movement is another prevalent symptom, making daily activities challenging. Impaired balance and coordination are often observed, which can increase the risk of falls. In addition to these main symptoms, individuals with Parkinson's disease may experience various other symptoms. These can encompass emotional changes such as depression, difficulties with swallowing, chewing, and speaking, as well as problems related to urinary function and constipation. Some individuals may also encounter skin problems as part of their Parkinson's symptoms [3].

1.1 Current Treatment Options and Their Limitations

Drug treatments for Parkinson's disease primarily involve the use of dopaminergic medications, such as dopamine agonists. These medications can be taken orally

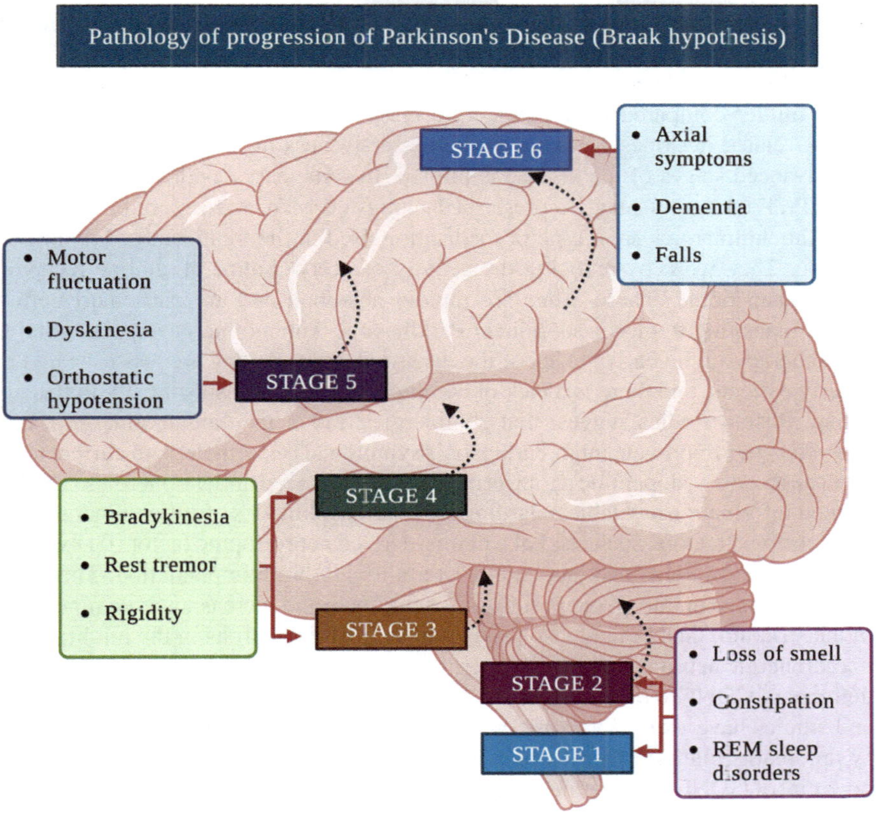

Fig. 1 Pathology of progression of Parkinson's Disease (Braak hypothesis) and symptoms at each stage

or administered through injection. They are considered the current "gold standard for treatment" and exhibit high responsiveness, particularly in cases of idiopathic Parkinson's disease. Dopamine agonists are often preferred for late-onset Parkinson's and may address both non-motor and motor symptoms. As the disease advances and other treatments become less effective, most patients eventually turn to dopamine agonists [4]. However, they are not as commonly used for early-onset Parkinson's due to the risk of levodopa-related dyskinesia. Levodopa, a medication that requires increasing dosage over time, can lead to "on–off" fluctuations when taken orally. In the case of the injection method, there can be irritation or problems at the pump site [5]. MAOIs (monoamine oxidase inhibitors) are a class of drugs used in the treatment of Parkinson's disease. They work by inhibiting the breakdown of levodopa and dopamine through oral administration. Unlike levodopa, which requires increasing dosage over time, MAOIs do not necessitate dose adjustments as the disease progresses. These medications may also positively impact cognitive decline in the later stages of Parkinson's. In terms of side effects, MAOIs tend to be milder compared to dopaminergic drugs. They may also help alleviate L-DOPA-related dyskinesia. However, their effectiveness in addressing symptoms in the advanced stages of the disease is limited. In some cases, additional drugs such as COMT inhibitors may be prescribed alongside MAOIs for certain treatments [6]. Anticholinergics are a type of medication used in the treatment of Parkinson's disease. They work by reducing the activity of acetylcholine at choline receptors when taken orally. These drugs are rapidly absorbed and are particularly effective in managing tremor-predominant Parkinson's. Anticholinergics can be used as monotherapy in the early stages of the disease. However, they are less tolerated by elderly patients, and there is a lack of comprehensive testing specifically in this age group. Recent studies suggest that cholinergics, rather than anticholinergics, may provide better improvement in Parkinson's symptoms. Nevertheless, in current treatment approaches, dopamine agonists have largely replaced anticholinergics. There is limited information available regarding the pharmacokinetics of anticholinergics [7]. Neurotrophic factors, such as glial cell line-derived neurotrophic factor (GDNF), are small natural proteins that can be delivered through brain implantation. They have shown promise in improving Parkinson's symptoms and increasing dopamine levels in the striatum. GDNF may also protect dopaminergic neurons in the midbrain and noradrenergic neurons in the locus coeruleus from neurotoxic damage. However, the delivery of GDNF to brain cells is challenging due to the blood–brain barrier (BBB), and studies have yielded varying outcomes regarding its effectiveness in providing symptomatic relief. Further research is needed to better understand and optimize the potential of GDNF as a treatment for Parkinson's disease [8]. Nanomedicine involves modifying existing drugs to enhance their delivery methods. This approach aims to enhance drug delivery across the blood–brain barrier or find alternative routes. By reducing drug loss in peripheral tissues, nanomedicine can enhance effectiveness while minimizing side effects. Ongoing research in this growing field focuses on developing protective factors and improving imaging techniques. However, further testing is needed before nanomedicine becomes a standard practice for Parkinson's disease treatment [9]. Surgical treatments for Parkinson's disease can provide high effectiveness and long-term results. Ablative surgery involves making an incision into the global pallidus, thalamus, or subthalamic nucleus, offering relief from rigidity, hypokinesia, and tremors. However, this procedure is irreversible and may lead to permanent side effects [10]. Deep brain stimulation (DBS) is a surgical alternative that involves the use of an implanted device to provide electrical stimulation to the basal ganglia, thereby activating and modulating its functions. Bilateral DBS is considered safer than bilateral ablative surgeries and is an established treatment for advanced Parkinson's. It can improve both non-motor and motor symptoms, with benefits lasting over 10 years in some cases. However, DBS may have limitations in speech symptoms, reducing gait and balance, and potential side effects include dyskinesia, imbalance, and dysarthria. Additionally, conventional DBS is open-loop and lacks patient adjustment, while limited battery life is a consideration

[11]. Transplanting stem cells into the striatum can lead to long-lasting improvement by replacing diseased neurons. Gene therapy aims to correct dopamine pathways at a genetic level. However, further research, particularly in human testing, is needed in these developing fields. On the other hand, therapy is a non-invasive treatment that can address multiple motor and non-motor symptoms. It often complements other forms of treatment for Parkinson's disease [12]. Physical therapy is a valuable approach to addressing mobility and motor-related symptoms in Parkinson's disease. It can greatly enhance the quality of life by treating multiple symptoms simultaneously through tailored physical training [13]. Occupational therapy aims to help patients maintain independence in work, leisure, and self-care activities, considering social and environmental factors [14]. Speech therapy focuses on improving speech through voice exercises, enhancing communication, and overall well-being [15]. Cognitive-behavioral therapy offers behavioral training methods as an alternative to medication, effectively managing symptoms such as insomnia with few side effects, but further testing is needed. Patient involvement and motivation are essential for the success of these therapies [16].

1.2 Need for Innovative Drug Delivery Systems in Parkinson's Disease Therapy

New drug delivery systems are required to treat Parkinson's disease and these systems play a crucial role in enhancing clinical outcomes and quality of life in patients with Parkinson's disease. Parkinson's disease is a neurodegenerative disorder that predominantly impacts motor functions. The mainstay of treatment for Parkinson's disease is medications such as levodopa that help reduce symptoms and control the condition. However, the method of delivery, such as oral tablets or capsules, can be limited by many factors [17]. One of the problems with oral drugs is changes in drug absorption and metabolism. This can cause changes in the body's chemistry, leading to poor control. In addition, the blood–brain barrier is a protective mechanism in the brain that can limit the use of additional drugs by preventing them from reaching their target. New drug delivery systems aim to overcome these limitations by providing more effective and controlled drug release. They can help make medications consistent and predictable, reduce medication changes, and improve symptoms. Additionally, technology could improve the way we use drugs that cross the blood–brain barrier that can treat specific areas of the brain affected by Parkinson's disease. Some examples of newer drugs being investigated to treat Parkinson's disease include intranasal administration through the nose directly into the brain. Intranasal administration can cross the blood–brain barrier and more effectively deliver the drug to the affected area [18]. Transdermal patches contain drugs that are absorbed through the skin and into the bloodstream. They provide a non-invasive method of drug delivery and provide sustained drug release, ensuring that the drug is gradually released over an extended duration. Implantable devices are surgically placed in the body and can deliver drugs directly to the brain. They can be designed to deliver specific doses at specific times and provide targeted and controlled drug release. One method of gene therapy is to alter genes in the brain to produce proteins. Gene therapy holds long-term promise and could be employed to treat Parkinson's disease by delivering genetic material directly to the brain. Therefore, innovation in drug delivery is essential for the treatment of Parkinson's disease. These systems have the potential to improve treatment outcomes, improve symptom management, and deliver treatments to certain parts of the brain. A new approach that overcomes the limitations of traditional drug delivery methods could pave the way for more effective and personalized treatments for Parkinson's patients [19].

1.3 Introduction to Nanomaterials as Promising Drug Delivery Vehicles

Nanomaterials have developed as highly favorable drug delivery vehicles on account of their exceptional capabilities and properties. These materials, which are typically in the range of 1 to 100 nm in size, offer numerous advantages in terms of drug encapsulation, targeted delivery, and controlled release. One key advantage is their large surface area-to-volume ratio, which facilitates efficient loading and encapsulation of drugs. Additionally, their small size enables them to penetrate various biological barriers and reach specific target sites within the body, such as tumors or infected tissues. Moreover, nanomaterials can be engineered to have specific surface properties, allowing for enhanced cellular uptake and improved drug release profiles. Overall, the use of nanomaterials as drug delivery vehicles holds great promise for improving therapeutic efficacy, reducing side effects, and enabling personalized medicine approaches [20].

Nanomaterials offer several advantages when it comes to targeted drug delivery, making them a highly attractive option. Firstly, their small size allows them to navigate through biological barriers and reach specific target sites within the body, such as diseased tissues or tumors. This precise targeting enhances the efficacy of the drug and reduces the risk of side effects by minimizing exposure to healthy tissues [21]. Secondly, nanomaterials can be engineered to have specific surface properties, enabling them to interact with target cells more effectively. This facilitates cellular uptake and improves the drug's bioavailability. Additionally, nanomaterials deliver a large surface area-to-volume ratio, allowing for efficient loading and encapsulation of drugs. This enables the controlled release of the drug, ensuring its prolonged and prolonged therapeutic effect. Overall, the implementation of nanomaterials for targeted drug delivery holds immense potential in improving treatment outcomes and advancing personalized medicine approaches [22].

1.4 Potential for Improved Therapeutic Outcomes and Reduced Side Effects

The utilization of nanomaterials in drug delivery holds significant potential for enhancing therapeutic outcomes while minimizing the occurrence of side effects. By utilizing nanomaterials as carriers, drug infusion is precisely to target sites inside the body, such as specific tissues or tumors. This targeted approach ensures that the drug is concentrated in the desired area, increasing its effectiveness while minimizing exposure to healthy tissues. As a result, the risk of adverse side effects is reduced, leading to a more favorable treatment experience for patients [23]. Furthermore, nanomaterials can be engineered to possess distinct surface features that empower them to interact more efficiently with target cells. This improved interaction enhances cellular uptake of the drug, promoting better drug delivery and bioavailability. With nanomaterials, drugs can be released in a controlled manner, allowing for sustained and prolonged therapeutic effects. This controlled release mechanism helps optimize the drug's concentration over time, improving its overall effectiveness and reducing the frequency of dosing. Overall, the incorporation of nanomaterials in drug delivery systems holds great promise for improving therapeutic outcomes. By achieving precise targeting, enhancing cellular uptake, and enabling controlled release, nanomaterial-based drug delivery systems possess the capability to revolutionize the field of medicine, offering improved interventions with minimal side effects [24].

2 Nanomaterials for Drug Delivery in Parkinson's Disease

2.1 Lipid-Based Nanocarriers

Lipid-based nanocarriers are a promising technology that holds great potential in various fields. These nanocarriers consist of lipids, which are fatty molecules, and they are designed to encapsulate and deliver a wide range of therapeutic agents, such as genes or drugs, to specific target sites in the body. The utilization of lipid-based nanocarriers in drug delivery has garnered considerable interest because of their capacity to enhance the bioavailability, solubility, and stability of poorly soluble drugs [25]. These nanocarriers can protect the encapsulated drugs from deterioration, enhance their circulation time in the bloodstream, and selectively release them at the desired site of action. This targeted drug delivery approach minimizes off-target effects and reduces systemic toxicity. Furthermore, lipid-based nanocarriers can be easily modified to enhance their functionality. For instance, the exterior of these nanocarriers can be modified with targeting ligands to enhance their specificity, such as peptides or antibodies, to precisely bind to receptors overexpressed on the surface of target cells [26]. This active targeting strategy allows for enhanced cellular uptake and improved therapeutic efficacy. Moreover to drug delivery, lipid-based nanocarriers have shown promise in other applications as well. They can be used in gene delivery to efficiently deliver therapeutic genes to specific cells or tissues for gene therapy. Moreover, these nanocarriers can be utilized in diagnostic imaging by incorporating contrast agents or imaging probes, enabling the visualization of specific tissues or pathological conditions. Ongoing research and development in this field continue to explore innovative approaches to enhance their efficiency, safety, and versatility [27].

2.1.1 Liposomes

Liposomes, which are lipid-based nanocarriers, have shown promise within the context of Parkinson's disease research. Parkinson's disease is a condition that involves the progressive degeneration of cells responsible for producing dopamine in the brain. One approach to treating Parkinson's disease is to administrate therapeutic agents directly to the affected regions of the brain using liposomes. Liposomes can be loaded with various drugs, including dopamine or its precursors, and can be designed to specifically target the brain regions impacted by Parkinson's disease [28]. By encapsulating these therapeutic agents within liposomes, their stability and bioavailability can be improved, facilitating for better drug delivery to the desired site of action. Furthermore, liposomes can safeguard encapsulated drugs from disintegration and facilitate their modulated release, which is crucial for maintaining therapeutic levels over an extended period. Moreover, for drug delivery, liposomes can also be utilized for gene therapy in Parkinson's disease [29]. They can be loaded with genes encoding therapeutic proteins and delivered to the brain to promote the production of these proteins. This approach holds the potential for addressing the underlying molecular mechanisms of Parkinson's disease and providing long-term benefits. Parkinson's disease therapies. Ongoing research in this area continues to explore and optimize the use of liposomes to combat this debilitating neurological condition [30].

2.1.2 Solid Lipid Nanoparticles (SLNs)

Solid lipid nanoparticles (SLNs) are a type of nanoscale drug delivery system that has gained significant attention in recent years. These nanoparticles are composed of solid lipids, which are biocompatible and biodegradable materials. SLNs offer several advantages over traditional drug delivery systems, making them a promising technology for various applications. One of the key benefits of SLNs is their ability to improve the durability and dissolvability of drugs with low water solubility [31]. By encapsulating these drugs within the lipid matrix, SLNs prevent their degradation and improve their bioavailability. This is particularly important for drugs with low aqueous solubility, as it enables their efficient delivery and uptake by the body. SLNs also offer controlled and sustained drug release profiles. The solid lipid matrix provides a barrier that slows down the release of the encapsulated drug, resulting in prolonged therapeutic effects. This feature is especially beneficial for drugs that require long-term treatment or have a restricted therapeutic margin [32]. Furthermore, SLNs can be easily adapted to selectively target particular tissues or cells. Surface modification with ligands or antibodies allows the nanoparticles to actively recognize and bind to target sites, increasing drug accumulation at the desired location. This targeted drug delivery approach improves therapeutic efficacy and minimizes systemic side effects. In addition to their drug delivery capabilities, SLNs have shown potential in various other applications. They can be used for the delivery of diagnostic agents, such as contrast agents for imaging techniques, enabling more accurate disease diagnosis [33]. SLNs also hold promise for gene therapy, as they can protect and deliver nucleic acids to target cells, facilitating gene expression modulation. Overall, solid lipid nanoparticles represent a versatile and promising technology for drug administration and other biomedical applications. Their exceptional properties, including improved drug solubility, controlled release, and targeted delivery, make them an attractive option for enhancing the efficacy and safety of various therapeutic interventions [34].

2.1.3 Nanostructured Lipid Carriers (NLCs)

Nanostructured lipid carriers (NLCs) are an advanced type of lipid-based nanocarrier system that has garnered considerable interest in recent years. These carriers are composed of a blend of solid and liquid lipids, creating a unique nanostructure with enhanced properties for various applications in drug delivery. The incorporation of both solid and liquid lipids in NLCs offers distinct advantages over conventional lipid-based carriers [35]. The presence of solid lipids helps to improve the physical robustness of the nanoparticles, preventing drug expulsion and maintaining a controlled release profile. On the other hand, the inclusion of liquid lipids enhances drug encapsulation capability and elevates the flexibility of the carrier, enabling efficient encapsulation of a wide array of therapeutic medications. One of the key benefits of NLCs is their ability to overcome the limitations associated with poorly water-soluble drugs. By utilizing the unique lipid matrix, NLCs can solubilize hydrophobic drugs and enhance their bioavailability. This is particularly important for drugs with low aqueous solubility, as it facilitates their effective delivery and improves therapeutic outcomes [36].

NLCs also exhibit improved stability during storage and transportation. The solid lipid component provides a protective barrier, shielding the encapsulated drug from environmental factors such as moisture, light, and heat. This helps to ensure the intactness and efficacy of the drug over an extended period. Moreover, NLCs offer the possibility of controlled and sustained drug release [37]. The arrangement of lipids in the nanostructured matrix impedes the diffusion of drugs and offers a reservoir for controlled release, leading to extended drug effects and decreased frequency of dosing. This prolonged release characteristic is particularly advantageous for drugs that require continuous therapeutic levels or exhibit a narrow therapeutic window. Additionally, NLCs can be surface-modified to achieve targeted drug delivery.

Through the attachment of ligands or targeting components to the surface of nanoparticles, NLCs can actively identify and bind to particular cells or tissues, thereby improving drug concentration at the intended location and reducing unintended impacts elsewhere [38]. This focused strategy has significant promise in enhancing the effectiveness and safety of therapeutic interventions. In summary, nanostructured lipid carriers (NLCs) represent an innovative and promising medium for drug transport. Their unique composition and structure enable enhanced drug solubility, improved stability, controlled release, and targeted delivery. These features make NLCs an attractive option for overcoming the challenges associated with various drugs and enhancing their therapeutic efficacy in a broad spectrum of possibilities [39].

2.1.4 Applications and Advantages of Parkinson's Disease Therapy

Specialized liposomes incorporating distinct constituents were created as vehicles for delivering resveratrol and epigallocatechin gallate, serving as drug carriers. These liposomes underwent alteration through the inclusion of leptin, with the purpose of bolstering their capacity to traverse the blood–brain barrier and effectively rejuvenate deteriorating dopaminergic neurons. The liposomes showed improved properties with increased mole percentage of certain components, leading to enhanced entrapment efficiency. The modified liposomes exhibited a higher ability to cross the blood–brain barrier and improved cell viability and target efficiency. The encapsulated compounds in the liposomes showed neural protective effects by reducing apoptosis and enhancing key proteins related to dopamine regulation. Overall, the modified liposomes present a promising delivery system for Parkinson's disease treatment [40]. In a study, nanostructured lipid carriers (RP-NLCs) and RP-loaded solid lipid nanoparticles (RP-SLNs) were developed and optimized. These formulations, along with hydrogel versions (RP-SLN-C and RP-NLC-C), showed sustained release and enhanced permeation. Pharmacokinetic studies demonstrated significant improvements in oral and topical delivery, while pharmacodynamic studies revealed enhanced dopamine and antioxidant levels, indicating the potential of these formulations for the effective treatment of Parkinson's disease [41]. In another study, nanostructured lipid carriers (NLCs) loaded with selegiline hydrochloride were prepared using hot homogenization. The optimized formulation showed high entrapment efficiency and sustained release of the drug. The pharmacological evaluation demonstrated that the NLCs restored behavioral parameters in rotenone-induced rats, suggesting their potential for the management of Parkinson's disease. Nasal administration of selegiline HCl-loaded NLCs holds promise as a therapeutic approach for Parkinson's disease [42].

2.2 Polymer-Based Nanocarriers

Polymer-based nanocarriers are a class of advanced nanoscale delivery systems that have garnered significant attention in drug delivery. These nanocarriers are composed of biocompatible polymers, which offer a wide range of advantages for various applications. The versatility of polymers allows for the design of nanocarriers with tailored properties, such as shape, size, and surface functionality, enabling efficient encapsulation and controlled release of drugs [43]. Polymer-based nanocarriers also provide protection to the encapsulated drug, preventing degradation and enhancing stability during storage and transportation. Additionally, the surface of these nanocarriers can be modified by targeting ligands or stimuli-responsive moieties, enabling active or triggered drug delivery to specific cells or tissues. With their tunable properties and versatile functionalities, polymer-based nanocarriers hold great promise for improving drug delivery systems and advancing therapeutic interventions [44].

2.2.1 Polymeric Nanoparticles

Polymeric nanoparticles, which are tiny particles at the nanoscale, consist of polymers that are both biodegradable and biocompatible. These nanoparticles have garnered considerable interest within the realm of nanomedicine. These nanoparticles offer several advantages for various applications in drug delivery and biomedical research. The unique properties of polymeric nanoparticles, such as their large surface area, small size, and tunable surface chemistry, these nanoparticles enable effective encapsulation and precise release of medications [44]. The polymeric matrix provides protection to the loaded drug, preventing its degradation and improving stability. Furthermore, the surface of polymeric nanoparticles can be modified by functional groups or targeting ligands, enabling specific interactions with target tissues, or cells, and enhancing the therapeutic efficacy of the encapsulated drug. The versatility and biocompatibility of polymeric nanoparticles make them a promising platform for targeted drug delivery, diagnostics, and other medical applications [45].

2.2.2 Dendrimers

Dendrimers are a class of highly branched macromolecules that have generated significant attention in diverse scientific areas and technological fields. These distinctive formations are distinguished by their tree-shaped design, featuring a central core and numerous branches or generations extending outward. Dendrimers offer numerous advantages that make them valuable in applications such as drug delivery, materials science, and diagnostics [46]. One of the key advantages of dendrimers is their precise control over size, shape, and surface functionality. Their highly branched nature allows for systematic modification and fine-tuning of their properties, making them versatile platforms for drug delivery systems. The ability to tailor dendrimers with specific functional groups on their surface enables targeted interactions with biological molecules, facilitating enhanced drug encapsulation, controlled release, and selective targeting to specific cells or tissues. This precise control over dendrimer structure and surface chemistry contributes to their potential in improving therapeutic outcomes and reducing side effects [47]. In addition to their role in drug delivery, dendrimers also find applications in diagnostics and imaging and their unique architecture provides a multitude of locations for the attachment of imaging agents or diagnostic probes, allowing for sensitive detection of disease markers or imaging of specific tissues. The controlled and predictable size of dendrimers offers advantages in terms of biodistribution, circulation time, and clearance from the body, further enhancing their utility in diagnostic applications [48]. Overall, dendrimers represent a fascinating class of macromolecules with immense potential in drug delivery, diagnostics, and materials science. Their precisely controlled structure, tunable surface functionality, and multifunctional properties make them promising candidates for a wide range of applications, contributing to advancements in various scientific and technological fields [49].

2.2.3 Polymer-Drug Conjugates

The polymer-drug conjugates have shown great promise in the treatment of Parkinson's disease, a neurological condition marked by the degeneration of dopaminergic neurons in the brain. These conjugates combine the therapeutic benefits of both polymers and drugs, offering advantages such as improved drug stability, prolonged circulation time, enhanced drug targeting, and reduced side effects. In Parkinson's disease, the delivery of therapeutic drugs to the brain is a significant challenge due to the blood–brain barrier [50]. Polymer-drug conjugates offer a viable solution by employing biocompatible polymers that can effectively penetrate the blood–brain barrier and transport the drug payload to the affected areas. By conjugating drugs with polymers, their stability is enhanced, shielding them from degradation and prolonging their presence in the bloodstream. This leads to prolonged drug release and sustained therapeutic effects, which is particularly important in the management of Parkinson's disease where continuous drug delivery is beneficial [51]. Furthermore, polymer-drug conjugates can be designed to target specific cells or tissues within the brain, maximizing therapeutic efficacy while minimizing off-target effects. Surface modifications or ligand conjugation on the polymer-drug conjugates can facilitate active targeting of the dopaminergic neurons or other relevant cells involved in Parkinson's disease. This targeted approach not only improves drug accumulation at the desired site but also reduces the required drug dosage, minimizing potential side effects. Overall, polymer-drug conjugates have shown great promise for the treatment of Parkinson's disease, offering innovative strategies for efficient drug delivery and improved therapeutic outcomes [52].

2.2.4 Examples of Their Use in Delivering Parkinson's Disease Drugs

Scientists have developed poly (ethylene glycol)-co-poly(ε-caprolactone) (PEG-PCL) nanoparticles encapsulating GB (GB-NPs) to enhance its efficacy for treating PD. These nanoparticles enable the sustained release of GB, which enhances its brain accumulation and therapeutic potential [53]. Phosphorus dendrimers and viologen dendrimers are highly promising macromolecular structures used in various fields including chemistry, materials science, biology, and nanomedicine. A new family of hybrid phosphorus-viologen dendrimers has emerged and these dendrimers combine the unique properties of phosphorus and viologen structures. They can be prepared in different forms, such as classical dendrimers, macromolecular asterisks, onion peel structures, and covalent polydendrimer frameworks. Preliminary studies show their potential in biological applications and in constructing organic–inorganic hybrid materials [54]. A novel idea for thermo-responsive drug delivery is proposed using copolymers of poly(2-oxazoline) that are conjugated with a hydrophobic drug. These copolymers are composed of two types: 2-n-propyl-2-oxazoline and 2-methoxycarbonylpropyl-2-oxazoline. The drug, benazepril, is attached to the copolymers through an ester linkage. The copolymer itself is safe and soluble at normal body temperature. However, when the drug is conjugated to the copolymer, its solubility decreases at lower temperatures. Once the drug is released from the copolymer, it becomes soluble again, allowing for controlled and slow drug release. This concept proposes the potential of using an injectable polymer-drug conjugate to create an insoluble depot, which can gradually release the drug over time [55].

2.3 *Inorganic Nanomaterials*

Inorganic nanomaterials are a class of nanoscale materials composed of non-organic elements or compounds, such as metals, metal oxides, or semiconductors. These nanomaterials have garnered significant attention due to their unique chemical and physical properties, making them valuable in a broad range of applications across various scientific and technological fields. The distinct characteristics of inorganic nanomaterials arise from their small size, typically in the range of 1 to 100 nm [56]. At this scale, quantum effects and surface properties become prominent, leading to altered optical, electrical, magnetic, and catalytic properties compared to their bulk counterparts. This provides opportunities for novel functionalities and applications. Inorganic nanomaterials find applications in diverse areas such as energy, electronics catalysis, sensing, and medicine. For example, in electronics, nanomaterials like quantum dots are used to enhance the performance of displays and photovoltaic devices due to their size-dependent optical properties [57]. In energy applications, nanomaterials are employed to improve the efficiency of solar cells, energy storage devices, and catalysts for renewable energy conversion. In the field of medicine, inorganic nanomaterials are utilized for targeted drug delivery, bioimaging, and therapeutics due to their unique surface properties and interactions with biological systems.

The wide-ranging applications of inorganic nanomaterials highlight their significance in advancing technologies and addressing global challenges. Continued research and development in this field are crucial for harnessing the potential of these materials and exploring new avenues for innovation and improvement in various industries [58].

2.3.1 Mesoporous Silica Nanoparticles (MSN)

Mesoporous silica nanoparticles (MSN) have acquired considerable attention in the field of nanotechnology and biomedical research. These nanoparticles possess a distinct structure characterized by an ordered arrangement of pores within their silica framework, resulting in a large surface area and pore volume. MSN offers several advantages, including their tunable pore size, biocompatibility, and versatile surface chemistry, making them highly attractive for a range of applications, including drug delivery, imaging, and catalysis. The tunable pore size of MSN allows for proper encapsulation and release of various drugs [59]. The mesopores serve as receptacles for drug loading, protecting the encapsulated drugs from degradation and improving their stability. Additionally, the controlled release from MSN can be precisely regulated by adjusting the pore size, structure, and surface modifications, enabling tailored and sustained drug release profiles. This feature is particularly beneficial for drugs that require controlled dosage or prolonged therapeutic effects. In addition to drug delivery, MSN has shown potential in medical imaging and diagnostics [60]. The large surface area of these nanoparticles facilitates the loading of imaging agents, such as contrast agents or fluorescent dyes, enhancing their detection sensitivity. Furthermore, the surface of MSN can be modified with targeting ligands or antibodies, enabling active targeting and specific interactions with diseased cells or tissues. This targeted imaging approach improves the accuracy of disease diagnosis and enables real-time monitoring of therapeutic interventions [61]. In summary, mesoporous silica nanoparticles (MSN) possess unique qualities that make them highly versatile and appropriate for drug delivery, imaging, and diagnostic applications. Their tunable pore size, biocompatibility, and versatile surface chemistry contribute to their potential in efficiently encapsulating drugs, providing controlled release, enhancing imaging capabilities, and enabling targeted interactions with specific cells or tissues. Continued research and development in this field will likely lead to further advancements and innovative applications of MSN in various biomedical and nanotechnology-related fields [62].

2.3.2 Magnetic Nanoparticles

Magnetic nanoparticles have emerged as a pioneering tool in the field of Parkinson's disease research and treatment. These nanoparticles possess magnetic properties that can be utilized for targeted drug delivery, imaging, and therapy. In the context of Parkinson's disease, magnetic nanoparticles can be used to enhance the delivery of therapeutic agents to the affected areas of the brain. Through surface modifications and functionalization, magnetic nanoparticles can be loaded with specific drugs and guided to the desired sites using external magnetic fields, thereby increasing the precision and efficiency of drug delivery [63]. Additionally, MNPs can be used as contrast agents in MRI allowing for improved visualization and assessment of disease progression. Furthermore, these nanoparticles can also be used in hyperthermia-based therapies, where heat is generated by the nanoparticles in response to an alternating magnetic field, providing a potential avenue for localized treatment of Parkinson's disease. The utilization of magnetic nanoparticles has shown great promise for advancing the management and understanding of Parkinson's disease through targeted drug delivery, imaging, and therapeutic interventions [64].

2.3.3 Carbon-Based Nanomaterials

Carbon-based nanomaterials have impressed considerable attention across multiple scientific disciplines and technological domains due to their exceptional properties and versatile applications. These nanomaterials, including carbon nanotubes, graphene, and fullerenes, exhibit unique structural arrangements and possess remarkable mechanical, electrical, and thermal characteristics. Carbon nanotubes feature cylindrical structures composed of rolled-up graphene sheets, offering exceptional tensile strength and electrical conductivity [65]. Graphene, a single layer of carbon atoms arranged in a two-dimensional lattice, is known for its excellent electrical conductivity and large surface area. Fullerenes, such as buckyballs, are spherical carbon molecules with fascinating electronic properties. Carbon-based nanomaterials find applications in diverse fields such as electronics, sensing, energy storage, and biomedical engineering. Their exceptional properties render them ideal candidates for enhancing device performance, enabling innovative sensor designs, and developing advanced drug delivery systems. The ongoing research and development in carbon-based nanomaterials hold tremendous promise for driving scientific advancements and revolutionizing a wide array of industries [66].

2.3.4 Unique Properties and Applications in Drug Delivery for Parkinson's Disease

Mesoporous silica nanoparticles (MSNs) were created using drug-structure-directing agents (DSDAs) that possess inherent therapeutic activity. The DSDA employed was L-Dopa, modified with fatty acids to form anionic surfactants capable of generating micelles as templates for silica framework assembly. This templating method allowed for the production of tunable MSNs with different sizes, shapes (spherical or elongated), and structures. By utilizing DSDAs, the need for surfactant removal and subsequent drug loading steps in conventional MSN synthesis can be avoided. The released L-Dopa from these MSNs was found to be influenced by the DSDA size, solubility, and surface chemical interactions with the MSN hosts. The sustained release of L-Dopa under intestinal conditions (pH 7.4) presents a potential application for treating Parkinson's disease, avoiding premature release in the stomach [67]. In a study, an ultrasensitive electrochemical immunosensor was developed that uses supramolecule-mediated AuNP composites (GNCs) on a gold electrode to detect nitrated α-syn. The GNCs offer high conductivity, abundant binding sites, and a large surface area. Anti-α-syn-modified magnetic nanoparticles (MNPs) were used as signal amplification tags in a sandwich assay. The combination of GNCs and MNPs improved the immunoassay performance, enhancing sensitivity and selectivity. This nitrated α-syn immunosensor demonstrates the potential for practical clinical applications due to its simplicity and sensitivity [68]. In another study conducted, a new immunosensor was developed to detect α-syno, an early biomarker in PD. The immunosensor uses a nanocomplex of poly(D-glucosamine)/gold nanoparticles/multi-walled carbon nanotubes/reduced graphene oxide to amplify the signal. The specific anti-α-syno antibody is then grafted onto the electrode surface. The immunosensor has a linear response range of 0.05 fM to 500.00 fM and a detection limit of 0.03 fM. It was successfully applied to analyze α-syno in human plasma samples [69].

3 Mechanisms of Drug Delivery by Nanomaterials

The mechanisms of drug delivery by nanomaterials are a subject of extensive research and exploration, aiming to enhance therapeutic outcomes and improve treatment strategies. Nanomaterials offer unique advantages in drug delivery due to their large surface area, small size, and tunable properties. One mechanism involves the encapsulation of drugs within the nanomaterials, protecting them from degradation and enabling controlled release at the target site [22]. Another mechanism involves the surface modification of nanomaterials by targeting ligands or functional groups, facilitating active or passive targeting of specific cells or tissues. Nanomaterials can also serve as carriers for drug conjugation, where the drug is chemically linked to the nanomaterial surface, enabling targeted delivery and controlled release. Furthermore, nanomaterials can exploit stimuli-responsive properties, such as pH or temperature, to trigger drug release in response to specific physiological conditions. Understanding and harnessing the diverse mechanisms of drug delivery by nanomaterials pave the way for the development of innovative and effective therapeutic measures with the potential to revolutionize the field of medicine [70].

3.1 Passive Targeting Strategies

Passive targeting strategies are a set of techniques utilized in drug delivery to elevate the accumulation of therapeutic agents at specific sites within the body (Fig. 2). These strategies exploit the natural physiological processes and properties of tissues to attain

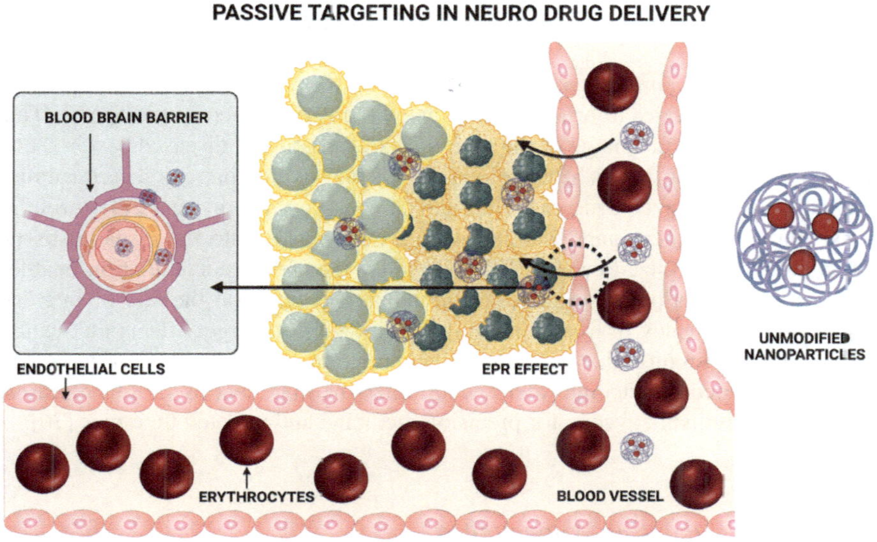

Fig. 2 Passive targeting approach in neuro drug delivery

targeted drug delivery without the need for active intervention. One of the common passive targeting approaches is the enhanced permeability and retention (EPR) effect, which takes advantage of the impaired lymphatic drainage and leaky vasculature of tumors [71]. Nanoparticles or macromolecular drug carriers can exploit these abnormal characteristics to accumulate preferentially in tumor tissues, leading to improved drug concentration at the site of interest. Additionally, passive targeting can also rely on the surface properties and size of drug carriers, as smaller particles can extravasate more easily through leaky blood vessels and accumulate in inflamed or diseased tissues. By harnessing these passive targeting strategies, drug delivery systems can optimize therapeutic efficacy, minimize off-target effects, and potentially revolutionize the cure of various diseases [72].

3.1.1 Enhanced Permeability and Retention (EPR) Effect

The EPR effect is a phenomenon that can be exploited in drug delivery strategies to target tumor tissues. The EPR effect capitalizes on the impaired lymphatic drainage and abnormal blood vessels found in tumors, resulting in increased vascular permeability and the retention of macromolecules or nanoparticles within the tumor microenvironment [73]. This effect allows for the selective accumulation of therapeutic agents at the tumor site while minimizing their distribution in healthy tissues. By leveraging the EPR effect, drug delivery systems can elevate the effectiveness of anticancer treatments by delivering a higher concentration of drugs directly to the tumor, thereby improving therapeutic outcomes and reducing side effects [74].

3.1.2 Size-Dependent Accumulation in Diseased Tissues

Size-dependent accumulation in diseased tissues is a phenomenon exploited in drug delivery strategies to bring about targeted delivery of therapeutic agents. This phenomenon takes advantage of the unique characteristics of diseased tissues, such as inflamed or tumor tissues, where blood vessels may exhibit increased permeability and gaps. Smaller-sized drug carriers, such as nanoparticles or nanoscale formulations, can exploit these gaps and extravasate more easily into the diseased tissue compared to larger-sized carriers [75]. This size-dependent accumulation enables a higher concentration of drugs to accumulate specifically at the site of interest, improving the efficacy of treatment while minimizing off-target effects on healthy tissues. By harnessing size-dependent accumulation, drug delivery systems can optimize therapeutic outcomes and revolutionize the treatment of various diseases, providing a promising avenue for precision medicine and targeted therapies [76].

3.2 Active Targeting Approaches

Active targeting approaches are innovative strategies used in drug delivery to better the specificity and efficiency of therapeutic interventions. These approaches involve the incorporation of functional groups or targeting ligands on the surface of drug carriers, allowing them to actively interact with specific cells or tissues. By attaching these targeting moieties, such as antibodies, aptamers, or peptides to the drug delivery system, active targeting can be achieved (Fig. 3) [77]. The targeting ligands identify and bind to biomarkers or specific receptors overexpressed on the top of target cells, enabling selective drug delivery. This active interaction enhances the deposition of therapeutic agents at the particular site, leading to reduced systemic toxicity and improved therapeutic efficacy. Active targeting approaches hold great potential for personalized medicine, as they allow for precise and targeted drug delivery, opening new avenues for the treatment of different diseases, including cancer, inflammatory disorders, and other pathological state [78].

3.2.1 Ligand-Mediated Targeting for Specific Receptor Recognition

Ligand-mediated targeting is a sophisticated strategy employed in drug delivery to achieve specific recognition of receptors and enhance the selectivity of therapeutic interventions. This approach involves the utilization of ligands, such as antibodies, aptamers, or peptides, that possess a high affinity for specific receptors on target cells or tissues. By attaching these ligands to drug delivery systems, precise and targeted binding to the receptors can be achieved, facilitating the efficient delivery of therapeutic agents [79]. The ligand-receptor interaction enables the drug carrier to specifically recognize and bind to the desired cells, enhancing the accumulation of therapeutic agents at the target site while reducing target effects. Ligand-mediated

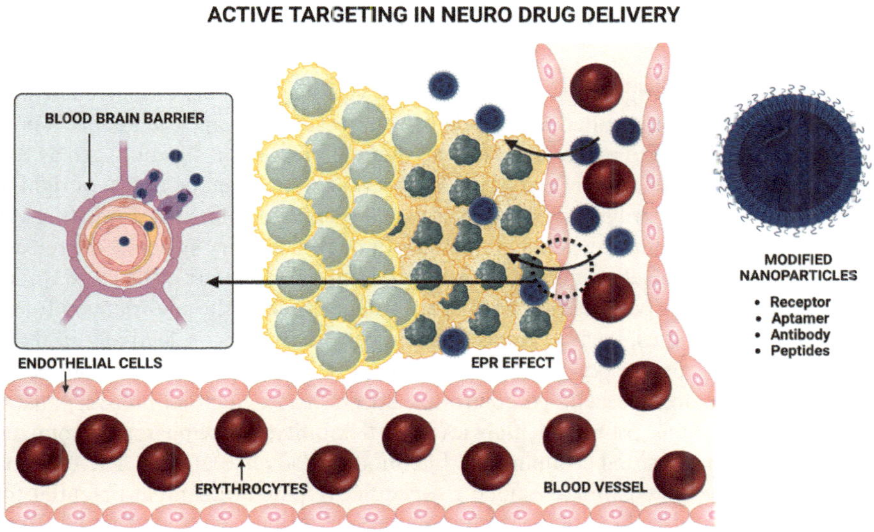

Fig. 3 Active targeting approach in neuro drug delivery

targeting shows immense potential for improving the efficacy and safety of drug delivery systems, enabling personalized medicine and laying the groundwork for treatments of various diseases, including cancer, autoimmune disorders, and other specific pathological conditions [80].

3.2.2 Receptor-Mediated Endocytosis for Targeted Drug Delivery

Receptor-mediated endocytosis is a highly effective strategy utilized in targeted drug delivery to elevate the specificity and internalization of therapeutic agents. This mechanism enforces the advantage of specific receptors expressed on the surface of target cells, which can selectively recognize and bind to ligands attached to drug carriers. Upon binding, the receptor-ligand complex triggers endocytosis, a cellular process that allows the uptake of the drug carrier into the target cell [81]. This targeted internalization enables the delivery of therapeutic agents directly into the cell's interior, enhancing their efficacy and minimizing their exposure to healthy cells. Receptor-mediated endocytosis shows great potential for various applications, including the treatment of cancers, genetic disorders, and infectious diseases. By exploiting this mechanism, targeted drug delivery systems can optimize therapeutic outcomes and revolutionize the field of medicine by providing more precise and efficient treatments [82].

3.3 Stimuli-Responsive Drug Release Systems

Stimuli-responsive drug release systems are innovative approaches employed in drug delivery to achieve controlled and on-demand release of therapeutic agents. These systems are designed to respond to specific internal or external stimuli, such as pH, temperature, glucose, protein, enzyme, DNA, redox, ion, magnetic fields, or light to trigger the release of drugs at desired locations or under specific conditions (Fig. 4). By incorporating stimuli-responsive elements into drug delivery systems, the release of drugs can be precisely regulated, ensuring optimal therapeutic efficacy [83]. For example, pH-responsive systems can take advantage of the acidic environment found in certain disease sites, such as tumors, to trigger drug release selectively in those regions. Temperature-responsive systems can exploit the temperature variations in specific body regions to achieve controlled drug release. Such stimuli-responsive drug release systems provide a high level of flexibility, allowing for customized drug delivery profiles and reducing the likelihood of adverse effects. The creation of drug delivery systems that respond to specific triggers holds great potential for advancing personalized medicine, improving treatment outcomes, and maximizing the therapeutic benefits for patients [84].

3.3.1 PH-Responsive Nanomaterials for Controlled Drug Release

pH-responsive nanomaterials represent a cutting-edge approach in drug delivery systems, enabling precise and controlled delivery of therapeutic agents. These nanomaterials are engineered to respond to changes in pH, particularly in specific physiological environments or disease sites. By incorporating pH-responsive components, such as pH-sensitive polymers or coatings, the release of drugs can be modulated based on the acidity or alkalinity of the surrounding environment [85]. In acidic conditions, commonly found in tumor tissues or inflamed regions, the nanomaterials undergo structural changes or disintegration, leading to the release of drugs at the target site. This pH-dependent drug release mechanism provides a high level of selectivity, ensuring that the therapeutic agents are predominantly released in the desired location while minimizing off-target effects. pH-responsive nanomaterials offer a favorable avenue for the growth of advanced drug delivery systems, enabling enhanced therapeutic outcomes, improved patient care and reduced side effects improved patient care [86].

3.3.2 Temperature-Responsive and Enzyme-Responsive Systems

Temperature-responsive and enzyme-responsive systems are innovative approaches in drug delivery that allow for the controlled inducing of therapeutic agents in response to specific stimuli. Temperature-responsive systems are designed to release drugs in a temperature-dependent manner, taking advantage of the variations in

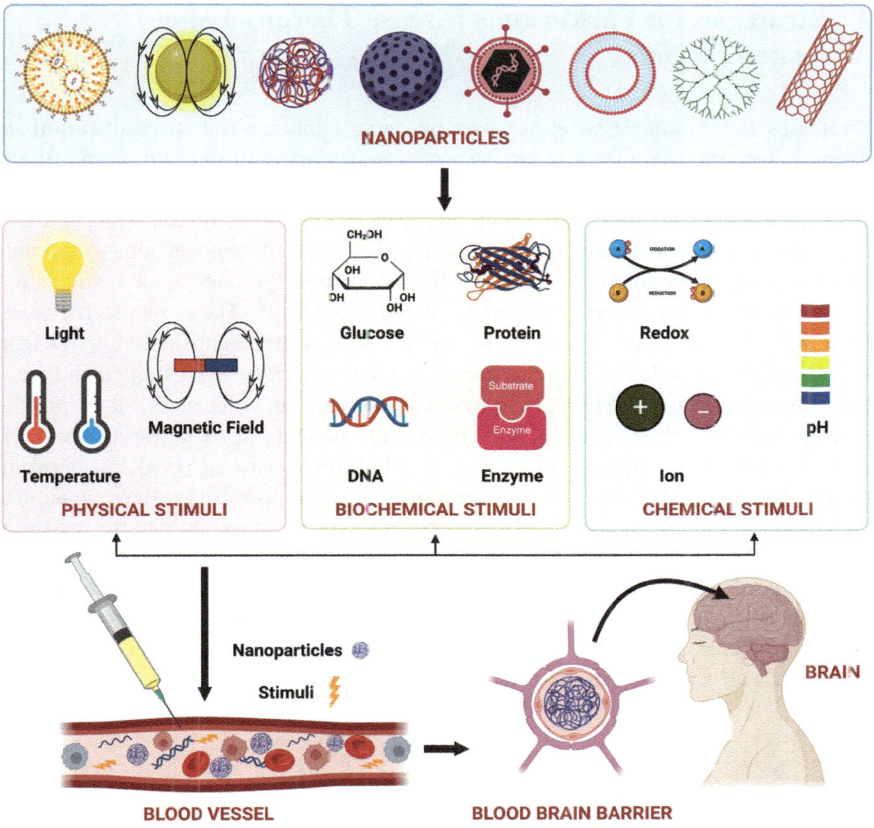

Fig. 4 Stimuli-responsive approach in neuro drug delivery

temperature within the body. These systems are engineered with materials that exhibit temperature-sensitive properties, such as polymers or liposomes, which undergo changes in structure or solubility upon temperature fluctuations [87]. Enzyme-responsive systems, on the other hand, respond to the presence of specific enzymes found in certain disease environments. By incorporating enzyme-sensitive components, such as peptide linkers or cleavable polymers, the drug release can be triggered in the presence of these enzymes, providing a targeted and timely delivery of therapeutic agents. Both temperature-responsive and enzyme-responsive systems offer precise control over drug release, ensuring optimal therapeutic efficacy while minimizing off-target effects. These innovative approaches hold significant potential in advancing the field of drug delivery, allowing for tailored treatments and improved patient outcomes [88].

4 Strategies for Parkinson's Disease Therapy Using Nanomaterials

Strategies for Parkinson's disease therapy using nanomaterials present promising avenues for improving treatment outcomes and managing the symptoms of this neurodegenerative disorder. Nanomaterials offer unique advantages in terms of drug delivery, neuroprotection, and tissue engineering, allowing for targeted and efficient therapies. One strategy involves the utilization of nanocarriers to enhance the transport of therapeutic agents, such as dopamine precursors or neuroprotective compounds, to the affected areas of the brain [89]. These nanocarriers can be designed to cross the blood–brain barrier, protect the encapsulated drugs from deterioration, and release them in a controlled manner, ensuring sustained and localized drug delivery. Additionally, nanomaterials can be functionalized to provide neuroprotective effects, such as scavenging free radicals or reducing neuroinflammation, which is incriminated in the growth of Parkinson's disease [90]. Furthermore, nanomaterial-based tissue engineering approaches hold promise for the regeneration and replacement of damaged or lost dopaminergic neurons, potentially restoring motor function and alleviating symptoms. By leveraging the unique properties of nanomaterials, these strategies aim to revolutionize Parkinson's disease therapy, offering new possibilities for targeted drug delivery, neuroprotection, and regenerative medicine approaches that could significantly improve the quality of life for individuals affected by this debilitating condition [91].

4.1 Dopamine Replacement Therapy

Dopamine replacement therapy plays a pivotal role in the treatment of Parkinson's disease, aiming to alleviate the motor symptoms associated with the deficiency of this neurotransmitter. This therapy involves the administration of exogenous dopamine or dopamine precursor drugs to compensate for the loss of cells that produce dopamine in the brain is a condition that can occur. By replenishing dopamine levels, the therapy helps restore proper neurotransmission and improve motor function in individuals with Parkinson's disease [92]. Various formulations and delivery methods, including oral medications, patches, and injections, are utilized to optimize drug delivery and achieve consistent dopamine levels in the brain. While dopamine replacement therapy provides symptomatic relief, it does not address the disease's underlying cause or slow disease progression. Nonetheless, this therapy remains a cornerstone in managing Parkinson's disease, allowing individuals to regain control over their movements and improve their quality of life [93].

4.1.1 Encapsulation and Controlled Release of Dopamine or Dopamine Agonists

The encapsulation and controlled release of dopamine or dopamine agonists in Parkinson's disease offer innovative strategies to optimize drug delivery and enhance therapeutic outcomes. These approaches involve encapsulating dopamine or dopamine agonist drugs within nanocarriers or drug delivery systems, allowing for targeted and sustained release at the desired site in the brain [94]. The encapsulation protects the drugs from degradation and facilitates their transport across the blood–brain barrier, ensuring efficient delivery to the affected regions. By controlling the release kinetics, these systems enable a continuous and controlled supply of dopamine or dopamine agonists, mimicking the natural release patterns and improving the efficacy of therapy [95]. This encapsulation and controlled release approach hold significant potential for improving the management of Parkinson's disease, minimizing side effects, and providing a more stable and consistent supply of dopamine to alleviate motor symptoms and enhance the quality of life for individuals living with this state [96, 97].

4.1.2 Strategies to Enhance Drug Stability and Bioavailability

There are various approaches to improve drug stability and bioavailability in Parkinson's disease. One strategy involves formulating the drug and enhances to safeguard it from deterioration and its absorption in the body. This can be achieved through the use of encapsulation techniques or the evolution of prodrugs, which are inactive compounds that are converted into active drugs within the body [98]. Another approach is to enhance the drug's solubility by using appropriate excipients or altering its chemical structure. Additionally, the use of targeted drug delivery systems, such as nanoparticles or liposomes, can improve drug distribution to the affected areas of the brain, increasing its efficacy while minimizing side effects. Furthermore, optimizing the dosing regimen and considering factors like food interactions can also contribute to enhancing bioavailability and drug stability in Parkinson's disease [99].

4.2 Neuroprotective Approaches

Neuroprotective strategies play a key role in managing Parkinson's disease. One approach involves the use of antioxidants, which assist in counteracting the damaging effects of free radicals and decreasing oxidative stress, a key factor in neurodegeneration. Antioxidant-rich diets, including fruits, vegetables, and omega-3 fatty acids, can be beneficial [100]. Another neuroprotective strategy involves targeting mitochondrial dysfunction, as impaired mitochondria contribute to neuronal damage. Mitochondrial enhancers, such as coenzyme Q10, have shown promise in enhancing mitochondrial function and protecting against Parkinson's progression. Additionally, anti-inflammatory agents can be utilized to counteract neuroinflammation, a process that exacerbates neuronal damage [101]. Medications like natural compounds or nonsteroidal anti-inflammatory drugs (NSAIDs) with anti-inflammatory properties may be considered. Furthermore, promoting neurotrophic factors, such as brain-derived neurotrophic factor (BDNF), can aid in maintaining and supporting the survival of dopaminergic neurons. Exercise, particularly aerobic exercise, has been found to increase BDNF levels and exhibit neuroprotective effects. Overall, these neuroprotective approaches hold the potential in decelerating the advancement of Parkinson's disease and preserving neuronal function [102].

4.2.1 Delivery of Antioxidant Agents to Combat Oxidative Stress

The effective delivery of antioxidant agents is crucial for combating oxidative stress in various conditions, including Parkinson's disease. One strategy involves the advancement of targeted drug delivery systems that can specifically deliver antioxidants to affected areas. Nanoparticles, liposomes, or microspheres can be utilized to encapsulate antioxidant agents, protecting them from degradation and facilitating their controlled release [103]. These delivery systems can be designed to selectively cross the blood–brain barrier, ensuring efficient delivery to the brain where oxidative stress is prominent. Furthermore, innovative techniques such as conjugating antioxidants to target ligands can enhance their specificity, allowing them to bind to specific receptors on affected cells. Another approach to increasing antioxidant levels in the body involves the use of prodrugs. Prodrugs are inactive compounds that are converted into active antioxidants once they enter the body. [104]. This approach can improve the solubility, stability, and absorption of the antioxidant agents. Additionally, the incorporation of antioxidants into functional foods or dietary supplements can provide a convenient and accessible means of delivering these agents to individuals with Parkinson's disease. By employing these delivery strategies, antioxidant agents can effectively combat oxidative stress and potentially slow down the development of Parkinson's disease [105].

4.2.2 Anti-inflammatory Drug Delivery for Neuroinflammation Modulation

Effective transport of anti-inflammatory drugs is essential for modulating neuroinflammation in various conditions, including neurodegenerative diseases like Parkinson's disease. One approach involves the development of targeted drug delivery systems that can deliver anti-inflammatory agents specifically to affected areas in the brain. Nanoparticles, liposomes, or micelles can be used to encapsulate these drugs, providing protection against degradation and enabling controlled release [106]. These delivery systems can be designed to cross the blood–brain barrier and accumulate in regions of neuroinflammation, ensuring optimal drug concentration at the site of action. Moreover, surface modifications or conjugation of targeting ligands can improve the specificity of drug delivery, allowing for precise binding to receptors on inflamed cells. One approach to reducing inflammation is the use of prodrugs. These are substances that are initially inactive, but are transformed into active anti-inflammatory agents once inside the body [107]. Prodrugs can improve drug stability, solubility, and bioavailability, enhancing their therapeutic effectiveness. Furthermore, implantable devices or sustained-release formulations can provide continuous and prolonged delivery of anti-inflammatory drugs, reducing the need for frequent administration. By employing these drug delivery approaches, effective modulation of neuroinflammation can be achieved, potentially mitigating the progression and symptoms of Parkinson's disease [108].

4.3 Gene Therapy Using Nanomaterials

Gene therapy utilizing nanomaterials offers a promising approach for treating various diseases, including Parkinson's disease. This innovative strategy involves the delivery of therapeutic genes using nanoscale materials, such as nanoparticles or viral vectors, to targeted cells in the body. These nanomaterials can be engineered to protect the therapeutic genes from degradation, facilitate their entry into cells, and promote their expression [109]. The nanocarriers can be surface-modified or functionalized with ligands to enhance cellular uptake and specific targeting to affected areas in the brain. Furthermore, the development of non-viral vectors, such as polymer-based nanoparticles or lipid-based nanoparticles, provides an alternative approach that offers advantages like reduced immunogenicity and the ability to carry larger DNA payloads. Through gene therapy with nanomaterials, it becomes possible to introduce therapeutic genes into target cells, regulate gene expression, and potentially restore or modulate cellular functions, providing a novel avenue for the treatment of Parkinson's disease [110].

4.3.1 Nanoparticle-Mediated Gene Delivery for Gene-Based Treatments

Nanoparticle-mediated gene delivery has emerged as a promising strategy for gene-based treatments in various diseases, including Parkinson's disease. This innovative approach involves the use of nanoparticles to efficiently deliver therapeutic genes to target cells. Nanoparticles, such as polymer-based or lipid-based carriers, can protect genetic material from degradation and facilitate its entry into cells [111]. Through surface modifications and functionalization, nanoparticles can be designed to improve their absorption by cells and specifically target affected areas in the body, including the brain in the case of Parkinson's disease. These nanoparticles' biocompatible and biodegradable nature ensures their safety and minimizes potential adverse effects. By utilizing nanoparticle-mediated gene delivery, it becomes possible to introduce therapeutic genes into target cells, regulate gene expression, and potentially correct or modulate underlying genetic abnormalities, providing a promising avenue for gene-based treatments in Parkinson's disease [112].

4.3.2 RNA Interference-Based Strategies for Targeted Gene Silencing

RNA interference (RNAi)-based strategies offer effective approaches for targeted gene silencing in various diseases, including Parkinson's disease. This innovative method involves the use of short hairpin RNA (shRNA) or small interfering RNA (siRNA) molecules to specifically target and degrade disease-causing messenger RNA (mRNA), thereby suppressing the expression of specific genes [113]. By designing siRNA or shRNA molecules complementary to the target gene sequence, they can be delivered to target cells using viral vectors, lipid-based nanoparticles, or other delivery systems. Once inside the cells, these RNA molecules engage with the cellular machinery to form RNA-induced silencing complexes (RISCs), leading to the deterioration of the target mRNA and subsequent reduction in protein production. This targeted gene silencing approach holds promise for selectively inhibiting disease-associated genes in Parkinson's disease, potentially providing therapeutic benefits by interfering with specific molecular pathways involved in the course of the disease [114].

5 Preclinical and Clinical Studies

5.1 Preclinical Studies with Animal Models

Preclinical studies in animal models of Parkinson's disease have provided valuable insights into the underlying mechanisms of the disease and potential therapeutic strategies. These studies have helped identify various neuroprotective agents, gene therapy approaches, and stem cell-based treatments for further investigation. Clinical trials have also been conducted to evaluate the safety and efficacy of novel therapies, such as deep brain stimulation, dopaminergic medications, and immunotherapies, in improving motor symptoms and overall quality of life in Parkinson's disease patients [115].

5.1.1 Evaluation of Nanomaterial-Based Drug Delivery Systems

The evaluation of drug delivery systems based on nanomaterials is a critical aspect of medical research aimed at enhancing therapeutic outcomes. The assessment of these innovative systems involves thorough investigations into their effectiveness, safety, and practicality. Clinical trials have a significant impact on evaluating nanomaterial-based drug delivery systems. These trials typically involve administering drugs encapsulated within nanomaterial carriers to patients and assessing their response to treatment. By measuring parameters such as drug release kinetics, targeted delivery, and therapeutic efficacy, researchers can determine the effectiveness of these systems in delivering drugs to specific sites within the body [116]. Safety evaluation is a crucial component of assessing nanomaterial-based drug delivery systems. Researchers closely monitor patients for any potential adverse effects or toxicities associated with the nanomaterial carriers. It is essential to understand the potential risks and side effects, such as immune responses, organ toxicity, or long-term complications, that may arise from the use of these systems. Rigorous safety evaluations ensure patient well-being and guide further improvements in the design and formulation of nanomaterial-based drug delivery systems. Practicality and feasibility assessments are also necessary to gauge the potential of nanomaterial-based drug delivery systems for clinical use. Factors such as scalability of production, stability of the formulations, and ease of administration are considered. These evaluations help determine the viability of translating these systems from the laboratory to real-world applications, considering factors such as cost-effectiveness, ease of manufacturing, and patient convenience. Various analytical techniques are employed to evaluate nanomaterial-based drug delivery systems [117]. These may include physicochemical characterization, in vitro studies, animal models, and clinical observations. By employing a multidisciplinary approach, researchers can gather comprehensive data on the performance, safety, and feasibility of these systems. Regulatory authorities have an essential impact in evaluating nanomaterial-based drug delivery systems. They ensure that rigorous guidelines and protocols are followed to protect patient rights and safety during clinical trials. Regulatory approval is necessary for the widespread implementation of these systems in clinical practice, underscoring the importance of robust evaluation. In conclusion, the evaluation of nanomaterial-based drug delivery systems is an essential step in advancing medical research and improving therapeutic outcomes. Through comprehensive assessments of effectiveness, safety, and practicality, researchers can ascertain the possibilities of these systems to revolutionize drug delivery and enhance patient care. Continued research, innovation, and collaboration among scientists, clinicians, and regulatory authorities are necessary to realize the full potential of nanomaterial-based drug delivery systems in clinical settings [118].

5.1.2 Assessment of Therapeutic Efficacy and Safety Profiles

The interdisciplinary progress in nanotechnology has greatly contributed to the advancement of nanomedicine, which holds the potential to enhance therapeutic effectiveness. The concept of delivering nanomedicine specifically to the affected area while mitigating harm to healthy tissues has positioned nanotechnology as a promising strategy for reducing toxicity associated with certain drugs. However, the toxicological assessment of nanomaterials has not kept pace with the rapid development of nanomedicine, leading to a lack of safety reports. In order to fully harness the potential of nanotechnology in nanomedicine development, it is crucial to obtain more toxicological data before any therapeutic substances can be used in humans [119]. One of the key advantages of nanomedicine over conventional counterparts is its extremely small size, resulting in a high surface area-to-volume ratio. The composition of these nanomedicine molecules can include hydrophilic or hydrophobic compounds with unique physicochemical properties, which can impact their physical and chemical characteristics, as well as their pharmacokinetics. Moreover, nanoparticles have the ability to traverse the blood–brain barriers due to their nanoscale dimensions. Changes in the physicochemical properties of nanomedicine can influence factors such as bioavailability, substance transport, cellular uptake, biotransformation, and elimination within the complex in vivo environment. A comprehensive evaluation of the safety profile is essential to acquire a comprehensive knowledge, of the toxicological implications of nanomedicine. Such an evaluation of safety profiles is indispensable and necessary for a thorough assessment of the therapeutic benefits and the development of a safer nanodrug delivery system [120].

5.2 Clinical Trials and Translational Research

5.2.1 Nanomaterial-Based Formulations in Clinical Trials

Nanomaterial-based formulations are currently being investigated in clinical trials for their potential therapeutic applications. These formulations utilize nanotechnology to manipulate and engineer materials at the nanoscale, enabling meticulous regulation of their characteristics and conduct. In these clinical trials, researchers are exploring various nanomaterials, such as nanoparticles, nanocapsules, and nanogels, as carriers for drug delivery systems. The distinctive characteristics of nanomaterials, like their high surface area-to-volume ratio and tunable surface chemistry, permit efficient encapsulation and targeted delivery of drugs to specific sites within the body [121]. Furthermore, nanomaterial-based formulations provide benefits such as enhanced bioavailability, prolonged drug release, and improved stability compared to traditional drug delivery systems. The nanoscale size of these formulations allows them to bypass biological barriers, such as the blood–brain barrier, and reach therapeutic targets that were previously inaccessible. Clinical trials involving nanomaterial-based formulations are being conducted in a diverse range of therapeutic areas, including neurology oncology, and cardiovascular disease [122].

For example, in cancer treatment, researchers are investigating the use of nanomaterials to deliver chemotherapy drugs directly to tumor cells while minimizing damage to healthy tissues. Moreover, for drug delivery, nanomaterial-based formulations are also being investigated for their diagnostic and imaging applications. By incorporating imaging agents into nanomaterials, researchers can develop targeted contrast agents for improved visualization of disease sites, enabling earlier detection and accurate monitoring of treatment response. While the field of nanomaterial-based formulations in clinical trials holds great promise, there are also challenges to address. Safety concerns, such as potential toxicity and long-term effects of these nanomaterials, need to be thoroughly evaluated. Regulatory approval and scalability of production are additional factors that require careful consideration. Overall, the ongoing clinical trials exploring nanomaterial-based formulations demonstrate the potential of nanotechnology in revolutionizing drug delivery and diagnostics. With further research and development, these formulations might open up additional possibilities, for effective and personalized treatments in various medical disciplines [123].

5.2.2 Evaluation of Clinical Outcomes, Safety, and Patient Compliance

The evaluation of clinical outcomes, patient compliance, and safety regarding the use of nanomaterials is of paramount importance in the field of medical research. Clinical trials play a vital role in assessing the efficacy and potential risks associated with these innovative materials. Clinical trials focusing on nanomaterials aim to gather empirical evidence regarding their effectiveness in treating various diseases and conditions. These trials typically involve administering nanomaterial-based formulations to patients and monitoring their response to treatment. The evaluation of clinical outcomes involves measuring parameters such as disease progression, symptom improvement, and overall patient well-being [124]. In addition to assessing clinical outcomes, the safety profile of nanomaterials is rigorously evaluated. Researchers examine potential adverse effects and toxicity associated with the use of these materials. This evaluation involves monitoring patients for any signs of allergic reactions, organ toxicity, or other harmful side effects. It is crucial to determine the dosage levels and administration routes that minimize risks while maximizing therapeutic benefits. Another critical aspect of clinical evaluation is patient compliance. It is important to understand whether patients are able to adhere to the prescribed treatment regimen involving nanomaterial-based formulations. Factors such as ease of administration, frequency of dosing, and patient acceptance of the treatment play a role in determining compliance [125].

Patient compliance is essential to ensure the validity and reliability of the clinical trial results. To evaluate clinical outcomes, safety, and patient compliance, clinical trials employ various methodologies. These may include randomized controlled trials, observational studies, and longitudinal assessments. By collecting comprehensive data on patient response, adverse events, and treatment adherence, researchers can draw conclusions about the efficacy, safety, and feasibility of nanomaterial-based formulations. Furthermore, regulatory authorities closely monitor clinical trials to ensure ethical considerations and patient safety. Stringent guidelines and protocols are in place to safeguard the rights and well-being of study participants [126]. The data collected during these trials serve as the basis for regulatory decision process and the approval of nanomaterial-based formulations for widespread use. In conclusion, the evaluation of clinical outcomes, safety, and patient compliance in clinical trials involving nanomaterials is a vital step in advancing medical and healthcare research. By conducting rigorous assessments, researchers can determine the efficacy, safety, and feasibility of these innovative materials, paving the way for their potential integration into mainstream medical practices [127].

6 Challenges and Future Directions

6.1 *Biocompatibility and Toxicity Considerations*

Regarding Parkinson's disease, the utilization of nanodrug delivery systems raises important considerations regarding biocompatibility and toxicity. These factors play a crucial role in ensuring the safety and effectiveness of these systems in delivering drugs to targeted areas. Nano drug delivery systems involve the use of nanoparticles, which are tiny particles ranging from 1 to 100 nm in size. These nanoparticles can be engineered to encapsulate medications and transport them to specific sites in the body, including the brain in the case of Parkinson's disease [128]. When designing nanodrug delivery systems, it is essential to carefully evaluate their biocompatibility. Biocompatibility pertains to the capacity of these nanoparticles to peacefully coexist and interact with biological systems without inducing negative responses. This assessment involves studying the interactions between nanoparticles and various components of the body, such as cells, tissues, and organs [129]. Toxicity considerations are equally important in the progression of nanodrug delivery systems. It is crucial to ensure that the nanoparticles used in these systems do not exert harmful effects on the body. This requires conducting rigorous toxicological studies to evaluate the potential adverse effects of nanoparticles, both in terms of acute toxicity and chronic toxicity. Several factors influence the biocompatibility and toxicity of nanodrug delivery systems. These include the surface properties, size, shape, and composition of the nanoparticles. For instance, nanoparticles with smaller sizes are more likely to penetrate tissues and cellular barriers, potentially affecting their functionality. Additionally, the surface properties of nanoparticles can determine their interactions with biological molecules and cells [96, 97]. To mitigate potential biocompatibility and toxicity concerns, researchers employ various strategies. Surface modifications of nanoparticles can be performed to boost their stability, reduce potential toxicity, and improve their interactions with the biological environment. Additionally, biodegradable nanoparticles that can break down over time and be eliminated from the body through natural processes are being explored to minimize long-term accumulation [130]. Robust preclinical testing is critical to evaluating the biocompatibility and toxicity of nanodrug delivery systems. In vitro studies using in vivo and cell culture experiments using animal models help assess the interactions and potential effects of nanoparticles in a controlled environment. These studies contribute to the identification of any adverse reactions and guide the optimization of nanodrug delivery systems for safe and effective use. By thoroughly assessing the interactions and potential adverse effects of nanoparticles, researchers can develop safe and effective systems that deliver medications to targeted areas, enhancing efficacy and minimizing the risks for individuals with Parkinson's disease [131].

6.2 Scalability and Manufacturing Challenges for Clinical Translation

When it comes to the clinical translation of innovative technologies, such as nanodrug delivery systems in the context of Parkinson's disease, there are significant challenges related to scalability and manufacturing. These challenges must be addressed to ensure the successful transition from research and development to large-scale production and clinical use. Scalability refers to the ability to efficiently and effectively increase the production of a technology or product to meet the demands of a larger population [132]. In the case of nanodrug delivery systems, it is essential to establish manufacturing processes that can produce these systems in sufficient quantities without compromising their quality and performance. This requires optimizing production techniques, ensuring consistency in the manufacturing process, and addressing any potential obstacles that may arise when scaling up. Manufacturing challenges are closely related to scalability and involve various considerations. One key challenge is the reproducibility of the manufacturing process. It is crucial to develop robust and standardized procedures that can consistently produce nanodrug delivery systems with the desired characteristics [133]. Variations in manufacturing can lead to inconsistencies in the performance of the systems, impacting their safety and efficacy. Another challenge is the selection and sourcing of materials for manufacturing. Nanodrug delivery systems often require specific materials with precise properties to achieve their intended functions. Ensuring a reliable supply chain for these materials, as well as addressing any issues related to material quality and availability, is vital for successful manufacturing and clinical translation [134].

Quality control and quality assurance are also critical aspects of manufacturing nanodrug delivery systems. Rigorous testing and evaluation throughout the manufacturing process are necessary to verify the performance, safety, and consistency of the systems. This includes assessments of the chemical and physical properties of the nanoparticles, as well as evaluating their stability and long-term behavior. Additionally, regulatory considerations and compliance with relevant standards pose challenges in the clinical translation of nanodrug delivery systems [135]. Meeting the requirements and guidelines set forth by regulatory authorities is essential to secure the well-being and efficiency of these systems for patients. This involves conducting appropriate preclinical and clinical studies, as well as addressing any specific regulatory hurdles associated with novel drug delivery technologies. Addressing scalability and manufacturing challenges requires collaboration between researchers, engineers, manufacturers, and regulatory bodies. Close partnerships can help identify and overcome potential obstacles, optimize manufacturing processes, and establish robust quality control measures. By addressing these challenges, the successful clinical translation of nano drug delivery systems can be achieved, ultimately benefiting individuals with Parkinson's disease and improving their treatment outcomes [136].

6.3 Regulatory Considerations and Approval Processes

In the realm of innovative drug delivery systems for Parkinson's disease and other medical applications, regulatory considerations and approval processes are of paramount importance. These factors ensure the safety, efficacy, and quality of these systems before they can be made available for clinical use. Regulatory considerations involve adherence to guidelines and regulations set by regulatory authorities, such as the European Medicines Agency (EMA) in Europe Food and Drug Administration (FDA) in the United States [137]. These guidelines outline the requirements and standards that must be met for a drug delivery system to obtain regulatory approval. They cover various aspects, including preclinical testing, clinical trials, manufacturing practices, labeling, and post-marketing surveillance. The approval process for drug delivery systems involves a rigorous evaluation of scientific data and evidence to exhibit the system's efficacy and safety. This process typically includes several stages, starting with preclinical studies in the laboratory and animal models, followed by clinical trials involving human subjects [138]. These trials assess the drug delivery system's performance, therapeutic benefits, and potential adverse effects. Regulatory authorities assess the data obtained from these studies to evaluate if the system meets the requisite standards for approval. Throughout the regulatory approval process, collaboration between researchers, manufacturers, and regulatory bodies is crucial [139]. Effective communication and adherence to regulatory guidelines help ensure that the drug delivery system is developed and evaluated according to established requirements. This collaboration also facilitates the exchange of information, addresses any regulatory concerns, and streamlines the approval process, ultimately leading to the availability of safe and effective drug delivery systems for Parkinson's disease and other medical states [140].

6.4 Personalized Medicine Approaches in Parkinson's Disease Therapy

In the field of Parkinson's disease therapy, personalized medicine approaches have gained significant attention. These approaches aim to tailor treatment strategies to individual patients based on their unique characteristics, such as genetic makeup, disease progression, and treatment response. By incorporating personalized medicine, healthcare providers can optimize therapy and improve outcomes for individuals with Parkinson's disease [141]. This approach entails utilizing various tools and techniques, including genetic testing, biomarker analysis, and advanced imaging, to better understand each patient's specific disease profile. With this information, treatment plans can be customized to target specific disease pathways, optimize medication dosages, and minimize adverse effects. Personalized medicine in Parkinson's disease therapy holds promise for more precise, individualized care that can enhance symptom management and potentially slow down disease progression [142].

6.5 Combination Therapies and Nanomaterial-Based Drug Delivery

The utilization of combination therapies along with nanomaterial-based drug delivery has arisen as an encouraging strategy in various fields, including Parkinson's disease treatment. Combination therapies involve the simultaneous or sequential use of multiple drugs or treatment modalities to enhance therapeutic outcomes. When combined with nanomaterial-based drug delivery systems, these therapies offer benefits including improved drug targeting, controlled release, and enhanced efficacy [116]. Nanomaterials can encapsulate multiple drugs within their structures, allowing for the precise co-delivery of different therapeutic agents. Furthermore, these nanomaterial-based systems can protect the drugs from degradation, enhance their stability, and facilitate their delivery to the desired sites in the body, including the brain in the case of Parkinson's disease. The integration of combination therapies and nanomaterial-based drug delivery holds great potential for synergistic effects, improved treatment outcomes, and personalized approaches in the management of Parkinson's disease and other complex conditions [143].

7 Conclusion

The use of nanomaterials as drug delivery vehicles holds great potential for improving therapeutic outcomes and reducing side effects in Parkinson's disease. These vehicles enable precise drug targeting, controlled release, and enhanced bioavailability. Passive targeting strategies, such as the enhanced permeability and retention (EPR) effect, exploit the physiological properties of diseased tissues for targeted accumulation. Ligand-mediated targeting and receptor-mediated endocytosis allow for specific recognition of receptors and internalization of drug carriers into target cells. Overall, nanomaterial-based drug delivery systems offer a promising approach for personalized medicine in Parkinson's disease therapy. Further research and development in this field hold the potential to revolutionize treatment strategies, improve patient outcomes, and provide new avenues for managing neurodegenerative diseases.

References

1. Funayama M et al (2022) Molecular genetics of Parkinson's disease: contributions and global trends. J Human Genet 68(3):125–130. https://doi.org/10.1038/s10038-022-01058-5
2. Bloem BR, Okun MS, Klein C (2021) Parkinson's disease. The Lancet 397(10291):2284–2303. https://doi.org/10.1016/s0140-6736(21)00218-x
3. Balestrino R, Schapira AHV (2019) Parkinson disease. Eur J Neurol 27(1):27–42. https://doi.org/10.1111/ene.14108
4. Szász JA et al (2019) A dopaminagonisták jelentősége a Parkinson-kór kezelésében a marosvásárhelyi ideggyógyászati klinikák 15 éves gyakorlatában - keresztmetszeti vizsgálat. Ideggyogyaszati Szemle-clinical Neuroscience. https://doi.org/10.18071/isz.72.0187
5. Lenka A et al (2022) Practical pearls to improve the efficacy and tolerability of levodopa in Parkinson's disease. Expert Rev Neurother 22(6):489–498. https://doi.org/10.1080/14737175.2022.2091436.
6. Tan YY, Jenner P, Chen S (2022) Monoamine oxidase-B inhibitors for the treatment of Parkinson's disease: past, present, and future. J Parkinson's Dis 12(2):477–493. https://doi.org/10.3233/jpd-212976
7. Barrett MJ et al (2021) Antimuscarinic anticholinergic medications in Parkinson disease: to prescribe or deprescribe? Mov Disord Clin Pract 8(8):1181–1188. https://doi.org/10.1002/mdc3.13347
8. Tong SY et al (2023) Serum glial cell line-derived neurotrophic factor (GDNF) a potential biomarker of executive function in Parkinson's disease. Front Neurosci 17. https://doi.org/10.3389/fnins.2023.1136499
9. Padilla-Godínez FJ, Ruiz-Ortega LI, Guerra-Crespo M (2022) Nanomedicine in the face of Parkinson's disease: from drug delivery systems to nanozymes. Cells 11(21):3445. https://doi.org/10.3390/cells11213445
10. Nemade D, Subramanian T, Shivkumar V (2021) An update on medical and surgical treatments of Parkinson's disease. Aging Dis 12(4):1021. https://doi.org/10.14336/ad.2020.1225
11. Little S, Brown P (2020) Debugging adaptive deep brain stimulation for Parkinson's disease. Mov Disord 35(4):555–561. https://doi.org/10.1002/mds.27996.
12. Prasuhn J, Brüggemann N (2021) Gene therapeutic approaches for the treatment of mitochondrial dysfunction in Parkinson's disease. Genes 12(11):1840. https://doi.org/10.3390/genes12111840
13. Mak MKY, Wong-Yu ISK (2019) Exercise for Parkinson's disease. Int Rev Neurobiol. Elsevier BV, pp 1–44. https://doi.org/10.1016/bs.irn.2019.06.001
14. Kim MY et al (2021) Occupational therapy interventions for instrumental activities of daily living for adults With Parkinson's disease: a systematic review. Am J OccupTher 75(3). https://doi.org/10.5014/ajot.2021.046581
15. Hidecker MJC et al (2022) Coordinated speech therapy, physiotherapy, and pharmaceutical care telehealth for people with Parkinson disease in rural communities: an exploratory, 8-week cohort study for feasibility, safety, and signal of efficacy. Rural Remote Health [Preprint]. https://doi.org/10.22605/rrh6679
16. Reynolds GO et al (2019) Cognitive-behavioral therapy for anxiety in Parkinson's disease. Behav Modif 44(4):552–579. https://doi.org/10.1177/0145445519838828
17. Park H, Otte A, Park K (2022) Evolution of drug delivery systems: from 1950 to 2020 and beyond. J Control Release 342:53–65. https://doi.org/10.1016/j.jconrel.2021.12.030
18. Peng H, Li Y, Ji W, Zhao R, Lu Z, Shen J, ... Zhang X (2022) Intranasal administration of self-oriented nanocarriers based on therapeutic exosomes for synergistic treatment of Parkinson's disease. ACS Nano 16(1):869–884
19. Chen W, Hu Y, Ju D (2020) Gene therapy for neurodegenerative disorders: advances, insights and prospects. Acta Pharmaceutica Sinica B 10(8):1347–1359. https://doi.org/10.1016/j.apsb.2020.01.015
20. Bhosale A et al (2023) Theoretical and applied concepts of nanocarriers for the treatment of Parkinson's diseases. OpenNano 9:100111. https://doi.org/10.1016/j.onano.2022.100111.

21. Asil SM et al (2020) Nanomaterial based drug delivery systems for the treatment of neurodegenerative diseases. Biomater Sci 8(15):4109–4128. https://doi.org/10.1039/d0bm00809e.
22. Baskin J, Jeon JY, Lewis SJG (2020) Nanoparticles for drug delivery in Parkinson's disease. J Neurol 268(5):1981–1994. https://doi.org/10.1007/s00415-020-10291-x
23. Vijiaratnam N et al (2021) Progress towards therapies for disease modification in Parkinson's disease. Lancet Neurol 20(7):559–572. https://doi.org/10.1016/s1474-4422(21)00061-2
24. Stoker TM, Barker RA (2020) Recent developments in the treatment of Parkinson's disease. F1000Research 9:862. https://doi.org/10.12688/f1000research.25634.1
25. Tambe VS, Wairkar S (2023) Lipid-based nanocarriers via nose-to-brain pathway for Alzheimer's and Parkinson's disease. Curr Nanosci 19(3):322–337. https://doi.org/10.2174/1573413718666220627140824
26. Ghazy E et al (2021) Nanomaterials for Parkinson disease: recent progress. J Mol Struct 1231:129698. https://doi.org/10.1016/j.molstruc.2020.129698
27. Paul A, Yadav KS (2020) Parkinson's disease: current drug therapy and unraveling the prospects of nanoparticles. J Drug Deliv Sci Technol 58:101790. https://doi.org/10.1016/j.jddst.2020.101790
28. Kumar B et al (2020) Liposomes: novel drug delivery approach for targeting Parkinson's disease. Curr Pharm Des 26(37):4721–4737. https://doi.org/10.2174/13816128266662000128145124.
29. Pandian SRK et al (2022) Liposomes: an emerging carrier for targeting Alzheimer's and Parkinson's diseases. Heliyon 8(6):e09575. https://doi.org/10.1016/j.heliyon.2022.e09575
30. Seo MW, Park TE (2021) Recent advances with liposomes as drug carriers for treatment of neurodegenerative diseases. Biomed Eng Lett 11(3):211–216. https://doi.org/10.1007/s13534-021-00198-5
31. Burnouf T et al (2021) Solid lipid nanoparticles (SLNs): an advanced drug delivery system targeting brain through BBB. Pharmaceutics 13(8):1183. https://doi.org/10.3390/pharmaceutics13081183
32. Costa C et al (2021) Intranasal delivery of nanostructured lipid carriers, solid lipid nanoparticles and nanoemulsions: a current overview of in vivo studies. Acta Pharmaceutica Sinica B 11(4):925–940. https://doi.org/10.1016/j.apsb.2021.02.012
33. Cometa S et al (2020) In vitro investigations on dopamine loaded solid lipid nanoparticles. J Pharm Biomed Anal 185:113257. https://doi.org/10.1016/j.jpba.2020.113257
34. Mohammed HA et al (2023) Solid lipid nanoparticles for targeted natural and synthetic drugs delivery in high-incidence cancers, and other diseases: roles of preparation methods, lipid composition, transitional stability, and release profiles in nanocarriers' development. Nanotechnol Rev 12(1):20220517. https://doi.org/10.1515/ntrev-2022-0517
35. Salvi VR, Pawar P (2019) Nanostructured lipid carriers (NLC) system: a novel drug targeting carrier. J Drug Deliv Sci Technol 51:255–267. https://doi.org/10.1016/j.jddst.2019.02.017
36. Tekade AR, Mittha PS, Pisal CS (2021) Nanostructured lipid carriers for nose to brain delivery targeting CNS: diversified role of liquid lipids for synergistic action. Adv Pharm Bull. https://doi.org/10.34172/apb.2022.078
37. Van NTH et al (2022) Nanostructured lipid carriers and their potential applications for versatile drug delivery via oral administration. OpenNano 8:100064. https://doi.org/10.1016/j.onano.2022.100064
38. Sakamula R, Yata T, Thong-Asa W (2022) Nanostructure lipid carriers enhance alpha-mangostin neuroprotective efficacy in mice with rotenone-induced neurodegeneration. Metab Brain Dis 37(5):1465–1476. https://doi.org/10.1007/s11011-022-00967-w
39. Nguyen TTL, Maeng HJ (2022) Pharmacokinetics and pharmacodynamics of intranasal solid lipid nanoparticles and nanostructured lipid carriers for nose-to-brain delivery. Pharmaceutics 14(3):572. https://doi.org/10.3390/pharmaceutics14030572
40. Kuo YC, Wang IH, Rajesh R (2021) Use of leptin-conjugated phosphatidic acid liposomes with resveratrol and epigallocatechin gallate to protect dopaminergic neurons against apoptosis for Parkinson's disease therapy. Acta Biomaterialia 119:360–374. https://doi.org/10.1016/j.actbio.2020.11.015

41. Dudhipala N, Gorre T (2020) Neuroprotective effect of ropinirole lipid nanoparticles enriched hydrogel for Parkinson's disease: in vitro, ex vivo, pharmacokinetic and pharmacodynamic evaluation. Pharmaceutics 12(5):448. https://doi.org/10.3390/pharmaceutics12050448
42. Mishra NK et al (2019) Development and characterization of nasal delivery of selegiline hydrochloride loaded nanolipid carriers for the management of Parkinson's disease. Cent Nerv Syst Agents Med Chem 19(1):46–56. https://doi.org/10.2174/1871524919666181126124846
43. Martano S et al (2022) Inorganic nanomaterials versus polymer-based nanoparticles for overcoming neurodegeneration. Nanomaterials 12(14):2337. https://doi.org/10.3390/nano12142337
44. Mahajan K et al (2022) Polymer based nanoparticles for BCS class II drugs— 'a mini review.' Mater Today Proc. https://doi.org/10.1016/j.matpr.2022.12.007
45. Annu N et al (2022) An insight to brain targeting utilizing polymeric nanoparticles: effective treatment modalities for neurological disorders and brain tumor. Front Bioeng Biotechnol 10. https://doi.org/10.3389/fbioe.2022.788128
46. Ordonio MB, Zaki RM, Elkordy A (2022) Dendrimers-based drug delivery system: a novel approach in addressing Parkinson's disease. Future Pharmacol 2(4):415–430. https://doi.org/10.3390/futurepharmacol2040027
47. Palan F, Chatterjee B (2022) Dendrimers in the context of targeting central nervous system disorders. J Drug Deliv Sci Technol 73:103474. https://doi.org/10.1016/j.jddst.2022.103474
48. Pérez-Carrión MD, Posadas I (2023) Dendrimers in neurodegenerative diseases. Processes 11(2):319. https://doi.org/10.3390/pr11020319
49. Morfill C, Pankratova S, Machado P, Fernando NK, Regoutz A, Talamona F, ... Kiryushko D (2022) Nanostars carrying multifunctional neurotrophic dendrimers protect neurons in preclinical in vitro models of neurodegenerative disorders. ACS Appl Mater Interfaces 14(42):47445–47460
50. Javia A et al (2022) Polymer-drug conjugates: design principles, emerging synthetic strategies and clinical overview. Int J Pharm 623:121863. https://doi.org/10.1016/j.ijpharm.2022.121863
51. Paipa-Álvarez HO, Delgado BM, Alvarado WP (2020) Nanotechnological applications of polymer-drug conjugate as oncological treatment. J Phys 1672:012010. https://doi.org/10.1088/1742-6596/1672/1/012010
52. Dadwal A et al (2023) Polymer-drug conjugates: origins, progress to date, and future directions. Elsevier eBooks, pp 221–248. https://doi.org/10.1016/b978-0-323-91248-8.00015-5
53. Zhao Y et al (2020) Polymeric nanoparticles-based brain delivery with improved therapeutic efficacy of ginkgolide B in Parkinson's disease. Int J Nanomed 15:10453–10467. https://doi.org/10.2147/ijn.s272831
54. Majoral JP et al (2021) Hybrid phosphorus–viologen dendrimers as new soft nanoparticles: design and properties. Org Chem Front 8(16):4607–4622. https://doi.org/10.1039/d1qo00511a
55. Park JR et al (2020) Drug–polymer conjugates with dynamic cloud point temperatures based on poly(2-oxazoline) copolymers. Polym Chem 11(32):5191–5199. https://doi.org/10.1039/d0py00602e
56. Wang F et al (2023) Chiral inorganic nanomaterials for biological applications. Nanoscale 15(6):2541–2552. https://doi.org/10.1039/d2nr05689e
57. Fan Y et al (2022) Biological applications of chiral inorganic nanomaterials. Chirality 34(5):760–781. https://doi.org/10.1002/chir.23428
58. Cong Y et al (2022) Penetration and translocation of functional inorganic nanomaterials into biological barriers. Adv Drug Deliv Rev 191:114615. https://doi.org/10.1016/j.addr.2022.114615
59. Attia MS et al (2023) Mesoporous silica nanoparticles: their potential as drug delivery carriers and nanoscavengers in Alzheimer's and Parkinson's diseases. Saudi Pharm J 31(3):417–432. https://doi.org/10.1016/j.jsps.2023.01.009

60. Mendiratta S et al (2019) Multidisciplinary role of mesoporous silica nanoparticles in brain regeneration and cancers: from crossing the blood–brain barrier to treatment. Part Part Syst Charact 36(9):1900195. https://doi.org/10.1002/ppsc.201900195
61. Swar S, Zajícová V, Stibor I (2019) Effectiveness of diverse mesoporous silica nanoparticles as potent vehicles for the drug L-DOPA. Materials 12(19):3202. https://doi.org/10.3390/ma12193202
62. Tzankov B et al (2019) Development of MCM-41 mesoporous silica nanoparticles as a platform for pramipexole delivery. J Drug Deliv Sci Technol 51:26–35. https://doi.org/10.1016/j.jddst.2019.02.008
63. Dhillon K et al (2022) Directional control of neurite outgrowth: emerging technologies for Parkinson's disease using magnetic nanoparticles and magnetic field gradients. J R Soc Interface 19(196). https://doi.org/10.1098/rsif.2022.0576
64. Chavan N et al (2022) Magnetic nanoparticles—a new era in nanotechnology. J Drug Deliv Sci Technol 77:103899. https://doi.org/10.1016/j.jddst.2022.103899
65. Erdem Ö et al (2021) Carbon-based nanomaterials and sensing tools for wearable health monitoring devices. Adv Mater Technol 7(3):2100572. https://doi.org/10.1002/admt.202100572
66. Owida HA, Turab NM, Al-Nabulsi J (2023) Carbon nanomaterials advancements for biomedical applications. Bull Electr Eng Inf 12(2):891–901. https://doi.org/10.11591/eei.v12i2.4310
67. Morales V et al (2021) l-Dopa release from mesoporous silica nanoparticles engineered through the concept of drug-structure-directing agents for Parkinson's disease. J Mater Chem B 9(20):4178–4189. https://doi.org/10.1039/d1tb00481f
68. Zhang Z et al (2021) The magnetic-nanoparticle-assisted sensitive detection of nitrated α-syn in blood based on a sensitizing electrochemical layer. Nanoscale 13(17):8107–8117. https://doi.org/10.1039/d1nr01415c
69. Tao D et al (2020) Ultrasensitive detection of alpha-synuclein oligomer using a PolyD-glucosamine/gold nanoparticle/carbon-based nanomaterials modified electrochemical immunosensor in human plasma. Microchem J 158:105195. https://doi.org/10.1016/j.microc.2020.105195
70. Anoop et al (2020) Approaches for encephalic drug delivery using nanomaterials: the current status. Brain Res Bull 155:184–190. https://doi.org/10.1016/j.brainresbull.2019.11.017
71. Chatterjee D, Kordower JH (2019) Immunotherapy in Parkinson's disease: current status and future directions. Neurobiol Dis 132:104587. https://doi.org/10.1016/j.nbd.2019.104587
72. Antonini A et al (2020) Immunization therapies for Parkinson's disease: state of the art and considerations for future clinical trials. Expert Opin Investig Drugs 29(7):685–695. https://doi.org/10.1080/13543784.2020.1771693
73. Ghosh S, Ghosh S, Sil PC (2019) Role of nanostructures in improvising oral medicine. Toxicol Rep 6:358–368. https://doi.org/10.1016/j.toxrep.2019.04.004
74. Ni N et al (2022) Inducible endothelial leakiness in nanotherapeutic applications. Biomaterials 287:121640. https://doi.org/10.1016/j.biomaterials.2022.121640
75. Pardo M et al (2021) Size-dependent intranasal administration of magnetoelectric nanoparticles for targeted brain localization. Nanomed Nanotechnol Biol Med 32:102337. https://doi.org/10.1016/j.nano.2020.102337
76. Smith IT et al (2022) Nanomedicine and nanobiotechnology applications of magnetoelectric nanoparticles. Wiley Interdisc Rev Nanomed Nanobiotechnol [Preprint]. https://doi.org/10.1002/wnan.1849
77. Mathew B et al (2019) Emerging therapeutic potentials of dual-acting MAO and AChE inhibitors in Alzheimer's and Parkinson's diseases. Archiv Der Pharmazie 352(11):1900177. https://doi.org/10.1002/ardp.201900177
78. Alavi M, Hamidi M (2019) Passive and active targeting in cancer therapy by liposomes and lipid nanoparticles. Drug Metab Pers Ther 34(1). https://doi.org/10.1515/dmpt-2018-0032
79. Van Gastel J et al (2021) Aging-related modifications to G protein-coupled receptor signaling diversity. Pharmacol Ther 223:107793. https://doi.org/10.1016/j.pharmthera.2020.107793

80. Mi P, Cabral H, Kataoka K (2019) Ligand-installed nanocarriers toward precision therapy. Adv Mater 32(13):1902604. https://doi.org/10.1002/adma.201902604
81. Tashima T (2020) Smart strategies for therapeutic agent delivery into brain across the blood–brain barrier using receptor-mediated transcytosis. Chem Pharm Bull 68(4):316–325. https://doi.org/10.1248/cpb.c19-00854
82. Anthony DP et al (2021) Targeting receptor-ligand chemistry for drug delivery across blood-brain barrier in brain diseases. Life Sci 274:119326. https://doi.org/10.1016/j.lfs.2021.119326
83. Das B et al (2023) Stimuli-responsive boron-based materials in drug delivery. Int J Mol Sci 24(3):2757. https://doi.org/10.3390/ijms24032757
84. Gowda BJ, Ahmed MG, Chinnam S, Paul K, Ashrafuzzaman M, Chavali M, ... Gupta PK (2022) Current trends in bio-waste mediated metal/metal oxide nanoparticles for drug delivery. J Drug Deliv Sci Tech 71:103305
85. Simão AR et al (2020) pH-responsive hybrid hydrogels: Chondroitin sulfate/casein trapped silica nanospheres for controlled drug release. Int J Biol Macromol 148:302–315. https://doi.org/10.1016/j.ijbiomac.2020.01.093
86. Beňová E et al (2021) pH-responsive mesoporous silica drug delivery system, its biocompatibility and co-adsorption/co-release of 5-Fluorouracil and Naproxen. Appl Surf Sci 561:150011. https://doi.org/10.1016/j.apsusc.2021.150011
87. Manouchehri S et al (2021) Advanced delivery systems based on lysine or lysine polymers. Mol Pharm 18(10):3652–3670. https://doi.org/10.1021/acs.molpharmaceut.1c00474
88. Shende P, Trivedi R (2021) Nanotheranostics in epilepsy: a perspective for multimodal diagnosis and strategic management. Nano Select 2(7):1277–1290. https://doi.org/10.1002/nano.202000141
89. Torres-Ortega PV et al (2019) Micro- and nanotechnology approaches to improve Parkinson's disease therapy. J Control Release 295:201–213. https://doi.org/10.1016/j.jconrel.2018.12.036
90. Sahu T et al (2021) Nanotechnology based drug delivery system: current strategies and emerging therapeutic potential for medical science. J Drug Deliv Sci Technol 63:102487. https://doi.org/10.1016/j.jddst.2021.102487
91. Chawla S et al (2020) Evolving nanoformulation strategies for diagnosis and clinical interventions for Parkinson's disease. Drug Discov Today 25(2):392–405. https://doi.org/10.1016/j.drudis.2019.12.005
92. Garcia-Pardo J et al (2021) Bioinspired theranostic coordination polymer nanoparticles for intranasal dopamine replacement in Parkinson's disease. ACS Nano 15(5):8592–8609. https://doi.org/10.1021/acsnano.1c00453
93. Karthivashan G, Ganesan P, Park SY, Lee HW, Choi DK (2020) Lipid-based nanodelivery approaches for dopamine-replacement therapies in Parkinson's disease: From preclinical to translational studies. Biomater 232:119704
94. Meng XT et al (2020) Vascular endothelial growth factor-loaded poly-lactic-co-glycolic acid nanoparticles with controlled release protect the dopaminergic neurons in Parkinson's rats. Chem Biol Drug Des 95(6):631–639. https://doi.org/10.1111/cbdd.13681
95. Liu L et al (2021) Encapsulation and pH-responsive release of bortezomib by dopamine grafted hyaluronate nanogels. Int J Biol Macromol 183:369–378. https://doi.org/10.1016/j.ijbiomac.2021.04.161
96. Wang J et al (2020) Molecular mechanisms of glutamate toxicity in Parkinson's disease. Front Neurosci 14. https://doi.org/10.3389/fnins.2020.585584
97. Wang S et al (2020) A novel photothermo-responsive nanocarrier for the controlled release of low-volatile fragrances. RSC Adv 10(25):14867–14876. https://doi.org/10.1039/c9ra10662f
98. Ma Z et al (2019) Pharmaceutical strategies of improving oral systemic bioavailability of curcumin for clinical application. J Control Release 316:359–380. https://doi.org/10.1016/j.jconrel.2019.10.053
99. Han HS, Koo SY, Choi K (2022) Emerging nanoformulation strategies for phytocompounds and applications from drug delivery to phototherapy to imaging. Bioact Mater 14:182–205. https://doi.org/10.1016/j.bioactmat.2021.11.027

100. Raza C, Anjum R, Shakeel NUA (2019) Parkinson's disease: mechanisms, translational models and management strategies. Life Sci 226:77–90. https://doi.org/10.1016/j.lfs.2019.03.057
101. Pérez-Segura I et al (2023) PPARs and their neuroprotective effects in Parkinson's disease: a novel therapeutic approach in α-Synucleinopathy? Int J Mol Sci 24(4):3264. https://doi.org/10.3390/ijms24043264
102. Sola P et al (2022) Neuroprotective approaches to halt Parkinson's disease progression. Neurochem Int 158:105380. https://doi.org/10.1016/j.neuint.2022.105380
103. Pinto ME et al (2020) Antioxidant therapy, oxidative stress, and blood-brain barrier: the road of dietary antioxidants. Elsevier eBooks, pp 125–141. https://doi.org/10.1016/b978-0-12-817780-8.00009-8
104. Percário S et al (2020) Oxidative stress in Parkinson's disease: potential benefits of antioxidant supplementation. Oxidative Med Cell Longev:1–23. https://doi.org/10.1155/2020/2360872
105. Martinelli C et al (2019) Antioxidants and nanotechnology: promises and limits of potentially disruptive approaches in the treatment of central nervous system diseases. Adv Healthc Mater 9(3):1901589. https://doi.org/10.1002/adhm.201901589
106. Talebi M et al (2021) An updated review on the versatile role of chrysin in neurological diseases: chemistry, pharmacology, and drug delivery approaches. Biomed Pharmacother 141:111906. https://doi.org/10.1016/j.biopha.2021.111906
107. Kalampokini S et al (2019) Nonpharmacological modulation of chronic inflammation in Parkinson's Disease: role of diet interventions. Parkinson's Dis:1–12. https://doi.org/10.1155/2019/7535472
108. Zhou M et al (2022) Apoptotic bodies for advanced drug delivery and therapy. J Control Release 351:394–406. https://doi.org/10.1016/j.jconrel.2022.09.045
109. Sayed N et al (2022) Gene therapy: comprehensive overview and therapeutic applications. Life Sci 294:120375. https://doi.org/10.1016/j.lfs.2022.120375
110. Saad JF, Saad FA (2023) Gene therapy for Alzheimer and Parkinson diseases. Curr Gene Ther 23(3):163–169. https://doi.org/10.2174/1566523223666230419101023
111. Spandana KMA et al (2020) A comprehensive review of nano drug delivery system in the treatment of CNS disorders. J Drug Deliv Sci Technol 57:101628. https://doi.org/10.1016/j.jddst.2020.101628
112. Wu L, Huang Z, Pan Z (2021) The spatiality and driving forces of population ageing in China. PLoS One 16(1):e0243559
113. Hyder SM, Chung JH, Ganguly K (2021) Are CRISPR/Cas9 and RNA interference-based new technologies to relocate crop pesticides? Elsevier eBooks, pp 47–63. https://doi.org/10.1016/b978-0-12-821910-2.00004-7
114. He A et al (2021) Targeting circular RNAs as a therapeutic approach: current strategies and challenges. Signal Transduct Target Ther 6(1). https://doi.org/10.1038/s41392-021-00569-5
115. Giuliano C et al (2021) Neuroprotective and symptomatic effects of cannabidiol in an animal model of Parkinson's disease. Int J Mol Sci 22(16):8920. https://doi.org/10.3390/ijms22168920
116. Singh AP et al (2019) Targeted therapy in chronic diseases using nanomaterial-based drug delivery vehicles. Signal Transduct Target Ther 4(1). https://doi.org/10.1038/s41392-019-0068-3
117. Rahmani M, Negro S, Hernández EB (2022) The potential use of tetracyclines in neurodegenerative diseases and the role of nano-based drug delivery systems. Eur J Pharm Sci 175:106237. https://doi.org/10.1016/j.ejps.2022.106237
118. Tan Q et al (2022) Getting drugs to the brain: advances and prospects of organic nanoparticle delivery systems for assisting drugs to cross the blood-brain barrier. J Mater Chem B. https://doi.org/10.1039/d2tb01440h
119. Montecucco F et al (2019) Apomorphine for Parkinson's disease: efficacy and safety of current and new formulations. CNS Drugs 33(9):905–918. https://doi.org/10.1007/s40263-019-00661-z

120. Li C et al (2020) Zonisamide for the treatment of Parkinson disease: a current update. Front Neurosci 14. https://doi.org/10.3389/fnins.2020.574652
121. Yadav K et al (2023) Biomedical applications of nanomaterials in the advancement of nucleic acid therapy: mechanistic challenges, delivery strategies, and therapeutic applications. Int J Biol Macromol 241:124582. https://doi.org/10.1016/j.ijbiomac.2023.124582
122. Song J et al (2021) Design and development of nanomaterial-based drug carriers to overcome the blood–brain barrier by using different transport mechanisms. Int J Mol Sci 22(18):10118. https://doi.org/10.3390/ijms221810118
123. Xie J et al (2019) Nanomaterial-based blood-brain-barrier (BBB) crossing strategies. Biomaterials 224:119491. https://doi.org/10.1016/j.biomaterials.2019.119491
124. Bianchini E et al (2022) Feasibility, safety, and effectiveness of telerehabilitation in mild-to-moderate Parkinson's disease. Front Neurol 13. https://doi.org/10.3389/fneur.2022.909197
125. Farr AC, Xiong MP (2020) Challenges and opportunities of deferoxamine delivery for treatment of Alzheimer's disease, Parkinson's disease, and intracerebral Hemorrhage. Mol Pharm 18(2):593–609. https://doi.org/10.1021/acs.molpharmaceut.0c00474
126. Bouça-Machado R et al (2021) Kinematic and clinical outcomes to evaluate the efficacy of a multidisciplinary intervention on functional mobility in Parkinson's disease. Front Neurol 12. https://doi.org/10.3389/fneur.2021.637620
127. Quintero JE et al (2022) Direct delivery of an investigational cell therapy in patients with Parkinson's disease: an interim analysis of feasibility and safety of an open-label study using DBS-Plus clinical trial design. BMJ Neurol Open 4(2):e000301. https://doi.org/10.1136/bmjno-2022-000301
128. Ashique S et al (2023) Strategic nanocarriers to control neurodegenerative disorders: concept, challenges, and future perspective. Int J Pharm 633:122614. https://doi.org/10.1016/j.ijpharm.2023.122614
129. Yang KH, Narayan RJ (2019) Biocompatibility and functionalization of diamond for neural applications. Curr Opin Biomed Eng 10:60–68. https://doi.org/10.1016/j.cobme.2019.03.002
130. Mogharbel BF et al (2022) Biodegradable nanoparticles loaded with levodopa and curcumin for treatment of Parkinson's disease. Molecules 27(9):2811. https://doi.org/10.3390/molecules27092811
131. Ghosh P, Bera A, De P (2021) Current status, challenges and future directions in the treatment of neurodegenerative diseases by polymeric materials. J Indian Chem Soc 98(1):100011. https://doi.org/10.1016/j.jics.2021.100011
132. Skidmore S, Barker RA (2023) Challenges in the clinical advancement of cell therapies for Parkinson's disease. Nat Biomed Eng 7(4):370–386. https://doi.org/10.1038/s41551-022-00987-y
133. Song J et al (2022) Multiplexed strategies toward clinical translation of extracellular vesicles. Theranostics 12(15):6740–6761. https://doi.org/10.7150/thno.75899
134. Kim TJ, Koo SM, Studer L (2020) Pluripotent stem cell therapies for parkinson disease: present challenges and future opportunities. Front Cell Develop Biol 8. https://doi.org/10.3389/fcell.2020.00729
135. Burnouf T, Agrahari V, Agrahari V (2019) Extracellular vesicles as nanomedicine: hopes and hurdles in clinical translation. Int J Nanomed 14:8847–8859. https://doi.org/10.2147/ijn.s225453
136. Desgres M, Menasché P (2019) Clinical translation of pluripotent stem cell therapies: challenges and considerations. Cell Stem Cell 25(5):594–606. https://doi.org/10.1016/j.stem.2019.10.001
137. Muheem A et al (2021) Recent patents, regulatory issues, and toxicity of nanoparticles in neuronal disorders. Curr Drug Metab [Preprint]. https://doi.org/10.2174/1389200221999201210213036
138. Wu LP, Wang D, Li Z (2020) Grand challenges in nanomedicine. Mater Sci Eng C, 106:110302. https://doi.org/10.1016/j.msec.2019.110302
139. Foulkes R et al (2020) The regulation of nanomaterials and nanomedicines for clinical application: current and future perspectives. Biomater Sci 8(17):4653–4664. https://doi.org/10.1039/d0bm00558d

140. Mohajerani A et al (2019) Nanoparticles in construction materials and other applications, and implications of nanoparticle use. Materials 12(19):3052. https://doi.org/10.3390/ma12193052
141. Kevadiya BD et al (2019) Neurotheranostics as personalized medicines. Adv Drug Deliv Rev 148:252–289. https://doi.org/10.1016/j.addr.2018.10.011
142. Tanga S (2022) Recent trends in precision drug and gene delivery. https://pubs.thescienceein.org/journal/index.php/nanomed/article/view/429
143. Cheng G et al (2022) Anti-Parkinsonian therapy: strategies for crossing the blood–brain barrier and nano-biological effects of nanomaterials. Nano-Micro Lett 14(1):105. https://doi.org/10.1007/s40820-022-00847-z

Nanoparticles for Brain Tumor Imaging and Therapy

Cleona Elizabeth Mary DCruz, Rupesh Kalidas Shirodkar, Yashwant Pathak, and Lalit Kumar

Abstract Nanoparticles have emerged as promising tools in the field of brain tumor imaging and therapy, offering unprecedented opportunities for precise diagnosis and targeted treatment. Over the years, researchers have explored the multifaceted applications of nanoparticles in addressing the complexities of brain tumors. Engineered nanoparticles, often coated with biocompatible materials, enable enhanced permeability across the blood-brain barrier, facilitating accurate imaging through various techniques such as magnetic resonance imaging (MRI) and fluorescence imaging. In imaging, nanoparticles serve as contrast agents, enhancing the resolution of imaging and enabling precise tumor localization and monitoring of therapeutic responses. In therapy, nanoparticles function as carriers for therapeutic agents, allowing delivery of therapeutic payloads directly to tumor sites, minimizing off-target effects and systemic toxicity. The ability to functionalize nanoparticles with targeting ligands further enhances specificity, ensuring selective interaction with tumor cells. The synergy of diagnostic and therapeutic functionalities in nanoparticle-based approaches not only improves treatment efficacy but also provides real-time monitoring of therapeutic responses. This chapter highlights the recent advancements in nanoparticle-based approaches, shedding light on their potential to revolutionize the diagnosis and treatment of brain tumors, ultimately paving the way for more effective and personalized healthcare strategies in neuro-oncology.

C. E. M. DCruz · R. K. Shirodkar
Department of Pharmaceutics, Goa College of Pharmacy, 18th June Road, Panaji-Goa 403001, India

Y. Pathak
USF Health Taneja College of Pharmacy, University of South Florida, Tampa, FL, USA

Faculty of Pharmacy (Adjunct Professor), Airlangga University, Surabaya, Indonesia

L. Kumar (✉)
Department of Pharmaceutics, National Institute of Pharmaceutical Education and Research, Hajipur, Bihar, Vaishali 844102, India
e-mail: lk.kundlas@gmail.com

S. K. Rath et al. (eds.), *Nanomaterials for Drug Delivery and Neurological Diseases Management*, Smart Nanomaterials Technology,
https://doi.org/10.1007/978-981-97-0308-1_14

Keywords Brain tumors · Nanoparticles · Quantum dots · Dendrimers · Carbon nanotubes · Fullerenes

1 Introduction

The mere thought of cancer conjures up a crushing sense of fatal despair, which is a testament to the ghastly disease and its harrowing ordeals. With genetics, lifestyle and environmental factors to blame, the incidence of cancer is steadily on the rise and around the world, nearly one in six persons has been gripped firmly in its deadly talons. And while most types of cancer present with serious risk, an uncontrolled and abnormal growth inside the brain; the very core of our existence, creates an extraordinarily profound threat to life. Despite the various surgical advances, the prognosis for patients with brain tumors particularly Glioblastoma multiforme (GBM) remains notably poor, carrying a high possibility of death within three years and the currently available therapeutic protocols and diagnostic approaches seem futile with genetic tumor heterogeneity, inconsistency in tumor tissue cellular architecture, uncontrolled and rapid proliferation, drug resistance, non-uniform expression of target receptors and tumor recurrence at the helm [1]. The existence of a physiological fence, the blood brain barrier (BBB), which denies entry of most blood plasma constituents, including circulating therapeutic agents across its highly restrictive boundary presents with another colossal hurdle to clinical therapy of neurological diseases.

Regardless of gadolinium (Gd)-based contrast-imaging, combination chemotherapy-radiation therapy and surgical resection being the prevalent standard protocol for brain tumor management, extensive research has steered ahead to navigate new waters. While diagnostic paths like computed tomography (CT), magnetic resonance imaging (MRI) and positron emission tomography (PET) are presently used to diagnose GBM, these tumor imaging strategies do not possess enough sensitivity to detect minute brain tumors and do not have the ability to differentiate residual glioma tumors from recurrent tumors. Although proving considerable effectiveness, the numerous limitations of conventional alkylating agents (Carmustine, Lomustine) and methylating agents (Temozolomide), their hepatic, neurologic and pulmonary toxicity, poor brain bioavailability owing to low permeation across the BBB, and non-targeted drug delivery leading to apoptosis of healthy cells pose a formidable challenge to treatment [2, 3]. As the incidence of malignant tumors keeps rising each year, to improve the treatment outcomes and survival rates, novel approaches for brain tumor imaging, early diagnosis, enhanced therapy and tracking of response to chemotherapy and radiotherapy are a pressing priority.

Fueled by the need for more efficient treatment options, clinical research hastened and deepened and successfully unlocked advancements in tumor diagnostics and therapeutics, taking clinical therapy from macroscale to microscale to nanoscale. Emanating from the ideas and concepts of renowned physicist Richard Feynman, nanoscience and nanotechnology have advanced rapidly over the decades, effected revolutionary changes in pharmacotherapy and have scaled infinite possibilities in every sphere imaginable. In the field of neuro-oncology, the development of diagnostic techniques and therapeutic paths went on for the win with nanocarriers on its team.

The array of superior properties that nanoparticles (NPs) offer including their small size, high surface area, physiological stability, ability to overcome BBB constraints, biocompatibility, enhanced bioavailability and delayed drug metabolism make them of versatile importance in disease targeting. The last decade demonstrated pivotal advances in brain tumor research, improved tumor imaging, targeted therapeutic agent delivery and radical diagnostic and therapeutic agents [4]. Nanotechnology latched on to play a paramount part in medical imaging, with nanodiagnostic techniques like MRI involving dendrimers and metallic NPs demonstrating improved sensitivity and specificity toward tumor cells that express the target receptors. Biocompatible NPs composed of gold, silver, iron oxide, lipids, dendrimers and magnetic nanomaterials can be manipulated by various techniques to conjugate with cancer targeting ligands, antibodies or entrap drugs, offer increased vascular permeability, increase drug solubility, have shown tremendous promise and are now in the forefront of clinical therapy. The emergence of nanoplatforms, integrating drugs with molecular imaging probes helped allay cytotoxicity, improved drug pharmacokinetics, and provided tissue targeting. Moreover, "Nanotheranostics" a system of NPs functioning as assets in diagnosis, treatment and as response markers to chemotherapeutics and radiotherapeutics, has also exhibited high applicability and exceptional treatment efficacy, marking it as a valuable resource in the future of tumor therapy [5].

2 Types of Nanoparticles

Nanoparticles surfaced with small and flexible structures (10 and 100 nm) as their fundamental asset. Owing to their noteworthy physical and chemical properties, a myriad of diagnostic and therapeutic agents established on the nanoplatform have been recently explored. Promising therapeutic approaches centering around multifunctional NPs and including metallic NPs, carbon nanotubes (CNTs), quantum dots (QDs), dendrimers, iron oxide NPs, superparamagnetic iron oxide NPs, lipid-based NPs, polymeric micelles and radiolabeled NPs shown in Fig. 1 have been reported with numerous advantages over conventionally used avenues [6].

2.1 *Gold NPs*

Nanoparticles based on colloidal gold have enkindled vital research for biomedical applications, diagnostic aids and drug and gene delivery. Gold NPs (AuNPs)

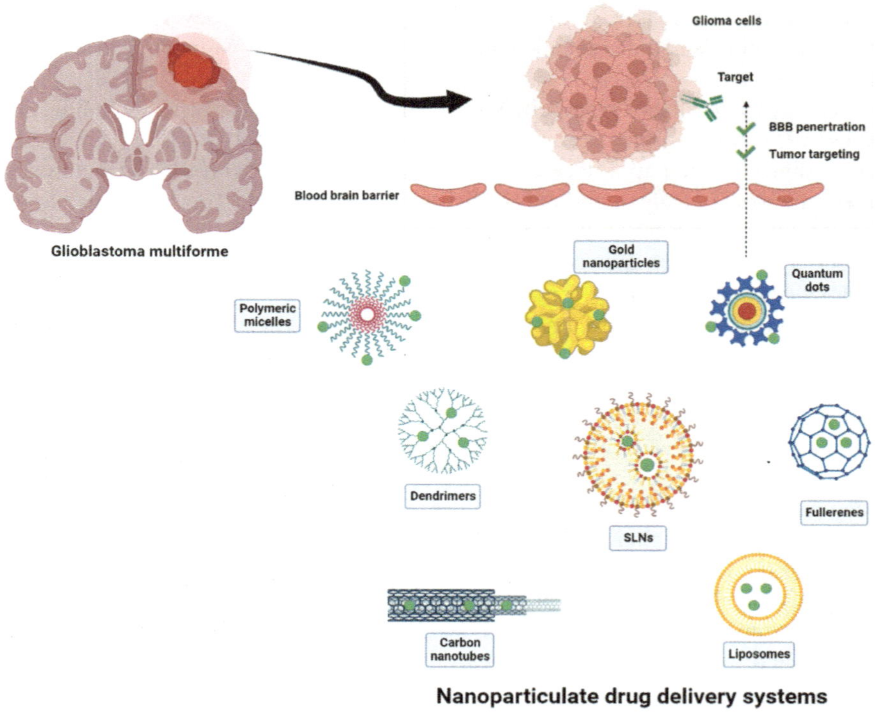

Fig. 1 Nanoparticulate drug delivery systems for brain tumor therapy

conceived from gold cores as spheres, rods, wires, cubes and cages are externally functionalized AuNPs which are modified to selectively interact with cells or biomolecules and targeted to specific diseases. With the currently available technologies and recent advances in synthetic methods and surface functionalization these nanosystems can be easily manipulated to aid in biomedical and therapeutic applications. They are biocompatible, and have shown negligible toxicity, with adjustable shapes and core sizes (1–150 nm), ease of ligand or antibody functionalization, marked optical properties, high X-ray absorption coefficient and overall good diagnostic properties [7]

AuNPs have been associated with various cellular targeting peptides to afford biological membrane permeability to NPs and adapted as tumor-targeted biomarkers and vehicles for drug delivery for diagnostic and therapeutic purposes. AuNPs have also been applied for photodynamic therapy (PDT) and photothermal therapy (PTT) for diagnostic purposes as well as in the management of oncological diseases because of the fluorescence quenching properties of the metal. In response to an exogenously applied laser light, AuNPs loaded with photosensitizer phthalocyanine 4 (Pc4) provoke photosensitization and cell death [8]. AuNPs have also been employed as conveyors for chemotherapeutic drugs that cannot navigate past the BBB under normal physiological settings. Doxorubicin (DOX) an extremely potent chemotherapeutic agent cannot cross BBB, but when conjugated with AuNPs, the AuNP-Dox shows a drastic change in pharmacokinetic properties, passes through the BBB, enters glioma cells, offers highly selective glioma cell death and causes no harm to healthy brain tissue.

AuNPs also afford non-covalent drug delivery which grants access to therapeutic agents without involving tumor cell uptake of the metallic NPs. AuNPs conjugated with polyethylene glycol (PEG) have been reported to be physiologically stable, biocompatible, exhibit prolonged systemic circulation and possess exceptional uniformity of size. Like all other inorganic NPs, the AuNPs trigger oxidative stress and subsequent cytotoxic effects. They also display anti-angiogenic properties with their ability to block vascular endothelial growth factor (VEGF) which predominantly governs angiogenesis, vasculogenesis and endothelial cell growth [9].

Recently, gold nanorods and nanoshells linked to antibodies are being promoted as photosensitizers for PTT that employ nanoparticle surfaces layered with a specific antibody to hone on cancer cells. When accumulated AuNPs at tumor sites are illuminated with near-IR light at a resonating frequency of the nanoshell, light absorption directs generation of heat that denatures proteins, nucleic acids and cellular membranes, which promotes cancer cell apoptosis. A variety of AuNPs have also been established as agents for thermotherapy which occurs when gold particles are heated with visible, Infrared (IR) or radiofrequency (RF) signals to induce localized tumor damaging effects, although this has not been extensively investigated yet.

In 2021, researchers explored a targeted combination therapy including DOX, YAP-siRNA and gold nanorods for the management of glioblastoma (Li et al., 2021). The study involved the development of a receptor-specific peptide; angiopep-2 modified cationic liposome laden with DOX, the Yes-associated protein (YAP) oncoprotein – siRNA and gold nanorods. The delivery system (D/R@Ang2-Lip+Au) showed high DOX encapsulation and high siRNA binding affinity. Fluorescence microscopy and flow cytometry analysis demonstrated increased uptake by glioblastoma cells while quantitative real-time Polymerase chain reaction (qPCR) and western blotting suggested that this novel system effectively resulted in the downregulation of the YAP oncoprotein expression thus resulting in curtailed YAP transcriptional activity and subsequently inhibiting proliferation and migration. The experimental analysis revealed that the D/R@Ang2-Lip+Au showed greater power to single out glioma cells when the angiopep-2 modification was used compared to non-targeted D/R@-Lip+Au. This synergistic complex of DOX, YAP-siRNA and gold nanorods could penetrate through the BBB, significantly inhibit tumor proliferation and furnish a novel concept for efficient delivery into glioblastoma cells and function as a brain targeting drug carrier.

In a recent study focused on glioblastomas Setua et al. investigated a combinatory chemo-radiotherapy approach using cisplatin-tethered gold nanospheres. Following intracellular uptake, the developed nanospheres cause DNA damage which triggers caspase mediated cell death. In an in-vitro model, the gold in the nanospheres and platinum in cisplatin upon irradiation behave as radiosensitizers and lead to emission of ionizing photoelectrons and Auger electrons, inducing intensive ablation of the tumorous glioma cells [10].

Targeting gold NPs with multiple receptor bound peptide chains was explored to focus on the tumor heterogeneity of glioblastomas. AuNPs associated with short chain amino acids against the mitogenic epidermal growth factor and transferrin receptors have been designed to investigate therapeutic activity. Meyers et al. reported a novel approach of peptide-targeted gold NPs for PDT of brain glioma. The study included a drug delivery system of gold NPs functionalized with epidermal growth factor peptide (EGF_{pep}) and modified with Phthalocyanine 4 (Pc 4), a well accepted PDT agent. The peptide-targeted gold NPs in combination with Pc 4 post in-vitro and in-vivo tests show increased specificity, elevated accumulation of fluorescence of Pc 4 in tumor cells as well as two-fold apoptotic activity compared to non-targeted gold NPs. In-vivo PDT with Pc 4 loaded EGF_{pep}-gold NPs also described inhibition in tumor growth thus demonstrating greater therapeutic efficacy of the targeted biomarkers [11]. In a similar study by Dixit et al., developed transferrin peptide (Tfpep) targeted gold NPs (Tfpep-AuNPs) complexed with photosensitizer Pc 4, to compare the delivery of Pc 4 via targeted AuNPs with non-targeted AuNPs. The in-vitro analysis with human glioblastoma cell lines (LN229 and U87) that highly express the transferrin receptor (TfR) revealed that the Tfpep-modified AuNP conjugates show a considerable increase in cellular uptake compared to unmodified AuNP conjugates. Additionally, the Pc 4 delivered from these Tfpep-AuNP conjugates accumulates within vesicles over a 4 h period and the consolidated results indicate that the Tfpep targeted AuNPs could be of biomedical relevance on the drug delivery and imaging platforms [8].

In 2016, a group of researchers investigated the use of gold NPs as radiosensitizers with the ability to diffuse electron and free radical prompted radiation damage to tumor cells. The study demonstrated the capacity of mixed gold and superparamagnetic iron oxide nanoparticle (SPION) micelles in the diagnosis and treatment of GBM. The gold and SPION micelles were developed by coating with polyethylene glycol-polycaprolactone (PEG-PCL) polymer [12]. The modified micelles were applied as imaging aids for CT and MRI in a syngeneic mouse model of glioblastoma and results suggested that MRI was more sensitive than CT to distinguish and define tumor thresholds after administration and localization of the developed micelles. The gold and SPION micelles were also assessed for radiosensitizing activity by quantifying the γ-H2AX foci as an indicator of DNA damage in glioma cell lines. The investigation revealed that the modified micelles possessed considerable radiosensitizing property and administration of this system along with radiation therapy resulted in a two-fold surge in the density of DNA double stranded breaks.

Exicure, Inc., a pioneer in gene regulation and immunotherapy agents applying spherical nucleic acid (SNA) technology directed an investigator-initiated trial for the treatment of glioblastoma using its licensed first generation gold NPs. In 2021, they successfully completed their first-in-human phase 0 clinical study (NCT03020017) to examine the safety of a study drug, NU-0129, based on brain-penetrant RNA interference-based SNAs. The system consisted of spirally structured and rigidly set small interfering RNA (siRNA) oligonucleotides arranged on the surface of gold nanoparticle cores. The study involved intravenously administering SNAs carrying siRNA distinct to the glioblastoma target oncogene Bcl2Like12 (Bcl2L12), one of the apoptosis regulators and quantifying the observations via inductively coupled plasma mass spectrometry (ICP-MS) and X-ray fluorescent microscopy. Based on prior preclinical evaluations and toxicological studies in non-human primates, a single-arm, open label phase 0 trial was performed to assess the safety, efficacy, pharmacokinetic parameters, tumoral localization and gene suppression [13]. The researchers reported that the siRNA-based SNAs pass through the BBB, accumulate in the GBM tumor cells and strongly engage with their target oncogene. The study results also revealed that no grade 4 or 5 treatment associated toxicities were observed and that NU-0129 absorption into glioblastoma cells enforced a decrease in tumor linked Bcl2L12 protein expression, thus establishing a brain-penetrating precision concept for systemic therapy of glioblastoma.

The AuNP conjugates have now been theoretically accepted as excellent tools with diagnostic and therapeutic capabilities, but there is immense need for multidisciplinary in-depth investigations and relevant clinical evidence to label them as effective treatment strategies.

2.2 Silver Nanoparticles

Over the past years, several other metal nanomaterial-based treatments have been translated into clinical trials and among these silver-based NPs (AgNPs) have shown favorable potential as therapeutic agents. They exhibit a broad spectrum of biological qualities depending on their size, shape, concentration and biological target. They can be synthesized by a number of methods such as laser ablation, evaporation–condensation, thermal decomposition, electrical irradiation, gamma irradiation, chemical reduction, lithography or microorganism-derived biological synthesis [14]. AgNPs came to be recognized in the biomedical sphere for their well known anti-microbial properties, but in addition to this because of their unparalleled physical, chemical and biological attributes, they have also been shown to have unique cytotoxic characteristics against mammalian cells. The therapeutic efficiency of nanoparticulate silver rests on its ability to trigger cell death. Ensuing their uptake into cells by endocytosis-linked mechanisms, the AgNPs are localized in cell endosomes, where the organelles direct lysosomal fusion. The lysosomal acidic conditions cause a marked increase in the release of Ag^+ ions from the AgNPs, which causes an unbalance in cellular homeostasis and ROS production leading to oxidative damage to DNA, proteins and lipid and resulting in apoptotic cell death. This cascade of events occurs by a "Trojan-horse" type mechanism where the cytotoxic features of AgNPs surface only after uptake by the cells. In addition to their silver-based cytotoxic property, the AgNPs also hold a nano size-related advantage and can be considered as a two-in-one therapeutic system [15].

Although AgNPs have shown tremendous medical potential they still appear to be toxic and thus to assure that the administered silver nanosystem preferentially accumulates only in target cancerous tissues, specific targeting approaches have been applied. Numerous studies have endorsed the abundant applications of AgNPs in cancer as drug delivery agents, cancer diagnosis, targeting and clinical therapy.

Locatelli and co-workers explored the targeted delivery of silver NPs and alisertib in glioblastoma. Multifunctional nanocomplexes formed by polymeric NPs were synthesized which contained two cytotoxic agents, i.e., the anti-neoplastic drug alisertib and AgNPs. The polymeric NPs were also linked with a targeting peptide chain, Chlorotoxin which specifically attaches to matrix metallopproteinase-2 (MMP-2) receptor in glioma cells. The individual and synergistic activity of the cytotoxic agents were tested in-vitro against human glioblastoma-astrocytoma epithelial-like cell line (U 87MG) and ^{99m}Tc radiolabeling of nanocarrier was used to study in-vivo biodistribution along with tumor reduction in tumor bearing rats [16]. The study revealed a synergic action of the Chlorotoxin-conjugated silver/alisertib nanocarriers with significant tumor reduction demonstrating that the targeted biocompatible silver nanoplatforms could present with multiple therapeutic applications and have potential in the management of brain cancer.

In 2015, a study evaluated the cytotoxic potential of AgNPs in GBM. They studied the cell propagation and incitement of the inherent apoptotic pathway of glioma cells in an *ovo* model, using human glioma cell line (U 87MG) in chicken embryo chorioallantoic membrane. Histological, immunohistochemical and cell apoptosis were adopted to assess the cell proliferation and tumor cell death. It was seen that AgNPs inhibit the proliferation of glioma cells and possess sufficient pro-apoptotic properties [17]

Research conducted in 2008 indicated that the uptake of AgNPs hindered mitochondrial cellular respiration and caused ROS production, resulting in programmed cancer cell death [18]. Additionally, a fivefold survival rate and combinatory antiproliferative and proapoptotic effect devoid of apparent systemic toxicity was reported when gliomas were treated with AgNPs with subsequent radiation therapy [19].

In a recent comprehensive investigation established a promising new "silver bullet" nanoparticle for the treatment of brain cancer. They synthesized and evaluated the properties of nanocomplexes composed of lanthanum manganite which were doped with silver atoms. The researchers ascertained that these NPs had possible clinical applications for their synergistic effects and could be employed in combination with radiotherapy, hyperthermia and their intrinsic toxicity to cancer cells [20]. The research elucidated that the doped silver NPs were small enough to penetrate the BBB and had the potential to kill cancer cells by producing high levels of ROS.

Although plenty of time and knowledge has been aimed at extensive research on metallic-based NPs, the major drawback for the vast application of these nanocarriers in-vitro and in-vivo is the cytotoxicity emanating from the degradation and release of toxic metal ions. Currently, the toxicity profiles and interactions of the AuNPs and AgNPs are not completely known, and an extensive understanding would be necessary to minimize the toxic effects on tissues and maximize brain tumor management.

2.3 Super Paramagnetic Iron Oxide Nanoparticles

Magnetic NPs were initially introduced as a promising nanomaterial in targeted drug delivery and subsequently emerged as a multifunctional clinical tool for MRI traceability. The core of magnetic NPs is generally made up of iron oxides, i.e., Magnetite (Fe_3O_4), hematite (α-Fe_2O_3) and maghemite (Fe_2O_3). They have been categorized as paramagnetic NPs (PMNPs) or superparamagnetic iron oxide NPs (SPIONs). SPIONs have been explored for their superior optical and magnetic properties and longer tumor retention periods. They are composed of an iron oxide core surrounded by a hydrophilic polymer coating fabricated from dextran, starch, PLGA (poly(lactic-co-glycolic acid)), PEG (polyethylene glycol) or alginate which impart stability, biocompatibility and prolong circulation time. SPIONs have exhibited excellent superparamagnetic properties, tuneable size, greater surface area-to-volume ratio and nontoxicity and are thus utilized as contrast agents for MRI [21]. They have been employed in preoperative and intraoperative imaging of brain tumors and MRI contrast agents that comprise these magnetic NPs which have the unique capability of MRI contrast enhancement.

SPIONs have also been developed for targeted therapy of brain tumors, by complexing peptides or antibodies to the surface which affords controlled targeting of the cancer cells and interruption in the active signaling pathways. SPIONs conjugated with human serum albumin (HSA) and polymeric materials have also been described for drug delivery, biodistribution and improvement in drug efficacy. Cui et al., investigated transferrin-conjugated magnetic silica (Fe_3O_4 magnetic beads coated with SiO_2) PLGA NPs loaded with DOX and paclitaxel (PTX) to overcome the poor transport across the BBB for brain glioma. Transferrin (Tf)-conjugated magnetic silica PLGA NPs were primed with DOX and PTX and their antiproliferative activity was analyzed in-vitro in U 87MG cell lines and in-vivo in tumor bearing rodents. Tf as a targeting ligand allowed an enhanced absorption of drug loaded NPs by glioma cells. Reduced tumor size was detected in the experimental mice, while a synergistic effect was observed using the DOX-PTX nanosystems, rather than free DOX or PTX. This indicated that the transferrin-conjugated DOX-PTX magnetic nanocarriers mediated motility of NPs across the BBB and improved the localization of the therapeutic agent in tumorous tissue [22].

A study was conducted to assist in observing gliomas by chlorotoxin-conjugated superparamagnetic nanoprobes. A physiologically compatible nanoprobe formed from a poly(ethylene glycol) (PEG) coated iron oxide NP was developed and was found to particularly target gliomas with the help of surface-bound targeting peptide chain, chlorotoxin (CTX). The magnetic NP system caused preferential accumulation within the gliomas and exhibited MRI contrast enhancing ability in-vitro in 9L gliosarcoma cells and in-vivo in tumors of a xenograft mouse model [23]. Histological assessment of tumor tissues also indicated that there was absence of toxic effects stemming from the nanoprobes. The high selectivity and benign biological response established these magnetic NPs as a convenient diagnostic and therapeutic tool for glioblastoma.

Hadjipanayis et al. explored EGFRvIII antibody-conjugated iron oxide NPs for MRI-guided convection-enhanced delivery (CED) and targeted therapy of glioma. Iron oxide NPs linked to a specific antibody that has affinity toward the epidermal growth factor receptor (EGFR) deletion mutant (EGFRvIII) prevalent on human glioma cells were synthesized and exploited for enhancing MRI contrast and drug targeting for GBM, both in-vitro and in-vivo, after CED. A considerable reduction in glioma cell survival was detected following magnetic NP treatment and absence of human astrocyte toxicity was noticed. A marked improvement in rodent survival was also noted after CED of magnetic NPs which indicated that iron oxide NPs complexed to an antibody specific to the EGFRvIII deletion mutant could provide contrast-enhanced MRI of tumorous glioma tissue and aid in achieving targeted cancer therapies [24].

2.4 Carbon-Based NPs

Carbon nanostructures represent a new class of carbon-based nanomaterials which have drawn significant interest in various spheres of research due to their distinct properties. Amid the commonly studied carbonaceous nanomaterials are graphene, nanodiamonds, carbon nanotubes, carbon-based quantum dots and fullerenes [25]. They are endowed with unique physico-chemical properties including thermal, optical, electrical, mechanical and structural characteristics compared to other NPs and many of them have been widely explored in numerous biomedical applications covering biosensing, drug delivery, bioimaging, diagnosis, cancer therapy, theranostics and tissue engineering.

2.5 Carbon Nanotubes

Carbon nanotubes are well-defined, hexagonally arranged, hollow, cylindrically shaped graphene nanostructures that have been highlighted as the building blocks of nanotechnology. They are one-dimensional carbon allotropes consisting of sp^2-bonded carbon atoms, fabricated from a thin graphitic layer rolled into a cylinder having a diameter in the nanometer (nm) size range. On the basis of their architecture and the number of graphene layers constituting the nanotube, they have been labeled as single-walled CNTs (SWCNTs), double-walled CNTs (DWCNTs) and multi-walled CNTs (MWCNTs) and several techniques have been adopted for their synthesis including chemical vapor deposition (CVD), carbon arc discharge, and laser ablation [26]. They have a combination of structural elasticity, strength and rigidity, electronic properties, broad surface area, high adsorption capacity, light weight, chemical inertness and distinguished thermal stability, high therapeutic efficacy, better specificity, low toxicity and offer pH-dependent and temperature-responsive therapeutic unloading and ease of functionalization rendering them as suitable candidates for imaging agents for tumor diagnosis and drug delivery. Being intrinsically hydrophobic and poorly soluble, the CNTs require functionalization of the sidechains by modifying the chemical structure. Various functionalization methods including covalent bonding, adsorption and electrostatic interaction have been utilized to alter the hydrophobicity of CNTs, increase solubility and avoid their tendency to agglomerate [27].

CNTs function as nanocontainers for effective delivery as they can load a larger amount of drug because of their inner hollow cylindrical framework, and suitably isolate the drug from the physiological environment. A myriad of studies have been conducted to investigate how anti-neoplastic drugs loaded into CNTs can be made to recognize target sites and one of the strategies to obtain targeted delivery is modifying the surface properties of the CNT with a particular protein specific to the target cancer cell. These innovative nanovehicles being modifiable with polymeric groups, carbohydrates, peptide chains and organic molecules can then function as a therapeutic route for targeting tumors. The intrinsic surface reactivity of the CNT also promotes bonding of auxiliary groups which improve the biocompatibility of CNTs. Owing to their natural morphology the CNTs offer the promise of facilitating non-invasive penetration across biological membranes, the ability to pass through the BBB, extended drug circulation and functionalization with targeting moieties [28, 29].

These carbon-based materials have long been explored as carriers for anticancer drugs, genes and proteins for chemotherapy. VanHandel et al. observed the uptake and toxic effects of MWCNTs in the GL261 murine intracranial glioma model. Upon intratumoral injection of labeled MWCNTs, they reported that roughly 10–20% of cells showed CNT accumulation and the CNT uptake took place by tumor-associated macrophages. Although a transient rise in the inflammatory cell infiltrates was detected after MWCNT administration, no considerable toxic effect was observed in rodents, while small variations in tumor cytokine expression were identified [30]. This initial study paved the way for further research to set up CNT technology as a potential non-toxic carrier targeting macrophages for brain tumor therapy.

A study aimed at evaluating CNTs as a CpG oligodeoxynucleotide (CpG) carrier in glioma models was conducted in 2011. The stimulation of Toll-like receptor-9 (TLR9); which induces antitumor immune responses, by CpG has been previously described to halt the immunosuppressive microenvironment and impede tumorous proliferation in glioblastoma models. Since TLR9 is intracellularly located, it was assumed that enhancing its localization could amplify the immunostimulatory response. Functionalized SWCNTs complexed with CpG (CNT-CpG) were developed and tested in-vitro and in a murine glioma model, GL261. Flow cytometry used to determine CNT-CpG uptake, showed an enhancement in uptake of CpG by tumor-associated phagocytic cells in both in-vitro and intracranial gliomas. The evaluation also demonstrated that the CNT-CpG complex was non-toxic and enhanced pro-inflammatory cytokine formation by primary monocytes. It was reported that the administration of a low dose intracranial injection of CNT-CpG not only obliterated intracranial gliomas via stimulation of natural killer (NK) and cytotoxic T lymphocyte (CD8) cells in half of tumor-bearing mice, but also displayed tumor-free remission in the surviving mice establishing long term anti-tumor immunity [31].

A similar study explored the likelihood of SWCNTs non-covalently modified with CpG (SWCNT/CpG) to selectively impede the extremely intrusive nature of glioma cells by stimulating the immune system [32]. They reported that the developed SWCNT/CpG helps preserve the immunostimulatory feature of the CpG, markedly inhibits the migratory property of tumor cells, reduced incitement of NF-κB in glioma cells and activates macrophages by initiation of the TLR9/ NF-κB pathway. It was observed that the suppression of glioma cell migration corresponded to the decline in the bulk of intracellular reactive oxygen species (ROS) implying that an antioxidant linked mechanism mediates this apoptotic process.

In 2014, Santos et al. used CNTs associated with near infrared radiation (NIR) producing hyperthermia to investigate its potential for non-ionizing radiotherapy for brain cancer and GBM. In-vitro tests included using human-derived glioma cell lines (U251, U87, LN229, T98G), by incubation of glioma cells with CNTs for 24 h after introduction to NIR for 10 min. It was reported that the glioma cells particularly localized CNTs, which on irradiation with NIR generated heat leading to necrotic glial death. In-vivo studies in the rat glioma model resulted in reduction in tumor size and absence of recurring tumors after a single treatment [33]. Additionally, this strategy effected necrosis to glioma stem cells as well as drug-resistant glioma cells and minimum effect of this sequential hypothermia therapy was observed to normal cells corresponding to the minimum uptake of CNTs. This study thus successfully demonstrates the therapeutic potential of hyperthermia-induced thermal ablation using the steady administration of CNT and NIR.

You et al. designed and synthesized a dual-functionalized carbon nanotube which functioned as a cancer targeting molecule. In orthotopic glioblastoma models, this novel nanosystem, which consisted of a cell penetrating peptide conjugated with a multi-walled carbon nanotube demonstrated high blood brain barrier permeability, reduced toxicity, enhanced cancer recognition and anticancer activity through increased ROS production thus marking it as an optimal strategy for management of glioblastoma [34].

2.6 *Quantum Dots*

Quantum dots (QDs) are artificially made semiconductor-based nanocrystals with sizes ranging between 2 and 10 nm. They represent an upcoming genre of fluorescent NPs for biological imaging with size-tuneable optical properties, high stability, strong resistance to degradation, ability to target tumors, high resistance to photo-bleaching compared to other fluorescent dyes or semiconductor QDs and afford remarkable photoluminescence owing to quantum confinement. When UV light hits these NPs, they emit light of various colors, and this particle size, shape and composition-dependent wavelength of fluorescence has thus found an application as fluorescent biological labels in medical imaging. They are mainly composed of a heavy metal core comprised of Cadmium selenide (CdSe) or Cadmium telluride (CdTe), that is coated with layers of an unreactive metallic shell typically Zinc sulphide (ZnS) [35].

In recent years, many CdSe/ZnS-QDs have been researched for their potential in cancer bioimaging, biosensing and drug delivery. In order to target a specific cancer site, further modification is necessary and QDs are covalently or non-covalently externally functionalized with bioactive molecules such as antibodies, peptide chains, nucleic acids, folate aptamers, cancer cell-specific ligands and other small molecules. The anti-neoplastic activity of QDs has been connected to heavy-metal discharge, intratumoral absorption, variations in immune response and generation of ROS.

In 2016, researchers studied the efficacy of Asparagine-Glycine-Arginine peptides (NGR) peptide-modified PEGylated QDs for navigating past the BBB and targeted fluorescent imaging of tumorous brain cells and associated vasculature. Cyclic NGR peptides have been described as aspiring targeting moieties for drug delivery to CD13-positive tumor cells and a drug complexed with an NGR peptide has even compelling cytotoxic behavior than a free drug. NGR-conjugated PEG-CdSe/ZnS QDs were developed by conjugating biotin tagged-NGR peptides to avidin-PEG-coated QDs and were characterized. Past research has identified that functional NGR peptide chains could target CD13-overexpressing tumors, which speculated that NGR could play a two-fold role in targeting brain cancer and its vasculature. The experimental studies revealed that the synthesized systems were stable, possessed the ability to successfully move across the BBB and target CD13-overexpressing glial cells and could thus aid in fluorescence imaging [36]. The study also demonstrated that the QDs highlight an innovative avenue for diagnosis and intraoperative imaging of glioma and could serve as potential more sensitive and specific methods of bio-imaging than conventional methods.

Currently, the potential toxicity associated with heavy metal content of the QDs limits their applicability and while researchers continue to develop newer formulations, further investigation is needed on the toxicity profile and physiological interactions before finally applying to clinical use.

2.7 *Carbon Quantum Dots*

In the last decade, newer members of the graphene family; Carbon quantum dots (CQDs) have garnered great attention. They have been widely synthesized, characterized and studied as likely nanovehicles for drug delivery holding the asset of their distinct features like miniature size (<5 nm) and ideal surface chemistry which aids in attaching chemotherapy drugs and target receptors. They possess exceptional optical properties, reduced toxic potential, improved photostability, excellent biocompatibility, allow easy surface modifications and are regarded as visionary fluorescent probes in numerous medical applications, bioimaging, phototherapy and biosensing.

The CQDs are currently being promoted as drug carriers to boost drug solubility, ameliorate localization at the target tumor site, reduce undesirable effects and enhance bioavailability and tolerance. The flexible surface functionalization also allows to build tumor targeting nanosystems. Several studies highlighting the efficiency of carbon dots and their modified complexes to take on the BBB have been described in recent years [37]. In 2014, a study demonstrated a simple technique to develop fluorescent carbon dots and investigated their probable use in non-invasive tumor imaging. They utilized a thermal handling approach on glycine (Gly) to generate carbon dots (C-dot/Gly) and explored their in-vitro cytotoxicity, tumoral absorption, tissue distribution and imaging characteristics in-vivo. The C6 rat glioma cell line in-vitro study showed that the C-dot/Gly possesses low cytotoxic ability, and a time- and concentration-dependent cell uptake occurs. The studies identified a large accretion of carbon dots in the glioma cells which presented a stronger fluorescence than the normal brain tissue concluding that the C-dots have the specific ability to target glioma cells [38].

A study by Li et al. included the formulation of transferrin-conjugated C-dots to examine the ability of the modified carbon dots to ferry therapeutic agents across the BBB. Carbon dots covalently conjugated with human Transferrin (Trans), or dye-labeled Transferrin (C-dot/Trans and C-dot//DyeTrans) were utilized and injected into the vasculature of zebrafish in-vivo to investigate its ability to cross the BBB via the Transferrin receptor-mediated delivery [39]. The studies established that the Transferrin linked C-dots gain access to the Central nervous system (CNS) via transferrin receptor-mediated endocytosis, by effectively penetrating the BBB, while unmodified C-dots do not.

Another parallel study conducted by the same group, in pediatric brain tumor cell lines verified that molecular complexes of C-dots, Transferrin and DOX (C-dot/Trans-DOX) display a higher drug absorption than simply DOX, implying the higher amount of transferrin receptors on these brain tumor cells. The results also revealed that the conjugated C-dot/Trans-DOX possessed higher chemotherapeutic activity than only DOX, suggesting an increased therapeutic efficacy when drug-carbon dot conjugates are applied [40].

Research conducted in 2015 examined self-targeting fluorescent carbon dots for the diagnosis of brain cancer. A novel form of C-dots (C-dot/Dex-Asp) focussed on gliomas, through the continuous pyrolysis of a blend of Dextrose (Dex) and L-aspartic acid (L-Asp) was synthesized by Zheng et al. The study reported exceptional biocompatibility and viable full-color emission as well as significant targeting capacity of C6 rat glioma cells without the use of any additional targeting molecules. Furthermore, a comparatively distinct signal and high-contrast biodistribution of the C-dot/Dex-Asp was detected in the glioma target site, 15 min after tail vein injection, which suggests the capacity of the C-dots to freely pass across the BBB and target the glioma tissue. While the developed C-dots exhibited the ability to act as fluorescent agents in imaging and targeting agents for diagnosis, the carbon dots constructed from pure Dextrose (C-dot/Dex), pure L-Aspartic acid (C-dot/l-Asp) or a blend of Dextrose and L-Glutamic acid (C-dot/Dex-Glu) possessed no or extremely poor specificity for gliomas, asserting its potential as nanomedicine for diagnostics and therapeutics [41].

These studies have established the clear ability of carbon dots to be used as theranostic tools and for the evolution of finer targeted therapies for brain tumors in the future and they have rightly gained the title of revolutionary brain cancer nanomedicine.

2.8 Fullerenes

The nanomedicine tide ushered in advancements in nanomaterials and one such acclamatory tool was the Fullerenes. Fullerenes (called Buckminsterfullerenes) are closed hollow spherical or ellipsoidal molecules comprising of carbon (C_{60}, C_{70}, C_{80} and C_{94}). The most established structure, the C_{60} fullerene is a spheroidal closed cage and has a highly stable icosahedral symmetry with C_5–C_5 single bonds forming twelve pentagons and C_5–C_6 double bonds forming twenty hexagons, thus resembling a soccer ball. Over the years various methods of fullerene production have been accepted including the Laser ablation method, Microwave method, Combustion of hydrocarbons with oxygen and argon and Chemical vapor deposition (CVD), although the Arc discharge method continues to remain a prominent process.

The distinct characteristic of C_{60} to readily accept free radicals, quench or generate cell damaging ROS along with its miniscule size, large surface area, inertness and outstanding physical, chemical, photodynamic and structural properties has paved the way for their extensive applications in biomedicine and clinical therapy. Being intrinsically inert, the fullerenes allow enclosing of various ionic molecules within its cage-like structure [42]. They are extremely hydrophobic in nature which contributes to aggregation of the nanostructures in medium, but this roadblock to the development process has been successfully overcome by derivatization of the fullerenes with polar groups. Modification of the parent structure by complexation with solubilizing agents or covalent functionalization of the fullerenes has obtained nanostructures with increased solubility and improved stability. Endohedral metallofullerenes (fullerenes with a metal atom(s) usually gadolinium, lanthanum, lutetium and scandium encapsulated) are modified forms of fullerenes which have attracted interest due to their wide application as diagnostic agents. Besides hindering immune responses and protecting the CNS tissues to a higher extent in comparison to gold-based NPs and CNTs, modified polyhydroxy fullerenes (PHFs) offer exceptional biocompatibility, biodegradability and exhibit remarkable antioxidant properties. PHFs also show notable inhibition in tumor growth and stimulate immune system upregulation. The dual characteristic of reactive free radical quenching combined with drug targeting property of fullerenes makes this carbon-based nano formulation therapeutically more effective. Functionalized fullerenes are endowed with characteristics that reinforce anti-cancer therapy in addition to its tumor inhibition properties and serve to combat systemic toxicity and drug resistance which are routinely associated with conventional chemotherapy.

Fullerenes and their derivatives have been widely studied in the medical field, and are gaining interest as contrast agents in imaging, drug delivery vehicles, diagnostic and therapeutic agents. Shultz et al., developed a theranostic agent based on a metallofullerene nanoplatform. The lutetium 177 (^{177}Lu) radiolabeled modified metallofullerene (^{177}Lu-DOTA-f-$Gd_3N@C_{80}$) was synthesized and conjugated with complexing agent 1,4,7,10-tetraazacyclododecane-1,4,7,10-tetraacetic acid (DOTA) to neutralize the toxicity of Gd^{3+} and the efficiency of this nanosystem was explored in orthotopic xenograft brain tumor models of GBM using human glioblastoma U87MG cells [43]. MRI and biodistribution studies of the developed agent were performed to evaluate gadolinium content. MRI studies showed extended tumor retention, which allowed for longitudinal tumor imaging and effective brachytherapy along with radiation-induced tumor damage and a dose-dependent improvement in survival rates.

In 2014, researchers investigated a novel approach based on gadofullerenes which could have diagnostic and therapeutic potential for glioblastoma. Aqueous gadofullerenes (Gd@Ful) comprised of $Gd@C_{82}(OH)_x$; $x \geq 20$ were developed. Analysis of magnetic relaxation time and MRI of a rodent with intracranially implanted C6 glioma cell line were conducted using Gd@Ful nanosuspensions. The developed Gd@Ful exhibited reduction in proton relaxation times and provided dual contrast of T1- and T2-weighted images in a rat brain tumor model following intravenous administration of the paramagnetic contrast agent (i.e., $Gd^{3+)}$. The introduction of Gd@Ful was found to promote the augmentation of tumor contrast enhancement because of the localization of the paramagnetic agent at the tumor site. The retention of the fullerene-based nanosuspension in the C6 glioma cells produces not only the enhancement in tumor contrast but is also therapeutically relevant. When intravenously administered with Gd@Ful nanosuspension, the researchers observed an increase in the survival rates in rats. The study demonstrated that Gd@Ful nanosuspension was found to have high anti-tumor therapeutic potential as well as contrast enhancing properties that could aid in bioimaging [44].

A study explored the potential of fullerene derivatives as cancer treatment focussing on the surface-dependent chemical properties. Aqueous C_{60} fullerene derivatives with various linkages (compounds 1–3: C–C bonds, compounds 4–5: C–S bonds, compound 6: C–P bonds, and compounds 7–9: C–N bonds) between the fullerene cage and the solubilizing agent utilizing various functional groups were synthesized. The results revealed that water-soluble fullerenes 1–6 induced neural stem cell (NSC) proliferation in-vitro and rescued the function of damaged CNS, while fullerene derivatives 7–9 were described to hinder glioma cell proliferation in-vitro and curtail the development of glioblastoma in zebrafish [45]. The study concluded that the presence of a specific functional group at the surface of fullerenes is a clear determinant of the characteristics and synergy of water-soluble C_{60} fullerenes with the NSCs and tumor cells thus bearing either a neuroprotective or antitumor property in the management of brain diseases.

Various other studies have stated that gadofullerenes have high anti-cancer activity (60%) in mice. The endohedral metallofullerenes were reported to have anti-angiogenetic characteristics and reduced toxic effects compared to conventional chemotherapeutic treatment. Studies also demonstrated that the count of tumor micro-vessels were found to decrease in tissues treated with fullerenol NPs due to reduction in the VEGF expression, which suggests that suitably modified fullerenes could be a suitable therapeutic approach countering angiogenesis for cancer [25].

Despite being described as greatly beneficial in numerous forms, studies show that fullerenes certainly present with substantial toxic effects controlled by their particle size, solubility, method of preparation and biological accumulation, and especially due to the production of reactive species thus prompting extensive investigations on their toxicity profiles before they are clinically applicable.

2.9 *Dendrimers*

Dendrimers are an emerging class of nanosized synthetic polymeric macromolecules characterized by hyper-branched, three-dimensional, well-defined globular structures resembling a tree or dendron. A typical dendrimer consists of a central core, and repeated branched units which permit dendrimer growth as geometrically arranged layers and abundant terminal functional groups at the surface. The most commonly studied dendritic nanomaterials include poly(amidoamine) (PAMAM) and poly(propylamine) (PPI) dendrimers [46]. The dendritic nanomaterials owing to their nano size, high aqueous solubility, compact globular shape, ease of surface multi-functionalization, low toxicity, and capacity for drug encapsulation within internal cavities have gained enormous attention as potential as drug delivery systems to improve biodistribution of drugs in the body and aid in controlled release of some drugs at a target site. The superior architectural structure of the dendrimer enables them with the flexibility to load therapeutic agents into its internal cavities non-covalently or by embedding them in the dendritic molecular framework by either covalent conjugation or electrostatic adsorption to surface groups. Studies suggest that complexation of a drug to dendrimers enables bypassing of the efflux transporter which leads to increased drug solubility and in turn improved bioavailability [47].

Dendrimers were among the many nanomaterials described as MRI contrast media and diagnostic tools. The unique dendritic structure enables the loading of a greater bulk of contrast agent either at the dendritic terminals or in the internal void, thus enhancing the imaging potential. The nano size of the dendrimers enables them to avert rapid renal excretion and exhibit a longer biological half-life. Moreover, suitably conjugating the dendritic structure with a targeting moiety could also offer specific imaging of tissues.

As the pioneer to exploring dendrimer-derived MRI contrast agents, Wiener et al. studied PAMAM dendrimers. A chelating agent diethylenetriaminepentaacetic acid (DTPA) was connected to the terminal amine of PAMAM dendrimers of generations G2 and G6, followed by coupling with $GdCl_3$ to transport the dendrimer contrast medium. The study reports higher longitudinal relaxivities by the modified dendrimers as opposed to the small molecular Gd-DTPA, because of their large molecular weight. These PAMAM dendrimer-based imaging contrasts also showed increased blood circulation half-lives and remarkable in-vivo imaging in comparison to other small molecular contrast agents [48].

In 2008, researchers investigated the delivery of PAMAM dendritic NPs past the BBB and into malignant brain tumor cells. They labeled PAMAM dendrimers of generation (G5–G8) with Gd-DTPA at the terminals and examined their delivery to tumors of mouse models using dynamic contrast-enhanced MRI [49]. The tests reported that the modified dendrimers possessed size in the nano range and functionalized dendrimers of G5–G7 (of sizes less than 12 nm) possessed the ability to permeate through the pores of the restrictive BBB. The study concluded that dendrimers with longer circulation half-lives were able to localize within tumor cells and that an optimum size of less than 12 nm was required for efficient delivery into malignant brain cancer cells.

Another study conducted by Bertin et al. developed dendritic Manganese (II) enhanced MRI (MEMRI) contrast agents for brain targeting. The Mn^{2+} conjugate exhibited higher aqueous solubility and demonstrated no in-vitro neuronal toxic responses at concentrations as high as 1 mM or any in-vivo toxic effects at 20 mM in a rat model (i.e., 100% rat survival). This exceptional safety profile of such a manganese-based dendritic contrast agent could be due to the slow diffusion and controlled discharge of the paramagnetic Mn^{2+} ions. Additionally, the relaxivity of the Mn^{2+} conjugate was greater compared to the commercially used MRI agent Mn-DPDP, which indicates that it could be used as a favorable candidate for brain targeting MRI in diagnosing and treating brain cancer and other neurodegenerative diseases [50].

Huang et al., explored a Chlorotoxin-linked macromolecular contrast agent for MRI tumor visualization. A dendrigraft poly-L-lysine dendrimer (DGLs) armed with Chlorotoxin (CTX) as a glioma targeting ligand and Gd-DTPA as the visualization cargo for MRI was synthesized. The study reported that this novel developed agent improved the tumoral absorption in C6 glioma cell line, but not in non-glioma cells. Furthermore, upon treatment with the modified dendrimer complex, the imaging contrast was found to be greatly amended in comparison with the unmodified complex and commercial contrast agent (control) and the heightened signal from the dendrigraft was suitably sustained longer than the control [36]. This study proved the remarkable potential of modified dendrimers for improving imaging and diagnosis.

With the pursuit of defeating the obstacles of BBB penetration, a study conducted by Dhanikula et al. demonstrated Methotrexate (MTX) loaded dendrimers for the management of glioma. MTX-loaded polyether-copolyester (PEPE) dendrimers, conjugated to D-glucosamine as the ligand for BBB permeation and tumor targeting, were developed and evaluated as drug carriers. Human derived glioma cell lines U-87MG and U-343MGa were used to assess the efficiency of the MTX-loaded dendrimers and permeability of the developed MTX dendrimers and rhodamine-labeled dendrimers across the BBB model and their distribution in vascularized glioblastoma model were studied in-vitro. Half-maximal Inhibitory concentration (IC_{50}) of MTX, used as a measure of the drug's efficacy was found to be less than the free MTX, indicating that loading MTX in PEPE dendrimers improved the drug's effectiveness. The MTX dendrimers also had the ability to kill MTX-resistant glioma cells thus suggesting their capacity to overcome MTX resistance. It was also reported that the amount of MTX transported across BBB was comparatively higher after loading the drug in dendrimers, while glycosylation of the dendrimers also enhanced drug potency and intratumoral transport [51]. These results indicate that glucosamine could be used for improving the permeation of agents across BBB and also as an effective ligand for targeting glioma tumor cells.

Dendrimers have also been reported to facilitate transport of various anti-neoplastic agents, small molecules, peptides and genes as well as passively target anti-cancer drugs to tumor tissues, to improve efficacy and diminish overall cytotoxicity. By perfecting drug carrier features like bioavailability, solubility and selectivity, these dendritic molecules could be promising vehicles and establish a new platform for brain drug delivery. In 2016, researchers examined a DOX loaded folic acid (FA) conjugated PAMAM for boosting BBB penetration of DOX. Dual targeting PEGylated PAMAM G5 dendrimers linked with tumor targeting FA to target tumor cells and Borneol (BO), to facilitate permeation across BBB and reduce toxic effects of naked PAMAM were synthesized. The CNS transportation and tumor targeting capacity were examined on a BBB model and C6 glioma cell line in-vitro along with pharmacokinetic and biodistribution studies on C6 glioma bearing rats in-vivo. The study reported that the modification of PAMAM dendrimers with BO effectively reduced the cytotoxicity and efficiently boosted BBB permeability. Moreover, conjugation of FA to the DOX dendrimers improved the total uptake by C6 glioma cells, enhanced DOX accumulation in glioma cells and exhibited higher tumor growth inhibition, marking this strategy as a promising novel targeting nanocarrier for glioblastoma therapy [52].

2.10 *Lipid Nanoparticles*

A plethora of lipid-derived nanocarriers have been introduced as drug delivery strategies that increase solubility, potentiate the bioavailability, circulation time and metabolic stability of the drug as well as encapsulate drugs and deliver them to target tissues thus leading to enhanced therapeutic effects, reduced side effects and providing controlled and targeted drug release. Some of the most widely studied lipid NPs include liposomes, solid lipid nanoparticles (SLNs), nanostructured lipid carriers (NLCs) and niosomes.

SLNs were presented as pioneers in lipid-based nanocarrier drug delivery. These submicron colloidal carriers are formulated from lipids, which are in solid phase at room temperature and are stabilized by emulsifiers. They possess unique properties of small size (50–1000 nm), large surface area and high drug loading capacity and are thus winning for their ability to improve the efficiency of therapeutic agents. Following the development of SLNs, nanostructured lipid carriers were introduced as lipid-based drug carriers. These novel drug delivery strategies created primarily to improve drug loading capacity and bioavailability are formed from a blend of solid and liquid lipids, but the final NPs are in solid state at physiological temperature [53]. On account of the presence of liquid lipids, the leakage of loaded drug after formulation and during the course of storage is reduced, thus furnishing higher stability as compared to SLNs. The release of therapeutic agents from the lipid particles arises by diffusion and concurrently by lipid particle degradation in the body.

Liposomes are colloidal carriers in the 80–300 nm size range and are small spherical vesicular structures constituted of self-associated bilayers of hydrated natural non-toxic phospholipids and steroids (e.g., Cholesterol). The distinct structural features of liposomes, i.e., an aqueous cavity surrounded by a lipid membrane, permit them to be carriers for both hydrophobic and hydrophilic compounds without any chemical modification [54]. Non-ionic surfactant-based vesicular drug delivery systems were termed Niosomes. These carriers have a closed bilayer vesicle structure and are formed from lipids and non-ionic surfactants in an aqueous medium. Niosomes have been currently applied as carriers for numerous therapeutic and diagnostic agents in anti-cancer drug delivery as well as targeted drug delivery. These exceptional drug carriers being non-ionic have excellent biocompatibility and low toxicity [55].

Numerous studies have described how drug carriers and their structural alterations exhibit greater bio-distribution in addition to increased bioavailability with a beneficial impact on BBB permeation and tumor uptake. Being primarily assembled from biocompatible organic substances and a blend of natural lipids, SLNs and NLCs involve safer biodegradation routes showing minimal toxic responses and also enable sustained release of the enclosed agent. Modifications with various ligands such as peptides, aptamers, antibodies, or small targeting biomolecules are also easily possible for any necessary application. Furthermore, SLNs and NLCs have been labeled as excellent vehicles for targeting brain diseases owing to their extremely biocompatible nature and low immunogenic capacity [56]. Over the years, extensive research focussed on these lipid-based nanocarriers has been directed along the lines of brain cancer therapy.

Song et al., developed a novel Arginine-glycine-aspartic acid peptide (RGD) containing temozolomide (TMZ) loaded NLCs for GBM chemotherapy. RGD-conjugated polyethylene glycol-b-distearoylphosphatidylethanolamine (PEG-DSPE) NLCs loaded with TMZ were synthesized. They were then evaluated for their particle size, zeta potential, drug encapsulation efficiency, drug release behavior, in-vitro cytotoxic effects in U 87MG glioma cells and in-vivo antitumor efficacy in mice bearing Glioma model. The results revealed that U 87MG tumor cells were successfully inhibited and that the developed formulation displayed the highest anti-tumor activity compared to other formulations. This study indicated that the RGD conjugated TMZ NLCs could be a selective and superior drug delivery nanocarrier for treating gliomas [57].

A research study examined the impact of niosomal drug entrapment on the pharmacokinetics of MTX. Niosomes formed by a non-ionic surfactant, cholesterol and dicetyl phosphate (DCP) enclosing MTX were administered to mice [58]. The results showed that the use of niosomal vesicles as carriers prolongs the levels of MTX in blood and increases uptake in brain cells because of the permeability characteristics of the niosomes, proving they could be efficiently used as lipid nanocarriers for brain tumor therapy.

Martina et al., studied the development of superparamagnetic liposomes as acceptable MRI contrast agents. Maghemite (γ-Fe_2O_3) nanocrystals were formed and enveloped within large unilamellar vesicles (LUV) composed of egg phosphatidylcholine (EPC) and distearoyl-SN-glycero-3-phosphoethanolamine-N-[methoxy(poly(ethylene glycol))-2000] (DSPE-PEG(2000). Evaluating the developed liposomes with cryogenic transmission electron microscopy (cryo-EM) and measuring the magnetization curves revealed that the magnetic-fluid-loaded liposomes (MFLs) were extremely stable, free from ferrofluid flocculation and exhibited no toxicity toward the J774 macrophage cell line. Mouse magnetic resonance studies demonstrated that the MFLs were efficient contrast agents for the diagnosis of brain tumors [59].

Another study investigated the potential of brain-targeted SLNs containing riluzole [60]. They synthesized SLNs containing riluzole using the warm oil-in-water microemulsion technique. Biodistribution and drug release studies were carried out in rodents after delivering riluzole loaded SLNs. The results indicated that the SLNs possessed colloidal size, increased drug loading capacity, higher efficacy and were able to suitably ferry riluzole into intracranial sites. The study established that the developed drug loaded SLNs have a great potential as therapeutic drug carriers for brain diseases.

Table 1 presents an outline of the various types of nanoparticles explored over the years for the treatment of brain tumors.

3 Limitations to Nanoparticle-Based Theranostics for Management of Brain Tumors

While nanocarriers are anticipated to eclipse current cancer management protocols of surgical removal, chemotherapy and radiotherapy in the near future, the underlying safety concerns and toxic effects of the nanomaterials in clinical research and patient care, their possible risks and benefits should be given due consideration.

The efficacy of NPs in brain tumor treatments as well as their toxicities differ with size, structural features, shape, biocompatibility, solubility, aggregation and degradation. While the larger lipid vesicles are selectively able to navigate across the BBB for tumor localization, the smaller sized ones may have unrestricted access across the BBB, which ensue the risk of uncontrolled embolisms. The larger structural surfaces of nanocarriers may result in their aggregation before and after permeation of the BBB. As the absorption of NPs by the reticuloendothelial system (RES) also depends on their size, there could be uncertain rates of nanoparticle uptake and clearance, and this could cause idiosyncratic treatment efficacy. Additionally, since NPs have dimensions similar to healthy living cells, their administration into the body may impede basic cellular functions [61]. The uncertainty of nanoparticle properties and functions being altered once in contact with biological fluids or specific microenvironments also arises and thus their characterization should be performed with multiple sensitive methods.

Another major obstacle to nanoparticle-based theranostics is the neurotoxicity resulting from nanomaterials. If the therapeutic levels are not strictly monitored, the

Table 1 Overview of therapeutic nanoparticles explored for brain tumor therapy

Type of therapeutic nanoparticle	Modification	Anti-cancer agent	Significance of study	Reference
SPIONs	Magnetic (Fe_3O_4) silica PLGA NPs conjugated with Transferrin	DOX-PTX	BBB penetration, tumor localization	[22]
Dendrimers	PEPE dendrimers, conjugated with D-glucosamine	MTX	BBB penetration, glioma targeting, overcomes MTX resistance	[51]
Dendrimers	PEGylated PAMAM G5 dendrimers conjugated with FA and Borneol	DOX	Reduced toxicity of PAMAM, BBB penetration, improved tumor localization, tumor growth inhibition	[52]
NLCs	RGD-conjugated PEG-DSPE NLCs	TMZ	Tumor inhibition	[57]
SLNs	–	Riluzole	High drug loading, improved permeability, brain targeting	[60]
Carbon dots	C-dots conjugated with Transferrin and DOX	DOX	Higher drug uptake, improved cytotoxicity	[40]
Carbon nanotubes	Functionalized SWCNTs conjugated with CpG	–	Enhanced uptake by tumor cells, Potentiation of pro-inflammatory cytokine production, Inhibition of tumor growth, long-term anti-tumor immunity	[31]
AgNPs	Lanthanum manganite doped silver atoms	Silver	BBB Penetration, Apoptotic activity by ROS generation	[20]

In above table terms are abbreviated as Ang-2—Angiopep-2; YAP—Yes-associated protein; siRNA—Small interfering Ribonucleic acid; SPIONs—Superparamagnetic iron oxide nanoparticles; PLGA—Poly(lactic-co-glycolic acid); PEPE—Polyether-copolyester; PEG—Polyethylene glycol; PAMAM—Poly(amidoamine); FA—Folic acid; RGD—Arginine-glycine-aspartic acid peptide; DSPE—Distearoylphosphatidylethanolamine; NLCs—Nanostructured lipid carriers; SLNs—Solid lipid nanoparticles; SWCNTs—Single walled Carbon nanotubes; CpG—5'—Cytosine—phosphate—Guanine—3' oligodeoxynucleotide; AgNPs—Silver nanoparticles; ROS—Reactive oxygen species; DOX—Doxorubicin; PTX—Paclitaxel; MTX—Methotrexate; TMZ—Temozolomide administered drug dosage may be altered in the body and result in permanent toxic effects. Neurotoxicity, a consequence of oxidative stress from the surplus generation of ROS and ensuing cytokine production impacts inflammatory responses and causes neuronal cell death. The use of NPs may also cause unsatisfactory irreversible structural modifications to the BBB, inducing ruinous ramifications like brain tissue edema and catering admission to external toxins and harmful molecules that are otherwise restricted.

While former generations of lipid-based NPs have not shown significant toxicity, their long-term effects are still unknown. Although these polymeric materials offer sustained release and tissue specificity, their biodegradation course has been linked with reasonable toxic events. Thus, the origin of the nanomaterial (naturally occurring or manufactured) is a major aspect in determining the latent toxic effects. Liposomes that were used to deliver drugs and diagnostic agents to the brain were found to exhibit increased neurotoxicity when conjugated with anti-neoplastic drug cisplatin [62]. CNTs show no conclusive proof of toxicity in humans but have been predicted to induce asbestos-like inflammation, while metallic nanomaterials could enter, accumulate and cause heavy-metal toxicity in tissues [63]. Other nanocarriers including gold, silver, iron oxide and silica in higher doses or on longer exposure may gradually accumulate in the brain over time, generate ROS and cause development of functional impairments because of low clearance rates. In pre-clinical and clinical trials, valid concerns have been raised due to anatomical and physiological variations between laboratory animals and humans, their distinct biological interactions and differences in toxicities as well as the metabolism of NPs. Thus, the pharmacokinetics, and delineation of safety of all nanocarriers ought to be accurately examined and documented [64]. Moreover, the complicated and multi-stage manufacturing process for large-scale production of nanocarriers, high cost of raw materials and lack of in-vitro/in-vivo correlation (IVIVC) of drug release profiles are a key obstacle. For efficient clinical therapy, the nanomedicines should exhibit enough long-term stability during clinical administration and suitable studies need to be conducted.

The use of nanomaterials for brain tumor management also stirs up apprehensions concerning environmental health, particularly because of the manufacturing processes and toxicological pollution in the environment due to uncertain size, shape and chemical compositions. Thus, the footprint on the environment resulting from the wide use of nanomaterials should be carefully determined. Thus, it is critical that the beneficial and detrimental significance of nanocarriers is plainly established, and efficient design and development schemes are employed before clinical translation. Rather than using a single strategy which might hinder or increase the time taken to achieve a therapeutic effect, adopting integrated nanotechnological advances and molecular processes, could yield a progressive approach for a superior way to manage brain tumors.

4 Conclusion

Owing to vast research and outstanding breakthroughs in the nanotechnology sphere and bioactive drug molecules numerous groups of nanocarriers are gaining momentum in the biomedical sphere. The progress in nanomedicine in the intraoperative visualization and therapeutics of brain cancer although recent, has exponentially grown and has exhibited immense potential.

The frontier of nanotheranostic medicine has also gained increasing interest, with small size, specificity, concomitant loading of drugs and contrast agents and targeted therapy improving diagnostic and therapeutic interventions. Considerable time and research has been devoted toward the development of multifunctional nanoparticulate systems for cancer imaging and therapeutics. Along with developments in the types of drug carriers better characterization approaches, pharmacokinetic studies and long-term toxicity studies are an urgent need. Gold, silver, iron oxide NPs, carbon-based NPs, dendrimers and lipid NPs hold an illustrious and wide array of medical applications of which controlled and targeted drug delivery, diagnosis and imaging tools and screening platforms have gained notoriety. A solid brain cancer management approach has been theoretically explored but to transcribe the preliminary research into comprehensive clinical trials, further extensive investigations are essential, particularly those relating to the drug loading capacity, methods to optimize tissue targeting and correctly evaluate toxicity to obtain the best clinical outcome. Diagnostic approaches like CT and MRI have begun to utilize novel modified nanoparticulate diagnostic agents with contrast enhancement, tissue targeting, and long circulation times thus enabling better visualization and marked delineation of healthy and tumorous tissues. The newer multifunctional NPs, with nano sizes, preferential drug accumulation, ease of BBB penetration, high specificity, reduced toxicity and intrinsic cytotoxic properties are proving to be a superlative form of cancer drug therapy. The overall goal of a better patient outcome and improved survival rates could be observed, by early and efficient diagnosis, constant monitoring prior and during treatment, effective treatment approaches and rehabilitation. Despite the wide expanse of uncharted territory, with the pace of research expeditiously picking up, the future of clinical cancer therapy certainly seems promising.

References

1. El Demerdash N, Kedda J, Ram N, Brem H, Tyler B (2020) Novel therapeutics for brain tumors: current practice and future prospects. Expert Opin Drug Deliv 17(1):9–21
2. Jain KK (2018) A critical overview of targeted therapies for glioblastoma. Front Oncol 8
3. Zhou Y, Peng Z, Seven ES, Leblanc RM (2018) Crossing the blood-brain barrier with nanoparticles. J Control Release 270:290–303
4. Ding S, Khan AI, Cai X, Song Y, Lyu Z, Du D, Dutta P, Lin Y (2020) Overcoming blood–brain barrier transport: advances in nanoparticle-based drug delivery strategies. Mater Today 37:112–125

5. Martins JP, das Neves J, de la Fuente M, Celia C, Florindo H, Günday-Türeli N, Popat A, Santos JL, Sousa F, Schmid R, Wolfram J, Sarmento B, Santos HA (2020) The solid progress of nanomedicine. Drug Deliv Transl Res 10(3):726–729
6. Bhaskaran NA, Kumar L (2021) Treating colon cancers with a non-conventional yet strategic approach: an overview of various nanoparticle systems. J Control Release 336:16–39
7. Meola A, Rao J, Chaudhary N, Sharma M, Chang SD (2018) Gold nanoparticles for brain tumor imaging: a systematic review. Front Neurol 9
8. Dixit S, Miller K, Zhu Y, McKinnon E, Novak T, Kenney ME, Broome A-M (2015) Dual receptor-targeted theranostic nanoparticles for localized delivery and activation of photodynamic therapy drug in glioblastomas. Mol Pharm 12(9):3250–3260
9. Kumar A, Zhang X, Liang X-J (2013) Gold nanoparticles: emerging paradigm for targeted drug delivery system. Biotechnol Adv 31(5):593–606
10. Setua S, Ouberai M, Piccirillo SG, Watts C, Welland M (2014) Cisplatin-tethered gold nanospheres for multimodal chemo-radiotherapy of glioblastoma. Nanoscale 6(18):10865–10873
11. Meyers JD, Cheng Y, Broome A-M, Agnes RS, Schluchter MD, Margevicius S, Wang X, Kenney ME, Burda C, Basilion JP (2014) Peptide-targeted gold nanoparticles for photodynamic therapy of brain cancer. Part Part Syst Charact 32(4):448–457
12. Sun L, Joh DY, Al-Zaki A, Stangl M, Murty S, Davis JJ, Baumann BC, Alonso-Basanta M, Kao GD, Tsourkas A, Dorsey JF (2016) Theranostic application of mixed gold and superparamagnetic iron oxide nanoparticle micelles in glioblastoma multiforme. J Biomed Nanotechnol 12(2):347–356
13. Kumthekar P, Ko CH, Paunesku T, Dixit K, Sonabend AM, Bloch O, Tate M, Schwartz M, Zuckerman L, Lezon R, Lukas RV, Jovanovic B, McCortney K, Colman H, Chen S, Lai B, Antipova O, Deng J, Li L, Tommasini-Ghelfi S (2021) A first-in-human phase 0 clinical study of RNA interference–based spherical nucleic acids in patients with recurrent glioblastoma. Sci Transl Med 13(584):eabb3945
14. De Matteis V, Cascione M, Toma C, Leporatti S (2018) Silver nanoparticles: synthetic routes, in vitro toxicity and theranostic applications for cancer disease. Nanomaterials 8(5):319
15. Kovács D, Igaz N, Gopisetty MK, Kiricsi M (2022) Cancer therapy by silver nanoparticles: fiction or reality? Int J Mol Sci 23(2):839
16. Locatelli E, Naddaka M, Uboldi C, Loudos G, Fragogeorgi E, Molinari V, Pucci A, Tsotakos T, Psimadas D, Ponti J, Franchini MC (2014) Targeted delivery of silver nanoparticles and alisertib: in vitro and in vivo synergistic effect against glioblastoma. Nanomedicine 9(6):839–849
17. Urbańska K, Pająk B, Orzechowski A, Sokołowska J, Grodzik M, Sawosz E, Szmidt M, Sysa P (2015) The effect of silver nanoparticles (AgNPs) on proliferation and apoptosis of in ovo cultured glioblastoma multiforme (GBM) cells. Nanoscale Res Lett 10(1)
18. Hsin Y-H, Chen C-F, Huang S, Shih T-S, Lai P-S, Chueh PJ (2008) The apoptotic effect of nanosilver is mediated by a ROS- and JNK-dependent mechanism involving the mitochondrial pathway in NIH3T3 cells. Toxicol Lett 179(3):130–139
19. Liu P, Huang Z, Chen Z, Xu R, Wu H, Zang F, Wang C, Gu N (2013) Silver nanoparticles: a novel radiation sensitizer for glioma? Nanoscale 5(23):11829
20. Khochaiche A, Westlake M, O'Keefe A, Engels E, Vogel S, Valceski M, Li N, Rule KC, Horvat J, Konstantinov K, Rosenfeld A, Lerch M, Corde S, Tehei M (2021) First extensive study of silver-doped lanthanum manganite nanoparticles for inducing selective chemotherapy and radio-toxicity enhancement. Mater Sci Eng C 123:111970
21. Marekova D, Turnovcova K, Sursal TH, Gandhi CD, Jendelova P, Jhanwar-Uniyal M (2020) Potential for treatment of glioblastoma: new aspects of superparamagnetic iron oxide nanoparticles. Anticancer Res 40(11):5989–5994
22. Cui Y, Xu Q, Chow PK-H, Wang D, Wang C-H (2013) Transferrin-conjugated magnetic silica PLGA nanoparticles loaded with doxorubicin and paclitaxel for brain glioma treatment. Biomaterials 34(33):8511–8520

23. Sun C, Fang C, Stephen Z, Veiseh O, Hansen S, Lee D, Ellenbogen RG, Olson J, Zhang M (2008) Tumor-targeted drug delivery and MRI contrast enhancement by chlorotoxin-conjugated iron oxide nanoparticles. Nanomedicine 3(4):495–505
24. Hadjipanayis CG, Machaidze R, Kaluzova M, Wang L, Schuette AJ, Chen H, Wu X, Mao H (2010) EGFRvIII antibody-conjugated iron oxide nanoparticles for magnetic resonance imaging-guided convection-enhanced delivery and targeted therapy of glioblastoma. Cancer Res 70(15):6303–6312
25. Fernandes NB, Shenoy RUK, Kajampady MK, DCruz CEM, Shirodkar RK, Kumar L, Verma R (2022) Fullerenes for the treatment of cancer: an emerging tool. Environ Sci Pollut Res (In Press). https://doi.org/10.1007/s11356-022-21449-7
26. Wong BS, Yoong SL, Jagusiak A, Panczyk T, Ho HK, Ang WH, Pastorin G (2013) Carbon nanotubes for delivery of small molecule drugs. Adv Drug Deliv Rev 65(15):1964–2015
27. Zhang W, Zhang Z, Zhang Y (2011) The application of carbon nanotubes in target drug delivery systems for cancer therapies. Nanoscale Res Lett 6(1)
28. Shapira A, Livney YD, Broxterman HJ, Assaraf YG (2011) Nanomedicine for targeted cancer therapy: towards the overcoming of drug resistance. Drug Resist Updates 14(3):150–163
29. Singh RP, Sharma G, Sonali SS, Kumar M, Pandey BL, Koch B, Muthu MS (2016) Vitamin E TPGS conjugated carbon nanotubes improved efficacy of docetaxel with safety for lung cancer treatment. Colloids Surf B: Biointerfaces 141:429–442
30. VanHandel M, Alizadeh D, Zhang L, Kateb B, Bronikowski M, Manohara H, Badie B (2009) Selective uptake of multi-walled carbon nanotubes by tumor macrophages in a murine glioma model. J Neuroimmunol 208(1–2):3–9
31. Zhao D, Alizadeh D, Zhang L, Liu W, Farrukh O, Manuel E, Diamond DJ, Badie B (2011) Carbon nanotubes enhance CpG uptake and potentiate antiglioma immunity. Clin Cancer Res 17(4):771–782
32. Alizadeh D, White EE, Sanchez TC, Liu S, Zhang L, Badie B, Berlin JM (2018) Immunostimulatory CpG on carbon nanotubes selectively inhibits migration of brain tumor cells. Bioconjug Chem 29(5):1659–1668
33. Santos T, Fang X, Chen M-T, Wang W, Ferreira R, Jhaveri N, Gundersen M, Zhou C, Pagnini P, Hofman FM, Chen TC (2014) Sequential administration of carbon nanotubes and near-infrared radiation for the treatment of gliomas. Front Oncol 4
34. You Y, Wang N, He L, Shi C, Zhang D, Liu Y, Luo L, Chen T (2019) Designing dual-functionalized carbon nanotubes with high blood–brain-barrier permeability for precise orthotopic glioma therapy. Dalton Trans 48(5):1569–1573
35. Onoshima D, Yukawa H, Baba Y (2015) Multifunctional quantum dots-based cancer diagnostics and stem cell therapeutics for regenerative medicine. Adv Drug Deliv Rev 95:2–14
36. Huang R, Han L, Li J, Liu S, Shao K, Kuang Y, Hu X, Wang X, Lei H, Jiang C (2011) Chlorotoxin-modified macromolecular contrast agent for MRI tumor diagnosis. Biomaterials 32(22):5177–5186
37. Jena L, McErlean E, McCarthy H (2019) Delivery across the blood-brain barrier: nanomedicine for glioblastoma multiforme. Drug Deliv Transl Res 10(2):304–318
38. Ruan S, Qian J, Shen S, Zhu J, Jiang X, He Q, Gao H (2014) A simple one-step method to prepare fluorescent carbon dots and their potential application in non-invasive glioma imaging. Nanoscale 6(17):10040–10047
39. Li S, Amat D, Peng Z, Vanni S, Raskin S, De Angulo G, Othman AM, Graham RM, Leblanc RM (2016) Transferrin conjugated nontoxic carbon dots for doxorubicin delivery to target paediatric brain tumor cells. Nanoscale 8(37):16662–16669
40. Li S, Peng Z, Dallman J, Baker J, Othman AM, Blackwelder PL, Leblanc RM (2016) Crossing the blood–brain–barrier with transferrin conjugated carbon dots: a zebrafish model study. Colloids Surf B: Biointerfaces 145:251–256
41. Zheng M, Ruan S, Liu S, Sun T, Qu D, Zhao H, Xie Z, Gao H, Jing X, Sun Z (2015) Self-targeting fluorescent carbon dots for diagnosis of brain cancer cells. ACS Nano 9(11):11455–11461
42. Shi J, Liu Y, Wang L, Gao J, Zhang J, Yu X, Ma R, Liu R, Zhang Z (2014) A tumoral acidic pH-responsive drug delivery system based on a novel photosensitizer (fullerene) for in vitro and in vivo chemo-photodynamic therapy. Acta Biomater 10(3):1280–1291

43. Shultz MD, Wilson JD, Fuller CE, Zhang J, Dorn HC, Fatouros PP (2011) Metallofullerene-based nanoplatform for brain tumor brachytherapy and longitudinal imaging in a murine orthotopic xenograft model. Radiology 261(1):136–143
44. Shevtsov MA, Nikolaev BP, Marchenko Ya Y, Yakovleva LY, Dobrodumov AV, Török G, Pitkin E, Lebedev VT (2014) Magnetic resonance imaging of Rat C6 glioma model enhanced by using water-soluble gadolinium fullerene. Appl Magn Reson 45(4):303–314
45. Hsieh F-Y, Zhilenkov AV, Voronov II, Khakina EA, Mischenko DV, Troshin PA, Hsu S (2017) Water-soluble fullerene derivatives as brain medicine: surface chemistry determines if they are neuroprotective and antitumor. ACS Appl Mater Interfaces 9(13):11482–11492
46. Kesharwani P, Jain K, Jain NK (2014) Dendrimer as nanocarrier for drug delivery. Prog Polym Sci 39(2):268–307
47. Gillies E, Fréchet J (2005) Dendrimers and dendritic polymers in drug delivery. Drug Discov Today 10(1):35–43
48. Wiener E, Brechbiel MW, Brothers H, Magin RL, Gansow OA, Tomalia DA, Lauterbur PC (1994) Dendrimer-based metal chelates: a new class of magnetic resonance imaging contrast agents. Magn Reson Med 31(1):1–8
49. Sarin H, Kanevsky AS, Wu H, Brimacombe KR, Fung SH, Sousa AA, Auh S, Wilson CM, Sharma K, Aronova MA, Leapman RD, Griffiths GL, Hall MD (2008) Effective transvascular delivery of nanoparticles across the blood-brain tumor barrier into malignant glioma cells. J Transl Med 6(1)
50. Bertin A, Steibel J, Michou-Gallani A-I, Gallani J-L, Felder-Flesch D (2009) Development of a dendritic manganese-enhanced magnetic resonance imaging (MEMRI) contrast agent: synthesis, toxicity (in vitro) and relaxivity (in vitro, in vivo) studies. Bioconjug Chem 20(4):760–767
51. Dhanikula RS, Argaw A, Bouchard J-F, Hildgen P (2008) Methotrexate loaded polyether-copolyester dendrimers for the treatment of gliomas: enhanced efficacy and intratumoral transport capability. Mol Pharm 5(1):105–116
52. Xu X, Li J, Han S, Tao C, Fang L, Sun Y, Zhu J, Liang Z, Li F (2016) A novel doxorubicin loaded folic acid conjugated PAMAM modified with borneol, a nature dual-functional product of reducing PAMAM toxicity and boosting BBB penetration. Eur J Pharm Sci 88:178–190
53. Seyfoddin A, Shaw J, Al-Kassas R (2010) Solid lipid nanoparticles for ocular drug delivery. Drug Deliv 17(7):467–489
54. Sercombe L, Veerati T, Moheimani F, Wu SY, Sood AK, Hua S (2015) Advances and challenges of liposome assisted drug delivery. Front Pharmacol 6(286)
55. Moghassemi S, Hadjizadeh A (2014) Nano-niosomes as nanoscale drug delivery systems: an illustrated review. J Control Release 185:22–36
56. Hou D, Xie C, Huang K, Zhu C (2003) The production and characteristics of solid lipid nanoparticles (SLNs). Biomaterials 24(10):1781–1785
57. Song S, Mao G, Du J, Zhu X (2015) Novel RGD containing, temozolomide-loading nanostructured lipid carriers for glioblastoma multiforme chemotherapy. Drug Deliv 23(4):1404–1408
58. Azmin MN, Florence AT, Handjani-Vila RM, Stuart JF, Vanlerberghe G, Whittaker JS (1985) The effect of non-ionic surfactant vesicle (niosome) entrapment on the absorption and distribution of methotrexate in mice. J Pharm Pharmacol 37(4):237–242
59. Martina M-S, Fortin J-P, Ménager C, Clément O, Barratt G, Grabielle-Madelmont C, Gazeau F, Cabuil V, Lesieur S (2005) Generation of superparamagnetic liposomes revealed as highly efficient MRI contrast agents for in vivo imaging. J Am Chem Soc 127(30):10676–10685
60. Bondì ML, Craparo EF, Giammona G, Drago F (2010) Brain-targeted solid lipid nanoparticles containing riluzole: preparation, characterization and biodistribution. Nanomedicine 5(1):25–32
61. Navya PN, Kaphle A, Srinivas SP, Bhargava SK, Rotello VM, Daima HK (2019) Current trends and challenges in cancer management and therapy using designer nanomaterials. Nano Converg 6(1):23

62. Huo T, Barth RF, Yang W, Nakkula RJ, Koynova R, Tenchov B, Chaudhury AR, Agius L, Boulikas T, Elleaume H, Lee RJ (2012) Preparation, biodistribution and neurotoxicity of liposomal cisplatin following convection enhanced delivery in normal and F98 Glioma bearing rats. PLoS ONE 7(11):e48752
63. Donaldson K, Poland CA, Murphy FA, MacFarlane M, Chernova T, Schinwald A (2013) Pulmonary toxicity of carbon nanotubes and asbestos - similarities and differences. Adv Drug Deliv Rev 65(15):2078–2086
64. Rosenblum D, Joshi N, Tao W, Karp JM, Peer D (2018) Progress and challenges towards targeted delivery of cancer therapeutics. Nat Commun 9(1)
65. Huang N, Cheng S, Zhang X, Tian Q, Pi J, Tang J, Huang Q, Wang F, Chen J, Xie Z, Xu Z, Chen W, Zheng H, Cheng Y (2017) Efficacy of NGR peptide-modified PEGylated quantum dots for crossing the blood–brain barrier and targeted fluorescence imaging of glioma and tumor vasculature. Nanomed Nanotechnol Biol Med 13(1): 83–93
66. Lihuang L, Qiuyan G, Yanxiu L, Mindan L, Jun Y, Yunlong G, Qiang Z, Benqiang S, Xiumin W, Liang-cheng L, Lei R (2020) Targeted combination therapy for glioblastoma by co-delivery of doxorubicin, YAP-siRNA and gold nanorods. J Mater Sci Technol 63
67. Wang Q, Zhang C, Shen G, Liu H, Fu H, Cui D (2014) Fluorescent carbon dots as an efficient siRNA nanocarrier for its interference therapy in gastric cancer cells. J Nanobiotechnol 12(1)

Polyphenols and its Nano Formulations as Therapeutic Agents Against Parkinson's and Alzheimer's Dementia

Abhishek Rawat, Sibasankar Sahu, Lakhveer Singh, Prashant Shukla, and Shashank Shekher Mishra

Abstract Polyphenolic compounds are the secondary metabolites of plants that have been studied for their potential to prevent or delay neurodegenerative disorders. Nowadays plant-derived natural products are gaining significant attention due to their medicinal potential. Therefore, there is an increasing interest in the therapeutic potential of plant polyphenols in neurodegenerative diseases. Due to the instability and low bioavailability of polyphenols, encapsulating bioactive compounds into micro and nano-systems has been effective in avoiding degradation, boosting bioactivity and bioavailability, and enabling targeted administration. The current review summarizes the nano-formulations of plant polyphenols in the context of relevance to neurodegenerative diseases

1 Introduction

The emergence of the common syndrome of dementia is significantly impacted by the aging of the world's population in terms of both its scope and global distribution. Dementia may be described as a "syndrome caused by neurodegeneration" in the 2014 World Alzheimer Report. As a leading cause of dependency, impairment, and mortality, it has emerged as one of the foremost health burdens of the twenty-first century. Though it primarily affects the elderly, it is thought that between 1 and 10% of cases start before age 65. After that, the frequency doubles every five years. There are many differences in the clinical spectrum of dementia. Primary degenerative dementias, such as vascular dementia (VaD), frontotemporal dementia (FTD), Alzheimer's disease (AD) and dementia with Lewy bodies (DLB), are distinguished

A. Rawat · S. Sahu · L. Singh · S. S. Mishra (✉)
School of Pharmaceutical & Population Health Informatics, Faculty of Pharmacy, DIT University, Dehradun, Uttarakhand, India
e-mail: Shashankmedchem09@gmail.com

P. Shukla
Department of Pharmacy, UPES School of Health Sciences and Technology, University of Petroleum & Energy Studies, Dehradun, Uttarakhand 248007, India

S. K. Rath et al. (eds.), *Nanomaterials for Drug Delivery and Neurological Diseases Management*, Smart Nanomaterials Technology,
https://doi.org/10.1007/978-981-97-0308-1_15

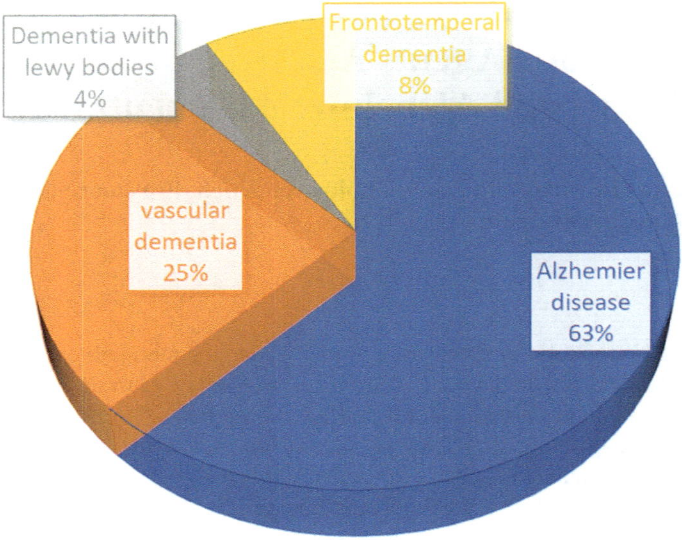

Fig. 1 Primary dementia subtype characteristics

from secondary dementias, such as those caused by AIDS, Huntington's disease or Parkinson's disease. Amyloid plaques and neurofibrillary tangles are the two key pathological characteristics of AD, the most prevalent of all cases. Additionally, there are occasional reports of mixed dementia with pathological features indicative of both vascular dementia and Alzheimer's disease. The term "mild cognitive impairment" (MCI) means people with some cognitive impairment who do not meet the criteria for dementia (Fig. 1).

Polyphenols are complexly arranged organic compounds that can be found in many plant-based diets. The phenolic ring, which is typically broken down into phenolic acids and phenolic alcohols, is the basic building component of polyphenols. Flavonoids, phenolic acids, stibines, lignans, and phenolic alcohols are the main categories of polyphenols. Depending on the strength of the phenolic ring, polyphenols can be divided into a number of classes. The bioactive phytochemicals that protect against chronic degenerative diseases support human health. Polyphenols may be described as a group of chemical compounds that have physiological effects and are present in plant-based diets [1]. The brain and central nervous system are affected by chronic, autoimmune diseases known as neurodegenerative disorders. Some typical examples of these conditions include Alzheimer's, Parkinson's, and Huntington's. Multiple processes, including protein aggregation, oxidative stress and mitochondrial failure, are responsible for the complexity of their etiology. Research is being conducted on natural bioactive compounds, such as turmeric, which have been used for centuries to treat inflammatory and autoimmune conditions. Polyphenolic compounds and their derivatives are currently being studied for their anti-inflammatory and antioxidant properties to combat neurodegenerative disorders effectively [2].

Polyphenolic compounds are natural compounds found in plants that have been studied for their potential to prevent or delay neurodegenerative disorders. With a molecular weight of 500 to 4000 Da, at least 12 phenolic hydroxyl groups, and 5 to 7 aromatic rings per 1000 Da, they are water-soluble phenolic compounds. Polyphenols have structural characteristics that make them therapeutically significant, notably in neuroprotection. These structural features include phenol rings, hydroxylation patterns, and conjugated double bonds. In order to prevent neuroinflammation, oxidative stress, iron toxicity, protein aggregation, and mitochondrial dysfunction in neurodegenerative illnesses, they can serve as metal chelators, fibril destabilizers, estrogens-like substances, enzyme binders, and antioxidants [3].

Polyphenols exhibit their neuroprotective actions by acting as scavengers of reactive oxygen and nitrogen species, and by modulating signaling pathways involved in neuronal survival, growth, and plasticity. The bioavailability of polyphenols varies widely, though, and even the polyphenols that are most prevalent in our diets may not produce the highest levels of active metabolites in the target tissues. Some polyphenols, such as isoflavones and gallic acid, are well-absorbed, while others, such as proanthocyanins and anthocyanins, are poorly absorbed. Various nanotechnologies have been introduced, such as liposomal-based nanoparticles, to overcome this challenge to improve the absorption and bioavailability of polyphenolic compounds [4].

Polyphenols, naturally occurring compounds found in plants, have been extensively studied for their neuroprotective properties. They possess antioxidant, anti-inflammatory, and anti-amyloidogenic effects, which are beneficial for reducing oxidative stress, inflammation, and protein aggregation in neurodegenerative diseases.

2 Classification of Polyphenols

Polyphenols occur in a variety of types, including broad, complex tannins, tiny, low-molecular-weight molecules, and derivative polyphenols. For redox reactions, one or more aromatic rings make up the chemical structure of phenols, and hydroxyl groups set in the ortho or para orientations are essential. Polyphenols are often water-soluble molecules in nature, yet they can also be volatile substances [24, 25]. An alternative method of producing polyphenols as secondary metabolites with biological significance is through enzymatic and nonenzymatic processes. For instance, the biotransformation required to create curcuminoids and stilbenes is catalyzed by the enzymes curcuminoid and stilbene synthase, respectively. Polyphenols can be classified into different groups as a function of the number of phenol rings that they contain and on the basis of structural elements that bind these rings to one another. These classes are flavonoids, stilbenes, phenolic acids, and lignans.

Phenolic acids are prevalent in foods and are classified into two types: benzoic acid derivatives and cinnamic acid derivatives. The hydroxycinnamic acids, which include p-coumaric, caffeic, ferulic, and sinapic acids, are more common than the hydroxybenzoic acids. Stilbenes consist of two phenyl moieties linked by a two-carbon methylene bridge. Stilbenes are quite rare in the human diet. Most stilbenes in plants act as antifungal phytoalexins, compounds that are synthesized only in response to infection or injury.

Two benzene rings may be linked together to form flavonoids by three carbon chains from a neighboring pyran ring. Furthermore, six groups of flavonoids—flavanones, flavanols, flavanols, isoflavones, flavones, and anthocyanidins—distinguish themselves from one another principally based on the variation in the type of heterocycle involved. Flavonoids are the most widely used polyphenols. Flavanols make up the majority of the flavonoids found in various food sources. These chemicals are primarily found in onions, though leeks and broccoli also contain them [5]. Quercetin, catechins, myricetin, etc., are some most common flavonoids. In addition, sources from plants have yielded the identification of over 4000 flavonoids. Based on the hydroxylation configuration, flavonoids are divided into four subclasses: flavanols, flavones, flavanones, and anthocyanidins [6] (Fig. 2).

Legumes are a rich source of these substances as well. Whereas soybeans are the main source of food, isoflavones have a superior impact on health. The most common types of isoflavone-aglycones are 7-O-glucosides and 6''-O-malonyl-7-O-glucosides. Dalbergin is the main neo-flavonoid found in plant-based meals. Along with glycitein, two more important isoflavones present in soy are daidzein and genistein. Such chemicals can also be found in red clovers. Flavanones are primarily found in citrus fruits; aromatic plants also contain these substances. The rigid parts of the fruits and covers contain flavanones, which are five times more abundant in whole meals than in juices. Because of the presence of OH between C4 and C7, which is identical to estradiol, isoflavones are a group of chemicals that are suspected to

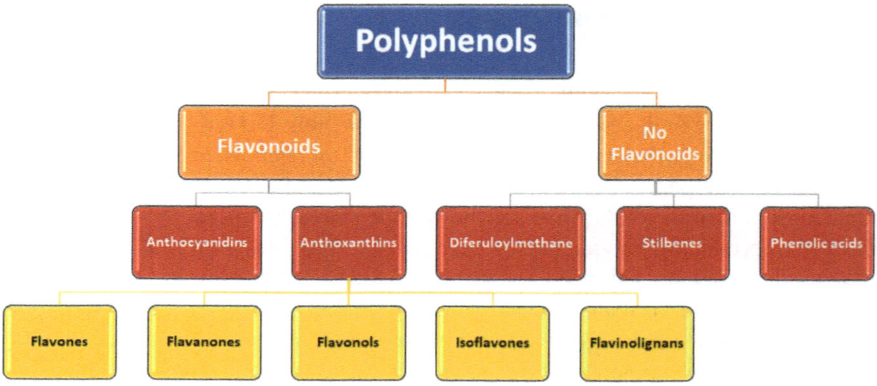

Fig. 2 Classification of polyphenols

be estrogens. Because they can connect to estrogen receptors, these substances are known as phytoestrogens [7].

3 Application of Polyphenols in Nanomedicine: Preclinical and Clinical Evidence

3.1 Polyphenols Containing Liposomes

The beneficial effects of curcumin and resveratrol on human health have been well documented, but their low solubility and stability limit their efficacy. Nanotechnology-driven delivery systems, such as polymeric micelles, nanostructured lipid carriers, and polymeric nanoparticles, have successfully resolved these issues and improved their therapeutic effects. Co-delivery systems for resveratrol and curcumin have also been explored, including lipid-core nanocapsules, oligo-hyalurosomes, and core–shell nanoparticles. However, these systems are still in development and require further improvement.

Liposomes are phospholipid bilayer membrane systems that can encapsulate a variety of nutraceuticals, including hydrophilic, hydrophobic, and amphiphilic compounds. They have been utilized as delivery systems for lutein, quercetin, kaempferol, carotenoids, EGCG, and quercetin. Liposomes also have a distinct lipid bilayer construction that allows for tenable orientation and location of encapsulated molecules. Various studies have shown that the association of carotenoids in the lipid bilayer significantly affects the characteristics of the liposomes. Additionally, it has been reported that resveratrol and curcumin preferentially locate in different regions of bilayer and can synergistically stabilize the liposomes to improve delivery performance. The method of preparing liposomes loaded with curcumin and/or resveratrol was described below.

The lipids Egg yolk phosphatidylcholine (EYPC) and Tween 80 were dissolved in ethanol together with the polyphenols and the resulting solution was dried using a rotary evaporator and vacuum-dried overnight. The thin film was then hydrated with phosphate-buffered saline and subjected to probe sonication processing to achieve homogeneous liposomes. Resveratrol liposomes have been designated R, curcumin liposomes C, and liposomes co-loaded with resveratrol and curcumin at mole ratios of 1:5, 1:1, and 5:1 were labeled CR1, CR3, and CR5, respectively.

The liposomal delivery system was characterized by its physicochemical stability and nanotechnological properties. The liposomes' size and polydispersity index (PDI) were measured. It was seen that the liposomes loaded with one or two polyphenols had a uniform size distribution, with a mean diameter between 75 and 90 nm, confirming that they were nano liposomal formulations. The particle size of the liposomes increased as the concentration of resveratrol increased. The coloaded liposomes showed a slight decrease in size compared to the liposomes loaded with a single polyphenol. The polyphenol encapsulating efficacy (EE) of the liposomal system was assessed, and it was observed that the liposomes coloaded with curcumin and resveratrol had the highest EE. Curcumin's incorporating capacity is explained by both its propensity to be lipophilic and its considerable impact on membrane structures [8].

4 Polyphenols Containing Nanoparticles

Curcumin-loaded lactoferrin nanoparticles

An effective natural polyphenol, curcumin is derived from the root of the turmeric plant (*Curcuma longa L.*). It was created to transport curcumin-loaded lactoferrin NPs into the SK-N-SH dopaminergic cells to prevent rotenone-induced neurotoxicity in Parkinson's Disease situations [9]. Curcumin has a low bioavailability, little absorption, and quickly leaves the body, making it unsuitable as a therapeutic agent [10]. Previous research has indicated that the mesencephalon of PD patients expresses higher levels of lactoferrin receptors, which are involved in the uptake of iron by cells [11]. Curcumin is encapsulated in this lactoferrin protein, which also offers the basic benefits of nanoparticles including ideal size for cellular absorption and enhanced intracellular localization [12]. The therapeutic effectiveness of nanoparticles depends on their size [13]. Immune cells are able to catch nanoparticles larger than 400 nm, which limits the biodistribution of these particles [14].

5 Resveratrol and Grape Extract-Loaded Solid Lipid Nanoparticles

Polyphenolic flavonoid resveratrol (3,5,40-trihydroxystilbene) occurs naturally as both cis and trans isomers, with the latter being the most prevalent and physiologically active [15]. Resveratrol has neuroprotective actions in neurological disorders by shielding neurons from oxidative stress and toxicity and by preventing apoptotic neuronal death. Red wine, mulberries, peanuts, rhubarb, grape seeds, and the skins of many other plants contain resveratrol [16]. Resveratrol's bioavailability limits were overcome by using SLN nanoparticles as a carrier. To produce nanoparticles, a middle ground between the high-shear homogenization method and the ultrasonication technique is used [17]. The SLNs are a dynamic system that holds promise for the targeted delivery of grape extracts to the brain as a natural resveratrol substitute to prevent the creation of amyloid-peptide (A) aggregates, potentially delaying or reducing the progression of Alzheimer's disease (AD) [18].

6 Gallic Acid Loaded onto Polyethyleneimine-Coated Human Serum Albumin Nanoparticles (PEI-HSA-GA NPs)

A-synuclein (aSN), a protein of 140 residues, aggregates and is a key player in the aetiology of several neurodegenerative diseases, including Parkinson's disease (PD) [19]. Many plants, including sumac, green tea, berries, and gallnuts contain gallic acid (GA), a phenolic antioxidant. Free radicals with a high oxidative potential can be diminished by GA. This has generated a great deal of interest in its potential application as a treatment for conditions linked to oxidative stress. By enhancing the brain's antioxidant defense, GA may prevent chronic cerebral hypoperfusion-related cognitive deficits [20]. In addition to having antioxidant capabilities, GA binds to and stabilizes a class of non-toxic aSN oligomers that mostly have an unfolded conformation and lack b-sheet structure, which is consistent with its ability to also stabilize the extended, naturally unfolded structure of monomeric aSN. The hydroxyl moieties' positions on the phenyl ring and their relationship to GA's inhibitory effect are related [21].

7 Dual-Drug Loaded Nanoparticles of Epigallocatechin-3-Gallate (EGCG)/Ascorbic Acid

The camellia sinensis green tea plant's most common polyphenol is EGCG [22]. Because of two gallocatechol rings in this catechin that have high effectiveness in directly removing free radicals, it possesses significant chelating and antioxidant properties [23]. Inducible nitric oxide synthase (iNOS), tumor necrosis factor (TNF), interleukin 6 (IL-6) or even safeguarding mitochondrial function are just a few of the numerous ways that EGCG can act. It can also reduce an accumulation, prevent TAU aggregation, inhibit TNF, iNOS or iNOS production, and suppress TNF [24, 25]. However, EGCG has many pharmacochemical disadvantages as well, including high instability, which decreases its bioavailability and, as a result, decreases its effectiveness. The oxidation of the polyphenolic structure is the main factor contributing to EGCG degradation. To counteract this impact, strong antioxidant molecules like ascorbic acid (AA) are usually added. In addition to scavenging oxygen and safeguarding double bonds, AA also gives the final compositions anti-inflammatory characteristics [26, 27]. One of the most popular polymers for the creation of NPs is poly (lactic-co-glycolic acid, or PLGA) [28]. Which has the properties of being biocompatible, biodegradable, and non-toxic. Additionally, polymeric NPs' surface PEGylation is frequently employed to extend their in vivo half-life. As a consequence of surface-tuning NPs with polyethylene glycol (PEG) chains, the immunogenicity and long-term stability of the nanosystem are clearly decreased, water solubility is improved, and opsonization is minimized [29]. When EGCG is loaded into PEGylated PLGA NPs, the molecule's physicochemical stability, as well as its bioavailability and therapeutic effectiveness, are improved [30].

8 Cyclodextrins

In a bioengineering facility, cyclic oligosaccharides called cyclodextrins (CDs) can be produced by the action of enzymes on starch-rich substrates [31–33]. or can develop naturally in the environment as a result of starch being fermented by bacteria [34, 35]. Normally referred to as "native CDs," naturally occurring cyclodextrins include -CD, -CD, and -CD, each of which has six, seven, or eight glucose units. The D-glucose units are connected by 1,4-bonds in their distinctive structure, which was initially characterized in 1948 [36]. The top and bottom edges of the ring are faced by the secondary and primary hydroxyls, and the internal cavity is lined with protons. Cyclodextrins are employed in the pharmaceutical, cosmetic, and food sectors for controlled administration, solubilization, and shelf-life extension of active components because of their shape as excellent solubilizing agents for non-polar molecules [37, 38]. Despite the fact that the former has more hydroxyl groups than the latter, β-CD is less soluble than α-CD because of the internal hydrogen-bond network that develops between the secondary hydroxyl groups. Water solubility rises as a result of molecular manipulation that breaks down hydrogen bonds. For instance, hydroxypropyl-β-CD (HPβCD) is at least 60% (w/w) soluble in water [39].

9 Combining Polyphenols with β-cyclodextrin

Unintentional protein misfolding, oligomerization, and aggregation are the root causes of a number of human degenerative diseases, such as Alzheimer's and Parkinson's [40]. Parkinson's disease and dementia (induced by synucleinopathies) are symptoms of Lewy bodies, which are macroscopic amyloid deposits of the protein-synuclein [41]. Polyphenols, a substantial class of chemicals, have been shown to inhibit and, in some cases, even deconstruct the amyloids that-synuclein and other proteins create [42, 43]. According to the process by which polyphenolic chemicals inhibit and break down α-synuclein amyloids, the presence of two or more "vicinal polyhydroxyphenyl groups" is much more significant than the total number of hydroxyl groups [44, 45]. Inhibition and amyloid disaggregation caused by these –OH groups have been linked to studies on molecular dynamics [42, 46]. Contrarily, the naturally occurring polyphenol curcumin, which is derived from the turmeric plant (Curcuma longa), is a unique molecule with simply mono hydroxyphenyl rings but is nonetheless a potent aggregation inhibitor [47, 48]. According to a theory, curcumin binds to the aliphatic amino acid residues found in the natural monomeric α-synuclein's middle hydrophobic stretch [49]. The aromatic rings then attach to adjacent hydrophobic α-synuclein residues following this first engagement. According to the same study, curcumin greatly inhibits α-synuclein's ability to form oligomers and fibrils by facilitating the protein's intramolecular transport. This reduces the amount of time that the hydrophobic patches are exposed by speeding up the reconfiguration rate of α-synuclein. According to different research, curcumin decreases the toxicity of α-synuclein by attaching to it and reducing the number of hydrophobic surfaces that are available [50].

In vitro, curcumin and β-cyclodextrin (β-CD) disaggregated -synuclein amyloids as well as prevented their formation [51]. Through its hydrophobic area and -OH groups, respectively, curcumin interacts with the hydrophilic residues and the middle hydrophobic region of -synuclein. By attaching to aromatic residues like the phenylalanine found in α-synuclein, β-CD then provides additional assistance. Seven glucose units make up the cyclic polysaccharide known as β-CD. It is a bucket-shaped molecule with an external hydrophilic surface and an inside hydrophobic hollow [51, 52]. The physiologically active molecule β-CD has been employed for a number of purposes, including catalysis [53], drug administration [54], cholesterol reduction [55], and preventing protein aggregation [56], to mention a few. It also functions as a pseudo-chaperone for protein folding [57]. In addition to interacting with polyphenols to assist them overcome their drawbacks, such as limited bioavailability, insolubility, and instability [58], β-CD also boosts their activity and effectiveness [59], as well as their anti-inflammatory and anti-proliferative capabilities [60].

10 Polyphenol Nanoencapsulation's: Stability and Bioavailability

When particles with diameters between one and one thousand nanometers are created, a science known as nanotechnology is used. The finished product displays characteristics or phenomena that can be attributed to the particle's size [61]. Today, nanoencapsulation is a successful method for increasing the solubility of polyphenols, minimizing the degradation process, lowering their toxicity, and controlling the active absorption and pharmacological response.

Nanoencapsulation refers to a broad range of methods based on chemical, physical, and physiochemical concepts. Chemical nanoencapsulation approaches (such as interfacial and in situ polymerization methods) call for the polymerization of monomers at the interface of two immiscible substances [62]. This is accomplished by introducing a cross-linker to the outer phase. Due to several intrinsic and extrinsic characteristics, such as their chemical composition and molecular weight, low hydro solubility, low stability in the gastrointestinal environment, substantial phase II metabolism, and quick elimination, polyphenols often have limited bioavailability [63]. Recently, a unique method to enhance the transport, distribution, and bioactivity of polyphenols has emerged: encapsulation in nano vectors such as cyclodextrins, matrix systems, solid dispersions, and liposomes [64].

11 Bioavailability Enhancements of Polyphenols Using Nano-encapsulation

Due to the instability and low bioavailability of polyphenols, encapsulating bioactive compounds into micro- and nanosystems has been effective in avoiding degradation, boosting bioactivity and bioavailability, and enabling targeted administration. More than 40 liposomal and polymeric nanoparticles are currently being explored in clinical trials; however, liposomal doxorubicin and albumin-bound paclitaxel have already been used there. Vector-mediated delivery methods have emerged as potential means of delivering bioactive compounds across the BBB at the moment [65].

12 Polymeric Nanoparticles' Encapsulation of Polyphenols

In order to create nanospheres or nanocapsules, polymeric nanoparticles (PNPs) were synthesized. Their architectures changed depending on the manufacturing technology employed (solvent evaporation, salting-out, super-critical fluid technology, dialysis procedures, utilizing the quick expansibility of a supercritical solution into solvent (liquid), etc.) [66]. PNPs are constructed using natural and synthetic polymers, such as albumin, chitosan, gelatin, sodium alginate, and poly(lactide coglycolides). Synthetic polymers include polylactides (PLA), polycapro-lactone (PCL), and polyethylene glycol (PEG). Due to their vesicular shape, nanocapsules specifically play a role in the storage of drugs. The remaining bioactive molecules are then kept in a liquid core that can be either aqueous or non-aqueous and is shielded by a rigid polymeric shell [67]. Oral administration, percutaneous approach, hypodermic injection, intramuscular injection, intravenous drip, mucosal adsorption, and other techniques can all be used to administer polyphenol-loaded polymeric nanoparticles with a typical type of colloidal dispersion into human bodies. PNPs carrying polyphenols crossed the BBB by receptor-mediated endocytosis, where they either released drugs into the endothelial cells or entered the brain. PNPs may cross the BBB using a variety of methods, including PNPs have the following capacities for drug release and transport through the BBB:

(i) Open direct or indirect tight junctions between endothelial cells;
(ii) Have a surfactant effect that can solubilize lipids in endothelial cell membranes and increase the permeability of drugs across the BBB; and
(iii) Release drugs into the brain after being endocytosed by endothelial cells. Additionally, all of these variables might interact in many ways to trigger the BBB [68].

13 Polyphenols Encapsulation by Liposomes

Liposomes are phospholipid vesicles that may encapsulate a variety of medications since they are made up of one or more concentric lipid bilayers that surround distinct aqueous regions. Most commonly, liposomes have been produced via reverse evaporation, high-pressure homogenization, emulsification, freeze-drying, centrifugation, pressure extrusion, and melting techniques [69].

The thin-film dispersion approach is the one that is most frequently utilized. In further detail, a sufficient amount of organic solvent is used to dissolve fat-soluble chemicals as well as membrane components like cholesterol and phospholipid. Vacuum rotation is used to extract the solvent, forming a thin layer that is later mechanically dispersed [70]. During these processes, hydrophilic molecules are confined in the aqueous core while hydrophobic molecules are introduced into the bilayer membrane. The four primary types of liposomal delivery methods are conventional liposomes, sterically stabilized liposomes, ligand-targeted liposomes, and combinations of the stated earlier. One of them is ligand-targeted liposomes, which have a huge potential for delivering bioactive compounds to certain cell types or organs in vivo that selectively express or overexpress particular ligands (such as receptors or cell adhesion molecules) at the site of illness [71]. The surface features of liposomes have received a lot of attention from researchers in an effort to enhance liposome targeting in vivo and in vitro [72]. Currently, ligands, polymers, peptides, and carbohydrates and their derivatives are the principal substances employed to change liposomes. Among these substances that can be created for the active targeting and increased bioavailability of bioactive chemicals include glycoproteins, glycolipids, and various oligosaccharides [73]. The liposome's unusual phospholipid bilayer structure has also made it more compatible with the BBB's lipoidal layer, which facilitates the passage of bioactive substances into the brain [74].

14 Future Perspectives

The therapeutic use of polyphenols and their nano formulations against neurodegenerative disorders including Parkinson's and Alzheimer's dementia is highly promising. In light of increased understanding over the past few decades, public interest in natural products has risen sharply. The food item polyphenols are recognized as an exceptional source of a number of chemicals with an extraordinarily diversified composition among other bioactive substances. Its biological activity and potential applications have been the subject of a sizable amount of experimentation. Due to its complexity and variety of manifestations, dementia is a disease that affects older people more frequently than other illnesses and is one of the foremost causes of mortality and impairment. Despite this, there are presently no viable treatments for dementia. By addressing the syndrome's modifiable risk factors, of which nutrition is one, it is feasible to avoid and/or treat this condition. Polyphenols exhibit in vitro anti-amyloid, anti-inflammatory, and antioxidant properties. One challenge with polyphenols is their low bioavailability, which limits their therapeutic efficacy. Nano formulations, such as nanoparticles, liposomes, micelles, and nanoemulsions, can improve the bioavailability and delivery of polyphenols to the brain. These nanosystems protect the polyphenols from degradation, enhance their solubility, prolong their circulation time, and facilitate their crossing of the blood–brain barrier (BBB). Nano formulations can be designed to selectively deliver polyphenols to specific brain regions affected by Parkinson's and Alzheimer's dementia. Functionalization of nanoparticles with ligands that bind to receptors overexpressed in these diseases can facilitate targeted delivery, enhancing their therapeutic potential while minimizing off-target effects. The extensively dispersed secondary metabolites of plant origin are called polyphenols. Due to their widespread presence in plant-based foods and strong evidence linking their consumption to cancer, diabetes, and cardiovascular disorders, these chemicals have gained prominence.

References

1. Dragovic-Uzelac V, Levaj B, Mrkic V, Bursac D, Boras M (2007) The content of polyphenols and carotenoids in three apricot cultivars depending on stage of maturity and geographical region. Food Chem 102(3):966–975
2. Laurindo LF, de Carvalho GM, de Oliveira Zanuso B, Figueira ME, Direito R, de Alvares Goulart R, Barbalho SM (2023) Curcumin-based nanomedicines in the treatment of inflammatory and immunomodulated diseases: an evidence-based comprehensive review. Pharmaceutics 15(1):229
3. Haslam E, Cai Y (1994) Plant polyphenols (vegetable tannins): gallic acid metabolism. Nat Prod Rep 11:41–66
4. Renaud J, Martinoli MG (2019) Considerations for the use of polyphenols as therapies in neurodegenerative diseases. Int J Mol Sci 20(8):1883
5. Hussain T, Gupta S, Adhami VM, Mukhtar H (2005) Green tea constituent epigallocatechin-3-gallate selectively inhibits COX-2 without affecting COX-1 expression in human prostate carcinoma cells. Int J Cancer 113(4):660–669
6. O'Leary KA, de Pascual-Tereasa S, Needs PW, Bao YP, O'Brien NM, Williamson G (2004) Effect of flavonoids and vitamin E on cyclooxygenase-2 (COX-2) transcription. Mutat Res/Fundam Mol Mech Mutagen 551(1–2):245–254
7. Tapiero H, Ba GN, Tew KD (2002) Estrogens and environmental estrogens. Biomed Pharmacother 56(1):36–44
8. Huang M, Liang C, Tan C, Huang S, Ying R, Wang Y, Zhang Y (2019) Liposome co-encapsulation as a strategy for the delivery of curcumin and resveratrol. Food Funct 10(10):6447–6458
9. Reddy VP et al (2020) Polyphenols in Alzheimer's disease and in the gut-brain axis. Microorganisms 8(2):199
10. Pandareesh M, Mythri R, Bharath MS (2015) Bioavailability of dietary polyphenols: factors contributing to their clinical application in CNS diseases. Neurochem Int 89:198–208
11. Faucheux BA et al (1995) Expression of lactoferrin receptors is increased in the mesencephalon of patients with Parkinson disease. Proc Natl Acad Sci 92(21):9603–9607

12. Bollimpelli VS et al (2016) Neuroprotective effect of curcumin-loaded lactoferrin nano particles against rotenone induced neurotoxicity. Neurochem Int 95:37–45
13. Davis S (1997) Biomedical applications of nanotechnology—implications for drug targeting and gene therapy. Trends Biotechnol 15(6):217–224
14. Wisse E, Davis S, De Leeuw A (1984) Structural elements determining transport and exchange processes in the liver. Microspheres Drug Ther
15. Neves RA et al (2012) Resveratrol in medicinal chemistry: a critical review of its pharmacokinetics, drug-delivery, and membrane interactions. Curr Med Chem 19(11):1663–1681
16. Markus MA, Morris BJ (2008) Resveratrol in prevention and treatment of common clinical conditions of aging. Clin Interv Aging 3(2):331–339
17. Neves AR et al (2013) Novel resveratrol nanodelivery systems based on lipid nanoparticles to enhance its oral bioavailability. Int J Nanomedicine 177–187
18. Loureiro JA et al (2017) Resveratrol and grape extract-loaded solid lipid nanoparticles for the treatment of Alzheimer's disease. Molecules 22(2):277
19. Mohammad-Beigi H et al (2016) Gallic acid loaded onto polyethylenimine-coated human serum albumin nanoparticles (PEI-HSA-GA NPs) stabilizes α-synuclein in the unfolded conformation and inhibits aggregation. RSC Adv 6(88):85312–85323
20. Korani MS et al (2014) Protective effects of gallic acid against chronic cerebral hypoperfusion-induced cognitive deficit and brain oxidative damage in rats. Eur J Pharmacol 733:62–67
21. Liu Y et al (2014) Gallic acid interacts with α-synuclein to prevent the structural collapse necessary for its aggregation. Biochim Biophys Acta (BBA)-Proteins Proteomics 1844(9):1481–1485
22. Schimidt HL et al (2017) Green tea supplementation produces better neuroprotective effects than red and black tea in Alzheimer-like rat model. Food Res Int 100:442–448
23. Braicu C et al (2013) The relationship between the structure and biological actions of green tea catechins. Food Chem 141(3):3282–3289
24. Wobst HJ et al (2015) The green tea polyphenol (−)-epigallocatechin gallate prevents the aggregation of tau protein into toxic oligomers at substoichiometric ratios. FEBS Lett 589(1):77–83
25. Mandel SA et al (2008) Cell signaling pathways and iron chelation in the neurorestorative activity of green tea polyphenols: special reference to epigallocatechin gallate (EGCG). J Alzheimers Dis 15(2):211–222
26. Zhang W et al (2018) Sparks fly between ascorbic acid and iron-based nanozymes: a study on Prussian blue nanoparticles. Colloids Surf, B 163:379–384
27. Dey S, Bishayi B (2018) Killing of S. aureus in murine peritoneal macrophages by ascorbic acid along with antibiotics chloramphenicol or ofloxacin: correlation with inflammation. Microb Pathog 115:239–250
28. Sharma S et al (2016) PLGA-based nanoparticles: a new paradigm in biomedical applications. TrAC, Trends Anal Chem 80:30–40
29. El-Hammadi MM et al (2017) Folic acid-decorated and PEGylated PLGA nanoparticles for improving the antitumour activity of 5-fluorouracil. Int J Pharm 516(1–2):61–70
30. Cano A et al (2019) Dual-drug loaded nanoparticles of Epigallocatechin-3-gallate (EGCG)/ Ascorbic acid enhance therapeutic efficacy of EGCG in a APPswe/PS1dE9 Alzheimer's disease mice model. J Control Release 301:62–75
31. Biwer A, Antranikian G, Heinzle E (2002) Enzymatic production of cyclodextrins. Appl Microbiol Biotechnol 59:609–617
32. Charoenlap N et al (2004) Optimization of cyclodextrin production from sago starch. Biores Technol 92(1):49–54
33. Ben Amara F et al (2022) Valorization of potato peels starch for efficient β-cyclodextrin production and purification through an eco-friendly process. Starch-Stärke 74(9–10):2200037
34. Villiers A (1891) Sur la transformation de la fécule en dextrine par le ferment butyrique. Compt Rend Fr Acad Sci 112:435–438
35. Freudenberg K, Jacobi R (1935) Über schardingers dextrine aus stärke. Justus Liebigs Ann Chem 518(1):102–108

36. Borchert W (1948) RONTGENOGRAPHISCHE UNTERSUCHUNGEN AN SCHARDINGER-DEXTRINEN. VERLAG Z NATURFORSCH POSTFACH 2645, pp 464–465. W-7400 Tubingen, Germany.
37. Jicsinsky L et al (1996) Comprehensive supramolecular chemistry, vol 3. by J. Szejtli and T. Osa, Pergamon, Oxford.
38. Davis ME, Brewster ME (2004) Cyclodextrin-based pharmaceutics: past, present and future. Nat Rev Drug Discovery 3(12):1023–1035
39. Qi ZH, Sikorski CT (1999) Controlled delivery using cyclodextrin technology. ACS Publications.
40. Eisenberg D, Jucker M (2012) The amyloid state of proteins in human diseases. Cell 148(6):1188–1203
41. Marques O, Outeiro TF (2012) Alpha-synuclein: from secretion to dysfunction and death. Cell Death Dis 3(7):e350–e350
42. Berhanu WM, Masunov AE (2010) Natural polyphenols as inhibitors of amyloid aggregation. Molecular dynamics study of GNNQQNY heptapeptide decamer. Biophys Chem 149(1–2):12–21
43. Hudson SA et al (2009) (−)-Epigallocatechin-3-gallate (EGCG) maintains κ-casein in its pre-fibrillar state without redirecting its aggregation pathway. J Mol Biol 392(3):689–700
44. Caruana M et al (2011) Inhibition and disaggregation of α-synuclein oligomers by natural polyphenolic compounds. FEBS Lett 585(8):1113–1120
45. Meng X et al (2009) Molecular mechanisms underlying the flavonoid-induced inhibition of α-synuclein fibrillation. Biochemistry 48(34):8206–8224
46. Berhanu WM, Masunov AE (2015) Atomistic mechanism of polyphenol amyloid aggregation inhibitors: molecular dynamics study of curcumin, exifone, and myricetin interaction with the segment of tau peptide oligomer. J Biomol Struct Dyn 33(7):1399–1411
47. BB A (2007) Curcumin: the Indian solid gold. Adv Exp Med Biol 595:1.
48. Arya P et al (2014) Selective interception of gelsolin amyloidogenic stretch results in conformationally distinct aggregates with reduced toxicity. ACS Chem Neurosci 5(10):982–992
49. Ahmad B, Lapidus LJ (2012) Curcumin prevents aggregation in α-synuclein by increasing reconfiguration rate. J Biol Chem 287(12):9193–9199
50. Singh PK et al (2013) Curcumin modulates α-synuclein aggregation and toxicity. ACS Chem Neurosci 4(3):393–407
51. Gautam S et al (2017) Polyphenols in combination with β-cyclodextrin can inhibit and disaggregate α-synuclein amyloids under cell mimicking conditions: a promising therapeutic alternative. Biochim Biophys Acta (BBA)-Proteins Proteomics 1865(5):589–603.
52. Del Valle EM (2004) Cyclodextrins and their uses: a review. Process Biochem 39(9):1033–1046
53. Hapiot F et al (2012) Functionalized cyclodextrins as first and second coordination sphere ligands for aqueous organometallic catalysis. Eur J Inorg Chem 2012(10):1571–1578
54. Zhang J, Ma PX (2013) Cyclodextrin-based supramolecular systems for drug delivery: recent progress and future perspective. Adv Drug Deliv Rev 65(9):1215–1233
55. Wehrmann ZT et al (2012) Quantitative comparison of the efficacy of various compounds in lowering intracellular cholesterol levels in Niemann-Pick type C fibroblasts. PLoS ONE 7(10):e48561
56. Qin X-R, Abe H, Nakanishi H (2002) NMR and CD studies on the interaction of Alzheimer β-amyloid peptide (12–28) with β-cyclodextrin. Biochem Biophys Res Commun 297(4):1011–1015
57. Machida S et al (2000) Cycloamylose as an efficient artificial chaperone for protein refolding. FEBS Lett 486(2):131–135
58. Fang Z, Bhandari B (2010) Encapsulation of polyphenols–a review. Trends Food Sci Technol 21(10):510–523
59. Gautam S, Sandipauthor K, Abhikauthor B (2015) -Cyclodextrin and curcumin, a potent cocktail for disaggregating and/or inhibiting amyloids: a case study with-synuclein
60. Yadav VR et al (2016) Cyclodextrin-complexed curcumin exhibits anti-inflammatory and antiproliferative activities superior to those of curcumin through higher cellular uptake (vol 80, vol 1021, 2010). Biochem Pharmacol

61. Etheridge ML et al (2013) The big picture on nanomedicine: the state of investigational and approved nanomedicine products. Nanomedicine: Nanotechnol, Biol Med 9(1):1–14
62. Reis CP et al (2006) Nanoencapsulation I. Methods for preparation of drug-loaded polymeric nanoparticles. Nanomedicine: Nanotechnol, Biol Med 2(1):8–21
63. Scalbert A, Williamson G (2000) Dietary intake and bioavailability of polyphenols. J Nutr 130(8):2073S-2085S
64. Lam WH et al (2004) A potential prodrug for a green tea polyphenol proteasome inhibitor: evaluation of the peracetate ester of (−)-epigallocatechin gallate [(−)-EGCG]. Bioorg Med Chem 12(21):5587–5593
65. Zhang Y, Lv C, Zhao G (2022) Ways to enhance the bioavailability of polyphenols in the brain: a journey through the blood-brain barrier. Food Rev Intl 38(sup1):812–828
66. Roney C et al (2005) Targeted nanoparticles for drug delivery through the blood–brain barrier for Alzheimer's disease. J Control Release 108(2–3):193–214
67. Khalid M, El-Sawy HS (2017) Polymeric nanoparticles: promising platform for drug delivery. Int J Pharm 528(1–2):675–691
68. Mozafari MR et al (2008) Encapsulation of food ingredients using nanoliposome technology. Int J Food Prop 11(4):833–844
69. Elhissi A et al (2006) A calorimetric study of dimyristoylphosphatidylcholine phase transitions and steroid–liposome interactions for liposomes prepared by thin film and proliposome methods. Int J Pharm 320(1–2):124–130
70. Hua S (2013) Targeting sites of inflammation: intercellular adhesion molecule-1 as a target for novel inflammatory therapies. Front Pharmacol 4:127
71. Chen ZL et al (2016) Transferrin-modified liposome promotes α-mangostin to penetrate the blood–brain barrier. Nanomedicine: Nanotechnol, Biol Med 12(2):421–430
72. Meng J, Agrahari V, Youm I (2017) Advances in targeted drug delivery approaches for the central nervous system tumors: the inspiration of nanobiotechnology. J Neuroimmune Pharmacol 12:84–98
73. Sihorkar V, Vyas S (2001) Potential of polysaccharide anchored liposomes in drug delivery, targeting and immunization. J Pharm Pharm Sci 4(2):138–158
74. Appeldoorn MM, Venema DP, Peters THF, Koenen ME, Arts ICW, Vincken J-P, Gruppen H, Keijer J, Hollman PCH (2009) Some phenolic compounds increase the nitric oxide level in endothelial cells in vitro. J Agric Food Chem 57:7693–7699

The Use of Microbial Nanoparticles to Treat Neurodegenerative Disorders

Lakhveer Singh, Saumya Rastogi, Priyanshu Kumar, and Shashank Shekher Mishra

Abstract Neurodegenerative disorders such as Alzheimer's disease, Parkinson's disease, Huntington's disease, amyotrophic lateral sclerosis (ALS), and multiple sclerosis mainly cause progressive damage to the neuronal cells and subsequently lead to reduced cognitive function, motor skills, and behavior. These disorders have a distinct pathophysiological mechanism and can be managed symptomatically with the available drugs. Although most of the drugs have shown promising results in managing this disorder majority of drugs face challenges in getting access to the target brain cells. Furthermore, due to their inability to cross the blood-brain barrier, these drugs accumulate in unwanted tissues and hence present significant toxic effects. Nanotechnology has revolutionized drug targeting especially the brain targeting of drugs. Nanosized formulations can easily penetrate the blood-brain barrier. Nanoparticles can be precisely synthesized in such a way as to target the specific area for higher efficiency which improves the treatments while minimizing side effects as well. The current book chapter focuses on the various limitations registered during managing and treating neurological disorders. The chapter also highlights the role of nanotechnology in improving the efficiency of drugs designed to fight neurological disorders like Parkinson's disease and Alzheimer's disease.

1 Introduction

Neurodegenerative disorders are a group of central nervous system (CNS) disorders that mainly the neurons in the brain and spinal cord. These disorders cause progressive damage to these cells and subsequently lead to reduced cognitive function, motor skills, and/or behavior [1].

Few of the well-known neurodegenerative disorders include Alzheimer's disease, Parkinson's disease, Huntington's disease, amyotrophic lateral sclerosis (ALS), and

L. Singh (✉) · S. Rastogi · P. Kumar · S. S. Mishra
School of Pharmaceutical & Population Health Informatics, Faculty of Pharmacy, DIT University, Dehradun, Uttarakhand 248009, India
e-mail: Lakhveer@dituniversity.edu.in

S. K. Rath et al. (eds.), *Nanomaterials for Drug Delivery and Neurological Diseases Management*, Smart Nanomaterials Technology,
https://doi.org/10.1007/978-981-97-0308-1_16

multiple sclerosis (MS). Each of these conditions has a unique set of symptoms and characteristics, but they all involve the degeneration of nerve cells in the CNS [2].

While the root cause of neurodegenerative disorders is still unknown, they are believed to be the result of composite factors like genetic, environmental, and lifestyle factors. Moreover, these disorders are known from years but permanent treatment of these disorders is still very difficult despite of enormous development in the medical field. However there are various treatments that can assist in symptom management and enhance the quality of life for individuals who are impacted by the condition [3].

The occurrence and prevalence of neurodegenerative diseases differ depending on the particular disease. Among the various neurodegenerative disorders, Alzheimer's disease stands out as the most prevalent cause of dementia among older individuals. The current estimate indicates that there are approximately 5.8 million Americans who are currently living with Alzheimer's disease, and this number is projected to increase to 14 million by the year 2050 [4]. As people age, the likelihood of developing Alzheimer's disease increases, and the majority of cases are seen in individuals over the age of 65. Additionally, studies suggest that women have a higher risk of developing Alzheimer's disease compared to men [5].

Parkinson's disease is a condition that impacts about 1% of individuals who are 60 years old or older. The likelihood of developing Parkinson's disease is known to increase with age, and the majority of cases are reported in people who are over 50 years of age. Additionally, men have a higher chance of developing Parkinson's disease than women [6].

Huntington's disease is a genetic condition that affects a small proportion of people, around 5–10 per 100,000. Symptoms usually begin to appear when individuals are between the ages of 30 and 50. Around 2 in every 100,000 people are affected by ALS. It mostly affects individuals aged 40 to 70 and men are more susceptible to it than women [7].

Overall, as people age, the likelihood of developing neurodegenerative disorders is expected to rise. The exact causes of neurodegenerative disorders are not yet fully understood, and more research is needed to develop effective treatments and preventions [1].

Currently, neurodegenerative disorders cannot be cured, and existing treatments focus on symptom management and disease progression prevention. Some of the current treatment options include:

Medications: Several medications are available to treat the symptoms of neurodegenerative disorders. For example, acetylcholinesterase inhibitors (donepezil, rivastigmine, and galantamine) are used to treat cognitive symptoms in Alzheimer's disease [8]. Dopamine agonists (levodopa, pramipexole, and ropinirole) are used to manage motor symptoms in Parkinson's disease [9].

Physical therapy: Improving muscle strength, flexibility, and balance can be achieved through physical therapy and exercise., which can help people with neurodegenerative disorders maintain their independence and quality of life [10].

Occupational therapy: Occupational therapy can help people with neurodegenerative disorders develop skills to perform daily activities and adapt to changes in their abilities [11].

Speech therapy: Speech therapy can help people with neurodegenerative disorders maintain their ability to communicate [12].

Surgery: In some cases, surgery may be an option to manage the symptoms of neurodegenerative disorders. For example, deep brain stimulation (DBS) can help improve motor symptoms in Parkinson's disease [13].

Supportive care: Palliative care and hospice care can assist individuals with neurodegenerative conditions in controlling symptoms and enhancing their quality of life.

Researchers are also investigating new treatments for neurodegenerative disorders, such as gene therapy, stem cell therapy, and immunotherapy. However, these treatments are still being developed and might not be readily accessible for a few years [14].

While there are drugs available to treat these disorders, they often have significant drawbacks. Here are some of the common drawbacks of drugs used in the treatment of neurodegenerative disorders [15, 16]:

Limited effectiveness: Many drugs used to treat neurodegenerative disorders can only slow down the progression of the disease, rather than reversing it. For example, drugs used to treat Alzheimer's disease may help to slow down the cognitive decline, but they cannot cure the disease.

Side effects: Several medications utilized for neurodegenerative disorders can produce adverse reactions, including nausea, vomiting, and dizziness. Some drugs may also interact with other medications, which can further complicate treatment.

Cost: Many drugs used to treat neurodegenerative disorders are expensive, which can make them inaccessible to those who cannot afford them. This can be particularly problematic for those with limited financial resources, as these individuals may not have access to the care they need.

Dependency: Some drugs used to treat neurodegenerative disorders can be habit-forming, which can lead to dependency and addiction. This is particularly true for drugs used to treat Parkinson's disease, which can cause dopamine dysregulation syndrome.

Disease progression: Some drugs used to treat neurodegenerative disorders can actually worsen the symptoms of the disease over time. For example, drugs used to treat Parkinson's disease can lead to dyskinesia, which is a movement disorder characterized by uncontrollable muscle movements.

It is important to note that not all drugs used to treat neurodegenerative disorders have these drawbacks, and the benefits of treatment often outweigh the risks. However, it's important that patients and caregivers know the possible downsides of these medications and collaborate with their healthcare providers to create a suitable treatment approach [17].

A major obstacle in treating neurodegenerative disorders is delivering drugs across the blood–brain barrier (BBB), a protective membrane that filters out harmful substances from entering the brain. Nanoparticles can help overcome this obstacle by bypassing the BBB and delivering drugs directly to the brain [18].

Nanoparticles can be created to target certain cells or areas in the brain, improving the treatment's efficiency while reducing any potential side effects. A practical example of this is coating nanoparticles with a protein that binds to a receptor on brain cell surfaces, allowing for selective targeting of those cells [18].

In addition to delivering drugs, nanoparticles can also be used for diagnostic purposes. Magnetic nanoparticles, one possible revision could be: magnetic resonance imaging (MRI) can be utilized to identify brain changes linked to neurodegenerative conditions [19].

However, while nanoparticles offer promising potential for the treatment of neurodegenerative disorders, there are still challenges that need to be addressed, such as optimizing the size and shape of the nanoparticles, ensuring their stability in the body, and minimizing their toxicity. Further research and development is needed to fully realize the potential of nanoparticles for treating neurodegenerative disorders [18].

2 Pathophysiology of Common Neurodegenerative Disorder

2.1 Alzheimer Disease

Alzheimer's disease is a brain disorder that gradually impairs memory, thinking, and behavior. It is the leading cause of dementia, responsible for 60–80% of all cases. The condition is triggered by the buildup of abnormal protein deposits in the brain that disrupt the normal functioning of neurons [4].

The symptoms of Alzheimer's disease typically begin with mild forgetfulness and progress to more severe cognitive and behavioral problems. Memory loss is one of the earliest and most common symptoms, followed by confusion, disorientation, and difficulty with language and communication. As the illness worsens, people may undergo mood and behavior alterations like depression, anxiety, and restlessness [4].

Alzheimer's disease cannot be cured, but its symptoms can be managed and its progression slowed down using medications and other therapies. Treatment may involve a combination of medication, behavioral therapy, and lifestyle changes. In addition, ongoing research is focused on developing new treatments that can address the underlying causes of the disease [20].

Pathophysiology: Alzheimer's disease is characterized by the buildup of unusual protein deposits in the brain. These include beta-amyloid plaques that form outside nerve cells and tau protein tangles that form inside nerve cells. Beta-amyloid is a sticky protein that clumps together to form plaques, while tau protein forms tangles [21].

Protein buildups can interfere with communication among nerve cells, leading to inflammation and damage to brain tissue. This damage can result in the death of nerve cells and shrinkage of the brain, particularly in areas responsible for memory, learning, and other cognitive functions [21].

Another important feature of Alzheimer's disease causes a decrease in important brain chemicals called neurotransmitters, specifically acetylcholine. These neurotransmitters are involved in the transmission of nerve impulses, and their depletion can contribute to the cognitive and behavioral symptoms of Alzheimer's disease [22].

It is possible that genetics may contribute to the development of Alzheimer's disease, as certain genetic mutations have been linked to an increased risk of developing the condition [23].

Overall, Alzheimer's disease is a complicated condition that has several root causes and mechanisms. Although available treatments can ease certain symptoms, there is still no cure for the disease.

2.2 *Parkinson's Disease*

Parkinson's disease affects movement and is caused by the loss of dopaminergic neurons in the brain's substantia nigra region, which results in low levels of dopamine. It leads to symptoms such as tremors, rigidity, bradykinesia (slowness of movement), and postural instability [24].

Parkinson's disease cannot be cured at present, but there are ways to manage its symptoms and improve quality of life. Doctors may prescribe medications like levodopa, which increase dopamine levels in the brain. Other treatment options include deep brain stimulation (DBS), physical therapy, and occupational therapy [24].

Pathophysiology: Parkinson's disease is a long-term and worsening condition. and its course can vary widely among individuals. The onset of symptoms typically occurs after age 50, but it can occur earlier in some cases. Around 1% of people who are 60 years old or older are affected by this disease [25].

The loss of dopaminergic neurons leads to a depletion of dopamine levels in the brain, which results in the motor symptoms of Parkinson's disease, including tremors, rigidity, bradykinesia (slowness of movement), and postural instability [26].

Parkinson's disease reduces the number of dopaminergic neurons in the brain, which results in lower levels of dopamine. This leads to various motor symptoms, including tremors, rigidity, bradykinesia (slow movement), and balance problems [26].

The cause of Parkinson's disease is not fully clear yet, but it's thought to be caused by a mixture of genetic and environmental factors. Certain genetic mutations have been linked to a higher chance of developing the disease [27].

Additionally, Parkinson's disease is characterized by the loss of dopaminergic neurons and the presence of clumps known as Lewy bodies. These Lewy bodies form due to the accumulation of alpha-synuclein protein in the brain and are believed to play a role in the neurodegeneration associated with Parkinson's disease [28].

Other neurotransmitter systems in the brain, including acetylcholine and noradrenaline, are also affected in Parkinson's disease and can cause non-motor symptoms such as cognitive problems, depression, and anxiety [29].

Overall, the pathophysiology of Parkinson's disease is a result of various genetic and environmental factors that interact and lead to the death of dopaminergic neurons., the accumulation of alpha-synuclein protein, and dysfunction in other neurotransmitter systems.

2.3 Huntington's Disease

Huntington's disease is a genetic condition that impacts the brain, resulting in the gradual and permanent destruction of nerve cells. The disease is inherited and caused by a mutation in the HTT gene, which creates a protein known as huntingtin. The mutated huntingtin protein accumulates in the brain and causes the death of brain cells [30].

Huntington's disease symptoms generally manifest in middle age, although onset may occur earlier or later in life. The symptoms include involuntary movements, such as jerking or twitching, and difficulties with balance and coordination. Other symptoms can include mood changes, cognitive decline, and difficulty with speech and swallowing [30].

At present, there is no known cure for Huntington's disease. Therefore, the treatment is focused on managing the symptoms of the disease. The treatment plan may consist of medications to manage movement and mood symptoms, as well as physical and occupational therapy to maintain independence and mobility. Genetic testing is available to identify people at risk of developing the disease, but it's not possible to prevent or slow down the progression of the disease [30].

Pathophysiology: We do not have a complete understanding of how the mutant huntingtin protein causes the degeneration of neurons. However, several pathological processes have been identified that are thought to contribute to the development of the disease [31]. These include:

Aggregation of mutant huntingtin protein: The mutant huntingtin protein has a tendency to aggregate and form insoluble clumps within neurons, which can disrupt cellular processes and lead to neuronal dysfunction.

Impaired protein degradation: The presence of the abnormal huntingtin protein can disrupt the proper operation of the ubiquitin–proteasome system and autophagy, two important mechanisms for protein degradation within cells. This leads to the accumulation of abnormal proteins, including mutant huntingtin, within neurons.

Mitochondrial dysfunction: Mutant huntingtin has been shown to impair mitochondrial function, leading to increased oxidative stress and energy depletion within neurons.

Excitotoxicity: The degeneration of neurons in the striatum can lead to an excess release of the neurotransmitter glutamate, which can activate receptors on neighboring neurons and cause them to become overexcited. This can lead to cell death through a process called excitotoxicity.

Inflammatory response: The degeneration of neurons in the striatum can also trigger an inflammatory response within the brain, which can further contribute to neuronal damage. The gradual deterioration of neurons in the striatum causes various symptoms like uncontrolled movements, coordination and balance issues, cognitive problems, and mental health conditions like depression and anxiety.

2.4 Amyotrophic Lateral Sclerosis

Amyotrophic lateral sclerosis (ALS), or Lou Gehrig's disease, is a disease that affects nerve cells in the brain and spinal cord and gradually leads to the loss of muscle control, making it difficult to speak, eat, move, and breathe. It is a progressive neurodegenerative disease [32].

The cause of ALS is not fully understood yet, but it's thought to be caused by a mix of genetic and environmental factors. Symptoms typically begin with muscle weakness and stiffness in the limbs, difficulty with speech and swallowing, and muscle twitching or cramping. As the disease progresses, the muscles used for breathing may also become affected, leading to respiratory failure and ultimately death [32].

ALS has no known cure at present. Therefore, the main goal of treatment is to alleviate symptoms and enhance the patient's quality of life. Treatment options may include medicines to slow the progression of the disease, physical therapy to help sustain mobility, and assistive tools to aid in daily activities and communication. Research is ongoing to better understand the disease and develop new treatments [32].

The exact reason behind ALS is uncertain, but it's believed to result from a mix of genetic and environmental factors. Mutations in numerous genes have been linked to the development of ALS, including the SOD1 gene, which produces an enzyme called superoxide dismutase that protects cells from damage caused by free radicals. In some cases, ALS is passed down in an autosomal dominant manner. It implies that a person may develop the disease by inheriting one mutated gene from one parent only [33].

The pathophysiology of ALS involves a complicated interaction of molecular and cellular processes that result in the deterioration of motor neurons. The accumulation of irregular proteins in motor neurons, including misfolded proteins and protein aggregates, is a significant feature of the disease. These abnormal proteins can interfere with normal cellular processes, leading to neuronal dysfunction and eventually cell death [34].

Another factor that contributes to the pathophysiology of ALS is inflammation. Inflammation is a natural defense mechanism of the immune system to injury or infection. However, long-term inflammation can harm neurons. In ALS, immune cells in the brain and spinal cord called microglia become activated and release pro-inflammatory cytokines. These cytokines can lead to the degeneration of motor neurons [35].

Pathophysiology: Excitotoxicity is another mechanism that plays a role in the pathophysiology of ALS. Excitotoxicity refers to the excessive activation of neurons by the neurotransmitter glutamate, which can lead to cell death. In ALS, the excess glutamate accumulates in the synapses between neurons, leading to overstimulation and eventual neuronal death [34].

Additionally, oxidative stress is considered to be a factor in the development of ALS. Oxidative stress arises from an inequality between the formation of reactive oxygen species (ROS) and the cells' capacity to neutralize them. ROS can harm cellular structures, such as DNA, proteins, and lipids, resulting in nerve cell malfunction and demise [34].

In summary, the pathophysiology of ALS is complex and involves a grouping of genetic, environmental, cellular, and molecular factors. While the exact mechanisms underlying ALS are not fully understood, research in this area is ongoing, and by gaining a better understanding of the disease, it is possible that more efficient treatments for the condition may be developed.

2.5 Prion Disease

Prion diseases, also called transmissible spongiform encephalopathies (TSEs), are rare and deadly neurodegenerative illnesses that impact both humans as well as animals. Prion diseases are caused by a misfolded protein called a prion, which is able to convert normal proteins into abnormal ones [36].

The abnormal buildup of proteins in the brain results in the creation of amyloid plaques and spongy changes in the brain tissue. These changes can lead to severe neurological issues like ataxia, myoclonus, and dementia[37].

Prion diseases can be sporadic, inherited, or acquired through exposure to contaminated tissue or food products. Examples of prion diseases in persons comprise Creutzfeldt-Jakob disease (CJD), variant CJD (vCJD), and Gerstmann-Straussler-Scheinker syndrome (GSS) [38].

At present, there is no known cure for prion diseases. The main approach to treatment is to provide support and alleviate symptoms. Preventative measures such as strict controls on the use of contaminated tissues in medical procedures and the testing of animals for the presence of prions in their tissues can help to reduce the risk of transmission.

Pathophysiology: The exact mechanism by which PrPSc leads to nerve cell damage is not fully understood, but it likely involves multiple stages:

Conversion of PrP into PrPSc: Prion diseases happen when the prion protein (PrPC) changes into an abnormal, disease-causing form (PrPSc) due to misfolding [39].

Accumulation of PrPSc: PrPSc is resistant to normal protein degradation mechanisms and accumulates in the brain over time, leading to the formation of insoluble protein aggregates [40].

Formation of plaques and fibrils: The accumulated PrPSc forms insoluble plaques and fibrils, which can interfere with normal neuronal function and cause damage to nerve cells.

Inflammatory response: The presence of abnormal prion proteins can trigger an inflammatory response in the brain, which can further damage nerve cells and exacerbate neurodegeneration.

Spread of disease: Prion diseases can be transmitted through contact with contaminated tissues or fluids, leading to the spread of disease between individuals.

The exact mechanisms by which PrPSc causes neurodegeneration are still being studied, but current research suggests that the accumulation of abnormal prion protein disrupts normal neuronal function, leading to the death of nerve cells and the development of clinical symptoms. The disease progression is usually slow and irreversible, and at present, there is no successful treatment available for prion diseases.

3 Treatment of Neurodegenerative Disorder

3.1 Drawback of Current Treatments

There are several drawbacks associated with current treatments for neurodegenerative disorders like Alzheimer's, Parkinson's, and Huntington's diseases [16]. These issues include:

Limited effectiveness: Most current treatments can only alleviate symptoms temporarily, but they do not cure the underlying disease. For example, medications for Alzheimer's disease may improve memory and cognitive function for a few months, but the benefits typically decline over time.

Side effects: Many of the medications used to treat neurodegenerative diseases have significant side effects that can be difficult to tolerate, especially for older adults who may be taking multiple medications.

Cost: The cost of medication and other treatments for neurodegenerative diseases can be prohibitive, particularly for those without adequate health insurance or financial resources.

Late diagnosis: In many cases, neurodegenerative diseases are not diagnosed until they have progressed significantly, making it more difficult to treat effectively.

Lack of disease-modifying therapies: There are currently no approved disease-modifying therapies for most neurodegenerative diseases. This means that treatments are focused on managing symptoms rather than addressing the underlying disease process.

Accessibility: Some treatments may not be available in all parts of the world, and even where they are available, not everyone may have access to them due to factors such as cost, distance, or limited healthcare infrastructure.

Overall, while current treatment approaches for neurodegenerative diseases can provide some relief for patients, there is still much work to be done to develop more effective, accessible, and affordable therapies that can slow or even halt disease progression.

4 Nanoparticles for Treatment of Degenerative Brain Disorder

Nanoparticles are very small particles that can be made from different materials such as metals, ceramics, polymers, and composites. Their size usually ranges from 1 to 100 nm in diameter and can have a wide range of physical and chemical properties. Nanoparticles have unique properties that make them useful in a wide range of applications, including medicine, electronics, and energy production [16].

For example, some nanoparticles have high surface area-to-volume ratios, which make them useful for catalysis and drug delivery. Others have unique magnetic, optical, or electrical properties that make them useful for sensors, imaging, and data storage [41].

However, the small size of nanoparticles also means that they can have different properties and behaviors than larger particles of the same material. For example, nanoparticles can penetrate cell membranes and tissues more easily than larger particles, which can have implications for their toxicity and environmental impact [41].

Research is ongoing to better understand the potential risks and benefits of nanoparticles, and to develop safe and effective ways to use them in various applications.

5 General Method for Synthesis of Nanoparticles

There are several general methods for synthesizing nanoparticles, including:

Chemical reduction: This involves reducing metal ions in a solution to form nanoparticles. For example, to create silver nanoparticles is by using a substance called silver nitrate and another substance called sodium borohydride to reduce it [42].

Sol–gel method: The Sol–gel method is a process that creates nanoparticles by combining metal alkoxides, hydrolysis, and condensation to form a gel. The gel is then dried and calcined to produce the final product. For example, silica nanoparticles can be synthesized by hydrolyzing tetraethyl orthosilicate (TEOS) in the presence of a base [43].

Microemulsion: This method involves the use of surfactants to form microemulsions, which are then used to synthesize nanoparticles. For example, gold nanoparticles can be synthesized by reducing gold salts in a microemulsion of water and oil [44].

Physical methods: Physical methods such as laser ablation, sputtering, and evaporation can also be used to synthesize nanoparticles. For example, silver nanoparticles can be synthesized by laser removal of a silver target in a liquid [45].

The method used for synthesizing nanoparticles depends on the type of nanoparticle and the desired properties. Each method has its advantages and disadvantages, and the selection of the method requires a thorough understanding of the underlying chemistry and physics.

Application of nanoparticles for treatment of neurodegenerative disorders:

Nanoparticles show promise in treating neurodegenerative disorders, like Alzheimer's and Parkinson's disease. These diseases cause misfolded proteins to accumulate in the brain and lead to neuron death.

Nanoparticles can be designed to target these misfolded proteins and prevent their aggregation, thereby reducing neurotoxicity and improving cognitive function. Additionally, nanoparticles can be used to deliver drugs and other therapeutic agents to specific regions of the brain, bypassing the blood–brain barrier and reducing side effects [41].

Scientists have studied various kinds of nanoparticles, such as liposomes, dendrimers, and metal nanoparticles, as possible treatments for neurodegenerative diseases. Liposomes, for example, are spherical lipid bilayer structures that can encapsulate drugs and protect them from degradation. Dendrimers are highly branched, nanoscale polymers that can carry multiple drugs and exhibit high biocompatibility. Metal nanoparticles, such as gold and silver nanoparticles, can be functionalized with biomolecules and used for imaging and drug delivery [46].

Although nanoparticles have the potential for treating neurodegenerative disorders, there are still challenges that need to be addressed. These include optimizing their size, shape, and surface chemistry, and ensuring their safety and effectiveness in clinical trials.

References

1. Holbrook JA, Jarosz-Griffiths HH, Caseley E, Lara-Reyna S, Poulter JA, Williams-Gray CH, Peckham D, McDermott MF (2021) Neurodegenerative disease and the NLRP3 inflammasome. Front Pharmacol 12(March):1–15. https://doi.org/10.3389/fphar.2021.643254
2. Tanaka M, Toldi J, Vécsei L (2020) Exploring the etiological links behind neurodegenerative diseases: inflammatory cytokines and bioactive kynurenines. Int J Mol Sci 21(7). https://doi.org/10.3390/ijms21072431
3. William Audeh M (2012) Genetic and environmental factors in cancer pathogenesis. In: Principles and practice of surgical oncology: a multidisciplinary approach to difficult problems, vol 512, pp 135–153. https://doi.org/10.29121/granthaalayah.v3.i9se.2015.3203
4. Association A (2013) 2013 Alzheimer's disease facts and figures. Alzheimer's Dement 9(2):208–245. https://doi.org/10.1016/j.jalz.2013.02.003
5. Hebert LE, Scherr PA, McCann JJ, Beckett LA, Evans DA (2001) Is the risk of developing Alzheimer's disease greater for women than for men? Am J Epidemiol 153(2):132–136. https://doi.org/10.1093/aje/153.2.132
6. Hughes RC (1994) Parkinson's disease and its management. Bmj 308(6923):281. https://doi.org/10.1136/bmj.308.6923.281
7. Skirton H, Glendinning N (1997) Using research to develop care for patients with Huntington's disease. Br J Nurs (Mark Allen Publ) 6(2):83–90. https://doi.org/10.12968/bjon.1997.6.2.83
8. Walczak-Nowicka ŁJ, Herbet M (2021) Acetylcholinesterase inhibitors in the treatment of neurodegenerative diseases and the role of acetylcholinesterase in their pathogenesis. Int J Mol Sci 22(17). https://doi.org/10.3390/ijms22179290
9. Antonini A, Tolosa E, Mizuno Y, Yamamoto M, Poewe WH (2009) A reassessment of risks and benefits of dopamine agonists in Parkinson's disease. Lancet Neurol 8(10):929–937. https://doi.org/10.1016/S1474-4422(09)70225-X
10. Mahalakshmi B, Maurya N, Lee SD, Kumar VB (2020) Possible neuroprotective mechanisms of physical exercise in neurodegeneration. Int J Mol Sci 21(16):1–17. https://doi.org/10.3390/ijms21165895
11. Rushanan SG, Nilsen DM, Grajo L (2021). Determining the initial content validity of the clinical competency assessment tool (CAT) for occupational therapists treating patients with neurodegenerative disease. Open J Occup Ther 9(4):1–11. https://doi.org/10.15453/2168-6408.1798
12. Farrajota L, Maruta C, Maroco J, Martins IP, Guerreiro M, de Mendonça A (2012) Speech therapy in primary progressive aphasia: a pilot study. Dement Geriatr Cogn Disord Extra 2(1):321–331. https://doi.org/10.1159/000341602
13. Eckenhoff RG, Planel E (2013) Anesthesia, surgery and neurodegeneration. Prog Neuropsychopharmacol Biol Psychiatry 47:121. https://doi.org/10.1016/j.pnpbp.2013.10.012
14. Wareham LK, Liddelow SA, Temple S, Benowitz LI, Di Polo A, Wellington C, Goldberg JL, He Z, Duan X, Bu G, Davis AA, Shekhar K, Torre AL, Chan DC, Canto-Soler MV, Flanagan JG, Subramanian P, Rossi S, Brunner T … Calkins DJ (2022) Solving neurodegeneration: common mechanisms and strategies for new treatments.Mol Neurodegener 17(1):129. https://doi.org/10.1186/s13024-022-00524-0
15. Deuschl G, Beghi E, Fazekas F, Varga T, Christoforidi KA, Sipido E, Bassetti CL, Vos T, Feigin VL (2020) The burden of neurological diseases in Europe: an analysis for the Global Burden of Disease Study 2017. The Lancet Public Health 5(10):e551–e567. https://doi.org/10.1016/S2468-2667(20)30190-0
16. Moradi SZ, Momtaz S, Bayrami Z, Farzaei MH, Abdollahi M (2020) Nanoformulations of herbal extracts in treatment of neurodegenerative disorders. Front Bioeng Biotechnol 8(April):1–20. https://doi.org/10.3389/fbioe.2020.00238
17. Cavalli A, Bolognesi ML, Mìnarini A, Rosini M, Tumiatti V, Recanatini M, Melchiorre C (2008) Multi-target-directed ligands to combat neurodegenerative diseases. J Med Chem 51(3):347–372. https://doi.org/10.1021/jm7009364

18. Poovaiah N, Davoudi Z, Peng H, Schlichtmann B, Mallapragada S, Narasimhan B, Wang Q (2018) Treatment of neurodegenerative disorders through the blood-brain barrier using nanocarriers. Nanoscale 10(36):16962–16983. https://doi.org/10.1039/c8nr04073g
19. Li KR, Wu AG, Tang Y, He XP, Yu CL, Wu JM, Hu GQ, Yu L (2022) The key role of magnetic resonance imaging in the detection of neurodegenerative diseases-associated biomarkers: a review. Mol Neurobiol 59(10). https://doi.org/10.1007/s12035-022-02944-x
20. Doniger GM, Beeri MS, Bahar-Fuchs A, Gottlieb A, Tkachov A, Kenan H, Livny A, Bahar Y, Sharon H, Ben-Gal O, Cohen M, Zeilig G, Plotnik M (2018) Virtual reality-based cognitive-motor training for middle-aged adults at high Alzheimer's disease risk: a randomized controlled trial. Alzheimer's Dement: Transl Res Clin Interv 4(March):118–129. https://doi.org/10.1016/j.trci.2018.02.005
21. Imbimbo BP, Lombard J, Pomara N (2005) Pathophysiology of Alzheimer's disease. Neuroimaging Clin N Am 15(4):727–753. https://doi.org/10.1016/j.nic.2005.09.009
22. Francis PT (2005) The interplay of neurotransmitters in Alzheimer's disease. CNS Spectr 10(11 SUPPL. 18):6–9. https://doi.org/10.1017/s1092852900014164
23. Tanzi RE (2012) The genetics of Alzheimer disease. Cold Spring Harb Perspect Med 2(10):294–296. https://doi.org/10.1101/cshperspect.a006296
24. Raza C, Anjum R, Shakeel NA (2019) Parkinson's disease: Mechanisms, translational models and management strategies. Life Sci 226:77–90.https://doi.org/10.1016/j.lfs.2019.03.057
25. Fahn S (2003) PDFlib PLOP: PDF linearization, optimization, protection page inserted by evaluation version description of Parkinson's Disease as a New York Academy of Sciences 991:1–14
26. Sveinbjornsdottir S (2016) The clinical symptoms of Parkinson's disease. J Neurochem:318–324.https://doi.org/10.1111/jnc.13691
27. Selvaraj S, Piramanayagam S (2019) Impact of gene mutation in the development of Parkinson's disease. Genes and Diseases 6(2):120–128. https://doi.org/10.1016/j.gendis.2019.01.004
28. Tompkins MM, Hill WD (1997) Contribution of somal Lewy bodies to neuronal death. Brain Res 775(1–2):24–29. https://doi.org/10.1016/S0006-8993(97)00874-3
29. Westerink BHC, Damsma G, Rollema H, De Vries JB, Horn AS (1987) Scope and limitations of in vivo brain dialysis: a comparison of its application to various neurotransmitter systems. Life Sci 41(15):1763–1776. https://doi.org/10.1016/0024-3205(87)90695-3
30. Novak MJU, Tabrizi SJ (2010) Clinical Review Huntington ' s disease. BMJ 341(july):34–40
31. Raymond LA, André VM, Cepeda C, Gladding CM, Milnerwood AJ, Levine MS (2011) Pathophysiology of Huntington's disease: time-dependent alterations in synaptic and receptor function. Neuroscience 198:252–273. https://doi.org/10.1016/j.neuroscience.2011.08.052
32. Hardiman O, Al-Chalabi A, Chio A, Corr EM, Logroscino G, Robberecht W, Shaw PJ, Simmons Z, Berg Van Den LH (2017) Amyotrophic lateral sclerosis. Nat Rev Dis Primers 3.https://doi.org/10.1038/nrdp.2017.71
33. Oskarsson B, Gendron TF, Staff NP (2018) Amyotrophic lateral sclerosis: an update for 2018. Mayo Clin Proc 93(11):1617–1628. https://doi.org/10.1016/j.mayocp.2018.04.007
34. Cunha-Oliveira T, Montezinho L, Mendes C, Firuzi O, Saso L, Oliveira PJ, Silva FSG (2020) Oxidative stress in amyotrophic lateral sclerosis: pathophysiology and opportunities for pharmacological intervention. Oxid Med Cell Longev. https://doi.org/10.1155/2020/5021694
35. Lyon MS, Wosiski-Kuhn M, Gillespie R, Caress J, Milligan C (2019) Inflammation, immunity, and amyotrophic lateral sclerosis: I etiology and pathology. Muscle Nerve 59(1):10–22. https://doi.org/10.1002/mus.26289
36. Ironside JW, Ritchie DL, Head MW (2018) Prion diseases. In: Handbook of clinical neurology, 1st edn, vol 145. Elsevier B.V. https://doi.org/10.1016/B978-0-12-802395-2.00028-6
37. Ritchie DL, Ironside JW (2017) Neuropathology of human prion diseases. In: Prion protein, 1st edn, vol 150. Elsevier Inc. https://doi.org/10.1016/bs.pmbts.2017.06.011
38. Barber C (2019) Rare health conditions 26 : fatal familial insomnia. Creutzfeldt-Jakob disease and Gerstmann-Sträussler- Scheinker syndrome 13(8)

39. Amyloids P, Groveman BR, Kraus A, Raymond LD, Dolan MA, Anson KJ, Dorward DW, Caughey B (2015) Charge neutralization of the central lysine cluster in prion protein (PrP) promotes PrP Sc -like folding of recombinant. 290(2):1119–1128. https://doi.org/10.1074/jbc.M114.619627
40. Lakkaraju AKK, Sorce S, Senatore A, Nuvolone M, Guo J, Schwarz P, Moos R, Pelczar P, Aguzzi A, Lakkaraju AKK, Sorce S (2022) 1 Introduction 2 Material and methods Mice 32(5):1–22
41. Sodhi RK, Madan J, Babu MA, Singh Y (2022) Chapter 16 - nanoformulations for neurodegenerative disorders, 2022–2023
42. Tadele M, Lemmens P, Bo L, Wulferding D, Yang J, Spende H (2019) Analytica Chimica acta preparation of silver nanoparticles coated ZnO/Fe_3O_4 composites using chemical reduction method for sensitive detection of uric acid via surface-enhanced Raman spectroscopy. Anal Chim Acta 1073:62–71. https://doi.org/10.1016/j.aca.2019.04.061
43. Parashar M, Kumar V, Ranbir S (2020) Metal oxides nanoparticles via sol–gel method: a review on synthesis, characterization and applications. J Mater Sci: Mater Electron:0123456789https://doi.org/10.1007/s10854-020-02994-8
44. Asgari S, Saberi AH, Mcclements DJ, Lin M (2019) Trends in Food Science & Technology Microemulsions as nanoreactors for synthesis of biopolymer nanoparticles. Trends Food Sci Technol 86(November 2018):118–130. https://doi.org/10.1016/j.tifs.2019.02.008
45. Eview R (2015) Methods of preparation of nanoparticles – a. 7(4):1806–1811
46. Disorders N, Bhattacharya T, Amanda G, Chopra H, Rahman M (2022) Applications of phyto-nanotechnology for the treatment of. 1–32

Aspects of Nanomedicines' Safety and Nanotoxicity for Brain-Targeted Drug Delivery

Amit Kumar Dubey, Niva Singh, Sneha Rani, Jyoti Kumari, and Shubhankar Kumar Singh

Abstract Nanoparticles (NPs) are escalating for the therapeutics, clinical investigations, and examining of ailment- or drug-induced mechanics in the human physiological micro and macro-system. Brain-targeted drug delivery is the most influential and promising approach in present decade. Smart nanomaterial-based targeted delivery in brain-specific loci will present a novel approach to target-delivery. Neurodegenerative diseases such as Alzheimer's, Parkinson's, and Huntington's diseases need safe and efficient therapeutics. Any changes in genome of brain lead to serious health issues. Genotoxic events and neurotoxic events sparked by nanoparticles lead to serious health issues and patient compliance. Nanomedicines safety and polymers/ionic toxicity profiling for brain-targeted drug delivery studies are required in present scenario. The neurotoxic outcome put forth by several traditional and advanced nano-constructs may be involved in pathophysiology of degeneration of neurons. Therefore, it is now a days crucial that an intensive information behind these mechanisms is required before taking nanomaterials as therapeutically value. In this present chapter, we systematically examine the pros and cons of nanocarriers in brain targeting theranostics.

Keywords Nanomedicines · Nanotoxicity · Brain targeting · Genotoxicity · Carcinogenicity

A. K. Dubey · N. Singh · Sneha Rani · J. Kumari · S. K. Singh (✉)
Parasite Immunology Lab, Division of Microbiology, Indian Council of Medical Research (ICMR)-Rajendra Memorial Research Institute of Medical Sciences (RMRIMS), Patna-800007, Bihar, India
e-mail: shubhankar30@gmail.com

A. K. Dubey
Department of Pharmaceutics, School of Pharmaceutical and Population Health Informatics (SoPPHI), DIT University, 248009, Dehradun, India

S. K. Rath et al. (eds.), *Nanomaterials for Drug Delivery and Neurological Diseases Management*, Smart Nanomaterials Technology,
https://doi.org/10.1007/978-981-97-0308-1_17

1 Introduction

Nanotechnology stands for a noble set of techniques that are used to synthesize nanometer structures/constructs within a dimension (size range) from 1 to 100 nm. This supports mercantile application all over the world. Nanoparticles such as silica, polymers, and quantum dots are of sizeable contribution to mankind but, ignoring its risks and assessment in terms of toxicity, the patient compliance will become diminished [1]. Changes in the genetic material can lead to serious human health defects, as mutations in somatic cells may cause cancer and can contribute to other chronic diseases. Genotoxic events can appear at both the DNA, chromosomal, or (during mitosis) whole genome level. The study of mechanisms leading to genotoxicity is crucially important, as well as the detection of potentially genotoxic compounds. The most crucial research zone (Toxicogenomics) can be signified as promising and effective for therapeutics assessment and recognizing molecular mechanisms and pathways. In addition to this, it enforces new insights of therapeutics into nanomolecular designs, and nano-constructs of wide applications [2–4].

In terms of very miniature size of nanoparticles, these have the potential to target neurological system. The noble nano-construct can cross the blood brain barrier. This nanodriven therapeutics can be utilized in neurology. Nanoparticle (NP)-driven drug carriers easily cross the labyrinth of vasculature, i.e. blood brain barrier and can be helpful in treating central neurological system disorder. Nanoparticles also help in axonal regenerations and neurotransmitter mechanistic bio-imaging. However, these nanoconstructs, and nanoparticles encapsulation may be hazardous to brain, i.e. toxicological signaling (nano-neurotoxicity). These may happen by any possible mechanisms such as overproduction in free radicals (ROS activity), autophagocytosis, deregulation in lysosome mechanism, and in certain activation in neuro-network pathways. In this book chapter, we discuss, possible toxicities and limitations of nanoparticles that are targeted to brain [5].

The nanotoxicology clinical examination is highly crucial to understand the safer sides. As a well-known fact that health impacts of particles (size range < 0.1 to $2.5\ \mu m$) have been researched in several studies. Therefore, before constructing the nanoparticles for CNS delivery, these measures should be under consideration. Most ignoring fact, mother to foetus transfer of genotoxicity (developmental toxicity) has been studied widely. Developmental toxicity is a transfer of mutated genetic variation from pregnant women to nascent child [6].

For safer and effective drug delivery, toxicological parameters should be considered. Neurotoxicity data obtained from clinical and preclinical studies were applied when brain-targeted delivery was prepared.

2 Neuro-Toxicological Aspects

A. Developmental Toxicity

Developmental toxicity of nanopolymers, nanoparticles, and nanocarriers targeted to CNS, PNS (brain), one of the sevenfold organs of sensory system, is to be considered for mental well-being. This will impact the quality of life. National toxicological program states that toxicity relates to developmental biology 'the entity which can interfere with healthy functioning/development and sometimes intervene to offspring in terms of side effects' [6, 7]. In most recent cases, the dose-dependent and size-dependent of transplacental nanocarrier+drug conjugates transferred to fetus, were published. It is most crucial to document the data related to direct toxic-effect and mechanism hindered via nanoparticles in fetus/offspring and indirectly processed from mother to fetus respectively. The reactive oxygen species (ROS) and genomic mutation that triggers inflammation in mother can sometimes be transferred to the foetus. It was reported in 2017, by Umezawa and Onada et al. They also reported locomotor activity, understanding, sub-conscious behavioral activity, signaling in memory, and completely in-social attitude due to nanocarrier (metallic) delivery in mother. These outcomes are neurobehavioral changes and few time targets. Few signaling points/targets in brain such as perivascular cells of hypothalamus, or first line of defense in brain (perivascular macrophages/PVM), and special glial cells (astrocytes), are toxicological targets of nanoparticles. They are highly susceptible targets to mother even at the low dose of nano-encapsulated therapeutics. The data revealed that preventive measures should be considered whenever nanocarrier delivery is provided to mothers. Clinical investigation to support that data was suggested by authors. This will help in safer design of nanoconstructs for brains and also impact on developmental pharmacology and delivery system.

B. Metallic Toxicity

Magnetic nanoparticles such as iron oxide NPs (IONPs) are suggested as target drug delivery of theranostics to brain (CNS). Indeed, it is used widely in diagnostics, still several times used for therapeutic delivery system. Iron oxide nanocarrier can potentially destroy neurons in brain. This can be possible via ionic charge accumulation, nuclei formation (aggregation of NPs), and ROS production. To overcome the toxicity of IONPs, quercetin-loaded NPs were proven safer for neuro-target delivery (dose-dependable) as suggested by [8]. Quercetin was found to be highly neuroprotective in recent times, because of its anti-oxidant characteristics. The only hurdle is its poor solubility in preparations and limited bioavailability. But, still quercetin-loaded neurodelivery was found safer to brain. In the study published in Nanobiotechnology, they synthesized QCSPIONs. It denotes the QCs conjugated IONPs or supermagnetic NPs. That nanoconstruct was used and found preventable in neurogenesis and much safer to CNS targeted delivery. It was found by researchers that quercetin inhibited the aggregation of neuronal proteins. QCs loaded carrier inhibits iron-overload to brain. QCs loaded nano-carrier impaired reactions such as Fenton/Haber–Weiss. It inhibits genetic toxicity via maintaining iron homeostasis, free radical monitoring activity, etc. QCSPIONs nanoconstruct was found helpful in dementia, and reduced neurotoxicity [8–10].

Silver nanoparticles (AgNPs) are most widely used in nano-research thrust. It is also an attractive nanocarrier for brain targeting. Therefore, possible toxicity, adverse effects, and toxicological interventions of AgNPs in regard to CNS or other nervous systems are needed to be studied. In another study by Janzadeh et al. 2022, they investigated and meta-analyzed the AgNPs neurotoxicity studies at the pre-clinical stage. They investigated 26 animal studies (AgNPs responses). The results they drew, suggested that silver NPs can able to trigger neurotoxicity and programmed cell death to neurons when delivered to brain. The standardized mean difference data was ~2.87 with a p-value of ~0.001. It was revealed that silver NPs ~10 nm size-range can harm neurons. However, it was found that continuous exposure for up-to 6 months triggered neuronal cell death. The developmental toxicity was observed when AgNPs were exposed to mother. It was revealed that newborn animals whose mother's brain were targeted by AgNPs, after 6 months of exposure, animals' memory and consciousness were inhibited and altered. Also, ROS activation was observed. Thus, silver NPs generate neurotoxicity. Also, apoptosis was showed in these animals after exposure to AgNPs. Silver NPs have long half-life and in prior to toxic effects they generate programmed cell death in CNS and harm blood brain barrier. Also, few side effects have also been reported in cerebral cortex. It was found optimum harm to frontal and temporal regions of brain. The root cause behind this may be Ag+ ions deposition in neuronal network in brain. Thus causing apoptosis [11].

However, the cytotoxicity in relation with silver NPs is still in question. Researchers are debating the mechanism behind hazardous risks in target delivery. In a study published in 2015, neurotoxicity was persuaded by silver ion (Ag+) via ROS production in rodents. The effective cells in brain were cerebral astrocytes. Sun and Yin investigated the neurotoxicological outcomes after AgNPs delivery to brain in rat's cerebral astrocytes. Alamar Blue assay generated the data that Ag+ ions are highly toxic to astrocytes. It triggered acute toxicity. Programmed cell death was also observed in pre-clinical studies. Cell necrosis, cytotoxicity, and de-integrity in plasma membrane were also been observed after Ag+ ionic target. Internal assembly of Ag+ ionic strength leads to hepatotoxicity; this is referred to as cellular internalization. When targeting AgNPs to brain, intracellular ROS production takes place. This happened via concentration and time-dependable in specialized glial cells, i.e. astrocytes. This triggered N-terminal kinases (JNK) phosphorylation and thus it stimulated the necrosis. One more result showed in cytokine assay that exponential activation in signaling molecules such as cytokines produced in specialized glial cells (astrocytes). Hence, it was proved that silver NPs involved in inflammation in neurons. Independently, AgNPs and Ag+ , both caused neurotoxicity. It concludes that silver NPs mediated carrier delivery is risk taking for brain [12–17]. Therefore accurate assessment is necessary before AgNPs delivery to neurons. From 2000 to 2020, silver nanoparticles are the prime focus of studies for target delivery. Green nanoparticle synthesis as silver NPs is of great effort because it lowers the toxic effects of metallic nanoparticles. A study published in scientific reports examined the green NPs on neuronal network in Rats. Tareq M, et al. performed and evaluated the green AgNPs on 34 Wistar male rats. Administration of AgNPs in a concentration of 0.5 to 10 mg/kg) upto fourteen days are given. The final results suggested that cortical and hippocampus zones in brain dis-functionalized. The biomarkers such as Malondialdehyde (MDA), nitric oxides, and glutathione (Glu) markers in neurodegenerative diseases triggered after exposure to silver NPs. Other neurotransmitters such as AchE and dopamines, nor-epinephrine, and serotonins were also investigated in that study. The data revealed that silver NPs triggered fewer effects in cortex with down-regulated ROS. But, serotonin and nor-adrenaline levels decreased, and acetylcholine activity was also inhibited after exposure to AgNPs in hippocampus and brain cortex zones. A potent transformation was observed at cellular level in neurons. Therefore, green synthesis lowers down the effects of silver ions neurotoxicity in brain. However, according to dose-dependent studies in regard to AgNPs for neurons, neurotoxicity was observed. Indeed, green nanoparticle delivery is little bit safer than silver ionic drug conjugated delivery to brain [17]. As a well-known fact that AgNPs induce antibacterial and antifungal features; but the less known toxic effect of silver ions or NPs designed from $AgNO_3$ researched. A study was investigated by [18] on SH-SY5Y cell line. The silver NPs exerted nano-neurotoxicity in solid tumor of ANS (autonomic nervous system) which can be seen in human neuroblastoma cell line. They designed two sized NPs (5 and 50 nm). Then, they observed the neurotoxicological parameters, genetic expressions such as amyloid genes, autophagic ferroptosis mechanism, ROS production, intracellular deposition of oxides, and molecular signaling pathways evaluated post 24 h treated cell line with AgNPs. The first data collected was of inhibition in cell proliferation, overexpression of amyloid-β peptides or BACE1 protein, and down-regulation of APP and ADAM10 genes. It was observed that silver nanoparticles blocked autophagy. Moreover, ferritinophagy was triggered, the over-activation of nuclear receptors. AgNPs activated the overproduction of DMT1 and SLC40A1 genes in tumor cell line. The GPX4 glutathione peroxidase-4 down-regulation was also observed in SH-SY5Y cells. In addition, malondialdehyde level was increased in cell line. This suggested that iron deposition at intracellular level is enhanced by silver NPs. Thus ROS overproduction is detected. In comparison, less sized AgNPs (5 nm) rather than 50 nm NPs, uptake efficiency enhanced and thus more exceedingly harmful effect seen in neuronal tumor cell lines. They reported that size dependable toxicity (AgNPs) in SH-SY5Y cells and it was mediated by ROS driven [18].

Zeman et al. [19] published a work on titanium oxide ((TiO_2). As we already know that TiO_2 has wide applications, its nanoparticle between a range of less than 100 nm, has proven in industrial applications such as colorants, cosmetics, paints, etc. It was reported that titanium oxide nanoparticle can be delivered via inhalation or GIT tract. Sometimes routes of administration may be at dermal level. But, it was found that TiO_2 deep perforation is restricted. However, active and passive targeting may vary according to EPR effect or tissue injury. It was found titanium oxide triggered free radical-related stress in brain phagocytic cells. It was observed that superoxide production enhanced after TiO2 exposure in brain (microglia). Thus, ROS production was escalated in microglia phagocytic cells. It directly harmed the blood brain barrier. Numerous studies supported this data that neuronal degradation or degeneration started after delivery of TiO_2 NPs and impairment was also shown in neurons. The dementia effect was also reported in these studies. Basically, these studies were experimented in rodents. After exposure to TiO_2 nanoparticles, rats learning capacity was disabled. Now, we can understand, TiO_2 wide applications raise a debate about its safety concern in terms of drug delivery/target delivery. It was observed that TiO_2 can easily penetrate through inhalation. It can cross BBB and directly accumulate in outermost structure-cortex. A few times, TiO_2 also accumulated in small extension of brain. That small area is called hippocampus. The nanotechnology-driven data (TiO_2) on microglia showed that TiO_2 activates these cells and ROS production increases, and it leads to programmed cell deaths at pre-clinical and clinical level. Overexposed or dose-dependable studies showed that TiO_2 leads to neuroinflammation in brain and sometimes, leads to severe neuronal damages and injury. Therefore, overall memory and recognition are impaired in this regard. Another study, five nanometer size- TiO_2 NPs targeted on SH-SY5Y cell line. SH-SY5Y cell line is of *Homo sapiens* neuroblastoma cells. TiO_2 NPs triggered ROS production in cell lines. Also Nrf2 nuclear localization was observed. The ER-mediated pathways directly affected after TiO_2 exposure to brain [19–21]. It has been noticed that P38-nuclear factor-E2-related factor-2 (Nrf-2) pathway that is triggered or over-activated by TiO_2 NPs is less understood. The dysregulation in this pathway leads to severe brain injury. Therefore, to examining the signaling cascade or molecular mechanism of TiO_2, Ze, Yuguan, et al. performed a series of experiments. They delivered TiO_2 intra-nasal delivery to mouse brain in order to understand oxidative stress level. They reported NF-kβ activation, Nrf-2 overexpression, HO-1 (regulated by Nrf-2 gene), and p38 activation after exposure to TiO_2 NPs in mouse brain. This leads to ROS production and moreover DNA damage has also been observed (DNA peroxidation). These results suggested that while designing the TiO_2 NPs, this caution should be taken into consideration [22]. Due to brain complexity, accumulation sites, and histological restrictions such as blood brain barrier, neurotoxicity yet not had been fully understood. Industrial-designed nanoparticles with full fledge not been relayed to brain activity. In this regard, a study investigated on silica NPs, food grade titanium dioxide NPs, and silver NPs on neurotoxicity. Similarly, polyacrylic acid (PAA) coated (CoFe2O4) NPs interaction analysis with brain functioning was examined because it has several biomedical applications. The researchers used neuro-tumor cell line (SH-SY5Y), and targeted it by NPs between a range of 2 and 50 μg/ml). The data revealed about brain toxicity after targeting by NPs, plasma membrane damage, cell-cycle arrests, reactive oxygen species generation, autophagosomes activations, etc. The studies told that dose-time dependable targeting or higher concentration of NPs leads to toxic particle deposition in sensitive zones of brain that regulate physiological function of our body. TiO_2 affects the autophagy and hindered the cellular activities within 3 days after TiO_2 target to brain [23–25].

Copper nanoparticles related data w.r.t brain is also less assembled. However, it is nephrotoxic is a well-known fact. Xu et al. [26] had studied nanosized copper NPs and its related cytotoxicity in rodents. They investigated in rat mesangial cells. The programmed cell death was examined. The caspase-3 activity was measured.

The autophagy was also examined and calculated statistically by acridine orange (AO) staining. The targeted genes Beclin-1, LC3B, and cell proliferation marker p62 were well examined for toxicological interventions of metallic NPs The final data revealed that at concentration higher or lower, it showed the above-mentioned effects. Thus, ROS activation and apoptosis happened in neuronal cells. They found acidic vesicular organelles overproduction due to copper NPs targeting delivery. The data signified that autophagy induced by copper NPs and thus neuro-toxicity generated in mesangial cells. The kind of toxicity data signified that safety guidelines are highly monitored before NPs industrial synthesis and then targeted to brain in-vivo [26, 27].

3 Neuronal Geno-toxicity

Genotoxic process is sometimes referred to as genetic mutations. It is a characteristic of mutagen to alter genomic code information. Genotoxic events may be reversible or irreversible. The DNA repair mechanism is involved in reversible transient changes. If mutagen alters the information at genomic level, it triggers cancer, thus potentially carcinogenic. Whenever genotoxicity examining was evaluated then, every aspect at genetic stage should be considered. Few points such as mutation at gene level, chromosome aberrations, etc., at larger scale aneuploidy is measured. The clastogenicity is also important data to be considered. The mutation triggered by nanomaterials was evaluated by micronucleus assay. The Ames test is not supported due to size variation estimation. Various noble biomarkers that lead to define genetic damage, i.e. genotoxicity such as epigenetic changes, omics, etc., cell lines (in-vitro toxicity) genotoxicity are need to be considered before NMs designed. Primary genotoxicity is related to genetic changes but secondary genotoxicity is related to inflammation. 3D bio-imprinting is established in recent years to model toxicology reliable data obtained without harming lives. The systemic exposure of NMs/NPs onto 3D models; assessment of genotoxicity is possible nowadays. Still novel genotoxicity test provides the necessary data for brain targeting.

A study was conducted by Mohamed HR and his team, with TiO_2NPs. Titanium dioxide nanoparticles were exposed to various organs for toxicological interventions data. Therefore, they administered TiO_2NPs to Male Swiss Webster mice. The dose was administered continuously for 5 days. Thereafter, the mice were sacrificed to obtain the data. The cytoarchitecture was slightly altered after exposure to TiO_2NPs in brain. The NPs administered and monitored in a dose-/time-dependent manner. The single cell comet assay data reported that DNA was fragmented. Point mutation was also examined in Presenilin-1. This is a crucial gene in Alzheimer's disease. Thus, these reports revealed that titanium dioxide NPs showed mutagenic and referred to as genotoxic to brain. This can lead to neurodegenerative diseases in later stages of life [28]. A study published in Journal of Biomedical Materials Research Part A, reported that TiO_2 NPs induce brain toxicity. They administered TiO_2 NPs via nasal delivery up-to 9 consecutive days at increasing concentrations such as 2.5 mg/

kg to 10 mg/kg-B.W. Afterwards neuron-related injury and overexpression/under-expression profile was examined. As predicted, they found accumulation of metallic NPs in brain areas. Thus induced ROS (oxidative stress), programmed cell death, specialized glial cells (astrocytes) were over-proliferated. The hippocampus area of brain was seriously hampered and necrosis was observed. The team of researchers found that more than 100 genes were overexpressed and similarly more than 100 genes were under-expressed after TiO_2 exposure of 10 mg/kg-BW nanoparticles. The DNA repair and cytoskeleton mechanism were inhibited. The signal transduction was altered. The regulatory genes such as Col1a1, AKT kinase, Ddit4, and Cyp2e1 were overexpressed. The dopaminic receptor gene D2 decreased after long-term TiO_2 exposure. Therefore, it induced genotoxic effects in rodents [29]. In 2016, a study was published by Qi L and his team, on crossing blood brain barrier and targeting ocular diseases. They tested biogenic magnetic (BM) nanocarrier of 30 nm. This is developed or synthesized by bacteria such as magnetotactic bacteria. The unique property of BM nanocarrier, it can pass through BBB. Therefore, various cytotoxicity and genotoxicity studies can be performed. It was reported that magnetic NPs have higher genotoxicity in comparison to BMs. A Bcl-2 gene overexpressed in case of BM exposure [30].

Now, we can understand that NPs can damage and activate adverse effects in dose-/time-dependent manner. They can trigger signaling cascade and inhibit them at molecular stage. Magnetite NPs investigated by a team of researchers were found to be genetic damaging agent. A study was conducted at pre-clinical level on female albino mice. The genotoxicity was proved by COMET assay in liver but, surprisingly genotoxicity was not detected in brain [31]

4 Carcinogenicity/Cytotoxicity

This data is highly significant for nanomaterial toxicity evaluation and assessment. The cell transformation assay is one of the major assays for carcinogenicity testing. It is generally applied for immune-compromised animals, most specifically for rodent embryos. But, this assay has a limitation as suggested in previous studies on Syrian hamster embryo. Fontana and team evaluated 4 variants of NPs (SiNPs) for genotoxic/carcinogenic evaluation. They synthesized 2 forms of silica nanomaterials by precipitation method and another 2 by pyrogenic method [32–34]. Another study was conducted by Hall et al., via poly(butylcyanoacrylate) (PBCA) NPs delivery. Dox drug was encapsulated inside NPs. It was designed for rat glioblastoma therapeutics. Still, cytotoxicity was not understood. The main aim of this study was to evaluate these NPs' behavior in BBB. The data reported was found to be potent. Cytotoxic bioassays showed PBCA-PS80-DOX NPs lower down the metabolic activities. A total of eighty four genes were tested. It was found that TNFR1 expression and programmed cell death lead to toxicity. Moreover PBCA-PS80 NPs were found safer in CNS targeting [35].

5 Long-Term Stability and in Vivo Toxicity

For the purpose of long-term stability assessment in brain targeting; lipid NPs were evaluated. 10 years back, Blasi P et al. synthesized and evaluated lipids NPs. They are synthesized by high pressure homogenization technique. Cetylpalmitate and polysorbate(®) 80 were examined by NMR technique. These well prepared NPs were evaluated on rodent's brain and chicken embryos. The assay they targeted was chorioallantoic membrane. They stored lipid NPs up to 4 °C (4 Yrs). They found only slight spread in size of NPs after a period of four years. NMR data revealed that lipid matrix was intact at 4 °C/4 Yr. The bioassay on membrane they performed reported that negligible or not visible toxic effects in rodent brain. Thus, lipid NPs can be the best choice for brain target delivery in terms of stability and efficacy. The colloidal lipids are highly safe for neuronal target delivery [36].

6 Neurotoxicity of E-cigarettes

In recent years, e-cigarettes based drug delivery was promoted for brain targeting. These electronic cigarettes are slighter toxic. These e-liquids and EC aerosols are in question nowadays because of prompt use of e-cigarettes by pregnant women leads to developmental mutagenesis, neurotoxicity, and threat to public health at the adolescent age [37].

References

1. Miyazaki K, Islam N (2007) Nanotechnology systems of innovation—an analysis of industry and academia research activities. Technovation 27(11):661–675. https://doi.org/10.1016/j.technovation.2007.05.009
2. Kohl Y, Rundén-Pran E, Mariussen E, Hesler M, El Yamani N, Longhin EM, Dusinska M (2020) Genotoxicity of nanomaterials: advanced in vitro models and high throughput methods for human hazard assessment—a review. Nanomaterials 10(10):1911. https://doi.org/10.3390/nano10101911
3. Ellinger-Ziegelbauer H, Aubrecht J, Kleinjans JC, Ahr HJ (2009) Application of toxicogenomics to study mechanisms of genotoxicity and carcinogenicity. Toxicol Lett 186(1):36–44. https://doi.org/10.1016/j.toxlet.2008.08.017
4. Magdolenova Z, Collins A, Kumar A, Dhawan A, Stone V, Dusinska M (2014) Mechanisms of genotoxicity. A review of in vitro and in vivo studies with engineered nanoparticles. Nanotoxicology 8(3):233–78. https://doi.org/10.3109/17435390.2013.773464
5. Feng X, Chen A, Zhang Y, Wang J, Shao L, Wei L (2015) Central nervous system toxicity of metallic nanoparticles. Int J Nanomed 10:4321. https://doi.org/10.2147/IJN.S78308
6. Umezawa M, Onoda A, Takeda K (2017) Developmental toxicity of nanoparticles on the Brain. Yakugaku Zasshi: J Pharm Soc Japan 137(1):73–78. https://doi.org/10.1248/yakushi.16-00214
7. https://ntp.niehs.nih.gov/whatwestudy/niceatm/test-method-evaluations/dev-tox/index.html#:~:text=Developmental%20toxicity%20tests%20evaluate%20the,uses%20large%20numbers%20of%20animals.

8. Bardestani A, Ebrahimpour S, Esmaeili A, Esmaeili A (2021) Quercetin attenuates neurotoxicity induced by iron oxide nanoparticles. J Nanobiotechnology 19:1–33. https://doi.org/10.1186/s12951-021-01059-0
9. Singh YP, Pandey A, Vishwakarma S, Modi G (2019) A review on iron chelators as potential therapeutic agents for the treatment of Alzheimer's and Parkinson's diseases. Mol Diversity 15(23):509–526. https://doi.org/10.1007/s11030-018-9878-4
10. Enteshari Najafabadi R, Kazemipour N, Esmaeili A, Beheshti S, Nazifi S (2018) Using superparamagnetic iron oxide nanoparticles to enhance bioavailability of quercetin in the intact rat brain. BMC Pharmacol Toxicol 19:1−2. https://doi.org/10.1186/s40360-018-0249-7
11. Janzadeh A, Behroozi Z, Saliminia F, Janzadeh N, Arzani H, Tanha K, Hamblin MR, Ramezani F (2021) Neurotoxicity of silver nanoparticles in the animal brain: a systematic review and meta-analysis. Forensic Toxicol 29:1–5. https://doi.org/10.1007/s11419-021-00589-4
12. Sun C, Yin N, Wen R, Liu W, Jia Y, Hu L, Zhou Q, Jiang G (2016) Silver nanoparticles induced neurotoxicity through oxidative stress in rat cerebral astrocytes is distinct from the effects of silver ions. Neurotoxicology 1(52):210–221. https://doi.org/10.1016/j.neuro.2015.09.007
13. Yin N, Liu Q, Liu J, He B, Cui L, Li Z, Yun Z, Qu G, Liu S, Zhou Q, Jiang G (2013) Silver nanoparticle exposure attenuates the viability of rat cerebellum granule cells through apoptosis coupled to oxidative stress. Small 9(9–10):1831–1841. https://doi.org/10.1002/smll.201202732
14. Zhang B, Liu N, Liu QS, Zhang J, Zhou Q, Jiang G (2020) Silver nanoparticles induce size-dependent and particle-specific neurotoxicity to primary cultures of rat cerebral cortical neurons. Ecotoxicol Environ Saf 15(198):110674. https://doi.org/10.1016/j.ecoenv.2020.110674
15. Kim SH, Ko JW, Koh SK, Lee IC, Son JM, Moon C, Kim SH, Shin DH, Kim JC (2014) Silver nanoparticles induce apoptotic cell death in cultured cerebral cortical neurons. Mol Cell Toxicol 10:173–179. https://doi.org/10.1007/s13273-014-0019-6
16. Skalska J, Strużyńska L (2015) Toxic effects of silver nanoparticles in mammals–does a risk of neurotoxicity exist? Folia Neuropathol 53(4):281–300. https://doi.org/10.5114/fn.2015.56543
17. Tareq M, Khadrawy YA, Rageh MM, Mohammed HS (2022) Dose-dependent biological toxicity of green synthesized silver nanoparticles in rat's brain. Sci Rep 12(1):22642. https://doi.org/10.1038/s41598-022-27171-1
18. Zhai X, Shan S, Wan J, Tian H, Wang J, Xin L (2022) Silver nanoparticles induce a size-dependent neurotoxicity to SH-SY5Y neuroblastoma cells via ferritinophagy-mediated oxidative stress. Neurotox Res 40(5):1369–1379. https://doi.org/10.1007/s12640-022-00570-y
19. Zeman T, Loh EW, Čierný D, Šerý O (2018) Penetration, distribution and brain toxicity of titanium nanoparticles in rodents' body: a review. IET Nanobiotechnol 12(6):695–700. https://doi.org/10.1049/iet-nbt.2017.0109
20. Czajka M, Sawicki K, Sikorska K, Popek S, Kruszewski M, Kapka-Skrzypczak L (2015) Toxicity of titanium dioxide nanoparticles in central nervous system. Toxicol In Vitro 29(5):1042–1052. https://doi.org/10.1016/j.tiv.2015.04.004
21. Ferraro SA, Domingo MG, Etcheverrito A, Olmedo DG, Tasat DR (2020) Neurotoxicity mediated by oxidative stress caused by titanium dioxide nanoparticles in human neuroblastoma (SH-SY5Y) cells. J Trace Elem Med Biol 1(57):126413. https://doi.org/10.1016/j.jtemb.2019.126413
22. Ze Y, Zheng L, Zhao X, Gui S, Sang X, Su J, Guan N, Zhu L, Sheng L, Hu R, Cheng J (2013) Molecular mechanism of titanium dioxide nanoparticles-induced oxidative injury in the brain of mice. Chemosphere 92(9):1183–1189. https://doi.org/10.1016/j.chemosphere.2013.01.094
23. Lojk J, Repas J, Veranič P, Bregar VB, Pavlin M (2020) Toxicity mechanisms of selected engineered nanoparticles on human neural cells in vitro. Toxicology 28(432):152364. https://doi.org/10.1016/j.tox.2020.152364
24. Gong JY, Holt MG, Hoet PH, Ghosh M (2022) Neurotoxicity of four frequently used nanoparticles: a systematic review to reveal the missing data. Arch Toxicol 96(5):1141–1212. https://doi.org/10.1007/s00204-022-03233-1

25. Athira SS, Prajitha N, Mohanan PV. Interaction of nanoparticles with central nervous system and its consequences. https://doi.org/10.5455/ajrms.20180717105137
26. Xu P, Cao M, Dong X, Yu Z, Liu J, Tan J, Wang Y, Li T, Zhao S (2022) Nanosized copper particles induced mesangial cell toxicity via the autophagy pathway. Braz J Med Biol Res 11:55
27. Xu P, Li Z, Zhang X, Yang Z (2014) Increased response to oxidative stress challenge of nano-copper-induced apoptosis in mesangial cells. J Nanopart Res 16:1–3. https://doi.org/10.1007/s11051-014-2777-4
28. Mohamed HR, Hussien NA (2016) Genotoxicity studies of titanium dioxide nanoparticles (TiO2NPs) in the brain of mice. Scientifica. https://doi.org/10.1155/2016/6710840
29. Ze Y, Hu R, Wang X, Sang X, Ze X, Li B, Su J, Wang Y, Guan N, Zhao X, Gui S (2014) Neurotoxicity and gene-expressed profile in brain-injured mice caused by exposure to titanium dioxide nanoparticles. J Biomed Mater Res Part A: Off J Soc Biomater, Jpn Soc Biomater, Aust Soc Biomater Korean Soc Biomater 102(2):470–478. https://doi.org/10.1002/jbm.a.34705
30. Qi L, Lv X, Zhang T, Jia P, Yan R, Li S, Zou R, Xue Y, Dai L (2016) Cytotoxicity and genotoxicity of bacterial magnetosomes against human retinal pigment epithelium cells. Sci Rep 6(1):26961. https://doi.org/10.1038/srep26961
31. Bassiony H, El-Ghor AA, Salaheldin TA, Sabet S, Mohamed MM (2022) Tissue distribution, histopathological and genotoxic effects of magnetite nanoparticles on Ehrlich solid Carcinoma. Biol Trace Elem Res 200(12):5145–5158. https://doi.org/10.1007/s12011-022-03102-z
32. Maser E, Schulz M, Sauer UG, Wiemann M, Ma-Hock L, Wohlleben W, Hartwig A, Landsiedel R (2015) In vitro and in vivo genotoxicity investigations of differently sized amorphous SiO_2 nanomaterials. Mutat Res/Genet Toxicol Environ Mutagen 1(794):57–74. https://doi.org/10.1016/j.mrgentox.2015.10.005
33. Decan N, Wu D, Williams A, Bernatchez S, Johnston M, Hill M, Halappanavar S (2016) Characterization of in vitro genotoxic, cytotoxic and transcriptomic responses following exposures to amorphous silica of different sizes. Mutat Res/Genet Toxicol Environ Mutagen 15(796):8–22. https://doi.org/10.1016/j.mrgentox.2015.11.011
34. Fontana C, Kirsch A, Seidel C, Marpeaux L, Darne C, Gaté L, Remy A, Guichard Y (2017) In vitro cell transformation induced by synthetic amorphous silica nanoparticles. Mutat Res/Genet Toxicol Environ Mutagen 1(823):22–27. https://doi.org/10.1016/j.mrgentox.2017.08.002
35. Hall AM, Hemmer R, Spaulding R, Wetzel HN, Curcio J, Sabel BA, Henrich-Noack P, Pixley S, Hopkins T, Boyce RL, Schultheis PJ (2016) Cytotoxicity and apoptotic gene expression in an in vitro model of the blood–brain barrier following exposure to poly (butylcyanoacrylate) nanoparticles. J Drug Target 24(7):635–644. https://doi.org/10.3109/1061186X.2015.1132222
36. Blasi P, Schoubben A, Traina G, Manfroni G, Barberini L, Alberti PF, Cirotto C, Ricci M (2013) Lipid nanoparticles for brain targeting III. Long-term stability and in vivo toxicity. Int J Pharm 15;454(1):316–23. https://doi.org/10.1016/j.ijpharm.2013.06.037
37. Ruszkiewicz JA, Zhang Z, Gonçalves FM, Tizabi Y, Zelikoff JT, Aschner M (2020) Neurotoxicity of e-cigarettes. Food Chem Toxicol 1(138):111245. https://doi.org/10.1016/j.fct.2020.111245